MOLECULAR PATHOLOGY LIBRARY

Philip T. Cagle, MD, Series Editor

For further volumes:
http://www.springer.com/series/7723

Matthias A. Karajannis • David Zagzag
Editors

Molecular Pathology of Nervous System Tumors

Biological Stratification and Targeted Therapies

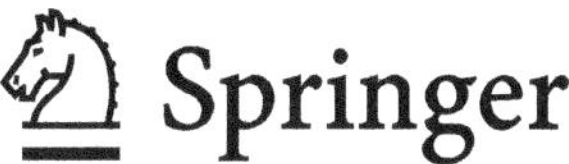

Editors
Matthias A. Karajannis
Associate Professor of Pediatrics and Otolaryngology
NYU Langone Medical Center
New York, NY, USA

David Zagzag
Professor of Pathology and Neurosurgery
NYU Langone Medical Center
New York, NY, USA

ISSN 1935-987X ISSN 1935-9888 (electronic)
ISBN 978-1-4939-1829-4 ISBN 978-1-4939-1830-0 (eBook)
DOI 10.1007/978-1-4939-1830-0
Springer New York Heidelberg Dordrecht London

Library of Congress Control Number: 2014955157

Printed on acid-free paper

Springer is part of Springer Science+Business Media (www.springer.com)

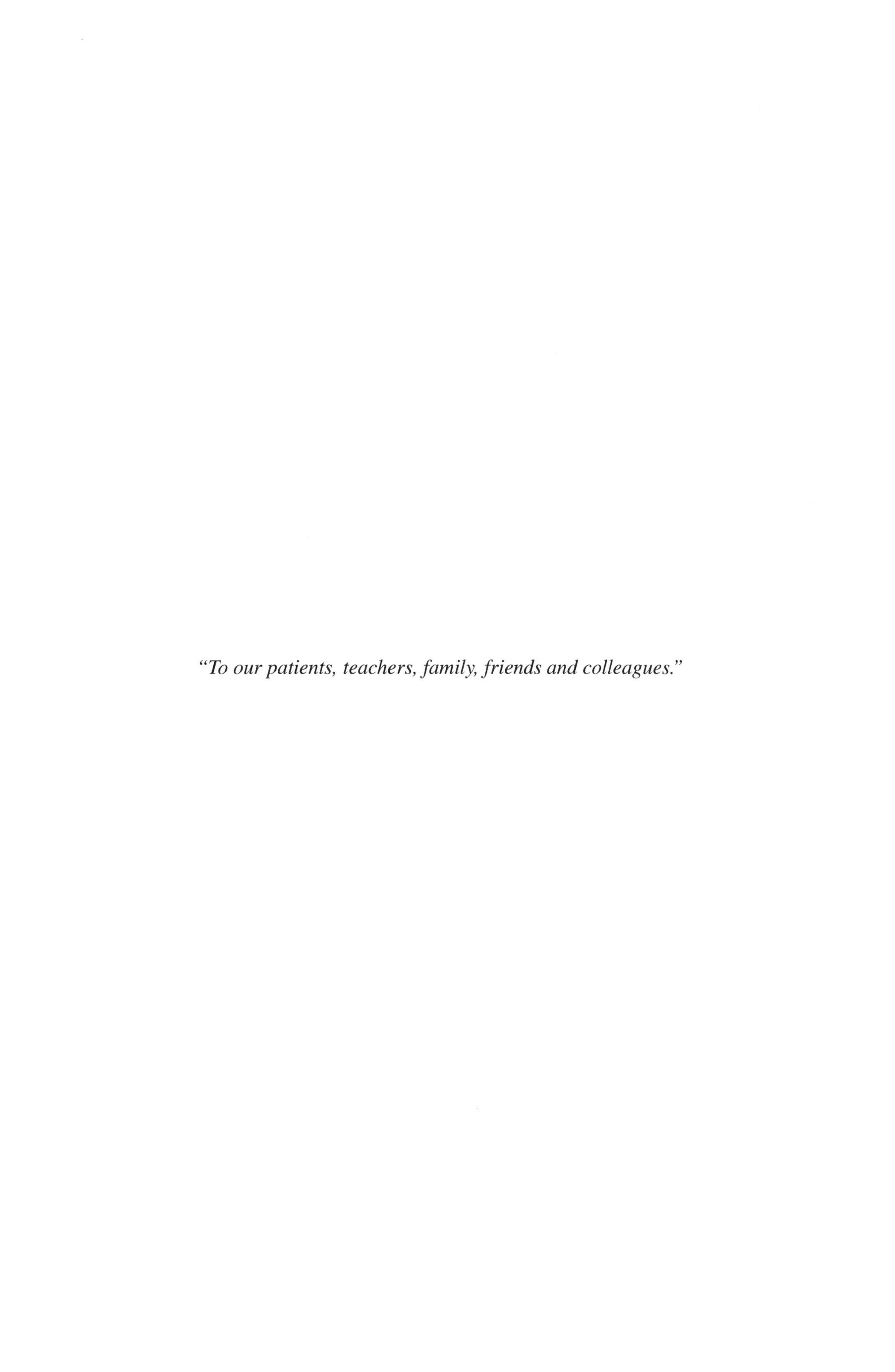

"To our patients, teachers, family, friends and colleagues."

Foreword

It is difficult to believe that in the space of my career so much progress has been made in the classification and treatment of CNS tumors. Beginning in an era when with diagnoses were determined almost solely by light microscopy of H&E-stained sections, and treatments were almost devoid of specificity, molecular features are increasingly instrumental to both diagnosis and treatment. Effective targeted approaches are now a reality for patients with some tumor types.

Prepared by an international panel of experts, this authoritative volume concisely and authoritatively delineates this current state of affairs. Obstacles to targeted treatments are freely acknowledged, but a refreshing vein of optimism pervades this book about a subject that in previous eras seemed to have so little promise. As such, this very readable work is highly recommended as an introduction to the new era of neuro-oncology with its potential for effective care of patients with tumors heretofore so difficult to control.

Peter C. Burger, M.D.

Preface

Recent advances in molecular biology and genetics have revolutionized our understanding of the biology that underlies the clinical diversity of nervous system tumors. The majority of these data have emerged from a number of large-scale genomic profiling projects and groups, and facilitated by the availability of ever more powerful next-generation sequencing and molecular profiling technologies. At the same time, functional studies have begun to characterize the biology of many of the molecular genetic alterations identified, including novel oncogenic driver mutations. In parallel, the advances in stem cell biology have provided valuable insight into the evolution and progression of brain tumors, including glioblastoma. Functional and preclinical studies are also aided by an increasing number and sophistication of genetically engineered mouse models that recapitulate the development of specific tumor subtypes.

Genomic profiling of disease entities that had been previously classified mainly through histomorphology and a limited set of immunohistochemical markers has revealed a diverse and complex biology of brain tumors. As a result, new molecular diagnostic tools are entering the field of neuropathology at a rapid pace. Newly defined sub-entities that are driven by divergent oncogenic pathways have been recognized to show distinctive clinical behavior and will likely require tailored risk-stratification and treatments. Molecular targeted therapies are increasingly entering clinical trials in neuro-oncology and hold promise for improving the outcome of patients with nervous system tumors, especially those that frequently recur despite aggressive multimodal therapy including surgery, radiotherapy, and chemotherapy. Molecular genetic testing that until very recently was limited to research labs is becoming increasingly available for routine clinical use.

This book is intended to be used as a comprehensive guide to the rapidly evolving field of molecular neuropathology of nervous system tumors, as well as the underlying biology and emerging molecular targeted therapies. We hope that it will serve as a useful resource for physicians as well as clinical and laboratory scientists involved with or interested in the up-to-date diagnosis and treatment of patients with brain tumors. Accordingly, the target audience includes neuropathologists, neuro-oncologists, neurosurgeons, radiation oncologists, neurologists, neuroradiologists, as well as residents and fellows, who diagnose and treat patients with nervous system tumors including tumors of the brain, spine, leptomeninges, and peripheral nerves.

Special emphasis was given to already established and emerging molecular diagnostic tests in neuropathology, as well as molecular targeted therapies. The book is organized by clinicopathologic disease entities, and each chapter has been prepared by a team of authors to cover a full spectrum of expertise including neuropathology, molecular biology, and clinical management, with a focus on practical diagnostic and clinical considerations.

New York, NY, USA

Matthias A. Karajannis, M.D., M.S.
David Zagzag, M.D., Ph.D.

Contents

Contributors

Kenneth Aldape, M.D. Department of Pathology, The University of Texas MD Anderson Cancer Center, Houston, TX, USA

Kelly L. Barton Division of Hematology–Oncology, Department of Pediatrics, Duke University Medical Center, Durham, NC, USA

N. Sumru Bayin, B.S., M.S. Department of Neurosurgery, NYU Langone Medical Center, New York, NY, USA

Oren Becher, M.D. Departments of Pediatrics and Pathology, Duke University Medical Center, Durham, NC, USA

Jaishri Blakeley, M.D. Department of Neurology, The Johns Hopkins Comprehensive Neurofibromatosis Center, The Johns Hopkins Hospital, Baltimore, MD, USA

Daniel C. Bowers, M.D. Division of Pediatric Hematology–Oncology, UT Southwestern Medical School, Dallas, TX, USA

Girish Dhall, M.D. Children's Hospital Los Angeles, Keck School of Medicine of University of Southern California, Los Angeles, CA, USA

Howard A. Fine, M.D. Perlmutter Cancer Center, NYU Langone Medical Center, New York, NY, USA

Sharon L. Gardner, M.D. Department of Pediatrics, NYU Langone Medical Center, New York, NY, USA

Kyle G. Halvorson, M.D. Division of Neurological Surgery, Department of Surgery, Duke University Medical Center, Durham, NC, USA

David H. Harter, M.D. Department of Neurosurgery, NYU Medical Center, New York, NY, USA

Martin Hasselblatt, M.D. Institute of Neuropathology, University Hospital Münster, Münster, Germany

Eyas M. Hattab, M.D. IU Health Pathology Laboratory, Indiana University School of Medicine, Indianapolis, IN, USA

Ashley A. Ibrahim, M.D. IU Health Pathology Laboratory, Department of Pathology and Laboratory Medicine, Indiana University School of Medicine, Indianapolis, IN, USA

David T. W. Jones, Ph.D. Division of Pediatric Neurooncology, German Cancer Research Center (DKFZ), Heidelberg, Germany

Alexander R. Judkins, M.D. Department of Pathology and Laboratory Medicine, Children's Hospital Los Angeles, Keck School of Medicine University of Southern California, Los Angeles, CA, USA

Michel Kalamarides, M.D., Ph.D. Department of Neurosurgery, Hospital Pitie-Salpetriere, Paris, France

Ganjam V. Kalpana, Ph.D. Departments of Genetics and Microbiology and Immunology, Albert Einstein College of Medicine, New York, NY, USA

Matthias A. Karajannis, M.D., M.S. Associate Professor of Pediatrics and Otolaryngology, NYU Langone Medical Center, New York, NY, USA

Andrey Korshunov, M.D. Clinical Cooperation Unit Neuropathology, German Cancer Research Center (DKFZ), Heidelberg, Germany

Christian Mawrin, M.D. Department of Neuropathology, Otto-von-Guericke University, Magdeburg, Germany

Roger McLendon, M.D. Department of Pathology, Duke University, Durham, NC, USA

Katharine McNeill, M.D. Departments of Medicine and Neurology, NYU Langone Medical Center, New York, NY, USA

Till Milde, M.D. Department of Pediatric Neurooncology and Department of Pediatric Hematology and Oncology, University Hospital Heidelberg, Heidelberg, Germany

German Cancer Research Center (DKFZ), Heidelberg, Germany

Aram S. Modrek, B.S. Department of Neurosurgery, NYU Langone Medical Center, New York, NY, USA

Paul A. Northcott, M.D. Division of Pediatric Neurooncology, German Cancer Research Center (DKFZ), Heidelberg, Germany

John G. Pappas, M.D., M.S. Division of Clinical Genetic Services, Department of Pediatrics, NYU Langone Medical Center, New York, NY, USA

Stefan M. Pfister, M.D. German Cancer Research Center (DKFZ), Department of Pediatric Neurooncology, and Department of Pediatric Hematology and Oncology, University Hospital Heidelberg, Heidelberg, Germany

Dimitris G. Placantonakis, M.D., Ph.D. Department of Neurosurgery, Kimmel Center for Stem Cell Biology, Brain Tumor Center, NYU Langone Medical Center, New York, NY, USA

Nancy Ratner, Ph.D. Department of Pediatrics, Cincinnati Children's Hospital, University of Cincinnati, Cincinnati, OH, USA

Fausto J. Rodriguez, M.D. Johns Hopkins University, Sheikh Zayed Tower, Baltimore, MD, USA

Amy Sheil, M.D. Department of Pathology, Cincinnati Children's Hospital Medical Center, Cincinnati, OH, USA

Jasmeet Chadha Singh, M.D. Division of Hematology and Oncology, Department of Medicine, NYU Langone Medical Center, New York, NY, USA

Matija Snuderl, M.D. Department of Pathology, NYU Langone Medical Center, New York, NY, USA

Anat Stemmer-Rachamimov, M.D., F.R.C.P(.C). Division of Neuropathology, Department of Pathology, Massachusetts General Hospital, Harvard Medical School, Boston, MA, USA

Uri Tabori, M.D. Department of Paediatrics, University of Toronto, Toronto, ON, Canada

Department of Haematology/Oncology, The Hospital for Sick Children, Toronto, ON, Canada

Michael D. Taylor, M.D., Ph.D., F.R.C.S(.C). Division of Neurosurgery and Labatt Brain Tumor Research Centre, Developmental & Stem Cell Biology Program, Department of Surgery, The Hospital for Sick Children, Toronto, ON, Canada

Department of Laboratory Medicine and Pathobiology, University of Toronto, Toronto, ON, Canada

Sriram Venneti, M.D., Ph.D. Cancer Biology and Genetics, Memorial Sloan Kettering Cancer Center, New York, NY, USA

Howard L. Weiner, MD, FACS, FAAP, FAANS. Division of Pediatric Neurosurgery, Department of Neurosurgery, NYU Langone Medical Center, New York, NY, USA

Brian Weiss, M.D. Neuroblastoma Program, Division of Oncology, Cincinnati Children's Hospital Medical Center, Cincinnati, OH, USA

Hendrik Witt, M.D. German Cancer Research Center (DKFZ), Department of Pediatric Neurooncology, and Department of Pediatric Hematology and Oncology, University Hospital Heidelberg, Heidelberg, Germany

Olaf Witt, M.D. German Cancer Research Center (DKFZ), Department of Pediatric Neurooncology, and Department of Pediatric Hematology and Oncology, University Hospital Heidelberg, Heidelberg, Germany

Johannes E. Wolff, M.D., Dr. Med., Dr. Med. Habil. Pediatric Hematology, Oncology and Blood and Marrow Transplantation, Cleveland Clinic, Cleveland, OH, USA

Stephen Yip, M.D., Ph.D. Department of Pathology & Laboratory Medicine, Vancouver General Hospital, Vancouver, BC, Canada

David Zagzag, M.D., Ph.D. Division of Neuropathology, Department of Pathology and Department of Neurosurgery, NYU Langone Medical Center, New York, NY, USA

Human Brain Tumor Bank, New York, NY, USA

Microvascular and Molecular Neuro-Oncology Laboratory, NYU Langone Medical Center, New York, NY, USA

1 Hereditary Predisposition to Primary CNS Tumors

Uri Tabori, Matthias A. Karajannis, and John G. Pappas

Primary central nervous system (CNS) tumors remain among the most devastating cancers in adults and children. Although the majority of CNS tumors occur in adults, brain tumors are the most common solid tumor of childhood and the dominant cause of morbidity and mortality in pediatric oncology. Although the majority of brain tumors are thought to arise sporadically, recent advancements in our understanding of the molecular genetics of brain tumors have resulted in an increased awareness for germline predispositions to these cancers.

While most adult CNS cancers are sporadic, as many as 50 % of childhood brain tumors are caused by germline mutations [1, 2]. In some cases, a specific pathological entity only exists in the context of a condition resulting from these germline mutations [3, 4]. Since in many cases tumors are only a part of the clinical manifestations of the mutation, the term cancer predisposition syndrome is used to define these conditions.

Cancer predisposition syndromes are monogenic disorders. Discovery of each single gene causing each syndrome was initially pursued by linkage studies and positional cloning. Germline mutation in one of these syndromic genes is the first hit in the associated tumors as well as the etiology of the developmental abnormalities associated with features of the syndrome i.e., malformations, dysmorphic features. Somatic mutation in one of these genes can also be the first hit or subsequent hit in sporadic tumors. Contemporary research interrogates the genetic contribution to brain tumors by gene expression arrays, whole genome sequencing in tumor and non-tumor tissues in human as well as animal models. Different sequences of genetic events leading to tumorigenesis as well as the associated molecular pathways were elucidated by the study of hereditary syndromes [5].

It is of great importance for physicians to be aware of and recognize these conditions in order to be able to offer appropriate referrals to clinical geneticists or other specialists. Affected individuals and families require counseling and may benefit from following specific treatment and surveillance plans or protocols. More recently, molecular targeted therapies have begun to emerge for some conditions, and will likely become increasingly available.

A good example for the above is tuberous sclerosis complex (TSC). This genetic syndrome is associated with seizures, developmental delay, brain tumors (subependymal giant cell astrocytomas, SEGAs), and other tumors. However, understanding the genetic causes of the syndrome allowed for development of surveillance protocol and targeted therapy for the brain cancers affecting these patients with dramatic change in the clinical approach to patients with the syndrome.

As can be seen in Fig. 1.1, the majority of these mutations involve tumor suppressors and affect key signaling pathways of cancer. Interestingly, while most of these are autosomal dominant, autosomal recessive syndromes, such as those involving Fanconi anemia genes and the mismatch repair genes, predispose the individual to a different tumor spectrum as compared to heterozygous carriers.

Cancer predisposing syndromes can be grouped in a variety of ways. Some syndromes will have many clinical manifestations, among which cancer is just a rare feature, while others have cancer as the only clinical manifestation. Other ways to divide these conditions include by pathogenesis or by age of onset. However, we will present the syndromes grouped by the specific tumors they cause, since this will allow clinicians involved in the care of patients with brain tumors to consider the appropriate differential diagnoses based on the specific tumor histology.

This chapter will focus on the most common tumor predisposition syndromes and will elaborate on the genetic background, pathogenesis, and clinical approach to these disorders. Details on additional syndromes are presented in Table 1.1.

Syndromes Associated with Glioma

Gliomas are by far the most common group of brain tumors associated with cancer predisposition syndromes. These syndromes should always be considered if an index patient presents

M.A. Karajannis and D. Zagzag (eds.), *Molecular Pathology of Nervous System Tumors: Biological Stratification and Targeted Therapies*, Molecular Pathology Library 8,
DOI 10.1007/978-1-4939-1830-0_1,

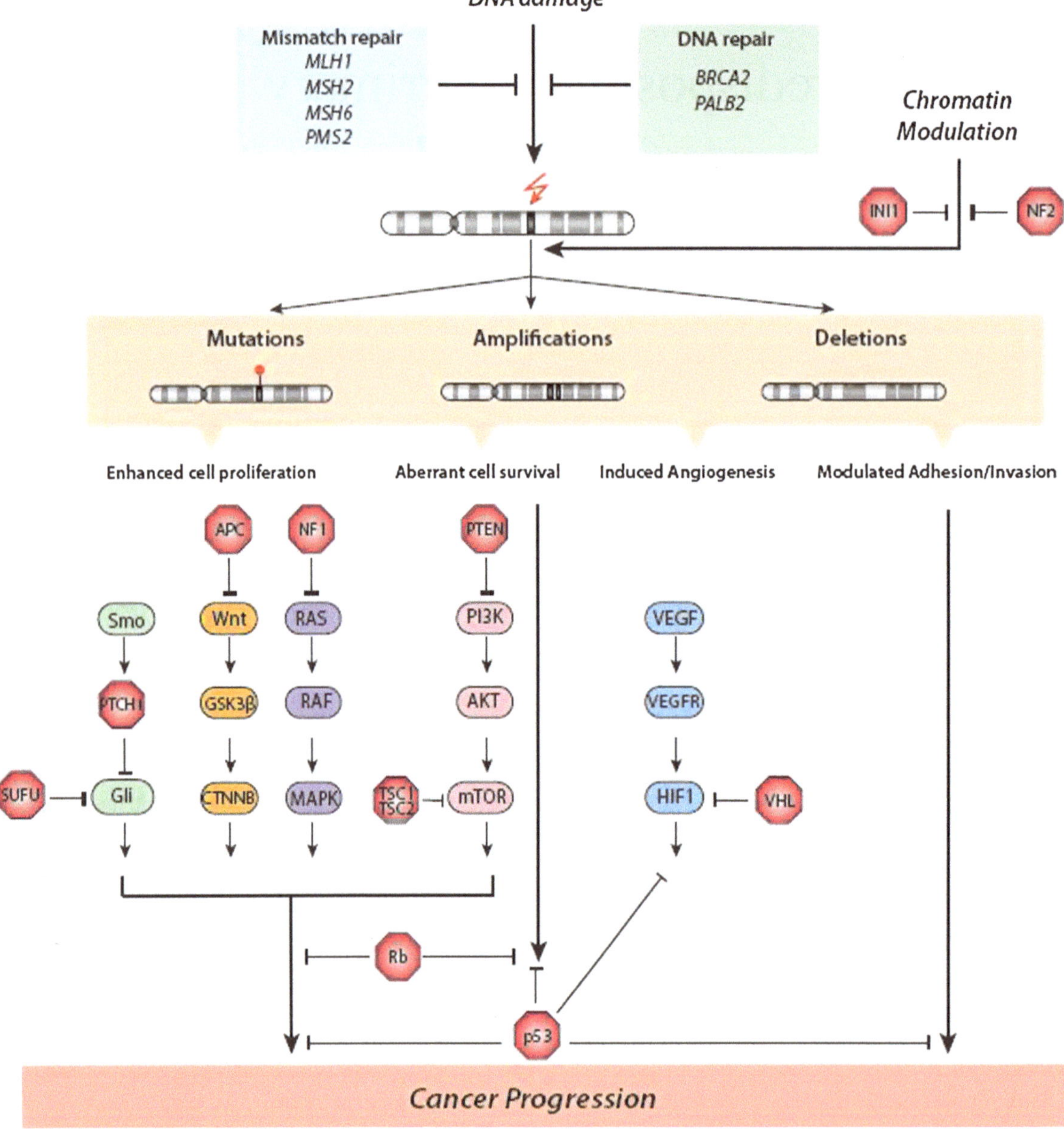

Fig. 1.1. Genes involved in predisposition to brain tumors.

with glioma. Each syndrome has unique features regarding clinical manifestations and personal or family history.

Neurofibromatosis Type I (NF1, von Recklinghausen's Disease)

NF1 is by far the most common CNS tumor predisposition syndrome. It is an autosomal dominant condition with a worldwide incidence of 1 per 2,500–3,000 individuals [6]. Importantly, this is a multisystem condition and diagnosis is generally made based on clinical criteria [6–8]. The following criteria are sensitive and specific in adults but affected children may not fulfil the criteria and genetic testing may aid the diagnosis [8]:

1. Six or more café-au-lait macules over 5 mm in greatest diameter in prepubertal individuals and over 15 mm in greatest diameter in postpubertal individuals
2. Two or more neurofibromas of any type or one plexiform neurofibroma
3. Freckling in the axillary or inguinal regions
4. Optic glioma

Table 1.1 Genetic syndromes not described in this chapter and associated with brain tumors.

Syndrome	Inheritance	Genetic abnormality	Cardinal features	Brain tumors	References
Aicardi syndrome	X-linked dominant lethal in males	Unknown	callosal agenesis, infantile spasms, chorioretinal lacunae	Choroid plexus papilloma	Frye RE, Polling JS, Ma LC. Choroid plexus papilloma expansion over 7 years in Aicardi syndrome. J Child Neurol. 2007 Apr;22(4):484-7. PubMed PMID: 17621535; PubMed Central PMCID: PMC2536525.
Distal 22q11.2 deletion syndrome	Autosomal dominant microdeletion usually sporadic	3.4 Mb deletion of chromosome 22q11.2, distal to the common DiGeorge syndrome (DGS) region encompassing the *INI1/ SMARCB1*	asymmetric face with preauricular sinuses and skin tags, cognitive disability	teratoid/rhabdoid tumor	Beddow RA, Smith M, Kidd A, Corbett R, Hunter AG. Diagnosis of distal 22q11.2 deletion syndrome in a patient with a teratoid/rhabdoid tumour. Eur J Med Genet. 2011 May-Jun;54(3):295-8. doi: 10.1016/j.ejmg.2010.12.007. Epub 2010 Dec 25. PubMed PMID: 21187175 Lafay-Cousin L, Payne E, Strother D, Chernos J, Chan M, Bernier FP. Goldenhar phenotype in a child with distal 22q11.2 deletion and intracranial atypical teratoid rhabdoid tumor. Am J Med Genet A. 2009 Dec;149A(12):2855-9. doi: 10.1002/ajmg.a.33119. PubMed PMID: 19938088 Jackson EM, Shaikh TH, Gururangan S, Jones MC, Malkin D, Nikkel SM, Zuppan CW, Wainwright LM, Zhang F, Biegel JA. High-density single nucleotide polymorphism array analysis in patients with germline deletions of 22q11.2 and malignant rhabdoid tumor. Hum Genet. 2007 Sep;122(2):117-27. Epub 2007 May 31. PubMed PMID: 17541642
Encephalocraniocutaneous lipomatosis	Isolated cases	unknown	Eye choristoma, nonscarring alopecia, nevus psiloliparus, subcutaneous fatty masses, nodular skin tags, and aplastic scalp defects, intracranial and intraspinal lipomas, congenital abnormalities of the meninges, seizures, developmental delays	low-grade glioma	Valera ET, Brassesco MS, Scrideli CA, de Castro Barros MV, Santos AC, Oliveira RS, Machado HR, Tone LG. Are patients with encephalocraniocutaneous lipomatosis at increased risk of developing low-grade gliomas? Childs Nerv Syst. 2012 Jan;28(1):19-22. doi: 10.1007/s00381-011-1601-z. Epub 2011 Oct 8. PubMed PMID: 21983849
Schimmelpenning-Feuerstein-Mims syndrome	Somatic mosaicism	*HRAS, KRAS*	sebaceous nevi, often on the face, associated with variable ipsilateral abnormalities of the central nervous system, ocular anomalies, and skeletal defects, seizures, developmental delays	Optic pathway glioma	Pavlidis E, Cantalupo G, Boria S, Cossu G, Pisani F. Hemimegalencephalic variant of epidermal nevus syndrome: case report and literature review. Eur J Paediatr Neurol. 2012 Jul;16(4):332-42. doi: 10.1016/j.ejpn.2011.12.004. Epub 2011 Dec 24. PubMed PMID: 22200538

(continued)

Table 1.1 (continued)

Syndrome	Inheritance	Genetic abnormality	Cardinal features	Brain tumors	References
Hypomelanosis of Ito	Somatic mosaicism	Chromsomal mosaicism	Skin macular hypopigmented whorls, streaks, and patches, developmental delays, seizures	choroid plexus papilloma	Morigaki R, Pooh KH, Shouno K, Taniguchi H, Endo S, Nakagawa Y. Choroid plexus papilloma in a girl with hypomelanosis of Ito. J Neurosurg Pediatr. 2012 Sep;10(3):182-5. doi: 10.3171/2012.5.PEDS11556. Epub 2012 Jul 13. Erratum in: J Neurosurg Pediatr. 2013 Jan;11(1):103. PubMed PMID: 22793165
Maffucci syndrome	Somatic mosaicism	*IDH1* or *IDH2*	multiple central cartilaginous tumors accompanied by soft tissue hemangiomas	Glioma, Pituitary adenoma, meningioma	Moriya K, Kaneko MK, Liu X, Hosaka M, Fujishima F, Sakuma J, Ogasawara S, Watanabe M, Sasahara Y, Kure S, Kato Y. IDH2 and TP53 mutations are correlated with gliomagenesis in a patient with Maffucci syndrome. Cancer Sci. 2014 Mar;105(3):359-62. doi: 10.1111/cas.12337. PubMed PMID: 24344754
Pai syndrome	Autosomal dominant	unknown	Median cleft lip, corpus callosum lipoma, skin polyps	Midline central nervous system lipomas	Mishima K, Mori Y, Minami K, Sakuda M, Sugahara T. A case of Pai syndrome. Plast Reconstr Surg. 1999 Jan;103(1):166-70. Review. PubMed PMID: 9915178.
Mupliple endicrine neoplasia type 1	Autosomal dominant	*MEN1*	tumors of parathyroids, pancreatic islets, duodenal endocrine cells, and the anterior pituitary	Meningioma and spinal cord ependymoma	Rogers L, Barani I, Chamberlain M, Kaley TJ, McDermott M, Raizer J, Schiff D, Weber DC, Wen PY, Vogelbaum MA. Meningiomas: knowledge base, treatment outcomes, and uncertainties. A RANO review. J Neurosurg. 2014 Oct 24:1-20. [Epub ahead of print] PubMed PMID: 25343186
Carney complex type 1	Autosomal dominant	*PRKAR1A*	cardiac, endocrine, cutaneous, and neural myxomatous tumors, as well as a variety of pigmented lesions of the skin and mucosae	Pituitary adenoma, schwannoma	Gadelha MR, Trivellin G, Hernández Ramírez LC, Korbonits M. Genetics of pituitary adenomas. Front Horm Res. 2013;41:111-40. doi: 10.1159/000345673. Epub 2013 Mar 19. Review. PubMed PMID: 23652674
Oral-facial-digital syndrome type VI	Autosomal recessive	*C5orf42, TMEM216*	Cerebellar malformations (molar tooth sign, tongue hamartoma, additional tongue frenula, upper lip notch, mesoaxial polydactyly of hands or feet	hypothalamic hamartoma	Lopez E, Thauvin-Robinet C, Reversade B, Khartoufi NE, Devisme L, Holder M, Ansart-Franquet H, Avila M, Lacombe D, Kleinfinger P, Kaori I, Takanashi J, Le Merrer M, Martinovic J, Noël C, Shboul M, Ho L, Güven Y, Razavi F, Burglen L, Gigot N, Darmency-Stamboul V, Thevenon J, Aral B, Kayserili H, Huet F, Lyonnet S, Le Caignec C, Franco B, Rivière JB, Faivre L, Attié-Bitach T. C5orf42 is the major gene responsible for OFD syndrome type VI. Hum Genet. 2014 Mar;133(3):367-77. doi: 10.1007/s00439-013-1385-1. Epub 2013 Nov 1. PubMed PMID: 24178751

Pallister-Hall syndrome	Autosomal dominant usually sporadic	*GLI3*	central polydactyly, anorectal malformations	hypothalamic hamartoma	Kang S, Graham JM Jr, Olney AH, Biesecker LG. GLI3 frameshift mutations cause autosomal dominant Pallister-Hall syndrome. Nat Genet. 1997 Mar;15(3):266-8. PubMed PMID: 9054938
Proteus syndrome	Somatic mosaicism	*AKT1*	disproportionate, asymmetric, and distorting overgrowth, bone abnormalities; characteristic cerebriform connective tissue nevus; epidermal nevi; vascular malformations of the capillary, venous, or lymphatic types; dysregulated adipose tissue; bullous lung alterations; intellectual disability; seizures; brain malformations	Meningioma	Cohen MM Jr. Proteus syndrome review: molecular, clinical, and pathologic features. Clin Genet. 2014 Feb;85(2):111-9. doi: 10.1111/cge.12266. Epub 2013 Oct 23. PubMed PMID: 23992099
Rubinstein-Taybi syndrome	Autosomal dominant usually sporadic	*CREBBP*	mental retardation, postnatal growth deficiency, microcephaly, broad thumbs and halluces, dysmorphic facial features	Meduloblastoma, meningioma	Roelfsema JH, Peters DJ. Rubinstein-Taybi syndrome: clinical and molecular overview. Expert Rev Mol Med. 2007 Aug 20;9(23):1-16. Review. PubMed PMID: 17942008
Short-rib thoracic dysplasia 12	Autosomal recessive	unknown	constricted thoracic cage, short ribs, shortened tubular bones, 'trident' appearance of the acetabular roof	Hypothalamic hamartoma	den Hollander NS, van der Harten HJ, Laudy JA, van de Weg P, Wladimiroff JW. Early transvaginal ultrasonographic diagnosis of Beemer-Langer dysplasia: a report of two cases. Ultrasound Obstet Gynecol. 1998 Apr;11(4):298-302. PubMed PMID: 9618859
Wiskott-Aldrich syndrome	X-linked recessive	*WAS*	Immunodeficiency, thrombocytopenia, eczema, and recurrent infections	Primary reticulum cell sarcoma of the brain	Model LM. Primary reticulum cell sarcoma of the brain in Wiskott-Aldrich syndrome. Report of a case. Arch Neurol. 1977 Oct;34(10):633-5. PubMed PMID: 334130
Xeroderma pigmentosum	Autosomal recessive	*XPA*, *ERCC1*, *ERCC3* (XP-B), *XPC*, *ERCC2* (XP-D), *DDB2* (XP-E), *ERCC4* (XP-F), *ERCC5* (XP-G), *POLH* (XPV)	severe sunburn with blistering, persistent erythema on minimal sun exposure, marked freckle-like pigmentation of the face, (photophobia, keratitis, atrophy of the skin of the eyelids, increased risk of cutaneous neoplasms	astrocytoma, medulloblastoma, schwannomas	Rapin I, Lindenbaum Y, Dickson DW, Kraemer KH, Robbins JH. Cockayne syndrome and xeroderma pigmentosum. Neurology. 2000 Nov 28;55(10):1442-9. Review. PubMed PMID: 11185579

5. Two or more Lisch nodules (iris hamartomas)
6. A distinctive osseous lesion such as sphenoid dysplasia or tibial pseudarthrosis
7. A first-degree relative (parent, sib, or offspring) with NF1 as defined by the above criteria

Individuals with NF1 can have significant morbidity unrelated to cancer predisposition [9]. The nervous system is commonly affected in NF1, and most cancers are of nervous system origin including gliomas, benign neurofibromas, and malignant nerve sheath tumors (MPNSTs). However, other cancers including chronic myelomonocytic leukemia, breast cancer, certain endocrine tumors, rhabdomyosarcoma, and neuroblastoma are reported with this condition [10].

Molecular Pathogenesis

NF1 results in loss of function of the tumor suppressor protein Neurofibromin. This large protein is a key negative regulator of the RAS pathway by catalyzing the hydrolysis of active guanosine triphosphate-bound RAS to inactive guanosine diphosphate-bound RAS [11]. Dysfunctional neurofibromin results in constitutive activation of downstream oncogenic pathways including MAPK and mTOR. Mutations or deletions in the *NF1*, gene can be identified in more than 95 % of individuals with NF1 [12]. However, since the gene is very large and difficult to analyze, diagnosis and management can be made based on clinical criteria. RAS/MAPK pathway activation is seen in almost all pediatric low-grade astrocytomas [13] and in 88 % of adult malignant gliomas [14]. Actual somatic mutations in *NF1* occur in 20 % of adult gliomas.

Mouse models of gliomas frequently alter the RAS/MAPK pathway. However, additional alterations in major tumor suppressor pathways such as TP53, RB, and PTEN are required to generate tumors [15].

Indeed, NF1 deficient mice do not have tumors but hyperplasia mimicking the optic pathway gliomas (OPG) commonly seen in these individuals [16]. Taken together, the benign nature of tumors seen in the CNS in patients with NF1 support the concept of oncogene induced senescence as a mechanism to explain the spontaneous growth arrest of these tumors when the RAS pathway is constitutively active [17].

Gliomas

The most common CNS tumor in NF1 are optic pathway gliomas (OPG) affecting up to 15 % of individuals with the syndrome. Conversely, up to a third of children with OPG have germline mutations in *NF1*. Bilateral optic nerve gliomas exist almost exclusively in children with NF1 (Fig. 1.2).

NF1 related OPG typically have an indolent course with spontaneous growth arrest. Indeed, the vast majority of these OPG will not progress after initial diagnosis. Up to 15 % of these tumors, however, do progress, resulting in visual loss or other symptoms and requiring intervention. High-grade gliomas are relatively uncommon, but have been reported and should be considered in patients whose tumors arise in an uncharacteristic location or demonstrate particularly aggressive behavior [18, 19].

Patients with NF1 often exhibit multiple lesions, mainly in the basal ganglia and brainstem which are difficult to assess. These include T2 bright lesions on MRI, without significant mass effect, termed FLAIR (fluid attenuated inversion recovery) associated sub-cortical intensities or FASCI (Fig. 1.2). These lesions tend to disappear spontaneously after initial growth and rarely cause symptoms. Differentiating between FASCI and low-grade gliomas in NF1 patients may be challenging.

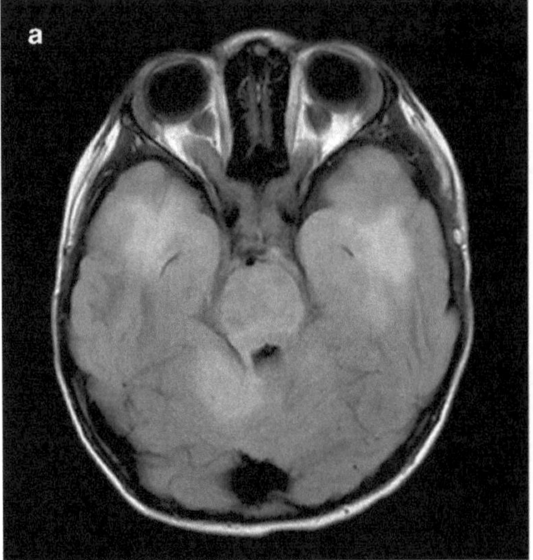

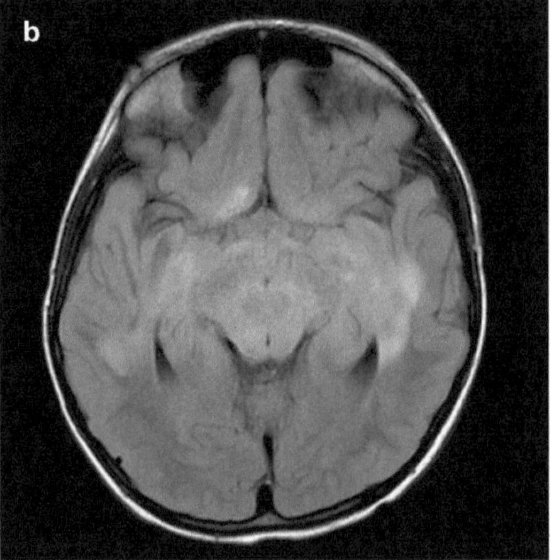

Fig. 1.2. Pathognomonic MRI findings in NF1. Bilateral optic nerve glioma (**a**) and FASCI (**b**) are almost exclusively seen only in children with NF1.

Clinical Implications

Since NF1 is a multisystem condition, careful monitoring is recommended in multidisciplinary clinics [6]. Due to the marked variability in clinical manifestations, including tumor occurrence, strategies for surveillance and follow-up must be tailored to each individual patient. Optic gliomas affecting both optic nerves and/or coexistence of FASCI should raise a suspicion of NF1 even in the absence of typical neurocutaneous findings such as café-au-lait macules, and genetic counseling is recommended.

Unfortunately, surveillance neuroimaging in asymptomatic children with NF1 has not been shown to reduce the incidence of visual loss in this population, and frequent neuro-ophthalmologic examination remains standard of care [20]. For FASCI and other atypical brain lesions, close monitoring is recommended and treatment should be reserved for patients with progressive clinical symptoms and in some cases, radiological progression.

Individuals with NF1 are particularly sensitive to the damaging effects of ionizing irradiation, leading both to an increased incidence of irradiation-induced cancers [21], as well as to cerebrovascular damage (Moyamoya syndrome) [22, 23]. Cranial irradiation in NF1 patients with OPG in particular and brain tumors in general, should be avoided as long as reasonable alternative treatment options exist.

Molecular Targeted Therapies

Inhibitors targeting the RAS and mTOR pathways are of great interest for the potential treatment of NF1 and NF1-related tumors, and are being investigated as novel therapeutic approaches in preclinical and clinical studies. Furthermore, targeting the microenvironment believed to be necessary for NF1 tumor growth may allow for additional NF1 specific therapies for these patients [24, 25]. For example, inhibition of c-KIT has shown encouraging efficacy for peripheral NF1 related neurofibromas in subsets of patients [26, 27], although it remains to be seen whether c-KIT represents a molecular target of value in NF1 related CNS tumors.

Li–Fraumeni Syndrome

The Li–Fraumeni syndrome (LFS) is the prototype cancer predisposition syndrome, causing cancer in multiple sites at different ages. LFS is an autosomal dominant condition affecting 1 in 5,000–10,000. Individuals with the disorder have a lifetime risk of 85–100 % of developing cancer. Originally described by Frederick Pei Li and Joseph F. Fraumeni, Jr. in 1969 [28] as a familial breast, soft tissue sarcoma and brain tumor predisposition syndrome, it is now known that these individuals have a risk of developing cancer in many additional organs, including rare tumors such as adrenocortical carcinomas, as well as hematologic malignancies [29].

According to Li et al. 1988 [30], who described the syndrome, the diagnosis is clinically established in families with a proband with a sarcoma diagnosed before age 45 years and a first-degree relative with any cancer before age 45 years and a first- or second-degree relative with any cancer before age 45 years or a sarcoma at any age. The association of LFS with germline mutations in the *TP53* prompted the formation of criteria to enhance the yield of *TP53* clinical genetic testing. The following criteria were published by Chompret et al. [31] and revised and evaluated by Gonzalez et al. [32], Tinat et al. [33], and Ruijs et al. [34] According to these studies the risk of a *TP53* mutation exceeds 20 % in any individual with:

1. A tumor belonging to the LFS tumor spectrum (e.g., soft tissue sarcoma, osteosarcoma, brain tumor, premenopausal breast cancer, adrenocortical carcinoma, leukemia, lung bronchoalveolar cancer) before age 46 years and at least one first- or second-degree relative with a LFS tumor (except breast cancer if the proband has breast cancer) before age 56 years or with multiple tumors; or
2. Multiple tumors (except multiple breast tumors), two of which belong to the LFS tumor spectrum and the first of which occurred before age 46 years; or
3. Adrenocortical carcinoma or choroid plexus tumor, regardless of family history.

Molecular Pathogenesis

In 1990 the association between LFS and germline mutations in the tumor suppressor gene *TP53* was made [35]. *TP53* is located at chromosome 17p13.1 and has been called the "gatekeeper of the genome," since it represents one of the key proteins that maintain genome integrity after DNA damage, hypoxia, and other stressors. *TP53* activation results in cell cycle arrest, senescence, and apoptosis. *TP53* is also involved in key metabolic pathways in the cell including cell metabolism and mitochondrial function [36]. *TP53* represents one of the most commonly mutated tumor suppressors known. Molecular genetic evidence of TP53 pathway disruption can be found in more than 50 % of tumors from adult cancer patients, as well as in 80 % of adult [13] and 50 % of pediatric high-grade gliomas [37].

Development of faithful preclinical models of LFS has been hindered by the fact that TP53 alteration in animal models generally fails to recapitulate the tumor phenotypes of the human disorder, and brain tumors are not a part of the phenotype even in some of the newer models [38]. Nevertheless, many glioma and medulloblastoma mouse models utilize TP53 alterations in conjunction with other cancer genes to mimic the human disease [39].

Three types of brain tumors are associated with LFS: high-grade gliomas, choroid plexus carcinoma, and medulloblastoma. Choroid plexus tumors affect LFS carriers in the first decade of life and medulloblastomas usually in the second, while malignant gliomas can occur throughout childhood, but more commonly in young adults.

Gliomas have been recognized as part of LFS from the earliest reports [28]. Although TP53 expression is associated with worse outcome in childhood glioblastoma [40], currently, no data exist regarding the significance of germline *TP53* mutations in pediatric high-grade gliomas. The surveillance protocol [41] developed by our group uncovered several low-grade gliomas suggesting that some of LFS associated glioblastomas arise as secondary glioblastomas and may benefit from early intervention.

Choroid plexus carcinomas are one of the most common presentations of LFS in young children and were recently added to the criteria for the diagnosis of the syndrome [33]. Furthermore, a significant number of patients with choroid plexus carcinoma will harbor germline *TP53* mutations. Somatic mutations in *TP53* are observed in up to 50 % of choroid plexus carcinomas, and this confers a poorer chance of survival for these patients [2]. This phenomenon may be caused by increased resistance of *TP53* mutant tumors to radiation and chemotherapy [42].

Medulloblastomas harbor somatic *TP53* mutations in 5–10 %, and appear strictly confined to the WNT (wingless-related integration site) and SHH (sonic hedgehog) subgroups of tumors [43]. Remarkably, *TP53* mutations do not alter the excellent survival of patients with WNT medulloblastomas, while *TP53* mutant SHH medulloblastomas are commonly seen in the second decade of life and have unfavorable outcome. Interestingly, these are commonly individuals with LFS. SHH medulloblastomas from LFS patients have a unique molecular genetic profile, suggesting chromothripsis ("chromosome shattering") as the initiating event [44].

Clinical Implications

Current recommendation is to screen for germline *TP53* mutations, i.e., LFS, in all individuals presenting either with a high-grade glioma and a family history of LFS tumors, or patients diagnosed with a choroid plexus carcinoma or medulloblastoma harboring somatic *TP53* mutations [33]. Cancer surveillance protocols developed specifically for individuals with LFS have revealed a high rate of early tumor detection [45]. Recently, a striking survival benefit for children has been observed using these protocols, mainly due to improved early detection of brain tumors (Fig. 1.3). Although no molecular targeted therapy for *TP53* mutated tumors is currently available, detection of a germline *TP53* mutation has significant prognostic and therapeutic implications for the patient. Both children and adults with LFS have been considered to be at an increased risk for developing radiation therapy-induced secondary malignant tumors [46, 47], as well as secondary myelodysplastic syndrome following specific chemotherapies [48].

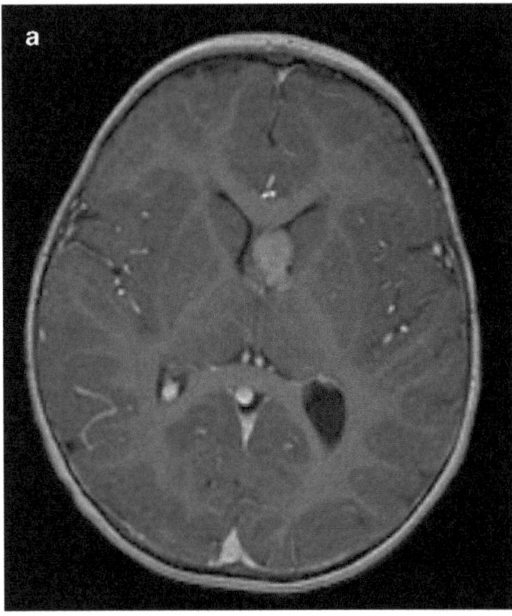

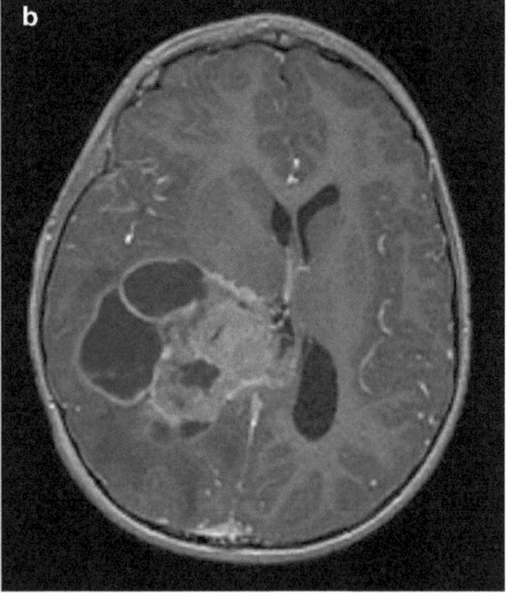

Fig. 1.3. Early detection of CPC after implementation of the surveillance protocol for LFS. Early detection of asymptomatic choroid plexus carcinoma in an LFS patient undergoing a surveillance protocol (**a**). A tumor from a patient with sporadic symptomatic choroid plexus carcinoma (**b**). The LFS patient underwent complete tumor resection followed by chemotherapy and is alive 7 years later. The patient with sporadic tumor did not survive despite radiation therapy and multiple courses of chemotherapy.

Constitutional Mismatch Repair Deficiency Syndrome

Constitutional Mismatch Repair Deficiency Syndrome (CMMR-D) is a rare familial cancer predisposition syndrome that has a unique clinical phenotype. This syndrome frequently presents with cafe-au-lait macules like NF1 [49, 50], resulting in occasional misdiagnosis and inappropriate management. CMMR-D is due to germline biallelic (homozygous or compound heterozygous) mutations in one of the mismatch repair (MMR) genes. Germline monoallelic mutations in MMR genes cause hereditary nonpolyposis colon cancer, Lynch syndrome and brain tumor-polyposis syndrome type 1 (BTPS1 or Turcot type 1) [51, 52]. The brain tumor in BTPS1 is glioblastoma multiforme.

Individuals with CMMR-D are predisposed to different and more aggressive cancers than Lynch syndrome. Children with CMMR-D are usually affected within the first two decades of life and present with hematological malignancies (most commonly T-cell lymphomas), malignant brain tumors, and gastrointestinal cancers.

Molecular Pathogenesis

Germline mutations in *MLH1*, *MSH2*, *MSH6*, and *PMS2* have been reported in association with CMMR-D. These mismatch repair genes are critical in repairing single base pair mismatches and misalignments [49]. In the absence of such genes, high mutation rates are observed, including in cancers which are described as "mutator phenotype" [14]. CMMR-D is inherited in an autosomal recessive fashion and is found mostly in consanguineous families. Some patients may have NF1 in addition to CMMR-D, which is thought to be caused by "secondary" early or germline mutations in the *NF1* gene as a part of the mutator phenotype [53].

Interestingly, mouse models of mismatch repair deficiency recapitulate cancers of the gastrointestinal tract and lymphomas, but fail to develop brain tumors [54, 55].

Brain Tumors

Malignant gliomas are the most common type of tumor observed in individuals with CMMR-D, usually presenting in the second decade of life. Some patients are initially diagnosed with low-grade gliomas, but these tend to transform to high-grade tumors. Medulloblastomas and PNETs (primitive neuroectodermal tumors) are also seen, but may have glial markers suggesting an earlier cell of origin. Some of these patients with high-grade gliomas have been reported as long-term survivors, possibly suggesting a somewhat more favorable prognosis compared to other adults and children with high-grade gliomas [56, 57].

Clinical Implications

Diagnosis of Lynch-related cancers can be made by evidence of microsatellite instability [58]. However, this method has not been shown to be sensitive in CMMR-D, especially in brain tumors and lymphomas. Immunostain of tumor tissue for the MMR proteins is almost universally negative in CMMR-D cancers, and has the unique diagnostic feature of negative stain in the corresponding normal tissue.

Any patient with gliomas, T-cell lymphoma and either café-au-lait macules, consanguinity or a family history of colon cancer should be screened for any of the four mismatch repair genes. Similarly, high index of suspicion should be raised for "NF1" patients with malignant gliomas and consanguinity.

Individuals with Lynch syndrome benefit from a strict surveillance protocol (www.NCCN.org) and from preventive colectomy. Therefore, early and accurate diagnosis may benefit parents and other family members. Since the risk of gliomas and lymphoma is extremely high for biallelic MMR patients, following a surveillance protocol may be beneficial for children with CMMR-D [59]. There are several reports of MMR tumors responding to specific agents including retinoic acid [60], which may be exploited for the treatment of these tumors.

Melanoma Astrocytoma Syndrome

In the mid-1990s, a syndrome of melanoma and other skin lesions associated with CNS malignancies was first described [61]. Since then, several other reports have delineated the association between familial melanoma and glioma. A common locus on the short arm of chromosome 9 was uncovered, and germline mutations were described in CDKN2A which codes for two proteins: p16(INK4) and p14(ARF) [62, 63]. Additional mutations in another gene in that location, *PTPRD*, were reported [64]. ARF and INK4A are major tumor suppressors in the TP53 and RB1 pathways respectively, and are altered in the majority of sporadic gliomas [14]. Further data, however, will be needed before specific screening and surveillance recommendations can be developed.

Syndromes Associated with Medulloblastoma

Medulloblastoma is the most common malignant brain tumor in children, but is also seen in adults. Several syndromes were first described to be associated with childhood medulloblastoma, but further data supports involvement of some of these syndromes in adult tumors as well [43]. We summarize here the most common syndromes, while others are described in Table 1.1.

Gorlin Syndrome (Basal Cell Nevus Syndrome)

Basal cell nevus syndrome (BCNS) is an autosomal dominant condition associated with multiple developmental anomalies and predisposition to benign and malignant tumors. The hallmark of BCNS is development of basal cell carcinomas and medulloblastomas. The association of multiple nevoid basal cell "epithelioma," jaw cysts and bifid ribs was first reported in 1960 [65].

Evans et al. [66] and Kimonis et al. [67] have published criteria for clinical diagnosis. Two major criteria and one minor or one major and three minor criteria are diagnostic of Gorlin syndrome. Some criteria require X-rays. Exposure to X-rays increases the risk for basal cell carcinoma and should be avoided.

Major Criteria

1. Falx calcification ascertained by AP skull X-rays.
2. Jaw keratocysts seen as translucencies on orthopantogram X-rays.
3. Two or more palmar/plantar pits.
4. Basal cell carcinoma before age 30 or multiple after age 30.
5. A first-degree relative with Gorlin syndrome.

Minor Criteria

1. Childhood medulloblastoma (primitive neuroectodermal tumor [PNET]).
2. Lympho-mesenteric or pleural cysts.
3. Macrocephaly (OFC >97th centile).
4. Cleft lip/palate.
5. Vertebral/rib anomalies (bifid vertebra), bifid/splayed/extra ribs ascertained by X-rays.
6. Preaxial or postaxial polydactyly.
7. Ovarian/cardiac fibromas.
8. Ocular anomalies (cataract, developmental defects, and pigmentary changes of the retinal epithelium).

Molecular Pathogenesis

The gene responsible for BCNS is *PTCH1* which is located on chromosome 9q22.3 [68]. PTCH1 is a protein that is a major suppressor of the sonic hedgehog (SHH) pathway by direct inhibition of SMO. Disruption of *PTCH1* leads to constitutive activation of the pathway and induction of *GLI* target genes and cell proliferation and survival. *SHH* is involved in neural development and midline segregation, which can explain some of the syndromatic manifestations of BCNS. Germline mutations in *SUFU*, which is a direct inhibitor of *GLI* have been reported in familial and sporadic medulloblastoma [69] in up to 50 % of desmoplastic tumors [70].

Most mouse models of medulloblastoma utilize alterations in the SHH pathway [71]. While alteration of PTCH1 only results in a tumor incidence of 10–20 %, its combination with other alterations results in very efficient formation of aggressive tumors.

Sequence analysis of *PTCH1* yields a mutation in 50–80 % of patients with Gorlin syndrome [72, 73]. Partial and whole-gene deletions are found in 6–21 % of patients [74]. In patients with mental retardation chromosome analysis and chromosomal microarray may reveal the 9q22.3 microdeletion. The 9q22.3 microdeletion syndrome is associated with cognitive impairment, metopic synostosis, obstructive hydrocephalus, macrosomia and seizures, in addition to the features of Gorlin syndrome [75].

Medulloblastoma

The first report of a brain tumor, medulloblastoma, in association with this hereditable syndrome [76] was published in 1963. The development of medulloblastoma in the setting of Gorlin syndrome occurs earlier compared to sporadic tumors. Most patients are younger than 3 years of age, and almost all tumors have a specific pathological subtype termed desmoplastic variant [77]. More specifically, desmoplasia with extensive nodularity (MBEN) is almost pathognomonic for the syndrome in young children [78, 79]. Of note, desmoplastic medulloblastomas in young children usually have a favorable outcome even without radiation therapy [80].

Meningioma

Several reports have documented the development of intracranial meningiomas in patients with Gorlin syndrome with or without prior craniospinal irradiation [81], although strength of association remains unknown.

Clinical Implications

Individuals with the clinical manifestations of BCNS, a family history of basal cell carcinomas, or other manifestations of the syndrome should be screened for germline mutations in *PTCH1 and SUFU*.

Patients with medulloblastoma and any of the above should also be screened, since radiation therapy is associated with an increased risk of developing basal cell carcinomas within the irradiated fields [82] in almost all patients. Furthermore, since the rate of germline mutations in the SHH pathway is extremely high in young children with desmoplastic medulloblastoma (Fig. 1.4) [70], children less than 3 years of age with desmoplastic tumors should be screened even without clinical manifestations of the syndrome. The current consensus recommends yearly brain MRI scans for all patients with BCNS until the age of 8 years [83].

The recent development of novel SHH pathway inhibitors [84] may lead to future targeted therapies for individuals with both Gorlin and SUFU syndromes, possibly including primary tumor prevention strategies.

Brain Tumor-Polyposis Syndrome 2 (BTPS 2 or Turcot Type 2; Familial Adenomatosis Coli)

Familial adenomatous polyposis (FAP) is an autosomal dominant cancer predisposition syndrome. Although the hallmark

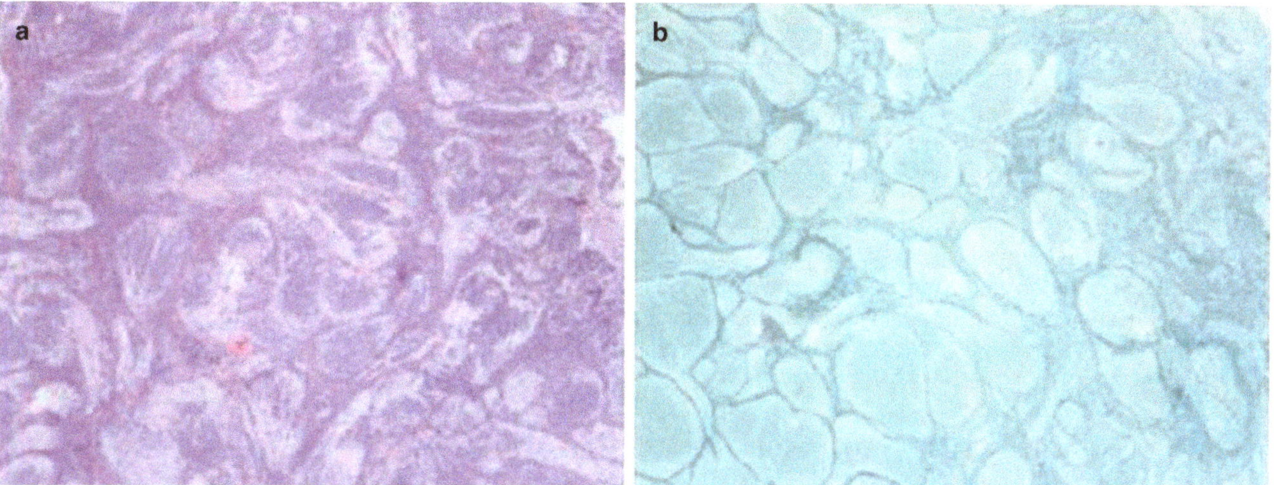

Fig. 1.4 Desmoplastic medulloblastoma. (**a**) Pale areas surrounded by densely packed hyperchromatic cells. (**b**) Same tumor reveals fine reticular areas with islands lacking reticulin

of this syndrome is the development of multiple gastrointestinal tract polyps and subsequent cancers, children with FAP are also at risk of developing medulloblastoma, hepatoblastoma, and aggressive fibromatoses.

The association between colorectal carcinoma and medulloblastoma was first reported in 1949 [85] and medulloblastoma is the only tumor observed in children with this syndrome. These patients and/or their family members display numerous (>100) small colonic polyps with later onset of malignant transformation to adenocarcinoma later in life. The pattern of inheritance here, distinct from BPTS type 1 (see glioma syndromes), is autosomal dominant and has been shown to be due to a heterozygous germline mutation in the adenomatous polyposis coli (*APC*) gene. Although the risk of developing medulloblastoma in patients with FAP is estimated 92-fold that of the general population [86], it is still a rare phenomenon among carriers.

Molecular Pathogenesis

FAP is caused by germline mutations in the gene *adenomatosis polyposis coli* (*APC*) [87]. *APC* is located on chromosome 5q21-22 and is a major regulator of the WNT pathway, which plays a paramount role in controlling embryonic development, stem cell viability and proliferation. Hyperactivation of the WNT pathway is reported in 5–10 % of medulloblastomas, usually as a result of mutations in *CTNNB1* [88, 89]. *APC* mutations are rare in sporadic medulloblastoma. Interestingly, no current mouse models exist for APC-driven medulloblastoma.

Clinical Implications

Since medulloblastoma is rare in FAP, carriers are not routinely screened for these tumors. However, a patient with medulloblastoma and FAP should undergo GI cancer surveillance, since the development of medulloblastoma in PBTS 2 may precede the development of colonic adenocarcinoma. Indeed, patients are reported with simultaneous diagnoses of medulloblastoma and colonic adenocarcinoma. It is important to note that *APC* mutated medulloblastomas are distinct from most *WNT* activated medulloblastomas. WNT tumors will have *CTNNB1* mutations that can be diagnosed by nuclear staining of the gene product. Although WNT pathway activation generally confers favorable survival in sporadic medulloblastomas, the prognosis of *APC* mutated tumors is still uncertain, and FAP patients therefore should not be treated with less aggressive protocols.

Fanconi Anemia Cancer Predisposition Disorders

Fanconi anemia is a cancer predisposition syndrome with bone marrow failure and characteristic malformations. The malformations are seen in about 60 % of affected individuals and include low birth weight, short stature, pigmentary abnormalities of the skin, abnormal thumbs, and hypoplastic radii [90]. There is genetic variability in Fanconi anemia (FA): patients may have mutations in one out of 15 known genes that cause the syndrome. One of the genes, FANCB, is associated with X-linked recessive inheritance and the rest with autosomal recessive [90].

The following features of FA suggest the clinical diagnosis and genetic testing [91]:

1. Characteristic congenital malformations as well as growth and developmental delays
2. Bone marrow failure in childhood which is usually progressive
3. Aplastic anemia in adults

4. Unexpected bone marrow failure after chemotherapy or radiation
5. Myelodysplastic syndrome or acute myelogenous leukemia
6. Solid tumors in young age including squamous cell carcinomas of the head and neck, esophagus, and vulva

If Fanconi anemia (FA) is clinically suspected the next step is chromosome breakage studies using diepoxybutane or mitomycin C as clastogenic agent [92]. If increased chromosome breakage is ascertained then DNA sequencing and deletion/duplication tests are available for all the known genes: *FNCA, FANCB, FANCC, BRCA2, FANCD2, FANCE, FANCF, FANCG, FANCI, BRIP1, FANCL, FANCM, PALB2, RAD51C*, and *SLX4* [93]. If the patient is Ashkenazi Jewish with no history of carrier testing in the patient or the parents then testing for the *FANCC* mutation (c.456+4A>C) should be the first step [94].

Bone marrow failure states and/or myeloid dysplasias or leukemias (median age for onset is 14 years) develop in most individuals with FA [91]. In addition, a variety of solid tumors have long been recognized to develop with increasing frequency, particularly liver adenomas (in association with prior androgenic steroid use for the bone marrow failure) [90], and gastrointestinal and gynecological carcinomas, with a median age at diagnosis of about 29 years [95]. The median age for onset of the leukemias is 14 years. It has been estimated that, by theoretically removing the competing risks of marrow failure and leukemias, individuals with FA have an estimated cumulative probability of developing a solid tumor of 76 % by the age of 45 years [96].

Although brain tumors in FA patients were reported in the past [97, 98], the involvement of medulloblastoma [99] and glioma [100] in specific germline mutations has not been suggested until recently.

Molecular Pathogenesis

FA is a genetically heterogeneous disorder associated with either biallelic mutations in any of the known 14 autosomal genes or a mutation in an X-linked gene [101]. Individuals in the FA complementation group *FANCD1* are estimated to represent no more than 3 % of all individuals with FA, and it is this group in whom biallelic mutations with *BRCA2* are found. *BRCA2* mutations are well known to be associated with familial predisposition to breast and ovarian cancer. Brain tumors have also been reported in such families [102]. These individuals may present a more severe phenotype with early onset of cancer. In particular, the cumulative probability of developing a brain tumor (almost always medulloblastoma) could be high as 85 % in the first decade [99]. This knowledge has prompted a search for other genes in the pathway and familial childhood cancers. Recently, germline mutations in *PALB2*, another gene in the Fanconi pathway, were reported to be associated with medulloblastomas and other pediatric cancers [103].

Mouse models of FA usually fail to produce the cancers and other organ damage seen in humans [104]. However, an increased incidence of tumors has been observed in *Fancd2* deficient mice [105]. This gene interacts with *BRCA2* and *PALB2*.

Clinical Implications

The rare individuals who develop medulloblastoma in the setting of FA do so at a very early age, often before a diagnosis of FA has been made. Individuals with FA undergoing treatment for cancer are known to be highly sensitive to both irradiation and chemotherapy, with increased susceptibility for treatment-associated toxicities, especially from alkylator-based chemotherapy [106]. Thus, any early onset pediatric brain tumor with cutaneous, skeletal, or neurological abnormalities consistent with a diagnosis of FA or in case of severe unexpected toxicity from chemotherapy, genetic counseling is recommended.

The concept of synthetic lethality is being exploited in the use of PARP inhibitors in BRCA1/2 deficient breast, ovarian, and pancreatic cancers [107, 108], which could be of value in FA as well. To date, however, no data exist on the use of PARP inhibitors in the treatment of FA-related medulloblastoma.

Meningioma

Meningiomas are slow growing CNS lesions accounting for roughly a third of CNS tumors in adults [109]. While most of these tumors are sporadic or occur as a result of prior radiation therapy, familial cases of meningiomas are well reported. The most common genetic syndrome associated with meningiomas is neurofibromatosis type 2 (NF2). This syndrome has additional clinical features, and will be discussed in the section of tumor specific syndromes. However, several kindreds with familial meningioma lack linkage to the NF2 locus [110] are diagnosed with other known syndromes such as Li–Fraumeni, Cowden, Gorlin, and multiple endocrine neoplasia (MEN) [111]. Recently, genetic analysis of familial meningiomas uncovered involvement of the SWI/SNF family members *SMARCB1* and *SMARCE1* in several families diagnosed with schwannomatosis [112] with meningiomatosis [113]. Furthermore, as described above, patients with Gorlin syndrome including *SUFU* mutations [114], carry an increased risk of meningiomas.

Indeed, several reports implicate the SHH pathway in a subset of sporadic meningiomas of non-NF2 origin, offering a potential molecular target for the treatment of these tumors [115, 116].

Tumor Specific Syndromes

These tumors are unique to a specific cancer predisposition syndrome. Whenever that specific pathology is recognized, a high index of suspicion for the corresponding cancer syndrome should exist, regardless of family of personal history.

Although we will elaborate on several specific syndromes, other cancers are highly suggestive of predisposition to cancer, and germline analysis is recommended. A good example is choroid plexus carcinoma [2], which is strongly associated with LFS.

Subependymal Giant Cell Astrocytoma

SEGA is seen almost exclusively in the context of patients with tuberous sclerosis (TS) complex and conversely, SEGA is the only CNS tumor seen in TS. TS is an autosomal dominant multisystem condition affecting both children and adults [3]. Tumors outside the CNS arising in these patients are generally slow growing and include cardiac rhabdomyoma, renal angiomyolipoma, and pulmonary lymphangioleiomyomatosis. Although these lesions are histologically benign, they can cause significant organ dysfunction resulting in morbidity and in some cases mortality. Additionally, individuals with TS can occasionally develop malignant renal cell carcinomas.

Molecular Pathogenesis

Linkage analysis enabled the discovery of two genes responsible for the TS syndrome. These are *TSC1*, also known as *Hamartin*, located on chromosome 9q34 [117] and *TSC2* or *Tuberin* on chromosome 16p13. These genes exert their tumor suppressor activity by inhibition of *RHEB*, which is the major activator of the mammalian target of rapamycin (mTOR) complex. The AKT/mTOR pathway is a key driver of tumorigenesis [118] in TS patients and an important therapeutic target.

SEGAs develop in 5–15 % of patients with TS complex, usually in the first two decades of life. Rarely, SEGAs may occur in patients without any other evidence of TS, typically in older adults. SEGAs are intraventricularly located tumors, usually in close proximity to the foramen of Monroe, are histologically benign (WHO grade I), but can nevertheless lead to significant morbidity and mortality due to development of hydrocephalus from obstruction of cerebrospinal fluid (CSF) flow at the foramen, as well as due to subependymal invasion into eloquent brain parenchyma.

Clinical Implications

In TS patients, brain MRI scans should be obtained at least annually during childhood and adolescence, when the risk for SEGA development is greatest [119].

TS represents a prototype disease in which biological discoveries have led to the successful development of effective targeted therapies, with profound consequences on clinical management. First-generation mTOR inhibitors (termed rapamycin analogs or rapalogs, including rapamycin) are mTOR complex 1 (mTORC1) specific inhibitors, acting downstream of TSC 1 and 2. As predicted by preclinical data, clinical trials using rapalogs have revealed striking tumor regression of virtually all SEGAs in treated TS patients [120–122] (Fig. 1.5), as well as improvement in pulmonary function for patients with lymphangioleyomyomatosis [123]. Additional evidence suggests that rapalogs can improve other aspects of the syndrome including neurological symptoms including seizures [124, 125]. As a consequence, everolimus was granted United States Food and Drug Administration (FDA) approval for the treatment of pediatric and adult TS patients with SEGA. In addition, prevention strategies and protocols for long-term therapy with rapalogs are currently being developed for these patients [126].

Atypical Teratoid Rhabdoid Tumor

This deadly pediatric embryonal tumor exists solely in the context of the *Rhabdoid Tumor Predisposition Syndrome* (*RTPS*).

Malignant rhabdoid tumor of the kidney was initially reported in 1978, but the association with second primary "embryonal" tumors in the brain was not recognized until much later [127]. Historically, these tumors were classified as medulloblastoma or PNET based on histologic resemblance, but recognized as a distinct clinico-pathologic entity in 1995 and termed CNS atypical teratoid/rhabdoid tumor (AT/RT) of infancy and childhood [128]. They were recognized to be highly lethal tumors, with virtually all children dying of progressive tumor within 6–12 months of diagnosis [128].

Cytogenetically, AT/RT commonly harbor monosomy of chromosome 22. In 1999, both germline (constitutional) and acquired mutations on chromosome 22q11.2 in children with CNS AT/RT were reported [129], and shortly thereafter the term "rhabdoid predisposition syndrome" was coined to define the newly recognized heritable syndrome predisposing to both renal or extra-renal malignant rhabdoid tumors and malignant brain tumors [130]. By 2008, the entity of "rhabdoid predisposition syndrome" was sufficiently well documented to merit inclusion within the "World Health Organization (WHO) Classification of Tumours of the CNS (4th Edition)" [131].

Molecular Pathogenesis

The *SMARCB1* gene, also known as *INI1/hSNF5*, was cloned in 1998 [132] and is located on chromosome 22q11. Heterozygous germline loss-of-function mutations in the gene were first described in 1999 [130]. This facilitated the definition and permitted assessment of the risk of germline mutations in individuals with AT/RT. Germline mutations occur in up to 35 % of AT/RT patients, are more common in younger patients, and can be invariably found in patients presenting with both CNS and extra-cranial tumors. The biologic function of *SMARCB1* remains poorly understood. However, it is thought to be involved in nucleosome modification [133] and disruption of the gene results in spindle checkpoint defects and a high rate of chromosomal instability [134].

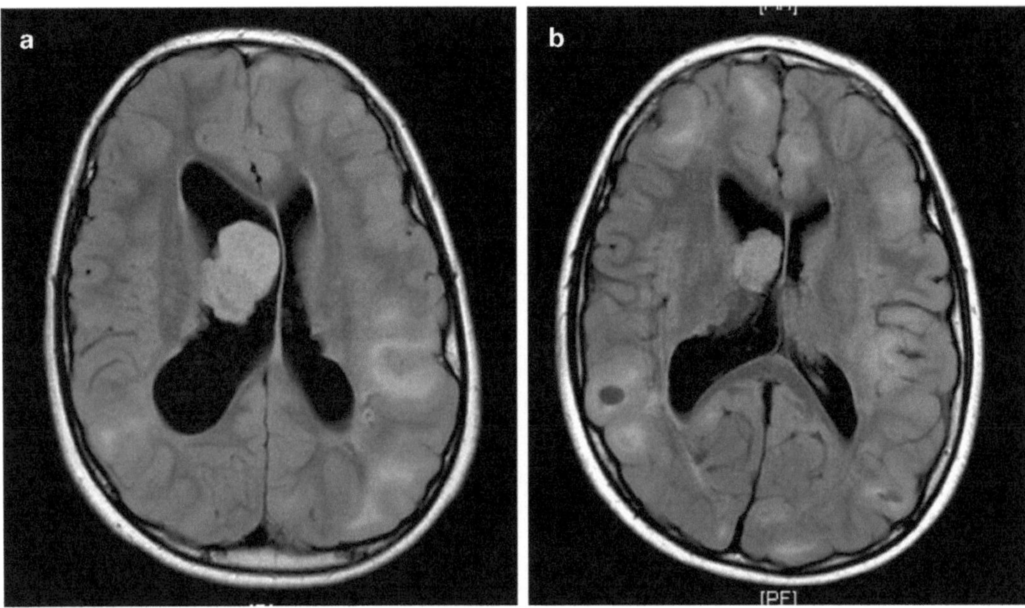

Fig. 1.5 Response of SEGA to oral treatment with sirolimus. Right ventricular SEGA causing mild hydrocephalus (**a**). The same lesion (**b**) after 3 months of oral therapy with sirolimus

Recent observation that loss of *SMARCB1* leads to activation of the *SHH* pathway is intriguing [135]. Mouse models using haploinsufficiency in Smarcb1 result in soft tissue sarcomas mimicking rhabdoid tumors but do not recapitulate AT/RT [136].

Clinical Implications

Patients with RTPS may present with synchronous or metachronous tumors. Known RTPS patients should undergo periodic surveillance imaging of both the abdomen (ultrasound or MRI) and the brain (MRI).

Until recently, CNS AT/RT was considered almost uniformly incurable and rapidly lethal. In recent years, however, the prognosis for young children with CNS AT/RT appears to have improved through better molecular diagnosis of the tumor and implementation of aggressive surgical resection of primary tumors followed by intensive chemotherapy [137–139]. It remains unclear whether the improved prognosis in older children with CNS AT/RT primarily reflects their ability to better tolerate radiation therapy, or rather is linked to differences in biology compared to the same tumors arising in infants. The outcome for children with CNS AT/RT specifically in the setting of the RTPS has not yet been reported.

The spectrum of tumors with *SMARCB1* somatic mutations is growing and includes other soft tissue sarcomas as well as schwannomas [140, 141]. Germline *SMSRCB1* mutations are the cause of familial schwannomatosis in about 40 % of the families with the condition [141, 142] and about 80 % of the remaining families with familial schwannomatosis have a mutation in *LZTR1* [143]. Because very few patients with recognized RTPS are long-term survivors, the cancer spectrum and lifetime risk of other malignancies in carriers remain unknown.

Hemangioblastoma

This tumor is the hallmark of the von Hippel–Lindau (VHL) syndrome, and patients diagnosed with hemangioblastoma require a genetic workup.

VHL syndrome is a tumor predisposition syndrome characterized by a variety of CNS and extraneural tumors. Von Hippel originally described retinal tumors as well as vascular tumors in the viscera, and the connection with the often fatal cystic vascular tumors of the cerebellum was first recognized by Lindau in 1926 [144].

The VHL syndrome is inherited as an autosomal dominant disorder with very high penetrance of over 90 % by age 65 years. The most common manifestation of the disease is CNS and retinal hemangioblastomas, which occur in 70 % and 60 % of patients, respectively [145]. The reduced life expectancy, however, is primarily linked to renal cell carcinomas that occur in up to 20 % of individuals.

The clinical diagnosis of VHL is considered in an individual without family history of VHL when two of the following are present [145–147]:

- Two or more hemangioblastomas of the retina, spine, or brain or a single hemangioblastoma in association with a visceral manifestation (e.g., multiple kidney or pancreatic cysts)
- Renal cell carcinoma

- Adrenal or extra-adrenal pheochromocytomas
- Less commonly, endolymphatic sac tumors, papillary cystadenomas of the epididymis or broad ligament, or neuroendocrine tumors of the pancreas

The clinical diagnosis of VHL is considered in an individual with a positive family history of VHL when one of the following is present:

- Retinal angioma
- Spinal or cerebellar hemangioblastoma
- Adrenal or extra-adrenal pheochromocytoma
- Renal cell carcinoma
- Multiple renal and pancreatic cysts

Clinical genetic testing for VHL is available with 72 % of the mutations being sequence variants and 28 % partial or whole-gene deletions [148–150]. Atypical presentation can be due to somatic mosaicism [151]. There is no genetic heterogeneity associated with the VHL phenotype.

Molecular Pathogenesis

The *VHL* gene is located on the short arm of chromosome 3 (3p25-26) and was first identified as the VHL tumor suppressor gene in 1993 [152]. VHL interacts with other proteins and forms a substrate recognition unit for ubiquitin ligase, which targets the hypoxia-inducible factor (HIF) genes 1 and 2 for degradation. Under normal circumstances, hypoxia results in HIF proteins to activate multiple metabolic and oncogenic pathways in the cell, including increased levels of VEGF, PDGF, erythropoietin and TGF. Abnormal VHL protein results in constitutive activation of HIF and other factors, leading to reduced apoptosis, increased proliferation, and increased angiogenesis [153], resulting in tumor formation [154].

Interestingly, mouse models using different alterations of *Vhl* resulted in erythrocytosis (polycythemia) and renal abnormalities [155], but did not produce a cancer phenotype or CNS lesions [156].

CNS Hemangioblastomas

These tumors arise, in order of diminishing frequency, in the cerebellum (44–72 % of all patients with VHL syndrome), the retina (25–60 %), intramedullary spinal cord (13–50 %), brainstem (10–25 %), supratentorial compartment (<1 %), and lumbosacral nerve roots (<1 %) [145]. CNS hemangioblastomas arising as single tumors outside of the posterior fossa are rarely sporadic, and multiple hemangioblastomas are virtually pathognomonic for the presence of a *VHL* germline mutation. The mean age of diagnosis of CNS hemangioblastomas is between 30 and 35 years. While CNS hemangioblastomas are considered "benign" tumors, these tumors were associated with significant morbidity and mortality prior to the recognition of their association with VHL and the establishment of screening guidelines for early detection.

Clinical Implications

All patients diagnosed with hemangioblastoma should be screened for germline mutations in *VHL*. De novo mutations are common and are detectable in up to 20 % of patients. Since mosaic mutations are reported, multiple hemangioblastomas, several tumors or family history of tumors compatible with the VHL spectrum can establish the diagnosis of VHL syndrome even in the absence of a detectable mutation in blood leukocytes. A surveillance protocol has been developed and it is aimed at not only improving survival, but also reducing morbidity from earlier interventions for VHL tumors [157, 158]. The suggested surveillance includes:

Starting at age 1 year: annual evaluation for neurologic symptoms, vision problems, and hearing disturbance; annual blood pressure monitoring; annual ophthalmology evaluation.

Starting at age 5 years: annual blood or urinary fractionated metanephrines; audiology assessment every 2–3 years; thin-slice MRI with contrast of the internal auditory canal in those with repeated ear infections. Starting at age 16 years: annual abdominal ultrasound and every other year MRI scan of the abdomen; MRI of the brain and total spine every 2 years.

Development of New Medications

The association of VHL and renal cell carcinoma has led the development of compounds which target VEGF receptor signaling, as VEGF is significantly overexpressed as a result of HIF activation in sporadic renal cell carcinoma. These "anti-angiogenic" drugs and others have been used in patients with hemangioblastomas with some success [159–161]. It is hoped that drugs that provide satisfactory long-term tumor control or are suitable for prevention will be developed for VHL patients in the future.

Cerebellar Dysplastic Gangliocytoma (Lhermitte–Duclos Disease)

This brain lesion is pathognomonic for Cowden syndrome or multiple hamartoma syndrome, "Cowden's disease." Cowden syndrome was first described in 1963 and named after the first reported patient, Rachel Cowden, who had multiple mucocutaneous hamartomatous abnormalities [162]. About 90 % of patients who develop Cowden Syndrome develop clinical manifestations before 20 years of age, although may not be diagnosed until the third decade of life. Women have between a 25 and 50 % lifetime risk of developing breast cancer as well as an increased risk of developing endometrial cancer, and both men and women have a 10 % lifetime risk of developing epithelial thyroid cancer. About 50 % of cases of Cowden syndrome are considered to be inherited.

Brain Tumors

The recognition that cerebellar dysplastic gangliocytoma (Lhermitte–Duclos Disease) might be a manifestation of

Cowden syndrome was first reported in 1991 [163]. While more commonly seen in adults [164] about 5–10 % occur during childhood.

Molecular Pathogenesis

Cowden syndrome is a member of the PTEN Hamartoma Tumor Syndrome (PHTS). This entity encompasses four major, clinically distinct syndromes associated with germline mutations in the tumor suppressor *PTEN*. These allelic disorders, Cowden syndrome, Bannayan–Riley–Ruvalcaba syndrome, and Proteus-like syndrome are associated with dysregulated cellular proliferation leading to the formation of hamartomas [165, 166]. Thus far, an increased risk of malignancy has only been documented in Cowden syndrome.

PTEN is located on chromosome 10q23 and is a phosphatase that competes with PI3K, a major protein kinase which acts by reducing PI3P levels in cells. Reduction of 3-phosphoinositides decreases activity of kinases downstream of PI3K such as Akt and mTOR, and is responsible for its tumor suppressor activity. The PI3K/Akt/mTOR pathway is a major oncogenic signaling pathway, which regulates cell metabolism, survival, proliferation, migration, and angiogenesis [167]. Although *PTEN* alterations are a major component of adult gliomagenesis [13], individuals with germline *PTEN* mutations do not have increased susceptibility for these tumors. Cowden syndrome has been associated with a germline mutation of the *PTEN* gene in about 80 % of cases, with an additional 10 % harboring mutations in the *PTEN* promoter region.

Clinical Implications

Overall, the incidence of cerebellar dysplastic gangliocytoma has been estimated to be 15 % among patients with Cowden syndrome undergoing magnetic resonance imaging surveillance scans, with additional patients revealing meningiomas (5 %) and other vascular malformations in 30 % [168]. Therefore, it is recommended that patients with Cowden syndrome undergo annual surveillance screening with brain MRI. Surveillance guidelines for individuals with Cowden syndrome are available (www.NCCN.org) and should be utilized for affected family members [167]. Recent observations of reduction in hamartomas for patients with PHTS after treatment with rapamycin [169], and the finding of excess levels of *mTOR* pathway expression in Lhermitte–Duclos disease (LDD) tumor tissue [170] suggest that medical prevention or treatment of LDD and other neoplasms in individuals with Cowden syndrome is feasible.

Vestibular Schwannomas (Acoustic Neuromas)

Bilateral vestibular schwannomas (VS), arising at the vestibular branch of the eighth cranial nerve, are pathognomonic for the tumor predisposition syndrome neurofibromatosis type 2 (NF2, Fig. 1.6). For historical reasons, NF2 has been grouped together with NF1 as phakomatoses (or "neurocutaneous syndromes"), but differs from neurofibromatosis type 1 with respect to the underlying genetic defect, disease biology, clinical manifestations, and tumor spectrum.

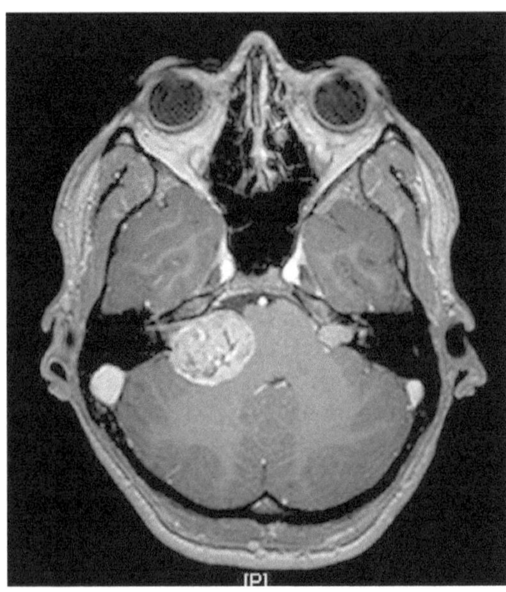

Fig. 1.6 Bilateral acoustic neuroma in NF2

Neurofibromatosis type II (NF2) is an autosomal dominant tumor predisposition syndrome characterized by the development of bilateral VS and schwannomas of other cranial, spinal, and peripheral nerves. Individuals with NF2 are also predisposed to developing intracranial, spinal, and optic nerve sheath meningiomas, as well as low-grade ependymomas of the CNS [171, 172].

The cardinal feature is bilateral vestibular schwannoma presenting clinically with any or the combination of hearing loss, tinnitus, and imbalance. One of the modified NIH criteria [173] is sufficient for the diagnosis:

1. Bilateral vestibular schwannomas
2. A first-degree relative with NF2 and (a) or (b)
   (a) Unilateral vestibular schwannoma
   (b) Any two of: meningioma, schwannoma, glioma, neurofibroma, posterior subcapsular lenticular opacities
3. Unilateral vestibular schwannoma and any two of: meningioma, schwannoma, glioma, neurofibroma, posterior subcapsular lenticular opacities
4. Multiple meningiomas and (a) or (b)
   (a) Unilateral vestibular schwannoma
   (b) Any two of: schwannoma, glioma, neurofibroma, cataract

Most affected have bilateral vestibular schwannomas by age 30. About 50 % of individuals have an affected parent. About 20–30 % of simplex cases (only case affected in a family) are mosaic for an *NF2* mutation. NF2 is due to all type of mutations in the *NF2* gene including all size deletions and chromosome abnormalities. The mutation detection rate approaches 72 % in simplex cases and exceeds 92 % for familial cases [66, 174–176].

Molecular Pathogenesis

The gene responsible for NF2 was discovered in 1993 as *Neurofibromin 2* or *Merlin* (HGNC Approved Gene Symbol: *NF2*), located on chromosome 22q12.2 [177, 178]. Despite intensive efforts, the physiologic role of Merlin, as well as its function as a tumor suppressor remains incompletely understood [179]. There is a high rate of mosaicism in individuals with a de novo mutation, termed "founders." Therefore the chance of transmission, which is autosomal dominant, may be less than 50 % in such individuals.

Intracranial Tumors

The hallmark of NF2 is the development of bilateral VS, with a lifetime penetrance of over 95 % in NF2 individuals. Although historically considered to be a syndrome mainly presenting in young adulthood, up to 20 % of patients will present prior to 15 years of age [180]. Alternatively, NF2 patients may first present with non-vestibular schwannomas (33 %), meningiomas (31 %), or spinal tumors (11.5 %). Over time, the majority if NF2 patients will develop bilateral VS, as well an increasing tumor burden including other intracranial schwannomas, as well meningiomas and ependymomas. Progressive VS result in neurological complications including hearing loss, facial weakness, and brainstem compression. Depending on location, other intracranial tumors may cause cranial nerve dysfunction, brain compression, and/or seizures.

Spinal Tumors

The incidence of spinal tumors in patients with NF2 may reach 89 % [181]. About one-third of spinal tumors in association with NF2 are intramedullary ependymomas. Of the extra-medullary tumors, schwannomas are most common, followed by meningiomas, with neurofibromas being very uncommon. These tumors are usually multifocal, and often asymptomatic. Progressive growth, however, can lead to pain, cord compression, myelopathy, and/or neurologic impairment.

Clinical Implications

A consensus meeting has produced surveillance guidelines for individuals with NF2 [182]. Asymptomatic children carrying the mutation should be followed expectantly and screened with MRI surveillance and audiograms beginning at age 10 years. Like other patients with rare diseases, NF2 are best managed by a multidisciplinary team with disease-specific expertise. Although surgery and supportive therapy have been the mainstay of treatment for NF2 patients, bevacizumab has recently emerged as a therapeutic option that can lead to tumor shrinkage and hearing improvement in a subset of NF2 patients with VS [182]. Other targeted therapies are under development and evaluation consensus recommendations for current treatments and accelerating clinical trials for patients with neurofibromatosis type 2 [183].

Implications of Molecular Tumor Testing on Genetic Counseling

Most patients are referred to genetic counseling due to combination of family history of cancer or other diseases and findings on clinical examination. This approach may change in the near future due to implementation of pathological and genetic tests as routine for tumor diagnosis. These may suggest cancer predisposition in the absence of the above clinical findings. Several examples are worth mentioning. A child diagnosed with desmoplastic medulloblastoma less than 3 years old has 50 % chance of having BCNS (Gorlin syndrome). ATRT and choroid plexus carcinomas mutated for *SMARCB1* and *TP53*, respectively, carry very high rate of germline mutations too. Furthermore, children older than 5 years with *TP53* mutant SHH medulloblastoma are most probably LFS patients. Since these molecular tests are routinely used and will be a part of all modern clinical trials, the indications for genetic counseling may change and the spectrum of tumors and clinical manifestations of some of these syndromes may change as a result.

Summary

This chapter does not aim at summarizing all clinical and molecular aspects of predisposition syndromes affecting brain tumors patients. Further information is available in the references provided. Furthermore, the relatively common syndromes were elaborated above while other less common syndromes are mentioned in Table 1.1. Nevertheless, the burden of cancer predisposition on neuro-oncology is significant and knowledge of the diagnosis, management, and appropriate treatment will impact the patient and family members. Recognizing hereditary conditions that predispose to brain tumors is important for providing the appropriate treatment and surveillance. Surveillance protocols have shown survival benefit and novel therapies exist for some specific genetic alterations.

In the research arena, detailed phenotyping and genotyping informs molecular pathophysiology with ensuing discovery of new genetic tests and new treatments. Individuals with germline mutations in cancer predisposing genes may benefit from early detection and personalized therapies for their cancer which will eventually offer improved morbidity and mortality.

References

1. Eaton KW, Tooke LS, Wainwright LM, Judkins AR, Biegel JA. Spectrum of SMARCB1/INI1 mutations in familial and sporadic rhabdoid tumors. Pediatr Blood Cancer. 2011;56:7–15.
2. Tabori U, Shlien A, Baskin B, et al. TP53 alterations determine clinical subgroups and survival of patients with choroid plexus tumors. J Clin Oncol. 2010;28:1995–2001.
3. Crino PB, Nathanson KL, Henske EP. The tuberous sclerosis complex. N Engl J Med. 2006;355:1345–56.
4. Evans DG. Neurofibromatosis 2 [Bilateral acoustic neurofibromatosis, central neurofibromatosis, NF2, neurofibromatosis type II]. Genet Med. 2009;11:599–610.
5. Testa JR, Malkin D, Schiffman JD. Connecting molecular pathways to hereditary cancer risk syndromes. Am Soc Clin Oncol Educ Book. 2013:81–90. doi:10.1200/EdBook_AM.2013.33.81.
6. Williams VC, Lucas J, Babcock MA, Gutmann DH, Korf B, Maria BL. Neurofibromatosis type 1 revisited. Pediatrics. 2009;123:124–33.
7. Szudek J, Evans DG, Friedman JM. Patterns of associations of clinical features in neurofibromatosis 1 (NF1). Hum Genet. 2003;112:289–97.
8. Ferner RE, Huson SM, Thomas N, et al. Guidelines for the diagnosis and management of individuals with neurofibromatosis 1. J Med Genet. 2007;44:81–8.
9. Rasmussen SA, Yang Q, Friedman JM. Mortality in neurofibromatosis 1: an analysis using U.S. death certificates. Am J Hum Genet. 2001;68:1110–8.
10. Brems H, Beert E, de Ravel T, Legius E. Mechanisms in the pathogenesis of malignant tumours in neurofibromatosis type 1. Lancet Oncol. 2009;10:508–15.
11. Rubin JB, Gutmann DH. Neurofibromatosis type 1—a model for nervous system tumour formation? Nat Rev Cancer. 2005;5:557–64.
12. Wimmer K, Yao S, Claes K, Kehrer-Sawatzki H, Tinschert S, De Raedt T, Legius E, Callens T, Beiglböck H, Maertens O, Messiaen L. Spectrum of single- and multiexon NF1 copy number changes in a cohort of 1,100 unselected NF1 patients. Genes Chromosomes Cancer. 2006;45(3):265–76. PubMed PMID: 16283621.
13. Jones DT, Hutter B, Jager N, et al. Recurrent somatic alterations of FGFR1 and NTRK2 in pilocytic astrocytoma. Nat Genet. 2013;45(8):927–32.
14. Cancer Genome Atlas Research Network. Comprehensive genomic characterization defines human glioblastoma genes and core pathways. Nature. 2008;455:1061–8.
15. Rankin SL, Zhu G, Baker SJ. Review: insights gained from modelling high-grade glioma in the mouse. Neuropathol Appl Neurobiol. 2012;38:254–70.
16. Thangarajh M, Gutmann DH. Review: low-grade gliomas as neurodevelopmental disorders: insights from mouse models of neurofibromatosis-1. Neuropathol Appl Neurobiol. 2012;38:241–53.
17. Sun P, Yoshizuka N, New L, et al. PRAK is essential for ras-induced senescence and tumor suppression. Cell. 2007;128:295–308.
18. Rosenfeld A, Listernick R, Charrow J, Goldman S. Neurofibromatosis type 1 and high-grade tumors of the central nervous system. Childs Nerv Syst. 2010;26:663–7.
19. Huttner AJ, Kieran MW, Yao X, et al. Clinicopathologic study of glioblastoma in children with neurofibromatosis type 1. Pediatr Blood Cancer. 2010;54:890–6.
20. Listernick R, Ferner RE, Liu GT, Gutmann DH. Optic pathway gliomas in neurofibromatosis-1: controversies and recommendations. Ann Neurol. 2007;61:189–98.
21. Sharif S, Ferner R, Birch JM, et al. Second primary tumors in neurofibromatosis 1 patients treated for optic glioma: substantial risks after radiotherapy. J Clin Oncol. 2006;24:2570–5.
22. Okuno T, Prensky AL, Gado M. The moyamoya syndrome associated with irradiation of an optic glioma in children: report of two cases and review of the literature. Pediatr Neurol. 1985;1:311–6.
23. Ibrahimi DM, Tamargo RJ, Ahn ES. Moyamoya disease in children. Childs Nerv Syst. 2010;26:1297–308.
24. Sun T, Gianino SM, Jackson E, Piwnica-Worms D, Gutmann DH, Rubin JB. CXCL12 alone is insufficient for gliomagenesis in Nf1 mutant mice. J Neuroimmunol. 2010;224:108–13.
25. Warrington NM, Gianino SM, Jackson E, et al. Cyclic AMP suppression is sufficient to induce gliomagenesis in a mouse model of neurofibromatosis-1. Cancer Res. 2010;70:5717–27.
26. Robertson KA, Nalepa G, Yang FC, et al. Imatinib mesylate for plexiform neurofibromas in patients with neurofibromatosis type 1: a phase 2 trial. Lancet Oncol. 2012;13:1218–24.
27. Yang FC, Ingram DA, Chen S, et al. Nf1-dependent tumors require a microenvironment containing Nf1+/− and c-kit-dependent bone marrow. Cell. 2008;135:437–48.
28. Li FP, Fraumeni Jr JF. Soft-tissue sarcomas, breast cancer, and other neoplasms. A familial syndrome? Ann Intern Med. 1969;71:747–52.
29. Olivier M, Hollstein M, Hainaut P. TP53 mutations in human cancers: origins, consequences, and clinical use. Cold Spring Harb Perspect Biol. 2010;2:a001008.
30. Li FP, Fraumeni JF, Mulvihill JJ, Blattner WA, Dreyfus MG, Tucker MA, Miller RW. A cancer family syndrome in twenty-four kindreds. Cancer Res. 1988;48:5358–62.
31. Chompret A, Abel A, Stoppa-Lyonnet D, Brugieres L, Pages S, Feunteun J, Bonaiti-Pellie C. Sensitivity and predictive value of criteria for p53 germline mutation screening. J Med Genet. 2001;38:43–7.
32. Gonzalez KD, Noltner KA, Buzin CH, Gu D, Wen-Fong CY, Nguyen VQ, Han JH, Lowstuter K, Longmate J, Sommer SS, Weitzel JN. Beyond Li-Fraumeni syndrome: clinical characteristics of families with p53 germline mutations. J Clin Oncol. 2009;27:1250–6.
33. Tinat J, Bougeard G, Baert-Desurmont S, Vasseur S, Martin C, Bouvignies E, Caron O, Bressac-de Paillerets B, Berthet P, Dugast C, Bonaiti-Pellie C, Stoppa-Lyonnet D, Frebourg T. 2009 Version of the Chompret criteria for Li Fraumeni syndrome. J Clin Oncol. 2009;27:e108–9.
34. Ruijs MW, Verhoef S, Rookus MA, et al. TP53 germline mutation testing in 180 families suspected of Li-Fraumeni syndrome: mutation detection rate and relative frequency of cancers in different familial phenotypes. J Med Genet. 2010;47:421–8.
35. Malkin D, Li FP, Strong LC, et al. Germ line p53 mutations in a familial syndrome of breast cancer, sarcomas, and other neoplasms. Science. 1990;250:1233–8.
36. Wang PY, Ma W, Park JY, et al. Increased oxidative metabolism in the Li-Fraumeni syndrome. N Engl J Med. 2013;368:1027–32.
37. Schwartzentruber J, Korshunov A, Liu XY, et al. Driver mutations in histone H3.3 and chromatin remodelling genes in paediatric glioblastoma. Nature. 2012;482:226–31.

38. Lang GA, Iwakuma T, Suh YA, et al. Gain of function of a p53 hot spot mutation in a mouse model of Li-Fraumeni syndrome. Cell. 2004;119:861–72.
39. England B, Huang T, Karsy M. Current understanding of the role and targeting of tumor suppressor p53 in glioblastoma multiforme. Tumour Biol. 2013;34:2063–74.
40. Pollack IF, Finkelstein SD, Woods J, et al. Expression of p53 and prognosis in children with malignant gliomas. N Engl J Med. 2002;346:420–7.
41. Villani A, Tabori U, Schiffman J, et al. Biochemical and imaging surveillance in germline TP53 mutation carriers with Li-Fraumeni syndrome: a prospective observational study. Lancet Oncol. 2011;12:559–67.
42. Krzyzankova M, Mertsch S, Koos B, et al. Loss of TP53 expression in immortalized choroid plexus epithelial cells results in increased resistance to anticancer agents. J Neurooncol. 2012;109:449–55.
43. Zhukova N, Ramaswamy V, Remke M, et al. Subgroup-specific prognostic implications of TP53 mutation in medulloblastoma. J Clin Oncol. 2013;31(23):2927–35.
44. Rausch T, Jones DT, Zapatka M, et al. Genome sequencing of pediatric medulloblastoma links catastrophic DNA rearrangements with TP53 mutations. Cell. 2012;148:59–71.
45. Masciari S, Van den Abbeele AD, Diller LR, et al. F18-fluorodeoxyglucose-positron emission tomography/computed tomography screening in Li-Fraumeni syndrome. JAMA. 2008;299:1315–9.
46. Kony SJ, de Vathaire F, Chompret A, et al. Radiation and genetic factors in the risk of second malignant neoplasms after a first cancer in childhood. Lancet. 1997;350:91–5.
47. Heymann S, Delaloge S, Rahal A, et al. Radio-induced malignancies after breast cancer postoperative radiotherapy in patients with Li-Fraumeni syndrome. Radiat Oncol. 2010;5:104.
48. Talwalkar SS, Yin CC, Naeem RC, Hicks MJ, Strong LC, Abruzzo LV. Myelodysplastic syndromes arising in patients with germline TP53 mutation and Li-Fraumeni syndrome. Arch Pathol Lab Med. 2010;134:1010–5.
49. Wimmer K, Etzler J. Constitutional mismatch repair-deficiency syndrome: have we so far seen only the tip of an iceberg? Hum Genet. 2008;124:105–22.
50. Durno CA, Holter S, Sherman PM, Gallinger S. The gastrointestinal phenotype of germline biallelic mismatch repair gene mutations. Am J Gastroenterol. 2010;105:2449–56.
51. Paraf F, Jothy S, Van Meir EG. Brain tumor-polyposis syndrome: two genetic diseases? J Clin Oncol. 1997;15(7): 2744–58.
52. Bakry D, Aronson M, Durno C, et al. Genetic and clinical determinants of constitutional mismatch repair deficiency syndrome: report from the constitutional mismatch repair deficiency consortium. Eur J Cancer. 2014;50(5):987–96. pii:S0959-8049(13)01070-8.
53. Wang Q, Montmain G, Ruano E, et al. Neurofibromatosis type 1 gene as a mutational target in a mismatch repair-deficient cell type. Hum Genet. 2003;112:117–23.
54. Edelmann W, Yang K, Umar A, et al. Mutation in the mismatch repair gene Msh6 causes cancer susceptibility. Cell. 1997;91:467–77.
55. Prolla TA, Baker SM, Harris AC, et al. Tumour susceptibility and spontaneous mutation in mice deficient in Mlh1, Pms1 and Pms2 DNA mismatch repair. Nat Genet. 1998;18:276–9.
56. Van Meir EG. "Turcot's syndrome": phenotype of brain tumors, survival and mode of inheritance. Int J Cancer. 1998;75:162–4.
57. Lusis EA, Travers S, Jost SC, Perry A. Glioblastomas with giant cell and sarcomatous features in patients with turcot syndrome type 1: a clinicopathological study of 3 cases. Neurosurgery. 2010;67(3):811–7; discussion 7.
58. Lynch HT, de la Chapelle A. Hereditary colorectal cancer. N Engl J Med. 2003;348:919–32.
59. Carol Durno CH, Aronson M, Holter S, Waltho S, Parkin P, Gallinger S, Farah R, Chan H, Bouffet E, Bartels U, Huang A, Druker H, Malkin D, Tabori U. Distinctive clinical, genetic and cancer features of children with mismatch repair cancer susceptibility and RAS/MAPK syndromes. Neuro Oncol. 2010;12:ii35.
60. Gottschling S, Reinhard H, Pagenstecher C, et al. Hypothesis: possible role of retinoic acid therapy in patients with biallelic mismatch repair gene defects. Eur J Pediatr. 2008;167:225–9.
61. Azizi E, Friedman J, Pavlotsky F, et al. Familial cutaneous malignant melanoma and tumors of the nervous system. A hereditary cancer syndrome. Cancer. 1995;76:1571–8.
62. Bahuau M, Vidaud D, Jenkins RB, et al. Germ-line deletion involving the INK4 locus in familial proneness to melanoma and nervous system tumors. Cancer Res. 1998;58:2298–303.
63. Randerson-Moor JA, Harland M, Williams S, et al. A germline deletion of p14(ARF) but not CDKN2A in a melanoma-neural system tumour syndrome family. Hum Mol Genet. 2001;10:55–62.
64. Solomon DA, Kim JS, Cronin JC, et al. Mutational inactivation of PTPRD in glioblastoma multiforme and malignant melanoma. Cancer Res. 2008;68:10300–6.
65. Gorlin RJ, Goltz RW. Multiple nevoid basal-cell epithelioma, jaw cysts and bifid rib. A syndrome. N Engl J Med. 1960;262: 908–12.
66. Evans DGR, Ramsden RT, Shenton A, Gokhale C, Bowers NL, Huson SM, Wallace A. Mosaicism in NF2 an update of risk based on uni/bilaterality of vestibular schwannoma at presentation and sensitive mutation analysis including MLPA. J Med Genet. 2007;44:424–8.
67. Kimonis VE, Mehta SG, Digiovanna JJ, Bale SJ, Pastakia B. Radiological features in 82 patients with nevoid basal cell carcinoma (NBCC or Gorlin) syndrome. Genet Med. 2004;6:495–502.
68. Johnson RL, Rothman AL, Xie J, et al. Human homolog of patched, a candidate gene for the basal cell nevus syndrome. Science. 1996;272:1668–71.
69. Taylor MD, Liu L, Raffel C, et al. Mutations in SUFU predispose to medulloblastoma. Nat Genet. 2002;31:306–10.
70. Brugieres L, Remenieras A, Pierron G, et al. High frequency of germline SUFU mutations in children with desmoplastic/ nodular medulloblastoma younger than 3 years of age. J Clin Oncol. 2012;30:2087–93.
71. Huse JT, Holland EC. Genetically engineered mouse models of brain cancer and the promise of preclinical testing. Brain Pathol. 2009;19:132–43.
72. Klein RD, Dykas DJ, Bale AE. Clinical testing for the nevoid basal cell carcinoma syndrome in a DNA diagnostic laboratory. Genet Med. 2005;7:611–9.
73. Marsh A, Wicking C, Wainwright B, Chenevix-Trench G. DHPLC analysis of patients with Nevoid Basal Cell Carcinoma Syndrome reveals novel PTCH missense mutations in the sterol-sensing domain. Hum Mutat. 2005;26:283.

74. Nagao K, Fujii K, Saito K, Sugita K, Endo M, Motojima T, Hatsuse H, Miyashita T. Entire PTCH1 deletion is a common event in point mutation-negative cases with nevoid basal cell carcinoma syndrome in Japan. Clin Genet. 2011;79:196–8.
75. Muller EA, Swaroop A, Atkin JF, Elliott AM, Chudley AE, Clark RD, Everman DB, Garner S, Hall BD, Herman GE, Kivuva E, Ramanathan S, Stevenson DA, Stockton DW, Hudgins L. Microdeletion 9q22.3 syndrome includes metopic craniosynostosis, hydrocephalus, macrosomia and developmental delay. Am J Med Genet A. 2012;158A:391–9.
76. Herzberg JJ, Wiskemann A. [The fifth phakomatosis. Basal cell nevus with hereditary malformation and medulloblastoma]. Dermatologica. 1963;126:106–23.
77. Amlashi SF, Riffaud L, Brassier G, Morandi X. Nevoid basal cell carcinoma syndrome: relation with desmoplastic medulloblastoma in infancy. A population-based study and review of the literature. Cancer. 2003;98:618–24.
78. Giangaspero F, Perilongo G, Fondelli MP, et al. Medulloblastoma with extensive nodularity: a variant with favorable prognosis. J Neurosurg. 1999;91:971–7.
79. Garre ML, Cama A, Bagnasco F, et al. Medulloblastoma variants: age-dependent occurrence and relation to Gorlin syndrome—a new clinical perspective. Clin Cancer Res. 2009;15:2463–71.
80. Rutkowski S, von Hoff K, Emser A, et al. Survival and prognostic factors of early childhood medulloblastoma: an international meta-analysis. J Clin Oncol. 2010;28:4961–8.
81. Pribila JT, Ronan SM, Trobe JD. Multiple intracranial meningiomas causing papilledema and visual loss in a patient with nevoid Basal cell carcinoma syndrome. J Neuroophthalmol. 2008;28:41–6.
82. Evans DG, Farndon PA, Burnell LD, Gattamaneni HR, Birch JM. The incidence of Gorlin syndrome in 173 consecutive cases of medulloblastoma. Br J Cancer. 1991;64:959–61.
83. Bree AF, Shah MR. Consensus statement from the first international colloquium on basal cell nevus syndrome (BCNS). Am J Med Genet A. 2011;155A:2091–7.
84. Rudin CM, Hann CL, Laterra J, et al. Treatment of medulloblastoma with hedgehog pathway inhibitor GDC-0449. N Engl J Med. 2009;361:1173–8.
85. Crail HW. Multiple primary malignancies arising in the rectum, brain, and thyroid; report of a case. U S Nav Med Bull. 1949;49:123–8.
86. Hamilton SR, Liu B, Parsons RE, et al. The molecular basis of Turcot's syndrome. N Engl J Med. 1995;332:839–47.
87. Kinzler KW, Nilbert MC, Su LK, et al. Identification of FAP locus genes from chromosome 5q21. Science. 1991;253:661–5.
88. Northcott PA, Korshunov A, Witt H, et al. Medulloblastoma comprises four distinct molecular variants. J Clin Oncol. 2011;29(11):1408–14.
89. Pfister S, Remke M, Benner A, et al. Outcome prediction in pediatric medulloblastoma based on DNA copy-number aberrations of chromosomes 6q and 17q and the MYC and MYCN loci. J Clin Oncol. 2009;27:1627–36.
90. Shimamura A, Alter BP. Pathophysiology and management of inherited bone marrow failure syndromes. Blood Rev. 2010;24:101–22.
91. Eiler ME, Frohnmayer D, Frohnmayer L, Larsen K, Olsen J, editors. Fanconi anemia: guidelines for diagnosis and management. 3rd ed. Eugene: Fanconi Anemia Research Fund Inc; 2008.
92. Auerbach AD. Fanconi anemia diagnosis and the diepoxybutane (DEB) test. Exp Hematol. 1993;21:731–3.
93. Ameziane N, Errami A, Léveillé F, Fontaine C, de Vries Y, van Spaendonk RM, de Winter JP, Pals G, Joenje H. Genetic subtyping of Fanconi anemia by comprehensive mutation screening. Hum Mutat. 2008;29:159–66.
94. Whitney MA, Saito H, Jakobs PM, Gibson RA, Moses RE, Grompe M. A common mutation in the FACC gene causes Fanconi anaemia in Ashkenazi Jews. Nat Genet. 1993;4:202–5.
95. Alter BP, Giri N, Savage SA, Peters JA, Loud JT, Leathwood L, Carr AG, Greene MH, Rosenberg PS. Malignancies and survival patterns in the National Cancer Institute inherited bone marrow failure syndromes cohort study. Br J Haematol. 2010;150:179–88.
96. Alter BP. Cancer in Fanconi anemia, 1927–2001. Cancer. 2003;97:425–40.
97. de Chadarevian JP, Vekemans M, Bernstein M. Fanconi's anemia, medulloblastoma, Wilms' tumor, horseshoe kidney, and gonadal dysgenesis. Arch Pathol Lab Med. 1985;109:367–9.
98. Alter BP, Tenner MS. Brain tumors in patients with Fanconi's anemia. Arch Pediatr Adolesc Med. 1994;148:661–3.
99. Alter BP, Rosenberg PS, Brody LC. Clinical and molecular features associated with biallelic mutations in FANCD1/BRCA2. J Med Genet. 2007;44:1–9.
100. Wilson BT, Douglas SF, Polvikoski T. Astrocytoma in a breast cancer lineage: part of the BRCA2 phenotype? J Clin Oncol. 2010;28:e596–8.
101. D'Andrea AD, Grompe M. The Fanconi anaemia/BRCA pathway. Nat Rev Cancer. 2003;3:23–34.
102. Offit K, Levran O, Mullaney B, et al. Shared genetic susceptibility to breast cancer, brain tumors, and Fanconi anemia. J Natl Cancer Inst. 2003;95:1548–51.
103. Reid S, Schindler D, Hanenberg H, et al. Biallelic mutations in PALB2 cause Fanconi anemia subtype FA-N and predispose to childhood cancer. Nat Genet. 2007;39:162–4.
104. Bakker ST, de Winter JP, te Riele H. Learning from a paradox: recent insights into Fanconi anaemia through studying mouse models. Dis Model Mech. 2013;6:40–7.
105. Houghtaling S, Timmers C, Noll M, et al. Epithelial cancer in Fanconi anemia complementation group D2 (Fancd2) knockout mice. Genes Dev. 2003;17:2021–35.
106. Ruud E, Wesenberg F. Microcephalus, medulloblastoma and excessive toxicity from chemotherapy: an unusual presentation of Fanconi anaemia. Acta Paediatr. 2001;90:580–3.
107. Carden CP, Yap TA, Kaye SB. PARP inhibition: targeting the Achilles' heel of DNA repair to treat germline and sporadic ovarian cancers. Curr Opin Oncol. 2010;22:473–80.
108. Leung K, Saif MW. BRCA-associated pancreatic cancer: the evolving management. JOP. 2013;14:149–51.
109. Choy W, Kim W, Nagasawa D, et al. The molecular genetics and tumor pathogenesis of meningiomas and the future directions of meningioma treatments. Neurosurg Focus. 2011;30:E6.
110. Pulst SM, Rouleau GA, Marineau C, Fain P, Sieb JP. Familial meningioma is not allelic to neurofibromatosis 2. Neurology. 1993;43:2096–8.
111. Asgharian B, Chen YJ, Patronas NJ, et al. Meningiomas may be a component tumor of multiple endocrine neoplasia type 1. Clin Cancer Res. 2004;10:869–80.
112. van den Munckhof P, Christiaans I, Kenter SB, Baas F, Hulsebos TJ. Germline SMARCB1 mutation predisposes to

multiple meningiomas and schwannomas with preferential location of cranial meningiomas at the falx cerebri. Neurogenetics. 2012;13:1–7.
113. Smith MJ, O'Sullivan J, Bhaskar SS, et al. Loss-of-function mutations in SMARCE1 cause an inherited disorder of multiple spinal meningiomas. Nat Genet. 2013;45:295–8.
114. Aavikko M, Li SP, Saarinen S, et al. Loss of SUFU function in familial multiple meningioma. Am J Hum Genet. 2012;91:520–6.
115. Clark VE, Erson-Omay EZ, Serin A, et al. Genomic analysis of non-NF2 meningiomas reveals mutations in TRAF7, KLF4, AKT1, and SMO. Science. 2013;339:1077–80.
116. Brastianos PK, Horowitz PM, Santagata S, et al. Genomic sequencing of meningiomas identifies oncogenic SMO and AKT1 mutations. Nat Genet. 2013;45:285–9.
117. van Slegtenhorst M, de Hoogt R, Hermans C, et al. Identification of the tuberous sclerosis gene TSC1 on chromosome 9q34. Science. 1997;277:805–8.
118. Sabatini DM. mTOR and cancer: insights into a complex relationship. Nat Rev Cancer. 2006;6:729–34.
119. Roach ES, Gomez MR, Northrup H. Tuberous sclerosis complex consensus conference: revised clinical diagnostic criteria. J Child Neurol. 1998;13:624–8.
120. Franz DN, Leonard J, Tudor C, et al. Rapamycin causes regression of astrocytomas in tuberous sclerosis complex. Ann Neurol. 2006;59:490–8.
121. Krueger DA, Care MM, Holland K, et al. Everolimus for subependymal giant-cell astrocytomas in tuberous sclerosis. N Engl J Med. 2010;363:1801–11.
122. Franz DN, Belousova E, Sparagana S, et al. Efficacy and safety of everolimus for subependymal giant cell astrocytomas associated with tuberous sclerosis complex (EXIST-1): a multicentre, randomised, placebo-controlled phase 3 trial. Lancet. 2013;381:125–32.
123. Paul E, Thiele E. Efficacy of sirolimus in treating tuberous sclerosis and lymphangioleiomyomatosis. N Engl J Med. 2008;358:190–2.
124. Ehninger D, Han S, Shilyansky C, et al. Reversal of learning deficits in a Tsc2+/– mouse model of tuberous sclerosis. Nat Med. 2008;14:843–8.
125. Wiegand G, May TW, Ostertag P, Boor R, Stephani U, Franz DN. Everolimus in tuberous sclerosis patients with intractable epilepsy: A treatment option? Eur J Paediatr Neurol. 2013;17(6):631–8.
126. Krueger DA, Care MM, Agricola K, Tudor C, Mays M, Franz DN. Everolimus long-term safety and efficacy in subependymal giant cell astrocytoma. Neurology. 2013;80:574–80.
127. Bonnin JM, Rubinstein LJ, Palmer NF, Beckwith JB. The association of embryonal tumors originating in the kidney and in the brain. A report of seven cases. Cancer. 1984;54:2137–46.
128. Rorke LB, Packer R, Biegel J. Central nervous system atypical teratoid/rhabdoid tumors of infancy and childhood. J Neurooncol. 1995;24:21–8.
129. Biegel JA, Zhou JY, Rorke LB, Stenstrom C, Wainwright LM, Fogelgren B. Germ-line and acquired mutations of INI1 in atypical teratoid and rhabdoid tumors. Cancer Res. 1999;59:74–9.
130. Sevenet N, Sheridan E, Amram D, Schneider P, Handgretinger R, Delattre O. Constitutional mutations of the hSNF5/INI1 gene predispose to a variety of cancers. Am J Hum Genet. 1999;65:1342–8.
131. Brat DJ, Parisi JE, Kleinschmidt-DeMasters BK, et al. Surgical neuropathology update: a review of changes introduced by the WHO classification of tumours of the central nervous system, 4th edition. Arch Pathol Lab Med. 2008;132:993–1007.
132. Versteege I, Sevenet N, Lange J, et al. Truncating mutations of hSNF5/INI1 in aggressive paediatric cancer. Nature. 1998;394:203–6.
133. Wilson BG, Roberts CW. SWI/SNF nucleosome remodellers and cancer. Nat Rev Cancer. 2011;11:481–92.
134. Vries RG, Bezrookove V, Zuijderduijn LM, et al. Cancer-associated mutations in chromatin remodeler hSNF5 promote chromosomal instability by compromising the mitotic checkpoint. Genes Dev. 2005;19:665–70.
135. Jagani Z, Mora-Blanco EL, Sansam CG, et al. Loss of the tumor suppressor Snf5 leads to aberrant activation of the Hedgehog-Gli pathway. Nat Med. 2010;16:1429–33.
136. Roberts CW, Galusha SA, McMenamin ME, Fletcher CD, Orkin SH. Haploinsufficiency of Snf5 (integrase interactor 1) predisposes to malignant rhabdoid tumors in mice. Proc Natl Acad Sci U S A. 2000;97:13796–800.
137. Chi SN, Zimmerman MA, Yao X, et al. Intensive multimodality treatment for children with newly diagnosed CNS atypical teratoid rhabdoid tumor. J Clin Oncol. 2009;27:385–9.
138. Gardner SL, Asgharzadeh S, Green A, Horn B, McCowage G, Finlay J. Intensive induction chemotherapy followed by high dose chemotherapy with autologous hematopoietic progenitor cell rescue in young children newly diagnosed with central nervous system atypical teratoid rhabdoid tumors. Pediatr Blood Cancer. 2008;51:235–40.
139. Tekautz TM, Fuller CE, Blaney S, et al. Atypical teratoid/rhabdoid tumors (ATRT): improved survival in children 3 years of age and older with radiation therapy and high-dose alkylator-based chemotherapy. J Clin Oncol. 2005;23:1491–9.
140. Rekhi B, Jambhekar NA. Immunohistochemical validation of INI1/SMARCB1 in a spectrum of musculoskeletal tumors: an experience at a Tertiary Cancer Referral Centre. Pathol Res Pract. 2013;209(12):758–66.
141. Plotkin SR, Blakeley JO, Evans DG, Hanemann CO, Hulsebos TJ, Hunter-Schaedle K, Kalpana GV, Korf B, Messiaen L, Papi L, Ratner N, Sherman LS, Smith MJ, Stemmer-Rachamimov AO, Vitte J, Giovannini M. Update from the 2011 International Schwannomatosis Workshop: from genetics to diagnostic criteria. Am J Med Genet A. 2013;161A(3):405–16.
142. Hadfield KD, Newman WG, Bowers NL, et al. Molecular characterisation of SMARCB1 and NF2 in familial and sporadic schwannomatosis. J Med Genet. 2008;45:332–9.
143. Piotrowski A, Xie J, Liu YF, et al. Germline loss-of-function mutations in LZTR1 predispose to an inherited disorder of multiple schwannomas. Nat Genet. 2014;46(2):182–7.
144. Melmon KL, Rosen SW. Lindau's disease. Review of the literature and study of a large kindred. Am J Med. 1964;36:595–617.
145. Lonser RR, Glenn GM, Walther M, et al. von Hippel-Lindau disease. Lancet. 2003;361:2059–67.
146. Butman JA, Linehan WM, Lonser RR. Neurologic manifestations of von Hippel-Lindau disease. JAMA. 2008;300:1334–42.
147. Maher ER, Neumann HP, Richard S. von Hippel-Lindau disease: a clinical and scientific review. Eur J Hum Genet. 2011;19:617–23.

148. Stolle C, Glenn G, Zbar B, Humphrey JS, Choyke P, Walther M, Pack S, Hurley K, Andrey C, Klausner R, Linehan WM. Improved detection of germline mutations in the von Hippel-Lindau disease tumor suppressor gene. Hum Mutat. 1998;12:417–23.
149. Hoebeeck J, van der Luijt R, Poppe B, De Smet E, Yigit N, Claes K, Zewald R, de Jong GJ, De Paepe A, Speleman F, Vandesompele J. Rapid detection of VHL exon deletions using real-time quantitative PCR. Lab Invest. 2005;85:24–33.
150. Banks RE, Tirukonda P, Taylor C, Hornigold N, Astuti D, Cohen D, Maher ER, Stanley AJ, Harnden P, Joyce A, Knowles M, Selby PJ. Genetic and epigenetic analysis of von Hippel-Lindau (VHL) gene alterations and relationship with clinical variables in sporadic renal cancer. Cancer Res. 2006; 66:2000–11.
151. Sgambati MT, Stolle C, Choyke PL, Walther MM, Zbar B, Linehan WM, Glenn GM. Mosaicism in von Hippel-Lindau disease: lessons from kindreds with germline mutations identified in offspring with mosaic parents. Am J Hum Genet. 2000;66:84–91.
152. Latif F, Tory K, Gnarra J, et al. Identification of the von Hippel-Lindau disease tumor suppressor gene. Science. 1993;260:1317–20.
153. Kaelin Jr WG. The von Hippel-Lindau tumour suppressor protein: O2 sensing and cancer. Nat Rev Cancer. 2008;8:865–73.
154. Clark PE, Cookson MS. The von Hippel-Lindau gene: turning discovery into therapy. Cancer. 2008;113:1768–78.
155. Inoue K, Fry EA, Taneja P. Recent progress in mouse models for tumor suppressor genes and its implications in human cancer. Clin Med Insights Oncol. 2013;7:103–22.
156. Fu L, Wang G, Shevchuk MM, Nanus DM, Gudas LJ. Generation of a mouse model of Von Hippel-Lindau kidney disease leading to renal cancers by expression of a constitutively active mutant of HIF1alpha. Cancer Res. 2011;71:6848–56.
157. Choyke PL, Glenn GM, Walther MM, Patronas NJ, Linehan WM, Zbar B. Von Hippel-Lindau disease: genetic, clinical, and imaging features. Radiology. 1995;194:629–42.
158. Rasmussen A, Alonso E, Ochoa A, et al. Uptake of genetic testing and long-term tumor surveillance in von Hippel-Lindau disease. BMC Med Genet. 2010;11:4.
159. Niemela M, Maenpaa H, Salven P, et al. Interferon alpha-2a therapy in 18 hemangioblastomas. Clin Cancer Res. 2001;7: 510–6.
160. Madhusudan S, Deplanque G, Braybrooke JP, et al. Antiangiogenic therapy for von Hippel-Lindau disease. JAMA. 2004;291:943–4.
161. Piribauer M, Czech T, Dieckmann K, et al. Stabilization of a progressive hemangioblastoma under treatment with thalidomide. J Neurooncol. 2004;66:295–9.
162. Lloyd 2nd KM, Dennis M. Cowden's disease. A possible new symptom complex with multiple system involvement. Ann Intern Med. 1963;58:136–42.
163. Padberg GW, Schot JD, Vielvoye GJ, Bots GT, de Beer FC. Lhermitte-Duclos disease and Cowden disease: a single phakomatosis. Ann Neurol. 1991;29:517–23.
164. Robinson S, Cohen AR. Cowden disease and Lhermitte-Duclos disease: an update. Case report and review of the literature. Neurosurg Focus. 2006;20:E6.
165. Lachlan KL, Lucassen AM, Bunyan D, Temple IK. Cowden syndrome and Bannayan Riley Ruvalcaba syndrome represent one condition with variable expression and age-related penetrance: results of a clinical study of PTEN mutation carriers. J Med Genet. 2007;44:579–85.
166. Hobert JA, Eng C. PTEN hamartoma tumor syndrome: an overview. Genet Med. 2009;11:687–94.
167. Blumenthal GM, Dennis PA. PTEN hamartoma tumor syndromes. Eur J Hum Genet. 2008;16:1289–300.
168. Lok C, Viseux V, Avril MF, et al. Brain magnetic resonance imaging in patients with Cowden syndrome. Medicine (Baltimore). 2005;84:129–36.
169. Marsh DJ, Trahair TN, Martin JL, et al. Rapamycin treatment for a child with germline PTEN mutation. Nat Clin Pract Oncol. 2008;5:357–61.
170. Abel TW, Baker SJ, Fraser MM, et al. Lhermitte-Duclos disease: a report of 31 cases with immunohistochemical analysis of the PTEN/AKT/mTOR pathway. J Neuropathol Exp Neurol. 2005;64:341–9.
171. Asthagiri AR, Parry DM, Butman JA, et al. Neurofibromatosis type 2. Lancet. 2009;373:1974–86.
172. Evans DG, Baser ME, O'Reilly B, et al. Management of the patient and family with neurofibromatosis 2: a consensus conference statement. Br J Neurosurg. 2005;19:5–12.
173. Baser ME, Friedman JM, Wallace AJ, Ramsden RT, Joe H, Evans DG. Evaluation of clinical diagnostic criteria for neurofibromatosis 2. Neurology. 2002;59(11):1759–65.
174. Wallace AJ, Watson CJ, Oward E, Evans DG, Elles RG. Mutation scanning of the NF2 gene: an improved service based on meta-PCR/sequencing, dosage analysis, and loss of heterozygosity analysis. Genet Test. 2004;8:368–80.
175. Kluwe L, Nygren AO, Errami A, Heinrich B, Matthies C, Tatagiba M, Mautner V. Screening for large mutations of the NF2 gene. Genes Chromosomes Cancer. 2005;42:384–91.
176. Evans DG, Kalamarides M, Hunter-Schaedle K, et al. Consensus recommendations to accelerate clinical trials for neurofibromatosis type 2. Clin Cancer Res. 2009;15:5032–9.
177. Trofatter JA, MacCollin MM, Rutter JL, et al. A novel moesin-, ezrin-, radixin-like gene is a candidate for the neurofibromatosis 2 tumor suppressor. Cell. 1993;72:791–800.
178. Rouleau GA, Merel P, Lutchman M, et al. Alteration in a new gene encoding a putative membrane-organizing protein causes neuro-fibromatosis type 2. Nature. 1993;363:515–21.
179. Li W, Cooper J, Karajannis MA, Giancotti FG. Merlin: a tumour suppressor with functions at the cell cortex and in the nucleus. EMBO Rep. 2012;13(3):204–15.
180. Evans DG, Birch JM, Ramsden RT. Paediatric presentation of type 2 neurofibromatosis. Arch Dis Child. 1999;81:496–9.
181. Mautner VF, Tatagiba M, Lindenau M, et al. Spinal tumors in patients with neurofibromatosis type 2: MR imaging study of frequency, multiplicity, and variety. AJR Am J Roentgenol. 1995;165:951–5.
182. Plotkin SR, Stemmer-Rachamimov AO, Barker 2nd FG, et al. Hearing improvement after bevacizumab in patients with neurofibromatosis type 2. N Engl J Med. 2009;361:358–67.
183. Blakeley JO, Evans DG, Adler J, Brackmann D, Chen R, Ferner RE, Hanemann CO, Harris G, Huson SM, Jacob A, Kalamarides M, Karajannis MA, Korf BR, Mautner VF, McClatchey AI, Miao H, Plotkin SR, Slattery 3rd W, Stemmer-Rachamimov AO, Welling DB, Wen PY, Widemann B, Hunter-Schaedle K, Giovannini M. Consensus recommendations for current treatments and accelerating clinical trials for patients with neurofibromatosis type 2. Am J Med Genet A. 2012;158A(1):24–41.

2 Brain Tumor Stem Cells

N. Sumru Bayin, Aram S. Modrek, and Dimitris G. Placantonakis

Primary brain tumors represent a challenging biological and clinical entity. The limited therapeutic options and high rates of morbidity and mortality associated with them highlight the need for a better understanding of their molecular and pathophysiological complexity [1]. In recent years, it has become clear that such tumors are highly heterogeneous, not just histologically but at the molecular level as well [2–5]. This heterogeneity raises the possibility that within each tumor exist different cell types, each with distinct roles in maintaining tumor heterogeneity and bearing unique combinations of signaling pathways and molecular markers.

One important question related to tumor heterogeneity is: Are the different cell types equally important for tumor growth or not? Over the past decade, accumulating evidence supports the theory that brain tumors are governed by a cellular hierarchy dominated by brain tumor stem cells (BTSCs). Indeed, small subpopulations of cells within such tumors possess stem-like properties and the enhanced ability to regenerate tumors in laboratory animals [6–13].

Cancer Stem Cell Definition

Although initially defined in liquid tumors, i.e., leukemias, some of the most compelling evidence for cancer stem cells in solid tumors originates in brain malignancies, and especially gliomas [14, 15]. BTSCs are very well defined by several functional criteria, which are borrowed from developmental biology. To be considered a stem cell, whether normal or cancerous, a cell should be able to *self-renew*, which refers to the limitless ability to proliferate and maintain the undifferentiated phenotype; and *differentiate* into different lineages, a property termed *multipotency*. Stem cells have the ability to undergo asymmetric division giving rise to a stem cell (self-renewal) and a lineage-restricted progenitor cell, which is limited in its differentiation potential and generates terminally differentiated mature cells after proliferating (Fig. 2.1).

It is hypothesized that variations in self-renewal and proliferative abilities generate a cellular hierarchy within brain tumors, with BTSCs at the apex of this hierarchy [6]. In addition to these obligate properties, BTSCs should be able to *initiate tumors* and phenocopy the original tumor when injected into animal models [7, 16]. The presence of BTSCs in brain tumors raises another important question: Do brain tumors arise from the oncogenic transformation of normal neural stem cells (NSCs) residing within the brain? Or can differentiated brain cells undergo mutations that lead to their dedifferentiation and tumorigenesis?

This chapter focuses on two aspects of stem cell biology in brain tumors. The first part will cover the role of NSCs and progenitor cells as candidates for the cell of origin in brain tumors. The second part will discuss molecular characteristics of BTSCs and their therapeutic implications. We believe that understanding cancer stem cell biology and its therapeutic implications will be crucial for developing fundamentally new, and hopefully more effective, treatments.

Brain Tumor Initiation

Mechanisms of brain tumor initiation are unclear; mouse models have revealed that a number of mutations are capable of initiating tumors and that the cell of origin may differ amongst different genetic subclasses of brain tumors or even within a given tumor type. Also, the question of how tumor cells acquire a BTSC phenotype during or after tumor initiation remains to be answered. Two dominant hypotheses have emerged to account for the presence of BTSCs within gliomas: (1) Brain tumors arise from the transformation of endogenous NSCs or progenitor cells that acquire aberrant self-renewal and differentiation properties; and (2) differentiated brain cells undergo oncogenic transformation, dedifferentiate and acquire stem cell characteristics. This section will provide background on neurogenesis and normal NSC biology, which will lay the foundation for understanding gliomagenesis and the molecular characteristics of BTSCs.

M.A. Karajannis and D. Zagzag (eds.), *Molecular Pathology of Nervous System Tumors: Biological Stratification and Targeted Therapies*, Molecular Pathology Library 8,
DOI 10.1007/978-1-4939-1830-0_2, © Springer Science+Business Media New York 2015

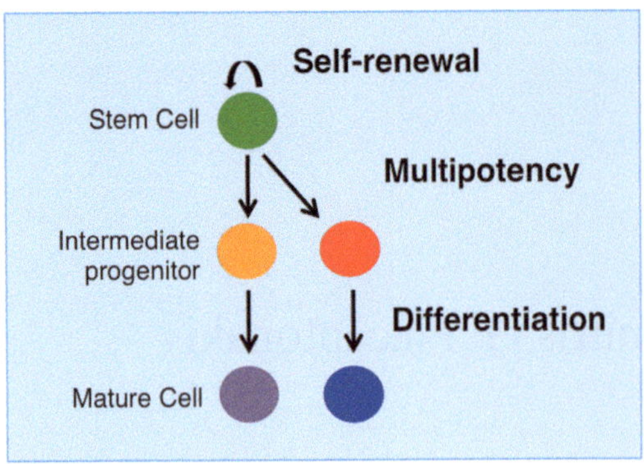

Fig. 2.1. Properties of stem cells. Stem cells have the ability to self-renew and differentiate to a mature cell through an intermediate progenitor. The ability to give rise to cells from different lineages is termed multipotency.

Neurogenesis in the Adult Brain

The cell of origin in brain tumors, including gliomas, is still a matter of debate [17]. However, there has been intense speculation that brain tumors may arise from neurogenic niches in the brain [18–27]. Since the discovery of adult neurogenesis, new insights have emerged about the mechanisms by which the brain maintains a small population of NSCs that can replenish both neurons and glia [28, 29]. Given the intrinsic ability of both BTSCs and NSCs to self-renew and differentiate, it is important to consider how cancer stem cells' ability to regulate their own function in the tumor deviates (or remains the same) from that of normal NSCs. NSCs in the adult brain actively generate both neurons and glia that contribute to the brain's cellular and functional homeostasis, as well as plasticity, remodeling, and response to injury [30–32]. In contrast to post-mitotic neurons, it is the cell types undergoing mitoses that are thought to harbor the greatest potential to give rise to brain tumors. Such mitotically active cells are found in neurogenic niches. Cells in the neurogenic niche perturbed by mutagenic events can theoretically serve as starting points for brain tumor formation and may harbor intrinsically higher oncogenic potential than other dormant neural cell types. Understanding neurogenesis and gliogenesis will allow us to explore concepts relevant to the cell-of-origin question in brain tumors and the regulation of BTSCs during tumorigenesis.

NSCs have been identified in at least two regions of the adult brain: the subventricular zone (SVZ) of the lateral ventricles, and the subgranular zone (SGZ) of the hippocampus [28, 33–35]. NSCs may also exist within the subcortical white matter [36]. During fetal life, radial glia, which are derived from neuroepithelium, are responsible for neurogenesis. Radial glia participate in neural organization; immature neurons that arise from radial glia move along their transcortical extensions for migratory guidance to their respective areas in the cortex, contributing to its stratified organization during the late embryonic stages [37]. With the transition to postnatal life, radial glia differentiate into many different cell types, including neurons, astrocytes, oligodendrocytes, ependymal cells, and the SVZ NSCs, which contribute to adult neurogenesis in the mammalian brain in postnatal life [28, 32, 34, 38, 39]. The adult SVZ NSCs, or type B cells, line the subependymal zone of the lateral ventricles. B cells give rise to intermediate progenitors termed transit-amplifying cells (or type C cells), which proliferate and have the ability to form immature neurons termed neuroblasts (type A cells). Neuroblasts migrate through the rostral migratory stream (RMS) to the olfactory bulb in rodents [40] and, additionally, through the medial prefrontal migratory stream in humans [41], eventually becoming mature post-mitotic neurons. Type B cells additionally give rise to oligodendrocyte precursor cells (OPCs) and astroglia depending on growth or inhibitory signals ([31, 42], see reviews [29, 43]).

In the hippocampal formation, the dentate gyrus SGZ houses radial astrocytes, which serve as a source of neurogenesis in the region [28, 33]. Radial astrocytes (type 1 cells) form intermediate progenitor cells (type 2 cells), which become immature granule cells (type 3 cells) and subsequently mature granule neurons [44–47]. The SGZ and SVZ house the two identified groups of stem cells responsible for formation of new neuronal and glial cell types in adult mammals. The majority of what we have learned about neurogenesis has emerged from studies conducted using rodent models. Some of these findings have been validated in post-mortem human brain samples [30, 35, 41], although such studies are limited in number. The discovery of active neurogenesis in the adult human brain has numerous implications for the pathobiology of brain tumor formation, neurodegenerative disorders, and response to injury.

Gliomagenesis

In the very beginning of brain tumorigenesis, the cellular composition is thought to differ drastically from that of a mature tumor. Given the known heterogeneity of fully developed tumors and the overwhelming possibility that the tumor began from a single cell type, an open question remains: How does this heterogeneity arise? To address this question, we will focus on gliomas, whose developmental biology is perhaps better understood than any other brain tumor.

We know that BTSCs from mature gliomas can phenocopy the tumors they were derived from in animal models. The BTSCs found in gliomas must have arisen from a tumor that lacked cells with stem cell properties or a tumor that arose from an endogenous NSC (Fig. 2.2). The cell of origin is defined as the cell type that has accumulated the correct combination of mutations that induces proliferation and eventually tumor formation (oncogenic transformation). Although not mutually exclusive, the cell of origin differs from the cell type that acquires mutations, which is referred to as the cell of mutation. This is because the cell of mutation, after acquiring the first oncogenic hit, may differentiate

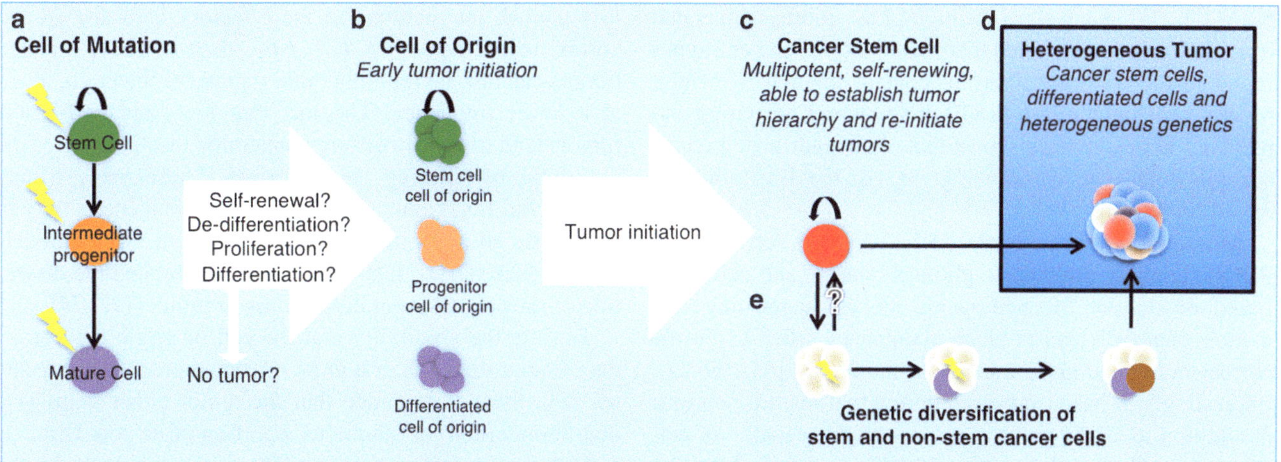

FIG. 2.2. Model of gliomagenesis. (**a**) Representation of a normal cellular hierarchy where the cell of mutation may give rise to the cell of origin (**b**). Cancer stem cells (**c**) are self-renewing and tumor re-initiating cells found in the tumor. Both cancer stem cells and non-stem cells experience genetic changes (**e**), contributing to the heterogeneous tumor (**d**). Different colors represent different cell types emphasizing intratumoral heterogeneity.

or dedifferentiate into another cell type before proliferating, so a distinction must be made for the cases where this happens (see reviews [17, 48]). An important concept to clarify is the difference between the cell of origin and BTSCs. Both can theoretically form the mature tumor, but the cell of origin is responsible for initiating the tumor and may or may not be a stem cell. The cell of origin is of interest in the discussion of BTSCs because evidence from mouse models has pointed to the possibility that NSCs within the brain may serve as the cells of origin. Given that BTSCs have stem cell properties, identifying the cell of origin may provide insight into how BTSCs are derived and how their ability to self-renew or differentiate differs from that of normal stem cells and the cell of origin. It is still unclear if multiple cell types within the brain can give rise to the same type of tumor and whether different types of tumors share the same cell of origin harboring different genetic mutations. To answer some of these questions, glioma models have been developed and used successfully to uncover key aspects of glioma biology.

Models of glioma aim to recapitulate human glioma pathology most commonly through two model systems: genetically engineered rodent models with mutations found in human gliomas, or xenografts of primary human glioma lines derived from patients. Other model systems also exist, including in vitro cultures of glioblastoma multiforme (GBM) cell lines, allografts of rodent glioma lines and virally mediated oncogenesis. These approaches have been used to provide reproducible platforms to study many aspects of tumor biology, including BTSCs, the cell of origin, and therapeutic implications [19, 21, 22, 49–54].

Primary lines derived from patient tumors carry a distinct advantage due to their genetic make-up, which most faithfully represents the disease [49]. The drawbacks of primary lines include: (1) the necessity to inject the mouse brain to create a xenograft, thus potentially altering the microenvironment; (2) the possibility that, in derivation of each culture, a subpopulation of the tumor is selected for; and (3) the fact that these tumors are grown in an immunodeficient background. Murine models have the disadvantage of a rodent genetic background and are limited in recapitulating the order and number of mutations that occur in a sporadic human glioma. Modeling efforts will likely continue to sample the phenotype produced by different combinations of mutations, location of the tumor, and the developmental point of induction of these mutations. In both cases, the tumor is grown in the mouse brain microenvironment, which raises an additional degree of separation from human glioma biology for both the mouse and xenograft model systems.

Experimental evidence from murine models of glioma suggests the cell of origin to be adult NSCs or proliferating progenitor/precursor cells, but not mature glia. However, this is highly controversial and remains an open question for the many different subtypes of glioma (see reviews [53, 55]). Following the discovery of adult neurogenesis, there was a paradigm shift in thinking about the origins of glioma, as the discovery of NSCs and their progenitor/precursor cell progeny became new candidates (Fig. 2.2). In a landmark effort to link the differentiation stage to tumor initiation, Holland et al. found that NSCs or neural progenitor cells expressing Nestin in the mouse brain were preferentially forming tumors with GBM characteristics after activation of the K-Ras/Akt pathway [25]. The same oncogenic insult did not produce tumors under the control of a GFAP promoter, suggesting that not all cell types within the same lineage could serve as the cell of origin [25]. Parada and colleagues have developed multiple tumor suppressor knockout models of gliomagenesis via inducible loss of p53, PTEN, and NF1, which are some of the most commonly mutated tumor suppressors in

GBM [56, 57]. Analysis of the high-grade gliomas generated from these models revealed that Nestin-expressing cell types found in the SVZ are likely to contain the cell of origin. More recent studies with PDGF-driven tumor formation and p53/NF1 knockout have shown that oligodendrocyte precursor cells (OPCs) are capable of giving rise to GBM tumors in mice [20, 58].

Mouse models using Ink4a-ARF loss, K-ras activation, or PDGF signaling give rise to gliomas in areas and cell types found outside of the neurogenic niches, suggesting that mature glial cells can produce malignancy when given the correct combination of oncogenic mutations [54, 59–62]. Interestingly, it has also been reported that mature neurons, in addition to GFAP-positive astrocytes, are capable of acting as the cell of mutation in a p53/NF1 model of glioma by undergoing dedifferentiation [24]. Some consideration should be given to the fact that some of these murine models represent functional genetic alterations that may or may not be the initiating events in glioma formation despite their oncogenic transforming abilities in this context. It remains an open question as to what the initial events in the different subtypes of glioma are, and how restricted the cell of origin truly is for any given tumor type, considering the unique combination of microenvironment, genetic changes, and organism.

It should be highlighted that in many of the aforementioned murine models, there is a propensity of early events in murine gliomagenesis to occur near the SVZ when the NSC population is targeted [56, 57, 63]. There is clinical evidence in humans that initiating events in glioma formation occur in or near the neurogenic zones of the brain. Human GBM has a propensity to occur most frequently in the periventricular area and less so in the surrounding cortex, albeit this evidence is controversial [63–65]. GBM also occurs infratentorially, but with much lower frequency [66]. The tendency for GBM to occur in the periventricular area within the cerebrum suggests that a cell-of-origin also resides within the same region; however, this correlation has not been directly linked to human neurogenesis. It is possible that tumors found far from neurogenic regions may be initiated by migrating cells that originated in the neurogenic niche. This is an interesting but unexplored hypothesis.

Grade II/III gliomas mutated for isocitrate dehydrogenase (IDH) tend to arise in different anatomic locations as compared to their grade IV GBM counterparts. Although IDH1 normally functions to convert isocitrate to α-ketoglutarate, the mutation leads to the production of oncometabolite 2-hydroxyglutarate (2HG) which stereo-chemically resembles α-ketoglutarate and is hypothesized to cause tumorigenic epigenetic changes [67–70]. In IDH-mutated gliomas, the cytosolic variant IDH1 is most frequently mutated, whereas mutations in IDH2 can be found less commonly [71]. Strikingly, the IDH1-mutated gliomas are most commonly found in the frontal lobe in an area that overlaps with the rostral and medial migratory streams used by neuroblasts to replenish interneurons in the olfactory bulb and frontal cortex, respectively [30, 63]. Nevertheless, IDH1-mutated tumors can also be found in other regions of the brain, albeit at a lower frequency. The fact that low- and high-grade tumors tend to arise in different anatomic locations raises the possibility of differing cells of origin. Alternatively, it may signify that IDH1 mutations promote gliomagenesis only in restricted cell types or lineages. The lack of mouse models that produce IDH1-mutated tumors has inhibited the dissection of the cell of origin in this class of tumors [72–74].

Despite the possibility that the cell of origin may originate from a stem cell or a more restricted progenitor/precursor cell, there is evidence that the tumor either gains (via dedifferentiation) or maintains a portion of its population as cells with stem cell properties. The continuum between the cell of origin and BTSCs is not well understood (Fig. 2.2). Murine models have allowed the detection and study of BTSCs in the context of gliomas and medulloblastomas primarily. Much of our understanding of BTSC biology has derived from the study of primary human GBM.

Identification of Brain Tumor Stem Cells

As mentioned earlier, the concept of cancer stem cells was initially developed in studies involving leukemias, where the cellular hierarchy is well established [14]. In such tumors, an abundance of lineage-specific cell surface markers made the isolation of distinct cell types within this hierarchy feasible. Some of the same surface markers were later used to isolate cancer stem cells in solid tumors. Before going into the details of surface markers and molecular characteristics of BTSCs, we will describe the main approaches used to identify them.

BTSCs, which are a subpopulation of cells within the tumor, are defined by their ability to *initiate tumors* in animal models that recapitulate patient tumor phenotype and heterogeneity [7, 8, 49]. As mentioned earlier, two critical properties of BTSCs are *self-renewal* and *multipotency* (Fig. 2.3). Self-renewal is tested with the following two standard assays. First, clonogenicity is assessed by in vitro tumor sphere formation ability over serial passaging [49, 75]. Briefly, cells that have been isolated according to their surface markers are seeded in suspension in low density or as single cells and the formation of spheres is analyzed. Serial sphere formation over time shows that cells have clonogenic potential, consistent with the ability of BTSCs to self-renew. A second critical assay is xenograft tumor formation, where these isolated cells form tumors when injected into immunodeficient or isogenic mice [15]. Such xenograft tumors are expected to recapitulate the original disease phenotype. Re-isolation of BTSCs from xenograft tumors and secondary tumor formation from those cells shows in vivo self-renewal.

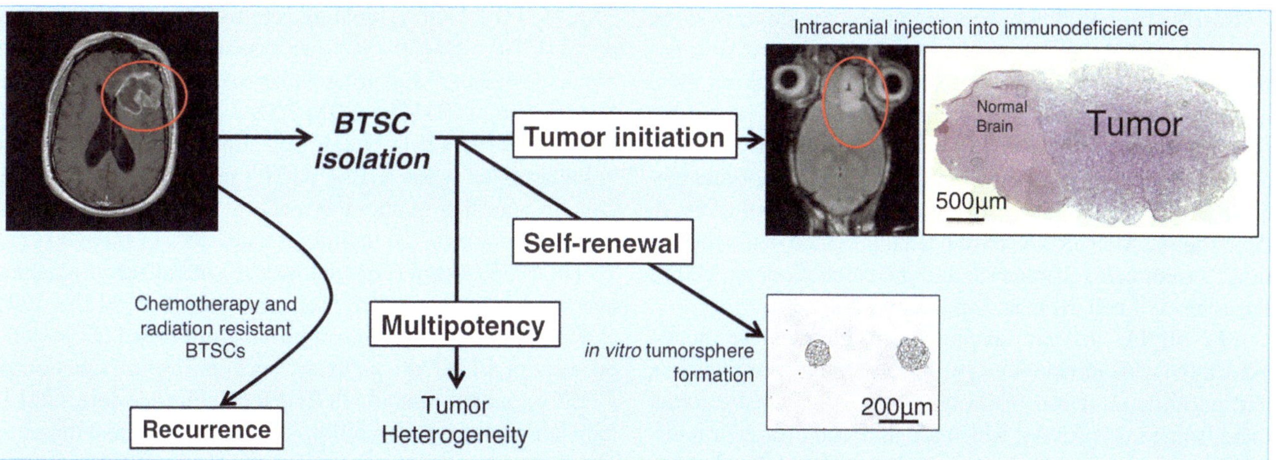

FIG. 2.3. Hallmarks of BTSC biology. Upon surgical resection and primary culture generation, BTSCs are isolated via expression of molecular markers. Isolated BTSCs are studied for their *tumor initiation*, *self-renewal*, and *multipotency*. Therapy-resistant BTSCs cause disease *recurrence*.

Differentiation potential, or multipotency, is another required functional property of BTSCs. In the case of gliomas, for example, BTSCs have been shown to give rise to glia, neurons, endothelium and pericytes [12, 13, 76–79]. These findings underscore the stem-like properties of BTSCs and provide a mechanism for BTSC-driven tumor heterogeneity.

By using these important assays, initial evidence for BTSCs came from pediatric brain tumors. Isolating cells by fluorescence-activating cell sorting (FACS) using cell surface markers originally found in human fetal brain, cells with tumorigenic properties were identified [80]. Shortly thereafter, Dirks and colleagues successfully isolated tumor-initiating cells in human GBM, the most malignant form of glioma, where they showed that CD133, a surface marker also expressed in embryonic NSCs and other adult stem cells, identifies cells with the ability to generate tumors when injected into immunodeficient animals [7, 8, 81]. After these seminal papers, the field of brain tumor stem cells expanded exponentially. However, we still need a better understanding of these cells in terms of their molecular signatures and niches, as well as their relevance to tumor growth and recurrence.

Molecular Characteristics of Brain Tumor Stem Cells

Molecular Markers

Functional similarities between BTSCs and NSCs directed researchers to analyze the expression of markers that were shown to be important for NSC biology and neural development. One of the best-defined molecular markers for brain tumors, including pediatric tumors, ependymoma, and especially GBM, is the cell surface marker CD133. CD133 is a pentaspan, glycosylated transmembrane protein. Apart from being expressed in fetal brain NSCs during embryonic development, its expression is highly associated with other tissue-specific stem cells and cancer stem cells of blood and solid malignancies [14, 81–85]. CD133-knockout murine models show photoreceptor degeneration, but the signaling functions of CD133 remain unknown [86]. In the context of GBM and medulloblastoma, it was shown that when injected into animals in limiting dilutions, CD133+ cells generate tumors more efficiently than their CD133− counterparts, suggesting that they have BTSC properties [87]. Furthermore, downregulation of CD133 via short hairpin RNA (shRNA) suppresses self-renewal of BTSCs in GBM [88].

Although CD133 is one of the best-studied markers in brain tumors, it is now well established that some CD133− cells do possess tumorigenic potential, suggesting that CD133 is not a universal marker and that CD133− BTSC populations exist as well [11, 89–91]. Furthermore, the fact that not all GBM tumors have CD133+ cells supports the hypothesis that CD133− BTSCs exist in these tumors [92–94]. Another important marker associated with BTSCs is the intermediate filament protein Nestin, a well-established NSC marker. Nestin+ cells were shown to have tumor-initiating ability in animal models and to generate tumor recurrence after chemotherapy [10, 61, 95]. BTSCs are also enriched for other NSC and stem cell markers, such as Nanog, Musashi-1, Bmi-1, Sox2, and Oct4 [96–98]. In addition, some BTSCs were shown to express other surface markers and transmembrane proteins, such as CXCR4, integrin α6, SSEA-1/CD15, L1CAM, and A2B5 [11, 99–101]. Finally, the side population (SP), defined as cells with the ability to extrude Hoechst dye via ABC-type transporters on the cell surface on flow cytometric analysis, has been shown to contain stem-like cells in a variety of brain tumors [102, 103].

Besides from traditional coding genes, the importance of noncoding RNAs in the regulation of gene expression has been increasingly recognized in recent years, making them important biomarkers in cancer biology. In particular, microRNAs are responsible for the posttranscriptional fine-tuning of gene expression by binding the 3′ UTR of messenger RNAs (mRNAs) and causing their translational arrest or degradation. MicroRNAs have been implicated in the regulation of stem cell self-renewal and differentiation, as well as the control of cell cycle and apoptosis [104].

MicroRNAs that are upregulated in gliomas are mostly associated with antiapoptotic, pro-proliferative, pro-invasion, and antidifferentiation pathways [105, 106]. On the other hand, some microRNAs, which are important for neural differentiation, were shown to be downregulated in gliomas, functioning as tumor suppressors [107]. An example of a microRNA critical to brain tumor biology is miR-124. Normally, miR-124 is known to promote neural differentiation in the brain. In gliomas, however, it was shown to be downregulated and its overexpression promotes differentiation [108, 109].

Many other microRNAs, whose targets include mRNAs encoding important survival and oncogenic molecules, such as PI3K, AKT, EGFR, and MAPK, were shown to play important roles in glioma and medulloblastoma [105, 108, 110].

Signaling Pathways

Dissecting major signaling pathways that are important for BTSC biology have been, and will continue to be, a challenge due to the complex interplay and cross talk between different signaling pathways. Besides molecular markers shared between NSCs and BTSCs, signaling pathways are also conserved between these two populations. This conservation has highlighted several signaling pathways in BTSC biology, some of which are described below.

Pathways Supporting Self-Renewal

Similar to NSC culturing, BTSCs are propagated as suspension culture, in serum-free media, under the influence of two mitogens, epidermal growth factor (EGF), and fibroblast growth factor (FGF), which are believed to induce self-renewal of BTSCs in vitro [49]. However, in the in vivo scenario, signals supporting self-renewal are dependent on the complex interplay of multiple pathways.

The Notch signaling pathway was originally identified by genetic screens in Drosophila as a master regulator of neural development [111–113]. Further investigation showed that Notch signaling is essential for maintaining NSCs in an undifferentiated state and represents a key component of fate decisions in neural and glial lineages [114, 115]. Apart from its critical role in neural development, Notch signaling has been highly associated with tumorigenesis, regulating both the self-renewal and differentiation of BTSCs in GBM [12, 77, 116–118]. Notch signaling is critical for the self-renewal of CD133+ GBM BTSCs, as evidenced by the fact that blockade of Notch signaling with γ-secretase inhibitors leads to depletion of CD133+ GBM BTSCs and decreases tumorigenicity [119, 120]. Notch signaling is activated in the vascular niche where GBM BTSCs reside [121]. More specifically, in this niche the endothelium provides Notch ligands to maintain the undifferentiated state of BTSCs [122].

The PI3K/Akt/mTOR pathway is critical for gliomagenesis and glioma BTSC self-renewal [2–5, 123, 124]. Commonly find mutations in gliomas are found in the components of PI3K/Akt pathway, such as loss of function of PTEN or gain of function of EGFR [3]. Furthermore, CD133 knockdown leads to inhibition of Akt activation and impaired self-renewal and tumorigenicity of glioma BTSCs, further confirming its crucial role in BTSC biology [123, 124].

Hedgehog-gli signaling has been implicated in medulloblastoma formation [125, 126]. It is important for BTSC clonogenicity, survival, tumorigenicity, and proliferation by operating through the key cell cycle regulators Cyclin D and Cyclin E [87, 127].

The Wnt/β-catenin signaling pathway functions by inducing progenitor cell proliferation and differentiation in gliomas [128]. Some reports also show that Wnt signaling is important for GBM BTSC self-renewal [91, 129].

Recent studies have shown that transforming growth factor-β (TGF-β) signaling regulates GBM BTSC biology [130–132]. TGF-β plays a role in regulating GBM BTSC self-renewal via acting through Sry-related HMG box factors (Sox2 and Sox4) [131]. Furthermore, inhibition of TGF-β in GBM tumors decreases perivascular $CD44^{high}/Id1^{high}$ BTSCs by repressing inhibitors of DNA-binding proteins Id1 and Id3 [130].

Another important signaling pathway relevant to BTSC self-renewal is mediated by hypoxia. GBM tumors are histologically heterogeneous and include regions that lack blood vessels and are highly necrotic and hypoxic [133]. Hypoxia has been previously shown to promote self-renewal of embryonic and adult stem cells [102, 134]. Along these lines, in gliomas hypoxia induces BTSC self-renewal via hypoxia-induced factors (HIF-1α and HIF-2α) [135–139]. These same factors also induce angiogenesis and neovascularization via upregulation of vascular endothelial growth factor (VEGF) [140]. Hypoxia is also known to reprogram CD133− BTSCs to become CD133+ [102]. Furthermore, hypoxia induces Notch signaling, whose importance in BTSC self-renewal was mentioned above [134]. Microscopic analysis has shown CD133 immunoreactivity around necrotic areas in GBM, a finding consistent with a hypoxic niche for BTSCs [141].

Pathways Promoting Differentiation

Bone morphogenetic protein (BMP) signaling functions as a strong differentiation signal. BMP4, important for astrocytic differentiation, induces GBM BTSC differentiation. BMP4 treatment was shown to block GBM BTSC self-renewal by suppressing asymmetric division, thereby depleting the stem cell compartment within tumors and leading to differentiation and proliferation block [76]. However, in a subset of glioma BTSCs, BMP-driven differentiation is impaired due to epigenetic silencing of the BMP receptor 1B (BMPR1B). This modification desensitizes glioma BTSCs to normal differentiation cues, thereby leading to their proliferation [142].

In GBM, some reports have suggested that the Notch pathway is critical for tumor-driven endothelial cell transdifferentiation of BTSCs [12, 13]. Similar to Notch signaling, TGF-β is known to regulate glioma progression by modulating the tumor microenvironment, including angiogenesis and immune response. TGF-β was also shown to induce differentiation of glioma BTSCs into vascular pericytes, which leads to further tumor growth by supporting vessel formation [78].

Stem Cell Niche and Tumor Microenvironment

Understanding the stem cell niche for BTSCs is highly important in unraveling the processes responsible for their self-renewal and signals inducing differentiation. Furthermore, the stem cell niche and microenvironment are highly critical in the context of drug design and delivery. Without understanding the different niches and signals provided within them, effective drug design is not possible.

Vascular Niche

NSCs were shown to reside within a vascular niche, adjacent to endothelial cells, which are believed to provide signals required for self-renewal [143]. BTSCs were also shown to reside closer to endothelial cells [144]. In medulloblastoma, CD133+ cells where shown to be in proximity to endothelial cells [121, 122]. Similarly, glioma BTSCs acquire a vascular niche, in which CD34+ endothelial cells present Notch ligands to BTSCs, keeping them in an undifferentiated state via activation of Notch signaling [122]. However, the complex architectural features of GBM suggest that BTSCs may also reside in relatively avascular microenvironments.

Hypoxic Niche

The importance of hypoxia in promoting self-renewal in embryonic stem cells and NSCs suggests that it may also regulate the self-renewal of BTSCs, especially in GBM, which is a highly hypoxic tumor. When considering this possibility, the question that arises is whether there are hypoxic areas within GBM. One such plausible histologic area is represented in pseudopalisading necrosis (PPN), in which densely packed cells surround necrotic regions [145]. The etiology and biological significance of PPNs is not well understood. However, others and we speculate that they may represent areas of active tumor growth and revascularization. A tantalizing hypothesis to explain such tumor growth and angiogenesis is, in turn, the presence of BTSCs within a hypoxic niche. Indeed, some studies have shown enriched CD133 immunoreactivity in PPNs, supporting this hypothesis [141]. Importantly, the putative presence of BTSCs in hypoxic areas devoid of blood vessels raises doubts about the effectiveness of systemic drug delivery methods.

Invasion

Invasion of glioma cells through the brain parenchyma represents perhaps their most malignant feature [146]. Single GBM cells have been shown to infiltrate normal brain tissue and travel more than several centimeters from the bulk of the tumor [147–149]. After surgical resection, the recurrent tumor occurs within the borders of the resection cavity, suggesting that these infiltrating cells have the capacity to regenerate tumors.

Although the mechanisms of invasion of BTSCs are not clear, C–X–C chemokine receptor type 4 (CXCR4) and its ligand, stromal-derived factor-1α (SDF-1α), which are highly important for vascularization, were shown to be crucial for the invasive behavior of GBM cells [140, 150]. Enrichment of SDF-1α/CXCR4 expression in glioma BTSCs highlights their invasive properties. This signaling was also shown to mediate recruitment of BTSCs toward endothelium, leading to further invasion and differentiation. Furthermore, this chemoattractant signaling induces endothelial proliferation via attracting tumor cells and inducing VEGF expression in gliomas and other systems, such as the gastrointestinal tract [151].

Therapeutic Importance of Brain Tumor Stem Cells

Besides understanding how tumors are formed and how the cellular hierarchy within the tumors is maintained, BTSCs are of particular interest because of their intrinsic resistance to current chemoradiotherapeutic approaches (Fig. 2.3). In GBM, postsurgical therapy consists of concomitant temozolomide administration and radiotherapy.

Therapy Resistance

Chemotherapy Resistance

The side population of GBM cells is believed to have the ability to actively transport chemotherapeutic agents to the extracellular space, due to the expression of ABC-type transporters on their plasma membrane [152]. Furthermore, analysis of cells that are resistant to lethal doses of chemotherapeutic drugs has revealed that they express stem cell markers, such as CD133, CD117, CD90, CD71, and CD45, and are able to regenerate tumors when injected into immunodeficient mice [153]. Gene expression analysis of CD133+ BTSCs in glioma showed increased expression of antiapoptotic genes. In relation to this finding, CD133 expression was shown to be significantly higher in recurrent tumors, further suggesting that BTSCs have intrinsic mechanisms of chemoresistance [99].

Recently, Parada and colleagues used a mouse model for GBM to demonstrate that upon treatment with temozolomide, an alkylating agent, which represents the standard of care in GBM, a restricted Nestin+BTSC population repropagated the tumor. Selective ablation of this population arrested tumor growth, suggesting that BTSCs are the reason for GBM recurrence [10].

Radioresistance

Besides their resistance to chemotherapy, BTSCs were shown to be highly resistant to radiation. Similar to chemoresistant populations, radioresistant GBM cells express BTSC markers. Molecular mechanisms involved in glioma BTSC self-renewal, such as Notch and TGFβ signaling, are thought to underlie such radioresistance [116, 154]. CD133+ BTSCs were also shown to have increased DNA repair capacity via selective activation of Chk1 and Chk2 kinases [155].

Most chemotherapeutic drugs target cycling cells. By the same token, response to radiation depends on cell cycle checkpoints. However, BTSCs are mostly dormant and quiescent, which spares them from cell cycle-dependent therapeutic approaches, and further highlights the importance of developing new therapies that directly target BTSCs [156].

Updates on Clinical Trials Targeting BTSCs

Because of their central role in promoting growth and recurrence of primary brain tumors, BTSCs are major candidates for targeted therapeutic approaches. In particular, signaling pathways promoting BTSC self-renewal and inducing therapy resistance represent critical drug targets.

As mentioned earlier in the chapter, the Notch pathway plays a crucial role in regulating self-renewal and therapy resistance in BTSCs [12, 77, 116–120, 122]. Therefore, inhibition of Notch signaling in a clinical setting has always been of major interest. Due its contribution to several other diseases processes as well, there are several Notch pathway inhibitors being tested in clinical trials. However, a major limitation of Notch inhibitors is its well-known role in normal tissue-specific stem cells and the risk of systemic toxicity [157]. In the context of brain tumors, there are active clinical trials testing the γ-secretase inhibitor RO4929097 (ClinicalTrials.gov NCT01269411, NCT01189240, NCT01122901).

Another important therapeutic target is the TGF-β signaling pathway, which plays a role in glioma BTSC self-renewal [130–132] and contributes to radioresistance of these cells as a part of the tumor microenvironment [151, 154]. Preclinical data with TGF-β receptor kinase inhibitors and neutralizing antibodies have shown that inhibition of TGF-β signaling sensitizes BTSCs to radiation [154]. TGF-β inhibition is being explored in clinical trials with high-grade glioma patients (ClinicalTrials.gov NCT00431561, NCT00761280).

Discussion

In this chapter, we summarized the current understanding of stem cell biology in brain tumors, as well as emerging concepts. We have approached the issue from two perspectives: the cell of origin of brain tumors and cancer stem cells in brain tumors (BTSCs). Throughout the chapter, we discussed the possibility of neurogenic niches in normal brain as the putative origin of brain tumors and we highlighted molecular signatures and signaling pathways implicated in BTSC biology.

Due to their intrinsic resistance to chemoradiotherapy and their highly tumorigenic nature, BTSCs represent attractive therapeutic targets. However, lack of universal molecular markers identifying BTSCs and complex interplay between signaling pathways regulating BTSC biology have thus far impaired the successful clinical implementation of directed therapeutics toward these cells. Furthermore, the overlap between molecular signatures in BTSCs and normal adult stem cells complicates the issue further due to putative toxicity. We believe that a better understanding of cellular heterogeneity and hierarchy in these tumors will be crucial to overcoming these issues and designing effective therapies against brain tumors and other malignancies.

References

1. Stupp R, et al. Radiotherapy plus concomitant and adjuvant temozolomide for glioblastoma. N Engl J Med. 2005;352(10):987–96.
2. Cancer Genome Atlas Research Network. Comprehensive genomic characterization defines human glioblastoma genes and core pathways. Nature. 2008;455(7216):1061–8.
3. Brennan C, et al. Glioblastoma subclasses can be defined by activity among signal transduction pathways and associated genomic alterations. PLoS One. 2009;4(11):e7752.
4. Phillips HS, et al. Molecular subclasses of high-grade glioma predict prognosis, delineate a pattern of disease progression, and resemble stages in neurogenesis. Cancer Cell. 2006;9(3):157–73.
5. Verhaak RG, et al. Integrated genomic analysis identifies clinically relevant subtypes of glioblastoma characterized by abnormalities in PDGFRA, IDH1, EGFR, and NF1. Cancer Cell. 2010;17(1):98–110.
6. Chen J, McKay RM, Parada LF. Malignant glioma: lessons from genomics, mouse models, and stem cells. Cell. 2012;149(1):36–47.
7. Singh SK, et al. Identification of human brain tumour initiating cells. Nature. 2004;432(7015):396–401.
8. Singh SK, et al. Identification of a cancer stem cell in human brain tumors. Cancer Res. 2003;63(18):5821–8.
9. Stiles CD, Rowitch DH. Glioma stem cells: a midterm exam. Neuron. 2008;58(6):832–46.

10. Chen J, et al. A restricted cell population propagates glioblastoma growth after chemotherapy. Nature. 2012;488(7412):522–6.
11. Son MJ, et al. SSEA-1 is an enrichment marker for tumor-initiating cells in human glioblastoma. Cell Stem Cell. 2009;4(5):440–52.
12. Wang R, et al. Glioblastoma stem-like cells give rise to tumour endothelium. Nature. 2010;468(7325):829–33.
13. Ricci-Vitiani L, et al. Tumour vascularization via endothelial differentiation of glioblastoma stem-like cells. Nature. 2010;468(7325):824–8.
14. Chao MP, Seita J, Weissman IL. Establishment of a normal hematopoietic and leukemia stem cell hierarchy. Cold Spring Harb Symp Quant Biol. 2008;73:439–49.
15. Clevers H. The cancer stem cell: premises, promises and challenges. Nat Med. 2011;17(3):313–9.
16. Prestegarden L, Enger PO. Cancer stem cells in the central nervous system—a critical review. Cancer Res. 2010;70(21):8255–8.
17. Visvader JE. Cells of origin in cancer. Nature. 2011;469(7330):314–22.
18. Hambardzumyan D, et al. The probable cell of origin of NF1- and PDGF-driven glioblastomas. PLoS One. 2011;6(9):e24454.
19. Hambardzumyan D, et al. Genetic modeling of gliomas in mice: new tools to tackle old problems. Glia. 2011;59(8):1155–68.
20. Lindberg N, et al. Oligodendrocyte progenitor cells can act as cell of origin for experimental glioma. Oncogene. 2009;28(23):2266–75.
21. Llaguno SA, et al. Neural and cancer stem cells in tumor suppressor mouse models of malignant astrocytoma. Cold Spring Harb Symp Quant Biol. 2008;73:421–6.
22. Marumoto T, et al. Development of a novel mouse glioma model using lentiviral vectors. Nat Med. 2009;15(1):110–6.
23. Zheng H, et al. Pten and p53 converge on c-Myc to control differentiation, self-renewal, and transformation of normal and neoplastic stem cells in glioblastoma. Cold Spring Harb Symp Quant Biol. 2008;73:427–37.
24. Friedmann-Morvinski D, et al. Dedifferentiation of neurons and astrocytes by oncogenes can induce gliomas in mice. Science. 2012;338(6110):1080–4.
25. Holland EC, et al. Combined activation of Ras and Akt in neural progenitors induces glioblastoma formation in mice. Nat Genet. 2000;25(1):55–7.
26. Jacques TS, et al. Combinations of genetic mutations in the adult neural stem cell compartment determine brain tumour phenotypes. EMBO J. 2010;29(1):222–35.
27. Wang Y, et al. Expression of mutant p53 proteins implicates a lineage relationship between neural stem cells and malignant astrocytic glioma in a murine model. Cancer Cell. 2009;15(6):514–26.
28. Doetsch F, et al. Subventricular zone astrocytes are neural stem cells in the adult mammalian brain. Cell. 1999;97(6):703–16.
29. Fuentealba LC, Obernier K, Alvarez-Buylla A. Adult neural stem cells bridge their niche. Cell Stem Cell. 2012;10(6):698–708.
30. Sanai N, et al. Corridors of migrating neurons in the human brain and their decline during infancy. Nature. 2011;478(7369):382–6.
31. Benner EJ, et al. Protective astrogenesis from the SVZ niche after injury is controlled by Notch modulator Thbs4. Nature. 2013;497(7449):369–73.
32. Rowitch DH, Kriegstein AR. Developmental genetics of vertebrate glial-cell specification. Nature. 2010;468(7321):214–22.
33. Eriksson PS, et al. Neurogenesis in the adult human hippocampus. Nat Med. 1998;4(11):1313–7.
34. Sanai N, Alvarez-Buylla A, Berger MS. Neural stem cells and the origin of gliomas. N Engl J Med. 2005;353(8):811–22.
35. Sanai N, et al. Unique astrocyte ribbon in adult human brain contains neural stem cells but lacks chain migration. Nature. 2004;427(6976):740–4.
36. Nunes MC, et al. Identification and isolation of multipotential neural progenitor cells from the subcortical white matter of the adult human brain. Nat Med. 2003;9(4):439–47.
37. Noctor SC, et al. Neurons derived from radial glial cells establish radial units in neocortex. Nature. 2001;409(6821):714–20.
38. Merkle FT, et al. Radial glia give rise to adult neural stem cells in the subventricular zone. Proc Natl Acad Sci U S A. 2004;101(50):17528–32.
39. Spassky N, et al. Adult ependymal cells are postmitotic and are derived from radial glial cells during embryogenesis. J Neurosci. 2005;25(1):10–8.
40. Lois C, Alvarez-Buylla A. Long-distance neuronal migration in the adult mammalian brain. Science. 1994;264(5162):1145–8.
41. Curtis MA, et al. Human neuroblasts migrate to the olfactory bulb via a lateral ventricular extension. Science. 2007;315(5816):1243–9.
42. Ahn S, Joyner AL. In vivo analysis of quiescent adult neural stem cells responding to Sonic hedgehog. Nature. 2005;437(7060):894–7.
43. Jackson EL, Alvarez-Buylla A. Characterization of adult neural stem cells and their relation to brain tumors. Cells Tissues Organs. 2008;188(1–2):212–24.
44. Kempermann G, et al. Early determination and long-term persistence of adult-generated new neurons in the hippocampus of mice. Development. 2003;130(2):391–9.
45. Seri B, et al. Astrocytes give rise to new neurons in the adult mammalian hippocampus. J Neurosci. 2001;21(18):7153–60.
46. Seri B, et al. Cell types, lineage, and architecture of the germinal zone in the adult dentate gyrus. J Comp Neurol. 2004;478(4):359–78.
47. Kuhn HG, Dickinson-Anson H, Gage FH. Neurogenesis in the dentate gyrus of the adult rat: age-related decrease of neuronal progenitor proliferation. J Neurosci. 1996;16(6):2027–33.
48. Nguyen LV, et al. Cancer stem cells: an evolving concept. Nat Rev Cancer. 2012;12(2):133–43.
49. Lee J, et al. Tumor stem cells derived from glioblastomas cultured in bFGF and EGF more closely mirror the phenotype and genotype of primary tumors than do serum-cultured cell lines. Cancer Cell. 2006;9(5):391–403.
50. Huszthy PC, et al. In vivo models of primary brain tumors: pitfalls and perspectives. Neuro Oncol. 2012;14(8):979–93.
51. Jones TS, Holland EC. Animal models for glioma drug discovery. Expert Opin Drug Discov. 2011;6(12):1271–83.
52. Candolfi M, et al. Intracranial glioblastoma models in preclinical neuro-oncology: neuropathological characterization and tumor progression. J Neurooncol. 2007;85(2):133–48.
53. Wee B, Charles N, Holland EC. Animal models to study cancer-initiating cells from glioblastoma. Front Biosci. 2011;16:2243–58.
54. Hambardzumyan D, et al. Modeling adult gliomas using RCAS/t-va technology. Transl Oncol. 2009;2(2):89–95.

55. de Almeida Sassi F, et al. Glioma revisited: from neurogenesis and cancer stem cells to the epigenetic regulation of the niche. J Oncol. 2012;2012, 537861.
56. Zhu Y, et al. Early inactivation of p53 tumor suppressor gene cooperating with NF1 loss induces malignant astrocytoma. Cancer Cell. 2005;8(2):119–30.
57. Kwon CH, et al. Pten haploinsufficiency accelerates formation of high-grade astrocytomas. Cancer Res. 2008;68(9):3286–94.
58. Liu C, et al. Mosaic analysis with double markers reveals tumor cell of origin in glioma. Cell. 2011;146(2):209–21.
59. Bachoo RM, et al. Epidermal growth factor receptor and Ink4a/Arf: convergent mechanisms governing terminal differentiation and transformation along the neural stem cell to astrocyte axis. Cancer Cell. 2002;1(3):269–77.
60. Dai C, et al. PDGF autocrine stimulation dedifferentiates cultured astrocytes and induces oligodendrogliomas and oligoastrocytomas from neural progenitors and astrocytes in vivo. Genes Dev. 2001;15(15):1913–25.
61. Uhrbom L, et al. Ink4a-Arf loss cooperates with KRas activation in astrocytes and neural progenitors to generate glioblastomas of various morphologies depending on activated Akt. Cancer Res. 2002;62(19):5551–8.
62. Uhrbom L, et al. Cell type-specific tumor suppression by Ink4a and Arf in Kras-induced mouse gliomagenesis. Cancer Res. 2005;65(6):2065–9.
63. Lai A, et al. Evidence for sequenced molecular evolution of IDH1 mutant glioblastoma from a distinct cell of origin. J Clin Oncol. 2011;29(34):4482–90.
64. Ellingson BM, et al. Probabilistic radiographic atlas of glioblastoma phenotypes. AJNR Am J Neuroradiol. 2013;34(3):533–40.
65. Drabycz S, et al. An analysis of image texture, tumor location, and MGMT promoter methylation in glioblastoma using magnetic resonance imaging. Neuroimage. 2010;49(2):1398–405.
66. Utsuki S, et al. Adult cerebellar glioblastoma cases have different characteristics from supratentorial glioblastoma. Brain Tumor Pathol. 2012;29(2):87–95.
67. Dang L, et al. Cancer-associated IDH1 mutations produce 2-hydroxyglutarate. Nature. 2009;462(7274):739–44.
68. Xu W, et al. Oncometabolite 2-hydroxyglutarate is a competitive inhibitor of alpha-ketoglutarate-dependent dioxygenases. Cancer Cell. 2011;19(1):17–30.
69. Figueroa ME, et al. Leukemic IDH1 and IDH2 mutations result in a hypermethylation phenotype, disrupt TET2 function, and impair hematopoietic differentiation. Cancer Cell. 2010;18(6):553–67.
70. Turcan S, et al. IDH1 mutation is sufficient to establish the glioma hypermethylator phenotype. Nature. 2012;483(7390):479–83.
71. Yan H, et al. IDH1 and IDH2 mutations in gliomas. N Engl J Med. 2009;360(8):765–73.
72. Sasaki M, et al. IDH1(R132H) mutation increases murine haematopoietic progenitors and alters epigenetics. Nature. 2012;488(7413): 656–9.
73. Sasaki M, et al. D-2-hydroxyglutarate produced by mutant IDH1 perturbs collagen maturation and basement membrane function. Genes Dev. 2012;26(18):2038–49.
74. Shih AH, Levine RL. IDH1 mutations disrupt blood, brain, and barriers. Cancer Cell. 2012;22(3):285–7.
75. Pastrana E, Silva-Vargas V, Doetsch F. Eyes wide open: a critical review of sphere-formation as an assay for stem cells. Cell Stem Cell. 2011;8(5):486–98.
76. Piccirillo SG, et al. Bone morphogenetic proteins inhibit the tumorigenic potential of human brain tumour-initiating cells. Nature. 2006;444(7120):761–5.
77. Hovinga KE, et al. Inhibition of notch signaling in glioblastoma targets cancer stem cells via an endothelial cell intermediate. Stem Cells. 2010;28(6):1019–29.
78. Cheng L, et al. Glioblastoma stem cells generate vascular pericytes to support vessel function and tumor growth. Cell. 2013;153(1):139–52.
79. Ying M, et al. Regulation of glioblastoma stem cells by retinoic acid: role for Notch pathway inhibition. Oncogene. 2011;30(31):3454–67.
80. Uchida N, et al. Direct isolation of human central nervous system stem cells. Proc Natl Acad Sci U S A. 2000;97(26):14720–5.
81. Coskun V, et al. CD133+ neural stem cells in the ependyma of mammalian postnatal forebrain. Proc Natl Acad Sci U S A. 2008;105(3):1026–31.
82. Pfenninger CV, et al. CD133 is not present on neurogenic astrocytes in the adult subventricular zone, but on embryonic neural stem cells, ependymal cells, and glioblastoma cells. Cancer Res. 2007;67(12):5727–36.
83. Shmelkov SV, et al. AC133/CD133/Prominin-1. Int J Biochem Cell Biol. 2005;37(4):715–9.
84. Gambelli F, et al. Identification of cancer stem cells from human glioblastomas: growth and differentiation capabilities and CD133/prominin-1 expression. Cell Biol Int. 2012;36(1):29–38.
85. Li Z. CD133: a stem cell biomarker and beyond. Exp Hematol Oncol. 2013;2(1):17.
86. Zacchigna S, et al. Loss of the cholesterol-binding protein prominin-1/CD133 causes disk dysmorphogenesis and photoreceptor degeneration. J Neurosci. 2009;29(7):2297–308.
87. Manoranjan B, et al. Medulloblastoma stem cells: where development and cancer cross pathways. Pediatr Res. 2012;71(4 Pt 2):516–22.
88. Paola B, et al. CD133 is essential for glioblastoma stem cell maintenance. Stem Cells. 2013;31(5):857–69.
89. Wang J, et al. CD133 negative glioma cells form tumors in nude rats and give rise to CD133 positive cells. Int J Cancer. 2008;122(4):761–8.
90. Beier D, et al. CD133(+) and CD133(-) glioblastoma-derived cancer stem cells show differential growth characteristics and molecular profiles. Cancer Res. 2007;67(9):4010–5.
91. Lottaz C, et al. Transcriptional profiles of CD133+ and CD133- glioblastoma-derived cancer stem cell lines suggest different cells of origin. Cancer Res. 2010;70(5):2030–40.
92. Yan X, et al. A CD133-related gene expression signature identifies an aggressive glioblastoma subtype with excessive mutations. Proc Natl Acad Sci U S A. 2011;108(4):1591–6.
93. Zarkoob H, et al. Investigating the link between molecular subtypes of glioblastoma, epithelial-mesenchymal transition, and CD133 cell surface protein. PLoS One. 2013;8(5):e64169.
94. Campos B, et al. Expression and regulation of AC133 and CD133 in glioblastoma. Glia. 2011;59(12):1974–86.
95. Reynolds BA, Weiss S. Generation of neurons and astrocytes from isolated cells of the adult mammalian central nervous system. Science. 1992;255(5052):1707–10.
96. Hemmati HD, et al. Cancerous stem cells can arise from pediatric brain tumors. Proc Natl Acad Sci U S A. 2003;100(25): 15178–83.

97. Venugopal C, et al. Bmi1 marks intermediate precursors during differentiation of human brain tumor initiating cells. Stem Cell Res. 2012;8(2):141–53.
98. Ikushima H, et al. Glioma-initiating cells retain their tumorigenicity through integration of the Sox axis and Oct4 protein. J Biol Chem. 2011;286(48):41434–41.
99. Liu G, et al. Analysis of gene expression and chemoresistance of CD133+ cancer stem cells in glioblastoma. Mol Cancer. 2006;5:67.
100. Lathia JD, et al. Integrin alpha 6 regulates glioblastoma stem cells. Cell Stem Cell. 2010;6(5):421–32.
101. Brescia P, Richichi C, Pelicci G. Current strategies for identification of glioma stem cells: adequate or unsatisfactory? J Oncol. 2012;2012:376894.
102. Bar EE, et al. Hypoxia increases the expression of stem-cell markers and promotes clonogenicity in glioblastoma neurospheres. Am J Pathol. 2010;177(3):1491–502.
103. Harris MA, et al. Cancer stem cells are enriched in the side population cells in a mouse model of glioma. Cancer Res. 2008;68(24):10051–9.
104. Gonzalez-Gomez P, Sanchez P, Mira H. MicroRNAs as regulators of neural stem cell-related pathways in glioblastoma multiforme. Mol Neurobiol. 2011;44(3):235–49.
105. Huse JT, et al. The PTEN-regulating microRNA miR-26a is amplified in high-grade glioma and facilitates gliomagenesis in vivo. Genes Dev. 2009;23(11):1327–37.
106. Kim H, et al. Integrative genome analysis reveals an oncomir/oncogene cluster regulating glioblastoma survivorship. Proc Natl Acad Sci U S A. 2010;107(5):2183–8.
107. Shi L, et al. hsa-mir-181a and hsa-mir-181b function as tumor suppressors in human glioma cells. Brain Res. 2008;1236:185–93.
108. Silber J, et al. miR-124 and miR-137 inhibit proliferation of glioblastoma multiforme cells and induce differentiation of brain tumor stem cells. BMC Med. 2008;6:14.
109. Godlewski J, et al. Targeting of the Bmi-1 oncogene/stem cell renewal factor by microRNA-128 inhibits glioma proliferation and self-renewal. Cancer Res. 2008;68(22):9125–30.
110. Kefas B, et al. microRNA-7 inhibits the epidermal growth factor receptor and the Akt pathway and is down-regulated in glioblastoma. Cancer Res. 2008;68(10):3566–72.
111. Artavanis-Tsakonas S, Delidakis C, Fehon RG. The Notch locus and the cell biology of neuroblast segregation. Annu Rev Cell Biol. 1991;7:427–52.
112. Hoppe PE, Greenspan RJ. Local function of the Notch gene for embryonic ectodermal pathway choice in Drosophila. Cell. 1986;46(5):773–83.
113. Poulson DF. Chromosomal deficiencies and the embryonic development of drosophila melanogaster. Proc Natl Acad Sci U S A. 1937;23(3):133–7.
114. Yoon K, Gaiano N. Notch signaling in the mammalian central nervous system: insights from mouse mutants. Nat Neurosci. 2005;8(6):709–15.
115. Mizutani K, et al. Differential Notch signalling distinguishes neural stem cells from intermediate progenitors. Nature. 2007;449(7160):351–5.
116. Wang J, et al. Notch promotes radioresistance of glioma stem cells. Stem Cells. 2010;28(1):17–28.
117. Kanamori M, et al. Contribution of Notch signaling activation to human glioblastoma multiforme. J Neurosurg. 2007;106(3):417–27.
118. Lino MM, Merlo A, Boulay JL. Notch signaling in glioblastoma: a developmental drug target? BMC Med. 2010;8:72.
119. Chen J, et al. Inhibition of notch signaling blocks growth of glioblastoma cell lines and tumor neurospheres. Genes Cancer. 2010;1(8):822–35.
120. Fan X, et al. NOTCH pathway blockade depletes CD133-positive glioblastoma cells and inhibits growth of tumor neurospheres and xenografts. Stem Cells. 2010;28(1):5–16.
121. Calabrese C, et al. A perivascular niche for brain tumor stem cells. Cancer Cell. 2007;11(1):69–82.
122. Zhu TS, et al. Endothelial cells create a stem cell niche in glioblastoma by providing NOTCH ligands that nurture self-renewal of cancer stem-like cells. Cancer Res. 2011;71(18):6061–72.
123. Gallia GL, et al. Inhibition of Akt inhibits growth of glioblastoma and glioblastoma stem-like cells. Mol Cancer Ther. 2009;8(2):386–93.
124. Eyler CE, et al. Brain cancer stem cells display preferential sensitivity to Akt inhibition. Stem Cells. 2008;26(12):3027–36.
125. Jones DT, et al. Dissecting the genomic complexity underlying medulloblastoma. Nature. 2012;488(7409):100–5.
126. Takezaki T, et al. Essential role of the Hedgehog signaling pathway in human glioma-initiating cells. Cancer Sci. 2011;102(7):1306–12.
127. Yang ZJ, et al. Medulloblastoma can be initiated by deletion of Patched in lineage-restricted progenitors or stem cells. Cancer Cell. 2008;14(2):135–45.
128. Karcher U, et al. Primary structure of the heterosaccharide of the surface glycoprotein of Methanothermus fervidus. J Biol Chem. 1993;268(36):26821–6.
129. Kim Y, et al. Wnt activation is implicated in glioblastoma radioresistance. Lab Invest. 2012;92(3):466–73.
130. Anido J, et al. TGF-beta receptor inhibitors target the CD44(high)/Id1(high) glioma-initiating cell population in human glioblastoma. Cancer Cell. 2010;18(6):655–68.
131. Ikushima H, et al. Autocrine TGF-beta signaling maintains tumorigenicity of glioma-initiating cells through Sry-related HMG-box factors. Cell Stem Cell. 2009;5(5):504–14.
132. Penuelas S, et al. TGF-beta increases glioma-initiating cell self-renewal through the induction of LIF in human glioblastoma. Cancer Cell. 2009;15(4):315–27.
133. Panchision DM. The role of oxygen in regulating neural stem cells in development and disease. J Cell Physiol. 2009;220(3):562–8.
134. Gustafsson MV, et al. Hypoxia requires notch signaling to maintain the undifferentiated cell state. Dev Cell. 2005;9(5):617–28.
135. Keith B, Johnson RS, Simon MC. HIF1alpha and HIF2alpha: sibling rivalry in hypoxic tumour growth and progression. Nat Rev Cancer. 2012;12(1):9–22.
136. Mendez O, et al. Knock down of HIF-1alpha in glioma cells reduces migration in vitro and invasion in vivo and impairs their ability to form tumor spheres. Mol Cancer. 2010;9:133.
137. Qiang L, et al. HIF-1alpha is critical for hypoxia-mediated maintenance of glioblastoma stem cells by activating Notch signaling pathway. Cell Death Differ. 2012;19(2):284–94.
138. Schwab LP, et al. Hypoxia-inducible factor 1alpha promotes primary tumor growth and tumor-initiating cell activity in breast cancer. Breast Cancer Res . 2012;14(1):R6.

139. Li Z, et al. Hypoxia-inducible factors regulate tumorigenic capacity of glioma stem cells. Cancer Cell. 2009;15(6): 501–13.
140. Zagzag D, et al. Hypoxia-inducible factor 1 and VEGF upregulate CXCR4 in glioblastoma: implications for angiogenesis and glioma cell invasion. Lab Invest. 2006;86(12):1221–32.
141. Heddleston JM, et al. The hypoxic microenvironment maintains glioblastoma stem cells and promotes reprogramming towards a cancer stem cell phenotype. Cell Cycle. 2009;8(20):3274–84.
142. Lee J, et al. Epigenetic-mediated dysfunction of the bone morphogenetic protein pathway inhibits differentiation of glioblastoma-initiating cells. Cancer Cell. 2008;13(1):69–80.
143. Tavazoie M, et al. A specialized vascular niche for adult neural stem cells. Cell Stem Cell. 2008;3(3):279–88.
144. Gilbertson RJ, Rich JN. Making a tumour's bed: glioblastoma stem cells and the vascular niche. Nat Rev Cancer. 2007;7(10):733–6.
145. Rong Y, et al. 'Pseudopalisading' necrosis in glioblastoma: a familiar morphologic feature that links vascular pathology, hypoxia, and angiogenesis. J Neuropathol Exp Neurol. 2006;65(6):529–39.
146. Teodorczyk M, Martin-Villalba A. Sensing invasion: cell surface receptors driving spreading of glioblastoma. J Cell Physiol. 2010;222(1):1–10.
147. de Groot JF, et al. Tumor invasion after treatment of glioblastoma with bevacizumab: radiographic and pathologic correlation in humans and mice. Neuro Oncol. 2010;12(3):233–42.
148. Sampetrean O, et al. Invasion precedes tumor mass formation in a malignant brain tumor model of genetically modified neural stem cells. Neoplasia. 2011;13(9):784–91.
149. Winkler F, et al. Imaging glioma cell invasion in vivo reveals mechanisms of dissemination and peritumoral angiogenesis. Glia. 2009;57(12):1306–15.
150. Onishi M, et al. Angiogenesis and invasion in glioma. Brain Tumor Pathol. 2011;28(1):13–24.
151. Hardee ME, Zagzag D. Mechanisms of glioma-associated neovascularization. Am J Pathol. 2012;181(4):1126–41.
152. Bleau AM, Huse JT, Holland EC. The ABCG2 resistance network of glioblastoma. Cell Cycle. 2009;8(18):2936–44.
153. Bao Z, et al. BMP4, a strong better prognosis predictor, has a subtype preference and cell development association in gliomas. J Transl Med. 2013;11:100.
154. Hardee ME, et al. Resistance of glioblastoma-initiating cells to radiation mediated by the tumor microenvironment can be abolished by inhibiting transforming growth factor-beta. Cancer Res. 2012;72(16):4119–29.
155. Bao S, et al. Glioma stem cells promote radioresistance by preferential activation of the DNA damage response. Nature. 2006;444(7120):756–60.
156. Pirozzi CJ, Reitman ZJ, Yan H. Releasing the block: setting differentiation free with mutant IDH inhibitors. Cancer Cell. 2013;23(5):570–2.
157. Hodges TR, et al. Isocitrate dehydrogenase 1: what it means to the neurosurgeon. J Neurosurg. 2013;118(6):1176–80.

3 Molecular Pathology Techniques

Matija Snuderl

The field of neuro-oncology has undergone a number of significant changes over the past decades. One of the most striking, however, has been the rapid pace of discovery in the field of molecular genetics, especially over the past few years. As a result, the genomic landscape of the most common entities has been defined, including a discovery of recurrent genetic alterations, leading to the establishment of diagnostic, prognostic, and predictive biomarkers. Some of these genetic markers, such as 1p/19q loss, O^6-methylguanine-DNA-methyltransferase (MGMT) promoter methylation, and isocitrate dehydrogenase 1 (*IDH1*) mutations, have already entered routine clinical diagnostics and are considered a standard of care. While the clinical utility of other molecular genetic biomarkers, such as epidermal growth factor receptor (*EGFR*) amplification, proto-oncogene B-Raf (*BRAF*) mutation/duplication, or molecular subclassification based on gene expression profile is not firmly established yet, some can be utilized for diagnostic purposes. Furthermore, given the development of targeted therapy, the molecular signature can be also utilized to identify the appropriate target population, substratify patients for clinical trials, and validate candidate predictive biomarkers. As in other tumors and diseases, advanced molecular diagnostics will not replace traditional histopathology, but provide valuable additional information to increase diagnostic accuracy and precision.

Given the limitations of standard cytotoxic therapies, such as chemotherapy and radiation therapy, in the treatment of brain tumors, it has become clear that major progress will require novel approaches. As a result, significant efforts are being made to develop more targeted or selective approaches, based on the specific molecular signature of the tumor. A variety of technical assays have been designed to analyze gene expression, as well as large chromosomal losses and gains, gene rearrangements, focal copy-number changes, point mutations, and epigenetic changes. Genome, transcriptome, and epigenome analyses will likely become a focus for diagnostics to identify new therapeutic targets.

Gliomas are the most common tumors of the central nervous system (CNS) and often require additional molecular work-up, either for diagnosis or biomarkers. In clinical practice, focused assays are usually performed. The most commonly used assays include analyses of 1p/19q loss, *MGMT* promoter methylation, and *IDH1* mutation status. Most commonly performed technical assays are fluorescence in situ hybridization (FISH), polymerase chain reaction (PCR) and its variants, variety of methylation specific assays and sequencing or immunohistochemistry (IHC). These assays are particularly useful in clinical management and diagnostics of adult diffuse gliomas. Although genetic changes and expression profiles have been well studied in other brain tumors as well, the routine clinical use of molecular testing in meningiomas, ependymomas, or medulloblastomas is not yet established. Whole genome expression profiling and DNA analysis of medulloblastomas have pioneered molecular and biological subclassification of a morphologically relatively uniform disease. Similar results were shown in gliomas and specific molecular classes have also been defined in meningioma and ependymoma using next-generation sequencing (NGS) and/or expression profiling. With the costs of whole genome approaches decreasing, we can expect a decline in number of single target assays in molecular laboratories in favor of broad genome-wide analyses in the future.

Molecular Techniques in Clinical Practice

Copy-Number Analysis

Fluorescence In Situ Hybridization

Fluorescence in situ hybridization (FISH) is one of the oldest and most commonly used techniques in molecular pathology [1]. FISH uses fluorescently labeled DNA probes which attach/hybridize to specific targets in the DNA, providing the

M.A. Karajannis and D. Zagzag (eds.), *Molecular Pathology of Nervous System Tumors: Biological Stratification and Targeted Therapies*, Molecular Pathology Library 8,
DOI 10.1007/978-1-4939-1830-0_3, © Springer Science+Business Media New York 2015

information on copy-number changes on the level of single cells while preserving the morphology of the underlying tissue. Using different fluorescent dyes enables the investigation of multiple DNA targets simultaneously. FISH can be used on formalin-fixed paraffin-embedded tissue (FFPE) and allows identification of genomic changes in situ. A disadvantage is that FISH probes/signals have to be relatively large to be detected by fluorescent-light microscopy and therefore are not useful for identifying small genomic changes, such as small insertions/deletions. Also, due to the relatively broad optical spectrum of fluorescent dyes, the number of dyes (and therefore, probes) is limited to four at most on a single slide.

FISH offers numerous applications for the routine detection of cytogenetic biomarkers. It can assess ploidy, large chromosomal gains and losses, focal amplifications/deletions, and large structural gene rearrangements. Because the assay is performed directly on the tissue, it allows for the detection of genetic changes even in a small biopsy, or when only a limited number of tumor cells are present among normal tissue. In contrast with whole genome assays, FISH also provides information of whether different genetic changes are present in the same tumor cell or in a different tumor subclone, i.e., genetic mosaicism.

Because of the diagnostic utility of FISH in clinical practice, its application for a variety of tumors is now considered standard of care, and standard protocols are well established. Therefore, any molecular pathology or neuropathology laboratory should be able to implement it. Probes are available commercially and automated systems are used in large laboratories. However, several issues and limitations have to be noted. The assay is labor intensive, with the maximum number of slides managed by a single technician ranging between 10 and 20 per single run, depending on the technician's experience. Larger sample volumes can be managed more efficiently with deparaffinization, protease digestion, and pre- and post-hybridization washes performed by an automated system. Automated systems also allow for standardized and uniform treatment of all specimens. Protease digestion is particularly important, since the brain tissue has a strong autofluorescence and insufficient digestion will result in strong background and weak hybridization signals. On the other hand, excessive digestion will damage the tissue and may lead to a technical failure. Also, the tissue fixation and processing can have a deleterious effect on the ability to perform FISH. Particularly heavy acid decalcification, which is fortunately rare in CNS specimens, almost always leads to FISH failure. The time required for scoring can vary greatly. While the 1p/19q assay, for example, is quite time-consuming and requires scoring ~100 nuclei and two slides, one for chromosome 1 and one for chromosome 19, EGFR and other amplification assays can be detected relatively quickly. However, in the light of recent observations about minor amplified subpopulations and the potential impact of different levels of EGFR amplification on survival, careful scoring of the entire tumor specimen is warranted [2].

For interpretation, appropriate cutoffs must be determined according to specificity and sensitivity for each test. The most common findings in neuropathology FISH are deletions, low-level copy-number gains/losses, and high-level copy-number gains, i.e., amplifications (Fig. 3.1). Gene rearrangements are less common. For 1p/19q deletions, one of the possible methods of interpretation is the median percentage of nuclei with two reference/control signals (e.g., 1q or 19p) and one test signal (e.g., 1p or 19q) plus three standard deviations as the cutoff values for deletion. Another possibility is to use the ratio of target versus reference signals, with most control specimens being near 1.0 and cutoff around 0.75–0.85, depending on the laboratory standards. In addition, there is increasing evidence in the 1p/19q literature that there are different clinical implications of absolute deletions with one target and two reference signals per nucleus compared to so-called relative deletions in tumors with polyploidy/aneuploidy. These tumors can show variable numbers of target and reference signals such as duplication with two target signals and four reference signals per nucleus, or 3:6, 4:8 ratios. This finding would be misinterpreted as absolute deletions by PCR loss of heterozygosity (LOH) methods. However, recent studies have shown that relative deletion, also known as a superloss, is an important prognostic marker and patients with relative deletion have shorter progression-free survival [3, 4].

Gene amplification testing is most commonly applied for *EGFR*, although the other two most commonly amplified receptor tyrosine kinase (RTK) genes platelet-derived growth factor receptor alpha (*PDGFRA*) and mesenchymal–epithelial transition factor (*MET*) RTK gene are gaining increasing attention, partly due to the increasing clinical availability of kinase inhibitors against these targets [5]. Also, while *EGFR* amplification is generally limited to adult GBMs, *PDGFRA* amplification is common in lower grade and pediatric gliomas [6]. Typically, RTK gene amplifications involve the majority of cells within a given tumor and with high levels of amplification. However, tumors with scattered amplified cells, which represent a minority of the tumor, are also encountered in clinical practice. This phenomenon is most commonly observed in *MET*-amplified GBMs, where cells with amplification can be rare and scattered throughout the tumor. Another recently described phenomenon is mosaic heterogeneity, where tumors are composed of subclones with mutually exclusive amplification of RTK genes [7–9]. Up to three coexisting subclones with amplifications of *EGFR*, *MET*, and *PDGFRA* within a single tumor have been described. More importantly, these studies have shown that during glioma progression, subclones have different propensities to infiltrate normal brain and genomic changes can vary widely among different parts of the same tumor [7]. In addition, studies have also shown that some GBM cells contain simultaneous amplification of different RTK genes. Although the significance of these findings is not clear, they emphasize the complexity of the disease and raise several

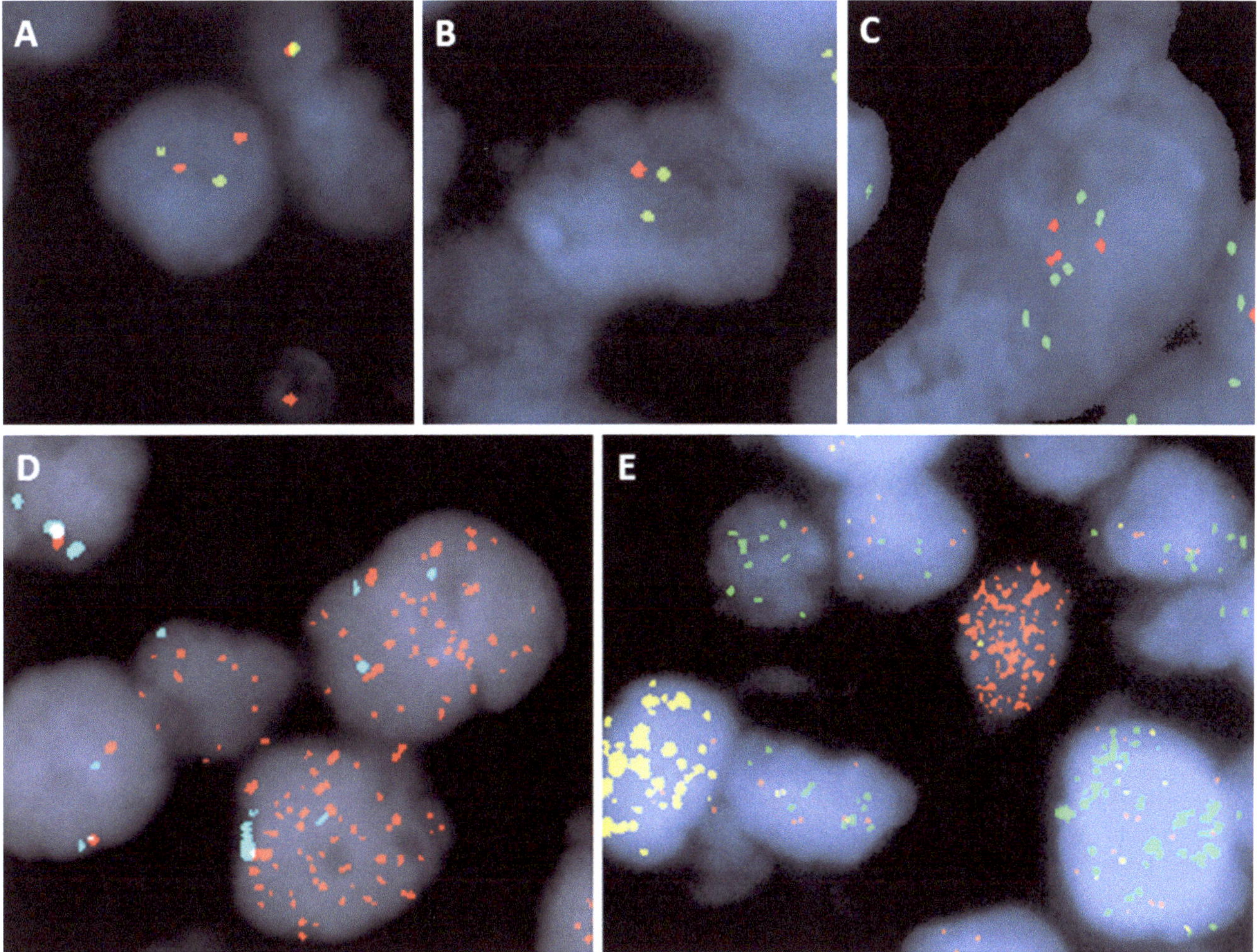

FIG. 3.1. Examples of FISH applications in molecular neuropathology: (**a–c**) 1p evaluation, 1p red, 1q green: (**a**) Maintenance of 1p (2:2 signals), (**b**) 1p loss (1:2 signals), (**c**) relative deletions/superloss (4:6). (**d**, **e**) RTK genes evaluation: (**d**) high level amplification of *EGFR* (*red*: *EGFR*, *blue*: CEP7), (**e**) mosaic heterogeneity with mutually exclusive amplifications of *EGFR* (*red*), *PDGFRA* (*green*), and *MET* (*yellow*) in subclones within a GBM. All panels: nuclei are counterstained with DAPI.

challenging implications for molecular pathology and clinical practice. This also raises an important practical question: whether the molecular analysis should be focused on a single target or multiplexed, i.e., analyzing several targets, or even the whole genome. This issue is also discussed in the section on array comparative genomic hybridization (aCGH) below. While specific criteria may differ among laboratories, it is reasonable to suggest that the presence of any subpopulation with gene amplification should be reported. Lastly, FISH can be used to evaluate for translocations. The most typical indication would be for *EWS* gene rearrangement in small, round blue cell tumors when Ewing's sarcoma/peripheral primitive neuroectodermal tumor (PNET) is in the differential.

The 1p/19q analysis can be performed by several techniques, most commonly by FISH, single nucleotide polymorphism (SNP) array, or PCR-based microsatellite LOH. However, FISH is the most commonly used assay and offers additional prognostic information compared to PCR LOH. Fluorescent test probes are commercially available and hybridize to so-called minimally deleted regions [10, 11]. The test probe localizes to 1p36 and a control/reference probe localizes on the opposite arm to 1q25. Target and control/reference probes for chromosome 19 localize to 19q13 and 19p13, respectively. One FFPE section cut at 4–5 μm is used for each chromosome. A few caveats apply for FISH 1p/19q. A normal copy-number LOH resulting from mitotic recombination would not be detected by FISH and could in theory result in false negatives [12]; however, this would be rare in 1p/19q co-deleted oligodendroglioma. More importantly, FISH cannot assess multiple markers to cover the entire arm of the chromosome. Therefore the observed loss might only represent a relatively small "probe-size" deletion on 1p or 19q. However, only the whole arm deletions are truly associated with a favorable prognosis. While the result would be read as positive technically, biologically this would represent a false-positive finding. Many tumors with these minimal deletions are in fact astrocytomas, rather than oligodendrogliomas, and are actually associated with a worse prognosis. GBMs in particular contain these minimal deletions, and a misdiagnosis of GBM with oligodendroglial component could be made based on a biologically false-positive finding. To avoid this pitfall, some laboratories avoid commercially available probes and choose home-brewed probes on 1p32 and 19q13.4, which are outside the minimal regions of deletion. Although the sensitivity is decreased, this strategy increases specificity of the assay.

The size of FISH probes, ~1 Mb, and staining with either a green or orange/red spectrum fluorescent dye, allows localization against the DAPI counterstained nucleus. As discussed above, four main patterns can be recognized: maintenance of 1p and 19q with two control probes and two target probes, absolute deletion with two control probes and one target probe, polysomy with several copies of target and control regions, and polysomy with deletion of target regions. This pattern known also as relative loss or superloss consists of four control signals and two target signals, for example. However, the ratio of signals can vary and show rations such as 6:3 or 8:4.

Multiple studies have confirmed high reproducibility between SNP/LOH analysis and FISH [13]. While SNP/LOH analysis has an advantage of analyzing multiple markers on chromosomal arms, FISH offers the ability of evaluating the tumor in situ, with small biopsies and without patient's matched normal blood. With growing evidence of implications of polysomy, FISH seems to offer additional prognostic value compared to PCR LOH. There is a strong association between histology and 1p/19q loss. Tumors with classic oligodendroglial features have a higher likelihood of 1p/19q codeletion [14, 15]. It is important to keep in mind that there is no need to select the most oligo-like area when choosing the best section for 1p/19q analysis. It seems that 1p19q codeletion is a very early event in the tumor development, and therefore is present in both oligodendroglial and astrocytic components of an oligoastrocytoma. Another interesting association exists between tumor site and genetics, with frontal oligodendrogliomas having a significantly higher likelihood of 1p/19q loss than temporal lobe tumors [3].

Array Comparative Genomic Hybridization

DNA arrays provide a whole genome analysis of copy number changes. Many arrays offer both copy-number variant and SNP content for LOH analysis in a single array. Genomic DNA can be isolated from FFPE tissue after deparaffinization and protease digestion. A normal male/female DNA standard is usually used for comparison. However, the patient's germline DNA from the peripheral blood can also be utilized. This is particularly useful for SNP analysis. The cancer arrays usually contain a high-resolution backbone with an average spacing approximately one oligo probe every 25–50 kb, which ideally avoid regions containing common copy-number variants (CNV) to minimize detection of benign CNVs. The probe density is usually higher: one every 5 kb in regions defined by International Standards of Cytogenomics Arrays (ISCA). Furthermore, some arrays contain an increased density of probes in known cancer-related genes with up to a single exon resolution, where the density of the probes can be up to one probe every 50 bp. This is particularly useful for genes with known specific deletions, duplications or mutations in cancer. One must keep in mind that although aCGH is a genome-wide technique, the distribution of probes highly depends on the purpose of the array. The design is specific for each clinical indication, and therefore laboratories performing aCGH testing for different clinical questions cannot use the same array for all of them. Although the backbones might be the same or very similar, DNA coverage distribution with highest probe density are significantly different based on whether the array was designed for autism, epilepsy, or cancer, for example.

While a simple PCR LOH does not provide a significant advantage, the aCGH + SNP arrays offer several advantages compared to FISH. The aCGH + SNP provides a whole genome view of the DNA (Fig. 3.2). The same reaction can be performed for all gliomas in the laboratory, regardless whether the diagnosis is GBM or oligodendroglioma, which decreases costs necessary for storing, optimizing, and running several different FISH probes. For example, in a small cell GBM variant where three separate FISH reactions, 1p, 19q, and EGFR, are needed, a single array can provide a definitive answer. In medulloblastoma, aCGH can be utilized for the subgroup classification since different subgroups carry characteristic chromosomal changes. In addition, the array provides information about other genomic changes in brain tumors such as *PTEN*, *CDKN2A/p16*, *PDGFRA*, *NF1*, and *MET*, which are not routinely tested. This information, while not utilized in current clinical care, will increasingly play a role for design of molecularly driven studies, including clinical trials. For example, clinical outcome predictions can be made by evaluating several loci of DNA rearrangements in medulloblastomas, where a number of FISH reactions could be replaced by a single aCGH [16]. If all potential targets are to be tested by FISH, the costs and labor intensity would be significantly higher than a single aCGH + SNP array. An additional advantage is the interpretation software which allows quick review of genomic changes and automated variant call. The software allows manually adjusting levels at which variants can be called and minimizes the possibility of false negatives. While the genome still has to be reviewed manually, the amount of time spent analyzing the array data seems to be equal or shorter in comparison with 1p/19q analysis, which is clearly the most labor-intensive assay in regard to data evaluation. A disadvantage of aCGH technique in comparison with FISH is that it might not be able to detect changes if only scattered infiltrating cells are present in the tissue [7] and might be challenging with small biopsies since approximately 1.5 μg of DNA is needed.

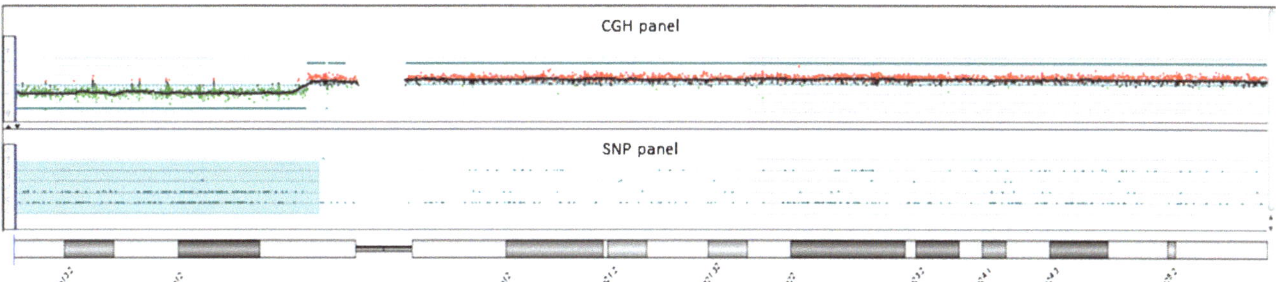

Fig. 3.2. Example of aCGH result in molecular neuropathology: view at chromosome 17 in a medulloblastoma shows a deletion of the short arm of the chromosome 17. This loss occurs in ~25–50 % of medulloblastoma. 17p loss has been associated with a poor survival in some studies suggesting that loss of a tumor suppressor gene located on 17p plays a role in the genesis or progression of medulloblastoma. A novel candidate gene, CTD nuclear envelope phosphatase 1 (*CTDNEP1*), was identified as a recurrent target of mutation in Group 3 and Group 4 medulloblastomas. *CTDNEP1* is located on chromosome 17p13.1 in a hotspot of deletion and LOH.

Mutation Analysis

Mutation-Specific Antibodies

Until recently, the only way to analyze point mutations was by Sanger sequencing. A truly revolutionary event was the introduction of mutation-specific IDH1 R132H antibody into clinical practice. That was quickly followed by a novel BRAF V600E mutation-specific antibody [17–20]. The advantage of using a mutation-specific antibody is undisputable. The staining can be performed in a clinical immunohistochemistry laboratory on FFPE on standard 5 μm sections (Fig. 3.3). Provided the antibody is robust and validated as being highly sensitive and specific, detection is fast, inexpensive, reliable, and allows identification of single infiltrating tumor cells. In comparison with rather nonspecific antibodies such as p53, the mutant protein is not expected to be present in any reactive or inflammatory conditions that may lead to overexpression of nonspecific markers. As a consequence, tumor mutation-specific antibodies are of great value in distinguishing not only reactive astrocytes from tumor cells but also oligodendroglioma/oligoastrocytoma from their morphological mimickers [21]. Although there is strong correlation between *IDH1* mutation and 1p/19q loss, the 1p/19q testing cannot be replaced by IDH1 antibody and several caveats must be noted. For IDH1, the antibody detects only one of several known mutations. While R132H is the most common mutation and represents ~90 % of *IDH1* mutations, other mutations at that site will not be detected by the antibody. Furthermore, mutations of *IDH2* at the residue R172 can also be found in gliomas, although rarely [22]. The R172 residue in *IDH2* is the exact analogue of the R132 residue in *IDH1*. The residue is located in the active site of the enzyme and forms hydrogen bonds with the isocitrate substrate [23]. Therefore, *IDH1* and *IDH2* sequencing provides a definitive answer in IDH1 R132H antibody-negative tumors.

BRAF V600E antibody can be used for the same purpose. However, it is most useful in supratentorial tumors. Although BRAF alterations in pilocytic astrocytoma of the cerebellum are common, they are usually due to a tandem repeat producing a fusion BRAF:KIAA1549 gene [24, 25], which would not be detected by the antibody. BRAF V600E is present in supratentorial pilocytic astrocytoma and pilomyxoid astrocytoma, pleomorphic xanthoastrocytoma (PXA), ganglioglioma and dysembryoplastic neuroepithelial tumor [26]. The antibody could be particularly useful in distinguishing between a PXA and a GBM on a small biopsy, since BRAF V600E mutation would be highly unusual in a GBM, but they are common in PXA [27].

Another example of a clinically important antibody detecting a molecular aberration is *INI1*. The loss of protein expression in an embryonal brain tumor is virtually diagnostic of atypical teratoid-rhabdoid tumor (AT/RT), a highly aggressive neoplasm of early childhood. Immunohistochemistry for INI1 should be performed on every medulloblastoma or primitive embryonal tumor in childhood to avoid misdiagnosis of the AT/RT [28].

Sequencing

Until recently, Sanger sequencing represented the most common way to investigate mutations in brain tumors. Considering that many genes commonly mutated in gliomas such as *TP53* and *NF1* are large and can be altered by several different mutations and the predictive value is unknown, sequencing played a minimal role in clinical laboratories for brain tumors. One of the relevant applications is *IDH1* and *IDH2* sequencing for tumors negative for IDH1 R132H by immunohistochemistry, when the suspicion for less common mutations is high based on clinical presentation. NGS methods are still mostly used in research. However, they are being adopted by clinical laboratories, usually as focused cancer gene panels (Fig. 3.4). As the cost of sequencing continues to decline, and the methods themselves including data analysis become easier to manage in the clinical setting, they will

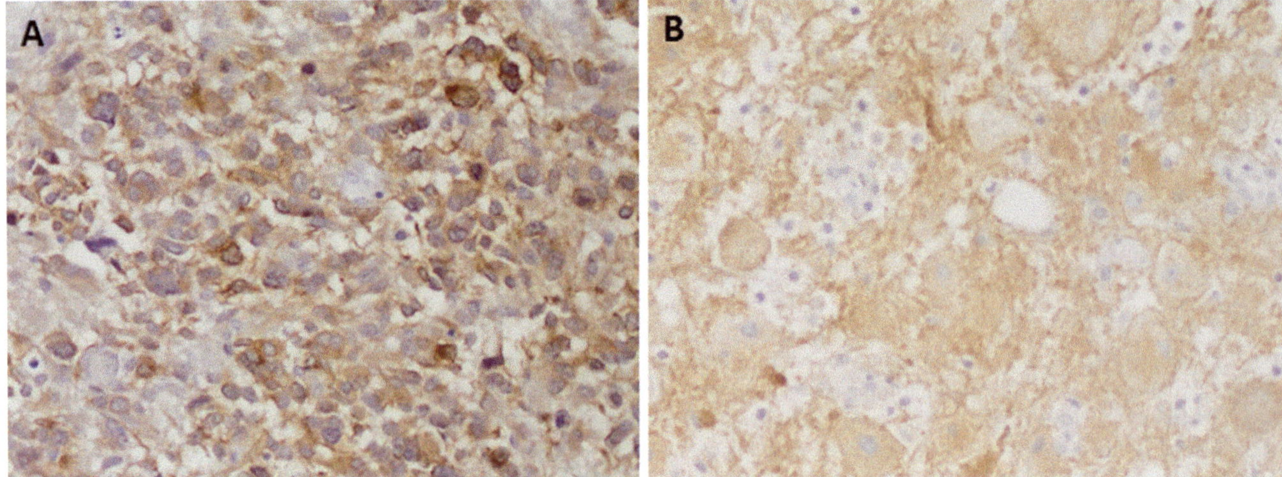

Fig. 3.3 Examples of utility of mutation specific antibodies in neuropathology: the immunohistochemistry with a specific antibody against (**a**) IDH1 R132H in a case of a diffuse astrocytoma and (**b**) BRAF V600E in a cerebellar ganglioglioma shows strong immunoreactivity specific for tumor cells. Reactive cells in the background are negative (**b**)

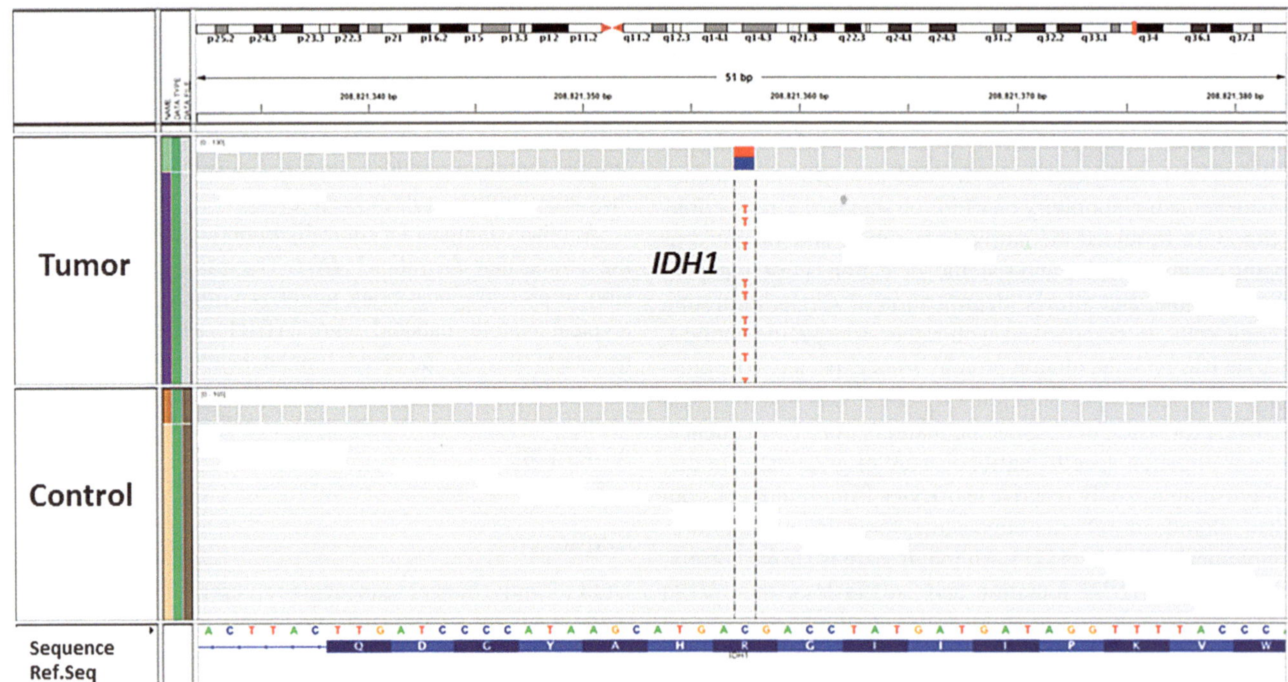

Fig. 3.4 Example of the next-generation sequencing in molecular neuropathology: in oligodendroglioma, whole genome sequencing (Illumina platform) identifies mutation in the IDH1 (c. 395 C>T, p.R132H) gene. The majority of *IDH1* mutations in gliomas are p.R132H. The example shown is in the form of the IGV browser view (Courtesy of Dr. Stephen Yip, BC Cancer Agency)

likely become increasingly available for routine use. In the future, NGS will most likely cover tens to hundreds of cancer-specific genes. However it is only the matter of time before the whole exome or whole genome sequencing cost will not be that much different from a focused panel. Additionally, whole exome/genome sequencing will allow identification of gene rearrangements, which were previously unappreciated phenomena in gliomas [29].

MGMT Testing

MGMT promoter methylation has been confirmed by several clinical studies as a biomarker in patients with gliomas. The MGMT gene is located on chromosome 10q26.34 and contains five exons, the first of which is noncoding. Transcription of the MGMT gene is initiated at a single site within a GC-rich, non-TATA box-containing promoter. Expression of the MGMT gene is epigenetically regulated by methylation-dependent silencing.

Temozolomide (TMZ) methylates DNA at position 6 of guanine nucleotides. The resultant O^6-methylguanine adducts pair with thymidine, and when DNA mismatch repair (MMR) enzymes attempt to excise O^6-methylguanine, they generate single- and double-strand breaks which lead to apoptosis. MGMT can rescue the cell by restoring the normal guanine, which leads to resistance to alkylating chemotherapy. Gliomas with MGMT promoter methylation are less capable to repair DNA and are more sensitive to TMZ.

Several methods have been established for detection of MGMT in glioma (reviewed in [30]). In general, they can be divided into methods requiring or not requiring bisulfite treatment. The three most common methods are methylation-specific PCR (MSP), real-time PCR or MethyLight PCR, and methylation-specific sequencing or pyrosequencing, and they all require bisulfite treatment of the tissue. Detection can be performed on FFPE tissue, as well as on the frozen tissue. For practical purposes, FFPE-based methods are preferable. Other methods that do not require bisulfite conversion and can be used in the clinical setting are methylation-specific multiplex ligation-dependent probe amplification (MS-MLPA) and IHC for MGMT protein expression.

There is a significant heterogeneity of MGMT expression and promoter methylation within a glioma. In contrast to 1p/19q testing, MGMT testing requires careful sample selection with a neuropathologist evaluating the case, providing an estimate of the percentage of neoplastic cells and selecting the section with the least amount of necrosis and contaminating non-tumor cells. If normal brain is present on the same section, microdissection of the tumor from the unstained slide is warranted. Many laboratories also require a minimum 50 % of a viable tumor in a given sample to perform testing.

DNA can be extracted from the FFPE tissue using available protocols and kits. The most common methods for MGMT promoter methylation require sodium bisulfite treatment of DNA, which converts unmethylated cytosine into uracil. Methylated cytosine in a CpG island remains unchanged. This bisulfite-modified DNA is used as a template for PCR and sequence differences between methylated and unmethylated DNA after bisulfite treatment allowing for the design of PCR primers that are specific for each template. Bisulfite treatment of DNA is the most difficult part of the assay since it causes further DNA fragmentation. Furthermore, partial conversion could lead to false-positive results. Therefore, appropriate methylated and unmethylated controls are necessary and must be treated in parallel to patient samples to ensure that complete conversion occurred.

MSP is the most commonly used method and allows for the evaluation of methylation status at 6–9 CpG sites. Two primer sets are usually used. One pair is used for amplification of sequences with converted cytosine after bisulfite treatment detects an unmethylated MGMT. A second pair of primers is used for sequences with unconverted cytosine (mC) and detection of a methylated MGMT. PCR product can be visualized by capillary gel electrophoresis, after fluorescent labeling, or by agarose gel electrophoresis (Fig. 3.5). With numerous established protocols available, this method can be easily established in a molecular laboratory and does not require specialized laboratory equipment. An advantage is an easy-to-read result; however a disadvantage is lack of the quantitative assessment of methylation. Another disadvantage is that this method does not include a control for bisulfite conversion, and incomplete conversion of unmethylated cytosines may be interpreted as methylation, leading to false-positive results.

The qMethylation-Specific RT-PCR-MethyLight assay is a simple, quantitative real-time PCR method to determine the methylation status of MGMT CpG islands. It utilizes the TaqMan PCR with forward and reverse primers. It also contains a fluorescent oligo probe, which emits only after it is degraded by the 5′–3′ exonuclease activity of Taq polymerase. It requires a second set of primers and a probe, for amplification of a housekeeping gene, which are used as amplification controls for quality and quantity of the DNA. Control gene primers and probes are designed for the regions with no CpG islands and complementary to the

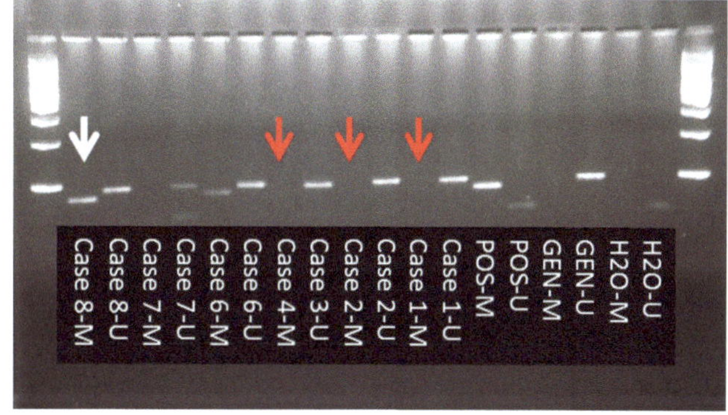

Fig. 3.5. Example of methylation specific PCR evaluation of MGMT in GBM: Agarose gel electrophoresis show examples of MGMT evaluation. *H_2O* water, *GEN* genomic control (negative for promoter methylation), *POS* positive control (positive for MGMT promoter methylation), *U* unmethylated primers, *M* methylated primers. Cases 1, 2, and 3 show no PCR product in the methylated lane and are examples of tumors without MGMT promoter methylation (*red arrows*). Case 6 shows a product in the methylated lane and is an example of a tumor with MGMT promoter methylation (*white arrow*).

bisulfite-converted sequence. This allows control for assessing the efficiency of bisulfite conversion and quantifying MGMT methylation.

The qRT-PCR assay is more specific, and rarely produces false-positive results. The assay is relatively easy to set up, but requires a real-time PCR instrument, which is available in most laboratories. The results are easy to interpret, and inclusion of the standard curve gives numerical values for copy numbers of methylated MGMT sequences, as well as housekeeping gene sequences. However, the percentage of contaminating stromal cells cannot be accurately assessed, and therefore quantitation of MGMT promoter methylation by qRT-PCR is not recommended.

Primers can be designed to cover both the upstream and downstream regions of CpGs, as well as methylated and unmethylated sequences. Sanger bidirectional DNA sequencing can be used to provide a semiquantitative measure of MGMT promoter. However, standard Sanger sequencing has not been established in MGMT analyses compared to methylation specific PCR. On the other hand, pyrosequencing, or sequencing by synthesis, has been used in some laboratories. Pyrosequencing also requires bisulfite treatment of genomic DNA and PCR amplification with primers surrounding CpGI, followed by pyrosequencing. The main advantage of pyrosequencing is the ability to quantify methylation at each CpG site and identify cases with low levels of methylation reliably. However, costs of equipment are high and it is therefore more appropriate for high volume laboratories. NGS methods are still mostly research applications; however, they will likely become available in clinical settings, and can be used for methylation analysis.

Methylation-specific MLPA utilizes unique approach with the ligation of oligonucleotide probes, followed by a digestion of the genomic DNA-probe hybrid complex with methylation-sensitive endonucleases. When the CpG locus is not methylated, methylation-sensitive restriction endonuclease cleaves its restriction site, resulting in lack of PCR amplification. When the CpG locus is methylated, the restriction site is protected from endonuclease digestion and PCR product is generated. The methylation-specific probes are designed so that the sequences detected contain a methylation-sensitive restriction site GCGC. The advantage of this semiquantitative method, in which the level of methylation at each site can be determined, is that it does not require bisulfite treatment. MLPA can detect changes in both CpG methylation and copy-number of up to 40 chromosomal sequences in a single reaction. Capillary electrophoresis is necessary to identify and quantify PCR products of the individual probes. The sample DNA is split and one part is subjected to a single ligation step, whereas for the other part ligation is combined with the methylation-sensitive digestion. Subsequent PCR reaction amplifies either total DNA or the methylated fraction. Comparison of the peaks of the ligated fraction and the fraction that is digested with endonuclease provides the methylation ratios. The disadvantage of this method is the need for special equipment and expensive reagents. However, for laboratories performing MLPA assays for other indications, the methylation-specific MLPA is easy to establish.

The use of IHC for the detection of MGMT has been investigated in a number of studies, with lack of concordance between MGMT expression by immunohistochemistry and MGMT promoter methylation. Furthermore, lack of MGMT expression by IHC was not as robust of a biomarker as MGMT promoter methylation. The conclusion from these studies is that MGMT promoter methylation and MGMT protein expression detected by immunohistochemistry cannot be used interchangeably to predict survival for patients with malignant gliomas [31]. Therefore, immunohistochemistry is not the method of choice for the detection of MGMT activity and its use should be discouraged.

Expression Profiling

Gene signatures have been shown to be capable of distinguishing molecular subtypes of tumors that appear indistinguishable histologically, but reflect different disease biologies as evidenced by differences in clinical presentation and/or outcomes. A number of groups have attempted to identify individual genes as well as signaling pathways from microarray data that are prognostic in malignant glioma and medulloblastoma [32–34]. Expression profiling was able to identify specific subgroups within each disease that were associated with improved or decreased survival. Despite some prognostic value [35], the application in clinical practice has been limited due to a variety of reasons such as costs, equipment requirement, and the need of frozen material for good-quality whole genome expression profile studies. Overall, as with all molecular tests in clinical practice, the use of FFPE-based assays is critical to the wide-scale acceptance of a biomarker due to the limited availability of fresh/frozen tissues. In GBM, a multigene profile compatible for FFPE samples is currently used as a stratification factor in a large Phase III clinical trial (RTOG-0825) [36]. The 9-gene set was validated with an independent sample set and was shown to be an independent predictor of clinical outcome after adjusting for clinical factors and MGMT status. Another approach is to use a selected set of genes that have been firmly associated with the subtype using FFPE samples on a platform such as NanoString® to molecularly classify brain tumors such as medulloblastoma or GBM (Fig. 3.6). RNA-based methods such as NanoString® that can utilize FFPE tissues are easier to implement in clinical laboratories than assays that require high-quality RNA from the frozen tissue, which will likely not be implemented in standard clinical practice.

Summary

Several well-established techniques are currently used in molecular neuropathology. Analyses include copy-number changes, mutations, and epigenetic modification assessed

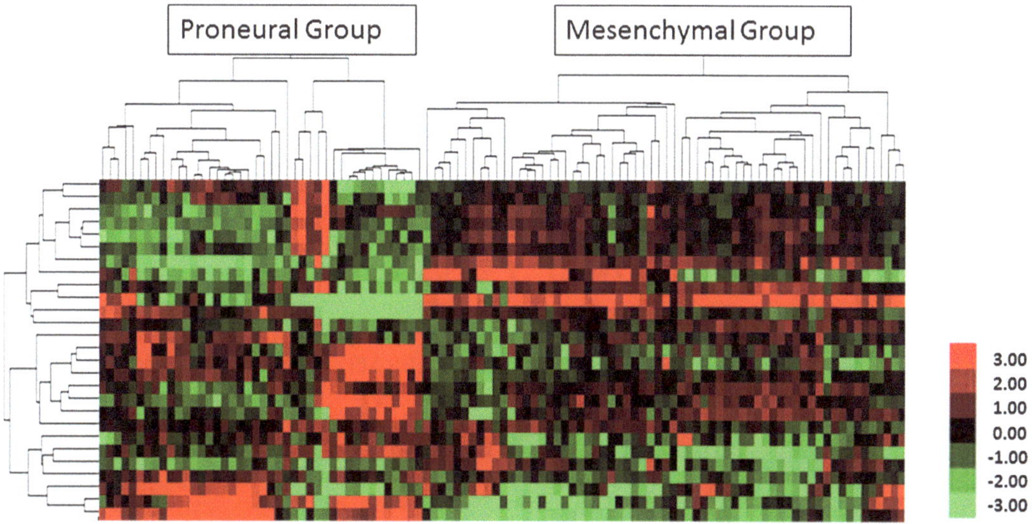

Fig. 3.6 Example of expression profile evaluation of GBM: RNA isolated from the FFPE tissues and can be used for the next-generation of expression profile techniques. Using an expression of a core of validated genes for GBM and unsupervised hierarchical clustering, tumors are segregating into different molecular subgroups such as Proneural and Mesenchymal. *Red–green* scale shows the change in the expression level (Figure created in collaboration with Dr. Stephen Yip, BC Cancer Agency)

most commonly by FISH, PCR, sequencing of mutation-specific antibodies. From the technical perspective, once validated, these techniques are robust and require minimal troubleshooting. The most commonly performed tests with the largest clinical impact include MGMT promoter methylation, 1p/19q status and *IDH1* mutation. These assays should be incorporated both within routine clinical care and within clinical trial designs. When used in the right clinical context after neuropathology review and with appropriate interpretation guidelines, they can provide diagnostic, prognostic, and predictive information that can help guide clinical management.

At the present time, the number of assays that can be performed on brain tumors and the information that can be obtained is significantly greater than what can be used for practical diagnostic and clinical purposes. Careful retrospective and prospective validation of molecular genetic alterations and profiles for prognostic and predictive value will be required in clinical studies before implementation into routine diagnostics and clinical care.

References

1. Horbinski C, Miller CR, Perry A. Gone FISHing: clinical lessons learned in brain tumor molecular diagnostics over the last decade. Brain Pathol. 2011;21(1):57–73.
2. Hobbs J, Nikiforova MN, Fardo DW, Bortoluzzi S, Cieply K, Hamilton RL, et al. Paradoxical relationship between the degree of EGFR amplification and outcome in glioblastomas. Am J Surg Pathol. 2012;36(8):1186–93.
3. Snuderl M, Eichler AF, Ligon KL, Vu QU, Silver M, Betensky RA, et al. Polysomy for chromosomes 1 and 19 predicts earlier recurrence in anaplastic oligodendrogliomas with concurrent 1p/19q loss. Clin Cancer Res. 2009;15(20):6430–7.
4. Wiens AL, Cheng L, Bertsch EC, Johnson KA, Zhang S, Hattab EM. Polysomy of chromosomes 1 and/or 19 is common and associated with less favorable clinical outcome in oligodendrogliomas: fluorescent in situ hybridization analysis of 84 consecutive cases. J Neuropathol Exp Neurol. 2012;71(7):618–24.
5. Chi AS, Batchelor TT, Kwak EL, Clark JW, Wang DL, Wilner KD, et al. Rapid radiographic and clinical improvement after treatment of a MET-amplified recurrent glioblastoma with a mesenchymal-epithelial transition inhibitor. J Clin Oncol. 2012;30(3):e30–3.
6. Paugh BS, Broniscer A, Qu C, Miller CP, Zhang J, Tatevossian RG, et al. Genome-wide analyses identify recurrent amplifications of receptor tyrosine kinases and cell-cycle regulatory genes in diffuse intrinsic pontine glioma. J Clin Oncol. 2011;29(30):3999–4006.
7. Snuderl M, Fazlollahi L, Le LP, Nitta M, Zhelyazkova BH, Davidson CJ, et al. Mosaic amplification of multiple receptor tyrosine kinase genes in glioblastoma. Cancer Cell. 2011;20(6):810–7.
8. Szerlip NJ, Pedraza A, Chakravarty D, Azim M, McGuire J, Fang Y, et al. Intratumoral heterogeneity of receptor tyrosine kinases EGFR and PDGFRA amplification in glioblastoma defines subpopulations with distinct growth factor response. Proc Natl Acad Sci U S A. 2012;109(8):3041–6.
9. Little SE, Popov S, Jury A, Bax DA, Doey L, Al-Sarraj S, et al. Receptor tyrosine kinase genes amplified in glioblastoma exhibit a mutual exclusivity in variable proportions reflective of individual tumor heterogeneity. Cancer Res. 2012;72(7):1614–20.
10. Barbashina V, Salazar P, Holland EC, Rosenblum MK, Ladanyi M. Allelic losses at 1p36 and 19q13 in gliomas: correlation with histologic classification, definition of a 150-kb minimal deleted region on 1p36, and evaluation of CAMTA1 as a candidate tumor suppressor gene. Clin Cancer Res. 2005;11(3):1119–28.

11. Smith JS, Alderete B, Minn Y, Borell TJ, Perry A, Mohapatra G, et al. Localization of common deletion regions on 1p and 19q in human gliomas and their association with histological subtype. Oncogene. 1999;18(28):4144–52.
12. Kuga D, Mizoguchi M, Guan Y, Hata N, Yoshimoto K, Shono T, et al. Prevalence of copy-number neutral LOH in glioblastomas revealed by genomewide analysis of laser-microdissected tissues. Neuro Oncol. 2008;10(6):995–1003.
13. Horbinski C. Practical molecular diagnostics in neuropathology: making a tough job a little easier. Semin Diagn Pathol. 2010;27(2):105–13.
14. Giannini C, Burger PC, Berkey BA, Cairncross JG, Jenkins RB, Mehta M, et al. Anaplastic oligodendroglial tumors: refining the correlation among histopathology, 1p 19q deletion and clinical outcome in Intergroup Radiation Therapy Oncology Group Trial 9402. Brain Pathol. 2008;18(3):360–9.
15. Perry A, Fuller CE, Banerjee R, Brat DJ, Scheithauer BW. Ancillary FISH analysis for 1p and 19q status: preliminary observations in 287 gliomas and oligodendroglioma mimics. Front Biosci. 2003;8:a1–9.
16. Pfister S, Remke M, Benner A, Mendrzyk F, Toedt G, Felsberg J, et al. Outcome prediction in pediatric medulloblastoma based on DNA copy-number aberrations of chromosomes 6q and 17q and the MYC and MYCN loci. J Clin Oncol. 2009;27(10): 1627–36.
17. Horbinski C, Kofler J, Kelly LM, Murdoch GH, Nikiforova MN. Diagnostic use of IDH1/2 mutation analysis in routine clinical testing of formalin-fixed, paraffin-embedded glioma tissues. J Neuropathol Exp Neurol. 2009;68(12):1319–25.
18. Horbinski C. To BRAF or not to BRAF: is that even a question anymore? J Neuropathol Exp Neurol. 2013;72(1):2–7.
19. Capper D, Preusser M, Habel A, Sahm F, Ackermann U, Schindler G, et al. Assessment of BRAF V600E mutation status by immunohistochemistry with a mutation-specific monoclonal antibody. Acta Neuropathol. 2011;122(1):11–9.
20. Capper D, Zentgraf H, Balss J, Hartmann C, von Deimling A. Monoclonal antibody specific for IDH1 R132H mutation. Acta Neuropathol. 2009;118(5):599–601.
21. Capper D, Reuss D, Schittenhelm J, Hartmann C, Bremer J, Sahm F, et al. Mutation-specific IDH1 antibody differentiates oligodendrogliomas and oligoastrocytomas from other brain tumors with oligodendroglioma-like morphology. Acta Neuropathol. 2011;121(2):241–52.
22. Yan H, Parsons DW, Jin G, McLendon R, Rasheed BA, Yuan W, et al. IDH1 and IDH2 mutations in gliomas. N Engl J Med. 2009;360(8):765–73.
23. Xu X, Zhao J, Xu Z, Peng B, Huang Q, Arnold E, et al. Structures of human cytosolic NADP-dependent isocitrate dehydrogenase reveal a novel self-regulatory mechanism of activity. J Biol Chem. 2004;279(32):33946–57.
24. Jones DT, Kocialkowski S, Liu L, Pearson DM, Backlund LM, Ichimura K, et al. Tandem duplication producing a novel oncogenic BRAF fusion gene defines the majority of pilocytic astrocytomas. Cancer Res. 2008;68(21):8673–7.
25. Sievert AJ, Jackson EM, Gai X, Hakonarson H, Judkins AR, Resnick AC, et al. Duplication of 7q34 in pediatric low-grade astrocytomas detected by high-density single-nucleotide polymorphism-based genotype arrays results in a novel BRAF fusion gene. Brain Pathol. 2009;19(3):449–58.
26. Chappe C, Padovani L, Scavarda D, Forest F, Nanni-Metellus I, Loundou A, et al. Dysembryoplastic neuroepithelial tumors share with pleomorphic xanthoastrocytomas and gangliogliomas BRAF(V600E) mutation and expression. Brain Pathol. 2013;23(5):574–83.
27. Dias-Santagata D, Lam Q, Vernovsky K, Vena N, Lennerz JK, Borger DR, et al. BRAF V600E mutations are common in pleomorphic xanthoastrocytoma: diagnostic and therapeutic implications. PLoS One. 2011;6(3):e17948.
28. Eberhart CG. Molecular diagnostics in embryonal brain tumors. Brain Pathol. 2011;21(1):96–104.
29. Frattini V, Trifonov V, Chan JM, Castano A, Lia M, Abate F, et al. The integrated landscape of driver genomic alterations in glioblastoma. Nat Genet. 2013;45(10):1141–9.
30. Cankovic M, Nikiforova MN, Snuderl M, Adesina AM, Lindeman N, Wen PY, et al. The role of MGMT testing in clinical practice: a report of the association for molecular pathology. J Mol Diagn. 2013;15(5):539–55.
31. Maxwell JA, Johnson SP, Quinn JA, McLendon RE, Ali-Osman F, Friedman AH, et al. Quantitative analysis of O6-alkylguanine-DNA alkyltransferase in malignant glioma. Mol Cancer Ther. 2006;5(10):2531–9.
32. Verhaak RG, Hoadley KA, Purdom E, Wang V, Qi Y, Wilkerson MD, et al. Integrated genomic analysis identifies clinically relevant subtypes of glioblastoma characterized by abnormalities in PDGFRA, IDH1, EGFR, and NF1. Cancer Cell. 2010;17(1): 98–110.
33. Northcott PA, Jones DT, Kool M, Robinson GW, Gilbertson RJ, Cho YJ, et al. Medulloblastomics: the end of the beginning. Nat Rev Cancer. 2012;12(12):818–34.
34. Northcott PA, Shih DJ, Peacock J, Garzia L, Morrissy AS, Zichner T, et al. Subgroup-specific structural variation across 1,000 medulloblastoma genomes. Nature. 2012;488(7409): 49–56.
35. Czernicki T, Zegarska J, Paczek L, Cukrowska B, Grajkowska W, Zajaczkowska A, et al. Gene expression profile as a prognostic factor in high-grade gliomas. Int J Oncol. 2007;30(1): 55–64.
36. Colman H, Zhang L, Sulman EP, McDonald JM, Shooshtari NL, Rivera A, et al. A multigene predictor of outcome in glioblastoma. Neuro Oncol. 2010;12(1):49–57.

4 Low-Grade Gliomas

Fausto J. Rodriguez and Daniel C. Bowers

Low-grade gliomas encompass multiple histological subtypes, including pilocytic astrocytomas (PA), pilomyxoid astrocytomas, diffuse astrocytomas (DA), oligodendrogliomas, subependymal giant cell astrocytomas (SEGA), pleomorphic xanthroastrocytomas (PXA), and others. Low-grade gliomas are grouped together because they share low mitotic rates, slow growth rates, and affected patients often achieve long-term survival with surgery alone. Also, upon instances of tumor progression, they are often treated with identical chemotherapy or radiation therapy regimens. Recent retrospective studies have suggested several genetic and molecular markers that are associated with specific tumor subtypes and may help with diagnostic and prognostic evaluation. Importantly, several of the identified molecular pathways involved are potentially targets for new chemotherapy agents, and their associated markers may also have predictive value in terms of therapeutic response.

However, except for PA arising in patients with neurofibromatosis type-1 (NF1) and SEGAs in children and young adults with tuberous sclerosis, little was known until recently about the molecular underpinnings of low-grade gliomas. Low-grade gliomas among patients without NF1 do not inactivate the *NF1* gene, and generally lack changes to the oncogenes and tumor suppressors altered in adult diffuse astrocytomas [1, 2]. Until recently, cytogenetic studies of pilocytic astrocytomas were notable for a lack of detectable chromosomal alterations, with largely normal karyotypes in the more than 100 cases initially studied [1].

Mutations in *IDH1* or *IDH2* have been identified in the majority of low-grade gliomas among adults, but interestingly are almost never detected in pediatric low- or high-grade glioma, and when present have mostly been reported in children at least 14 years old [3–5]. This suggests that adolescents with *IDH*-mutant tumors may represent the youngest patients with "adult" low-grade gliomas.

The purpose of this chapter is to describe the histopathology, cytogenetics, gene expression profiles, and molecular genetics of low-grade gliomas. This information will be useful in identifying molecular signaling pathways, defining prognostic groups and ultimately leading to the development of novel, molecularly targeted therapies for low-grade gliomas.

Pathology

Low-grade gliomas represent a spectrum of neoplasms that may be broadly separated into circumscribed and diffuse groups. Circumscribed gliomas encompass pilocytic astrocytoma (PA), SEGA, and PXA (Figs. 4.1 and 4.2). These tumors usually have discrete borders at the imaging and gross pathology levels, which allow for gross total resection and cure by surgery depending on anatomic location (Table 4.1). The diffuse glioma group includes diffuse astrocytoma and oligodendroglioma (Figs. 4.3 and 4.4). They demonstrate a more infiltrative pattern of growth on both imaging and histologic sections. Compared with the circumscribed group, the diffuse gliomas have a higher propensity for histologic progression to higher grade tumors and therefore more aggressive behavior.

Circumscribed Gliomas

Pilocytic Astrocytoma

PAs represent the most frequent glioma subtype in children. They are characterized by elongated, bipolar astrocytes usually with bland nuclear features. The classic architecture is a biphasic pattern, with alternating Rosenthal fiber-rich compact areas and loose, microcyst rich regions. Eosinophilic granular bodies may be present in these regions and even abundant. Additional variable features include hyalinized or glomeruloid vessels, hemosiderin deposition, and degenerative nuclear pleomorphism or multinucleated cells. Monotonous oligodendroglial-like cells may predominate in some examples. Occasional mitoses and non-pseudopallisading necrosis may be present, but they have an inconsistent relation with clinical outcome [6, 7]. As other astrocytomas, these

M.A. Karajannis and D. Zagzag (eds.), *Molecular Pathology of Nervous System Tumors: Biological Stratification and Targeted Therapies*, Molecular Pathology Library 8,
DOI 10.1007/978-1-4939-1830-0_4,

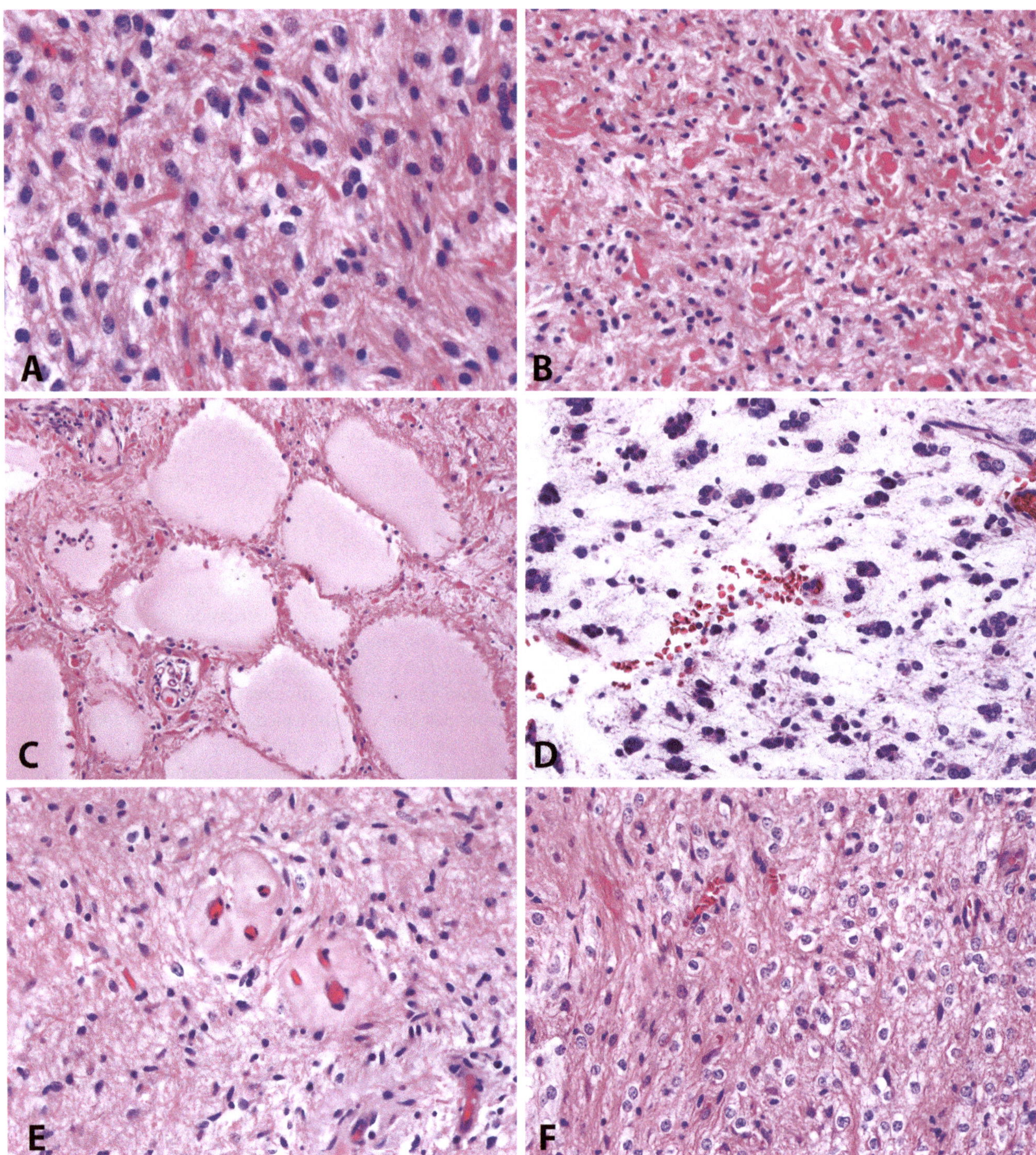

Fig. 4.1. Pathologic features of pilocytic astrocytoma (PA). PA is histologically characterized by the presence of neoplastic bipolar astrocytes in compact areas (**a**). Rosenthal fibers are a frequent feature of pilocytic astrocytomas and may be numerous (**b**). The second architectural pattern of PA is characterized by loose stroma, containing microcysts (**c**) and occasionally multinucleated cells and clusters of small nuclei (**d**). Microvascular hyalinization is frequent in PA (**e**), as it is typical of long standing, slow growing tumors. A variable component of round cells with perinuclear halos may be present in a subset of PA (**f**), and raises the important differential diagnosis with oligodendroglial neoplasms.

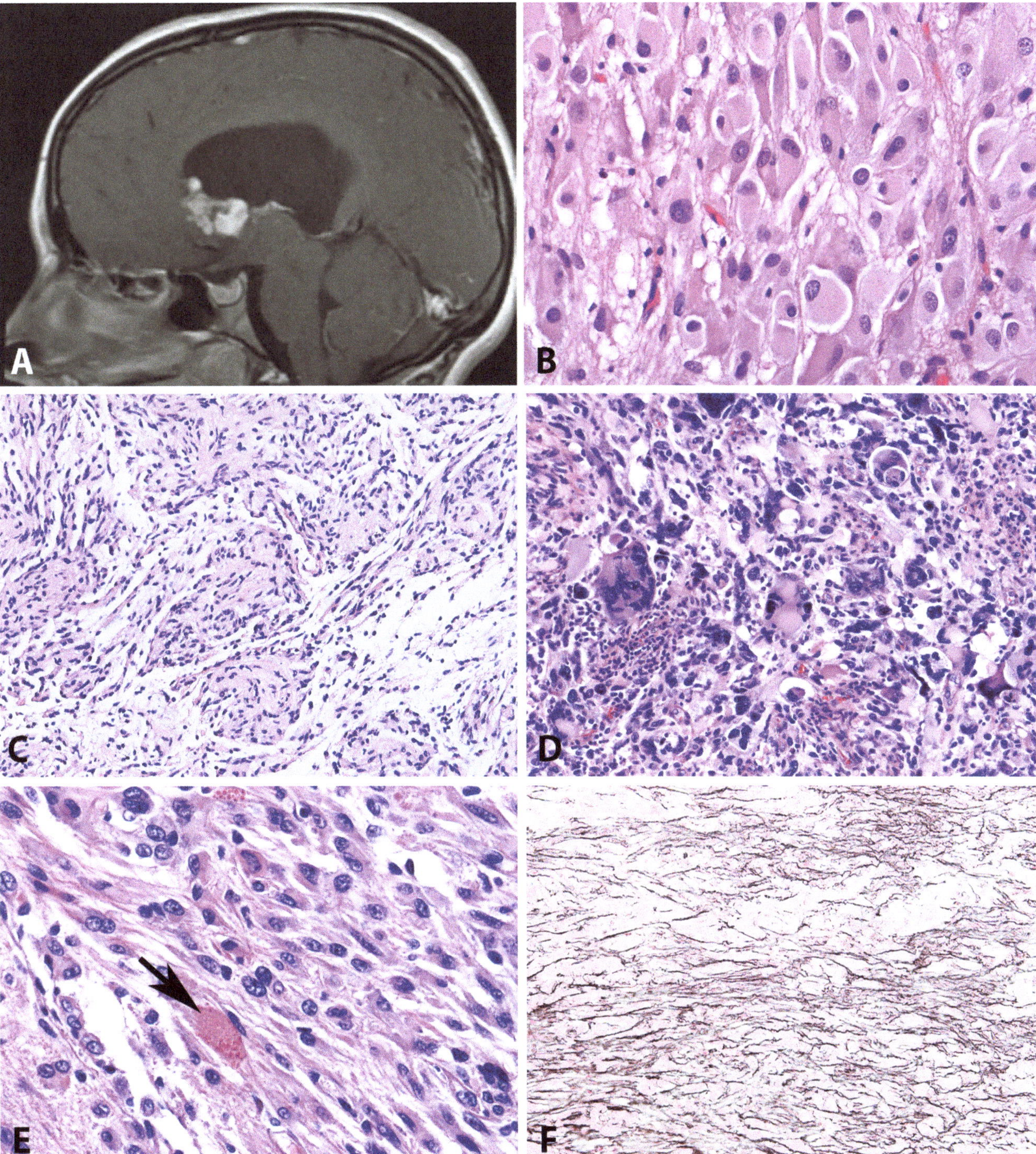

Fig. 4.2. Pathologic features of circumscribed gliomas. Subependymal giant cell astrocytoma (SEGA) develops within the lateral ventricle, almost always near the Foramen of Monro (T1-weighted MR image post-contrast) (**a**). The histology of SEGA is distinctive, containing large cells with voluminous eosinophilic cytoplasm and prominent nucleoli (**b**). Pilomyxoid astrocytoma is a distinctive variant of pilocytic astrocytoma, usually developing in the hypothalamus of young children, characterized by perivascular arrangements in a loose myxoid stroma (**c**). Pleomorphic xanthoastrocytoma is another distinctive astrocytoma characterized by conspicuous pleomorphic cells (**d**), usually with low proliferative activity, as well as a fascicular arrangement and eosinophilic granular bodies (*arrow*) (**e**). Unlike other gliomas, PXAs tend to be reticulin-rich, particularly in superficial regions juxtaposed to the leptomeninges (**f**).

Table 4.1. Histopathology and molecular features of low-grade gliomas.

Tumor type	Location	Histology	Grade	IHC	Cytogenetics	Molecular genetics	Signaling pathways
Pilocytic astrocytoma	Cerebellum > optic pathways, brainstem, supratentorial, spinal cord	Bipolar cells, compact and microcystic areas, Rosenthal fibers, eosinophilic granular bodies	I	GFAP, OLIG2+, p53–	7q34 duplication, whole Ch7 or 8 gain	*BRAF-KIAA1549* fusion, *BRAF* (V600E) mut, *RAF1* fusions, *NF1* inactivation (syndrome associated cases)	MAPK, mTOR
Pilomyxoid astrocytoma	Hypothalamic region > brainstem, hemispheres, spinal cord	Monomorphic spindle cells, myxoid stroma, perivascular pseudorosettes	II	GFAP+	Similar to PA	Similar to PA	Similar to PA
SEGA	Lateral ventricle (near foramen of Monro)	Large cells, round nuclei, macronucleoli, amphophilic cytoplasm	I	S100, GFAP+++, synaptophysin, neurofilament+	–	*TSC1* and *TSC2* mutations	mTOR
Angiocentric glioma	Cortex (temporal lobe)	Monotonous spindle cell with perivascular arrangement	I	GFAP+, EMA + (dot-like)	6q23.3 gain/ deletion	*MYB* alterations	Cell cycle regulation
Pleomorphic xanthoastrocytoma	Hemispheric (temporal lobe)	Cellular pleomorphism, xanthic change, fascicular arrangement, eosinophilic granular bodies	II	S100 > GFAP+, CD34, synaptophysin +/–, p53–	–	*BRAF* (V600E) mut; mTOR pathway (*NF1*, *TSC2*, *PI3R1*), *TP53* (rare)	MAPK, mTOR
Diffuse astrocytoma	Throughout CNS	Infiltrative pleomorphic cells, rare to absent mitotic activity	II	GFAP+++, OLIG2+++, IDH1 (R132H) (frequent), p53 (frequent)	7q, 8q gain	*IDH1/2*, *TP53*, *ATRX*, *PTEN*, *CDKN2A*, mutations	MAPK, PI3K/mTOR, cell cycle regulation
Low-grade oligodendroglioma/ oligoastrocytoma	Hemispheric (frontal > temporal, parietal, occipital)	Round cells with perinuclear halos, chicken-wire microvasculature	II	S100+++, OLIG2+++, IDH1 (R132H) (frequent), p53–	1p19q co-deletion	*IDH1/2*, *CIC*, *FUBP1* mutations; *TERT* promoter mutations	
Pediatric diffuse astrocytoma		Same as adult	II	GFAP, OLIG2+++, IDH (R132H) (usually –), p53+	8q13.1 gain/ deletion; 6q23.3 gain/deletion	*FGFR1*, *MYB*, *MYBL1*, *BRAF* (V600E) alterations	MAPK, PI3K/mTOR, cell cycle regulation
Pediatric low-grade oligodendroglioma	Hemispheric (frontal–temporal lobes)	Same as adult	II	S100, OLIG2+++, IDH1 (R132H) (usually –), p53–	1p19q co-deletion (rare)	*FGFR1*, *MYB* alterations; IDH1 (R132H) (rare)	MAPK, PI3K/mTOR, cell cycle regulation

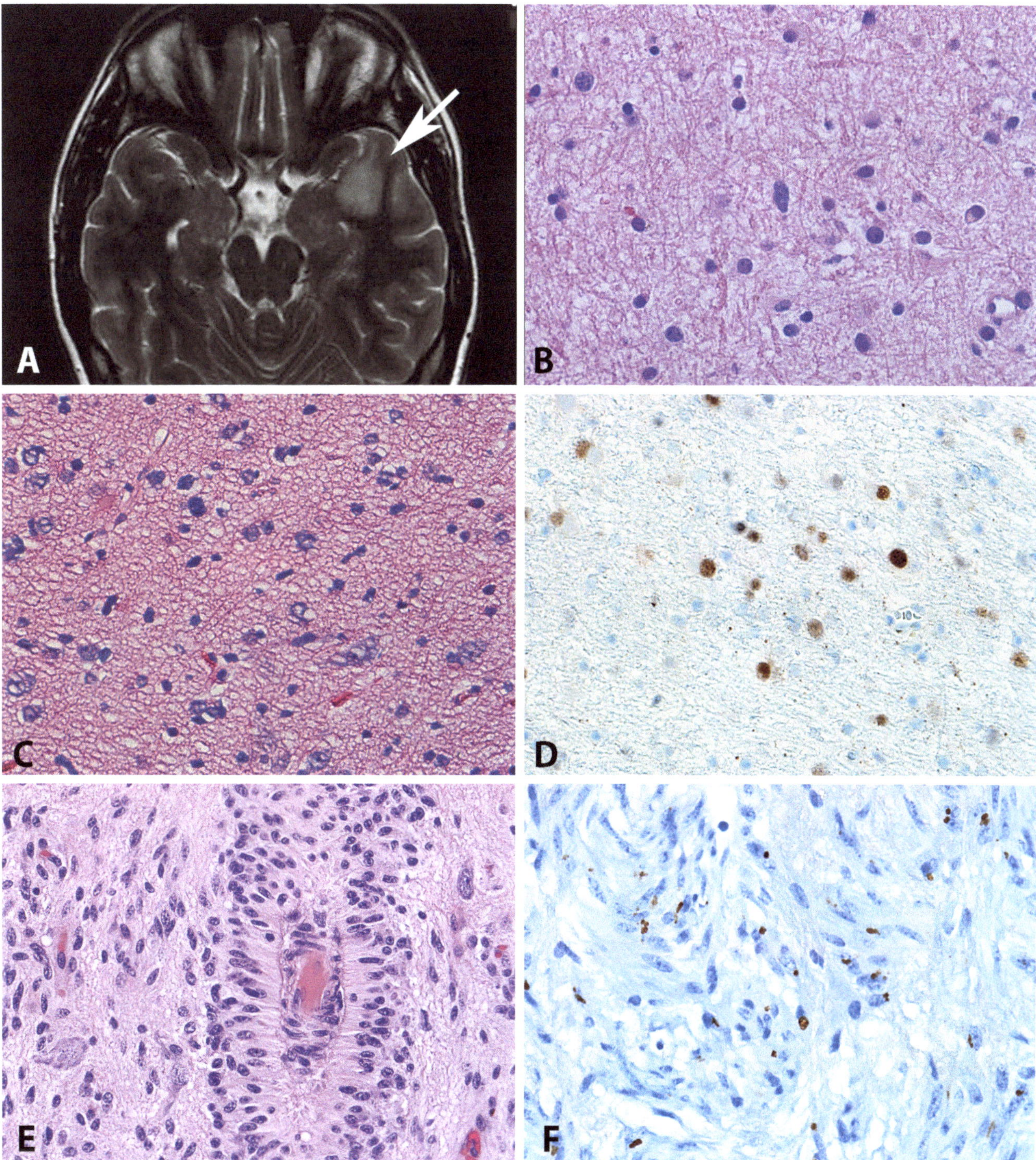

Fig. 4.3. Pathologic features of diffuse astrocytomas and angiocentric gliomas. Diffuse astrocytomas (WHO grade II) present as areas of hyperintensity in T2 weighted MR images (*arrow*, **a**). As the histologic level, diffuse astrocytomas usually have low cellularity but have definite atypia manifesting by irregular nuclear contours and hyperchromasia (**b**). Some diffuse astrocytomas may show obvious hypercellularity, but by definition mitotic activity is rare to absent (**c**). Immunohistochemistry frequently demonstrates strong p53 immunolabeling, a surrogate for *TP53* mutations (**d**). Angiocentric glioma is a distinctive low-grade neoplasm characterized by monotonous cells with elongated nuclei infiltrating cortex but also arranged around vessels (**e**). Despite their infiltrative nature, angiocentric glioma shares biologic properties with ependymomas, including the presence of microlumens highlighted by EMA immunohistochemistry (**f**).

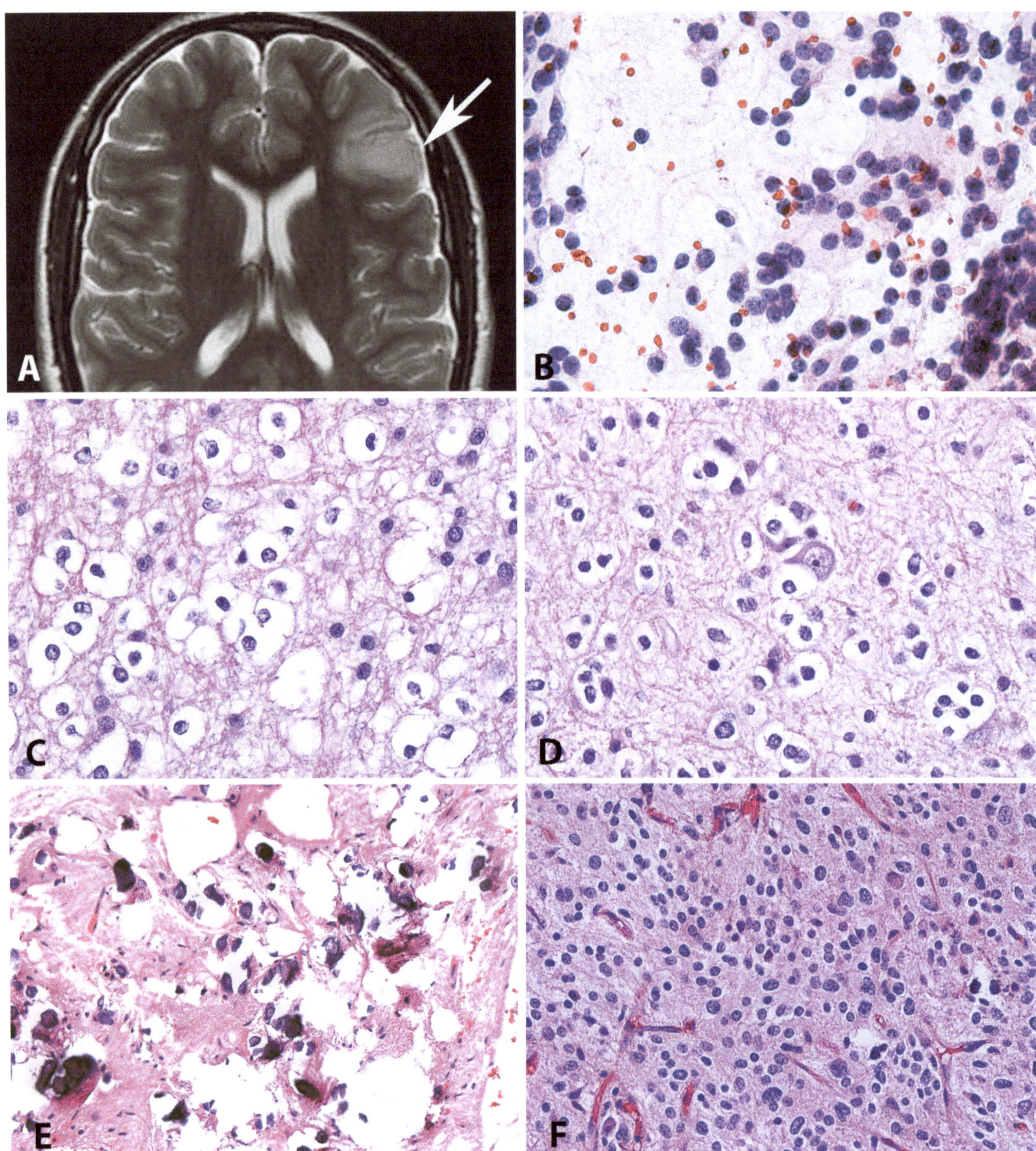

Fig. 4.4. Pathologic features of low-grade oligodendrogliomas. Oligodendrogliomas frequently involve the frontal cortex, with expansion of infiltrated gyri (Axial T2 weighted MR) (**a**). On cytologic preparations, oligodendrogliomas demonstrate round cells with a small nucleolus (**b**). The nuclear uniformity and characteristic halos are best appreciated in formalin-fixed paraffin-embedded sections (**c**). Perineuronal satellitosis is a characteristic feature of infiltrating gliomas, particularly oligodendroglioma (**d**). Microcalcifications are not uncommon in oligodendroglial neoplasms (**e**). The designation of oligoastrocytoma is reserved for tumors that have areas with astrocytic and oligodendroglial morphology. Most of these tumors are morphologically ambiguous as this H&E shows (**f**), and lead to prominent interobserver variability.

tumors express GFAP and OLIG2. P53 and Ki-67 show low labeling indices. Elevated Ki-67 labeling indices have been associated with worse outcome in some studies [8] but not in others [9, 10]. Unlike the category of diffuse gliomas, the development of anaplasia/histologic malignancy in PA is a very rare event (<2 %), and has been defined as the presence of brisk mitotic activity with or without necrosis [11].

Pilomyxoid Astrocytoma

Pilomyxoid astrocytoma (PMA) is considered a variant of PA, characterized by monophasic morphology within a myxoid background and conspicuous aggregates around blood vessels [12]. Unlike conventional PA, PMA lacks a biphasic pattern and Rosenthal fibers. Eosinophilic granular bodies are rare to absent. The classic presentation of PMA is the hypothalamic region of young children. Because of its higher likelihood for aggressive behavior and leptomeningeal dissemination [13], the WHO assigns a grade II to this variant. Morphologic and molecular overlap occurs with conventional PA, which is supported by the recognition of tumors with intermediate features between PMA and PA or PMAs that mature into PA over time [14].

Subependymal Giant Cell Astrocytoma

SEGA is a unique astrocytoma subtype that arises almost always within the lateral ventricles near the foramen of Monro in tuberous sclerosis patients. It is composed of large cells with voluminous eosinophilic cytoplasm, round nuclei and prominent nucleoli. The mitotic activity is very low. At an immunohistochemical and ultrastructural level, these tumors demonstrate evidence of neuronal differentiation in addition to a glial phenotype, which is more accurately consistent with a glioneuronal neoplasm [15]. This includes immunoreactivity for synaptophysin and neurofilament protein in addition to GFAP.

Pleomorphic Xanthoastrocytoma

PXA is a rare neoplasm with distinctive histology. It is composed of spindle neoplastic cells with often conspicuous pleomorphism, sometimes including giant cell forms. Mitotic activity is very low in most cases, and this disconnect between the cellularity and pleomorphism of the tumor and its relative lack of mitoses is one of the first clues to the diagnosis. Eosinophilic granular bodies, particularly large pale forms, are also frequent.

PXA may also demonstrate immunoreactivity for neuronal markers in addition to S100 and GFAP. P53 immunolabeling is typically weak or negative, while CD34 expression is relatively frequent [16]. An additional characteristic finding is the presence of pericellular staining with reticulin special stains, particularly in areas juxtaposed to leptomeninges.

Although PXA is low grade (WHO grade II) by definition, among the circumscribed gliomas it has the highest propensity for recurrence and biologic aggressiveness. A subset develops anaplastic features in the form of brisk mitotic activity and/or necrosis and microvascular proliferation [17]. However, these changes do not consistently predict an adverse outcome, and pending more definite data, a grade III is not yet allowed under the WHO classification.

Diffuse Gliomas

Angiocentric Glioma

Angiocentric glioma is a distinctive neoplasm that was added to the WHO 2007 classification [18, 19]. It is slow growing, frequently associated with epilepsy and therefore shares many clinical properties with dysembryoplastic neuroepithelial tumor. Despite gross circumscription, it is histologically infiltrative. The most characteristic feature of angiocentric glioma is the presence of thin elongated nuclei with little pleomorphism and a perivascular aggregation in a parallel and perpendicular pattern (Fig. 4.3). GFAP expression is a constant feature by immunohistochemistry, but in addition EMA frequently stains in a dot-like fashion, and microlumina may be present on electron microscopy, which suggests a dual astrocytic/ependymal phenotype.

Diffuse Astrocytoma

Diffuse astrocytoma (DA) is a specific subtype characterized by neoplastic astrocytes with nuclear hyperchromasia, atypia, usually low cellularity and rare to absent mitotic figures (Fig. 4.3). Unlike the circumscribed glioma group, DA demonstrates an exquisite infiltration of underlying brain parenchyma, making them surgical challenges. They also have a strong tendency for progression to higher grade neoplasms (anaplastic astrocytoma, glioblastoma), particularly in adults.

Oligodendroglial Tumors

Oligodendroglial tumors include oligodendrogliomas and mixed oligoastrocytomas. They may be low (grade II) or high grade (grade III) (Fig. 4.4). Oligodendroglial morphology is defined by round nuclei with perinuclear halos and little internuclear variability. A delicate "chicken-wire" type microvasculature may be present. Limited mitotic activity may be present, but brisk mitotic activity, endothelial hypertrophy and necrosis define higher grade tumors. Adult oligodendroglioma in particular has classic molecular alterations involving chromosomal arms 1p and 19q, and has almost become a combined pathologic/molecular diagnosis.

Pediatric Diffuse Gliomas

Prior observations have hinted that morphologically similar neoplasms in the adult and pediatric populations may have different clinical behavior. DA, for example, may not always have the same predictable progression to anaplasia in children as in adults. This has been confirmed by molecular studies [20]. Diffuse intrinsic pontine gliomas represent a distinct subset of diffuse gliomas in children, and are essentially defined by their anatomic development within the brainstem. Although in theory, a subset of these may be identified as grade II early in their course, high-grade histologic features are almost always present postmortem [21]. Oligodendrogliomas in children for example lack 1p19q codeletion and *IDH1/2* mutations in contrast to adult tumors [22–24]. Furthermore, the mutational landscape uncovered by recent, large scale sequencing efforts is different, and simpler, in pediatric diffuse gliomas.

New and Unclassifiable Entities

After accounting for well-defined histopathologic categories, a subset of low-grade gliomas remain diagnostic challenges, particularly in the pediatric population. In fact, approximately 20 % of pediatric brain tumors are unclassifiable according to traditional schemes, most of which involve low-grade gliomas (Burger PC, personal communication). One particular entity that has been recognized for a while, but has been the recent focus of several larger series is a low-grade oligodendroglioma-like tumor that remains indolent despite widespread superficial CNS dissemination [25–28]. This tumor has frequent 1p chromosome arm loss but lacks IDH1 (R132H) mutations. There is also a rare subset of pediatric low-grade tumors that have been termed descriptively "massively calcified low-grade glioma" that lack alterations associated with other low-grade gliomas [29].

Gene Expression Profiling

Global gene expression profiling studies have provided important biologic insights into the biology of gliomas in general and low-grade gliomas in particular. In PA, gene expression profiling studies have highlighted differential gene expression signatures related to anatomic regions and NF1 vs. sporadic occurring tumors [30]. These studies have also uncovered possible biomarkers associated with worse clinical outcome in PA including overexpression of *Matrilin-2* [31], and underexpression of *ALDH1L1* [32] and myelin basic protein (*MBP*) [33].

Analogous studies focusing on DA have also provided important insights particularly highlighting phenotypic and genetic differences between adult and pediatric DA. These included expression changes in genes involved in neural stem cell maintenance, CNS development, DNA replication, and cell cycle [20], which may explain in part the more aggressive behavior of these tumors when occurring in adults. Integration of mutation, copy number, and transcriptome analysis has also allowed the separation of distinct molecular subgroups of grade II and III diffuse gliomas with biological and prognostic relevance. Using this approach, Gorovets et al. classified diffuse astrocytic tumors into three molecular classes denoted "preglioblastoma" (PG), "neuroblastic" (NB), and "early-progenitor-like" (EPL) [34]. The NB and EPL subclasses were associated with a higher frequency of *IDH* and *TP53* mutations and 8q gains, as well as better clinical outcome compared with the PG class. Interestingly, 8q gain is one of the most frequent cytogenetic abnormalities of diffuse astrocytoma [35].

Molecular Genetics and Signaling Pathways

Genetic Predisposition to Low-Grade Glioma

The earliest insights into the molecular alterations contributing to glioma formation have evolved from the study of inherited tumor syndromes. Neurofibromatosis type 1 (NF1) is associated with germline mutations in the *NF1* gene that encodes for the protein neurofibromin, a negative regulator of RAS signaling. These patients are predisposed to gliomas of various grades, particularly PA of the optic pathways. Furthermore, biallelic *NF1* inactivation is a feature of these patients tumors [36]. Tuberous sclerosis complex is associated with germline mutations in *TSC1* or *TSC2*, which leads to increased mTOR activity and a predisposition to SEGA. Conversely, Li–Fraumeni syndrome is associated with *TP53* mutations, which predisposes to a variety of tumors, including infiltrating astrocytomas [37]. These early observations suggested that the pathways deregulated by these germline alterations were important for gliomagenesis.

More recent studies have also highlighted a role for germline polymorphisms that predispose to diffuse glioma development. For instance, genotyping efforts have uncovered single nucleotide polymorphisms (SNP) variants at 8q24.21 (near the *MYC* gene) to be associated with an increased risk for gliomas with *IDH1/2* mutations, both astrocytic and oligodendroglial [38].

Circumscribed Gliomas

BRAF and MAPK Alterations

One of the most remarkable discoveries in pediatric neurooncology in the recent years has been the identification of *BRAF* duplications in the majority (53–77 %) of PA tumors [39–44]. Subsequent studies demonstrated that this tandem duplication always involves the kinase domain of BRAF and leads to a novel fusion (usually *BRAF-KIAA1549*) [42, 45]. This novel fusion has oncogenic properties resulting in ERK/MAPK pathway activation (Fig. 4.5). Furthermore, it induces glioma-like lesions in mice when introduced into neural stem cells [46]. This alteration is almost always restricted to PA, particularly those arising in the cerebellum or optic

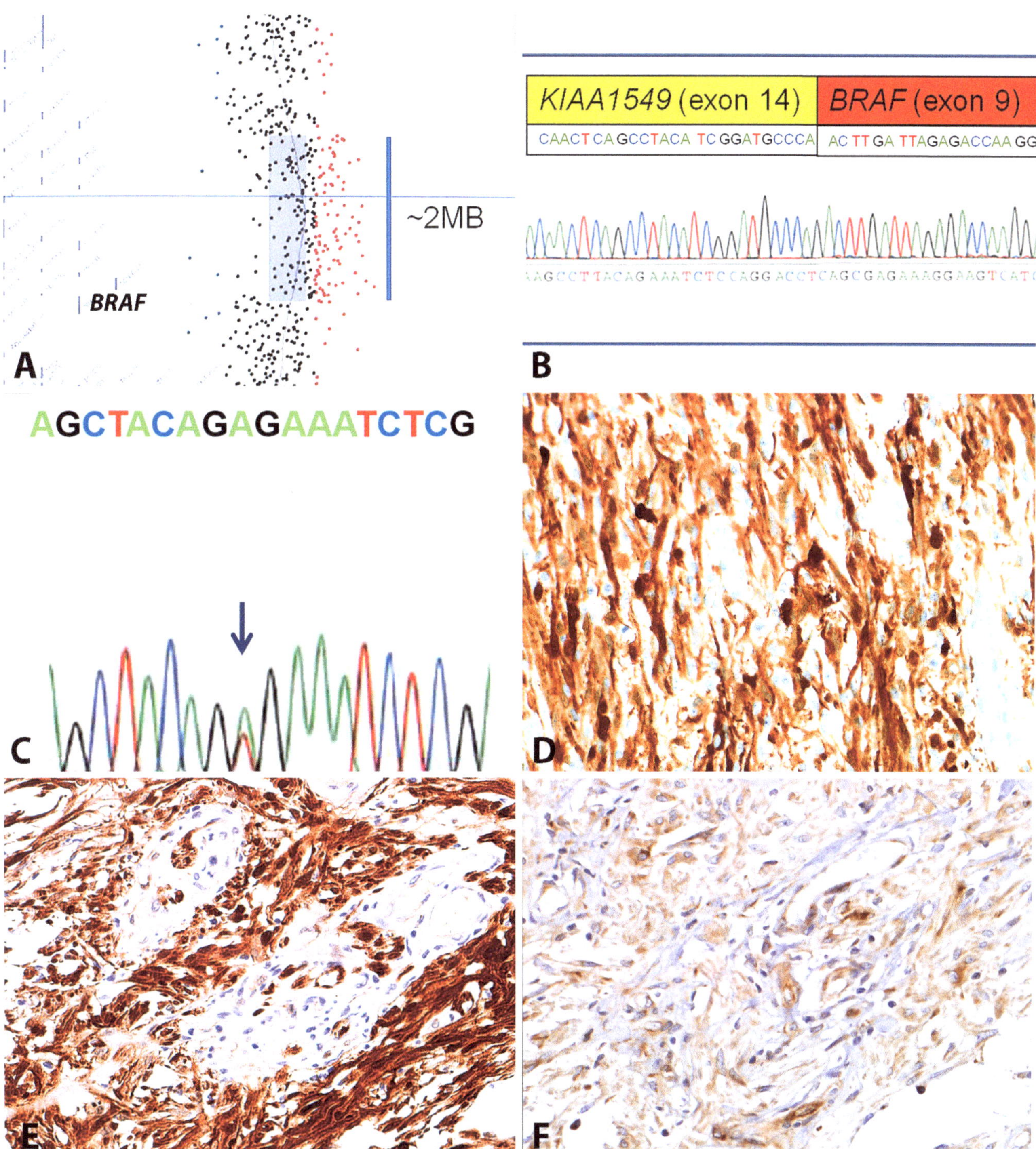

Fig. 4.5. Molecular features of circumscribed gliomas. The most frequent molecular alteration in PA is a *BRAF* duplication that may be identified by array CGH (**a**). This duplication usually leads to a gene fusion, usually involving the neighboring gene *KIAA1549* (**b**). In contrast, most pleomorphic xanthoastrocytomas contain a *BRAF* (V600E) mutation resulting from a single nucleotide change (**c**). Activating *BRAF* alterations may result in induction of the phenomenon of oncogene-induced senescence, and associated with increased p16 expression (**d**), which may explain the low proliferation rates in many of these tumors. The genetic alterations present in PA and other circumscribed gliomas result in near universal activation of the MAPK and mTOR signaling pathways, which may be identified by detection of phospho-ERK (**e**) and phosphor-S6 (**f**) protein, respectively.

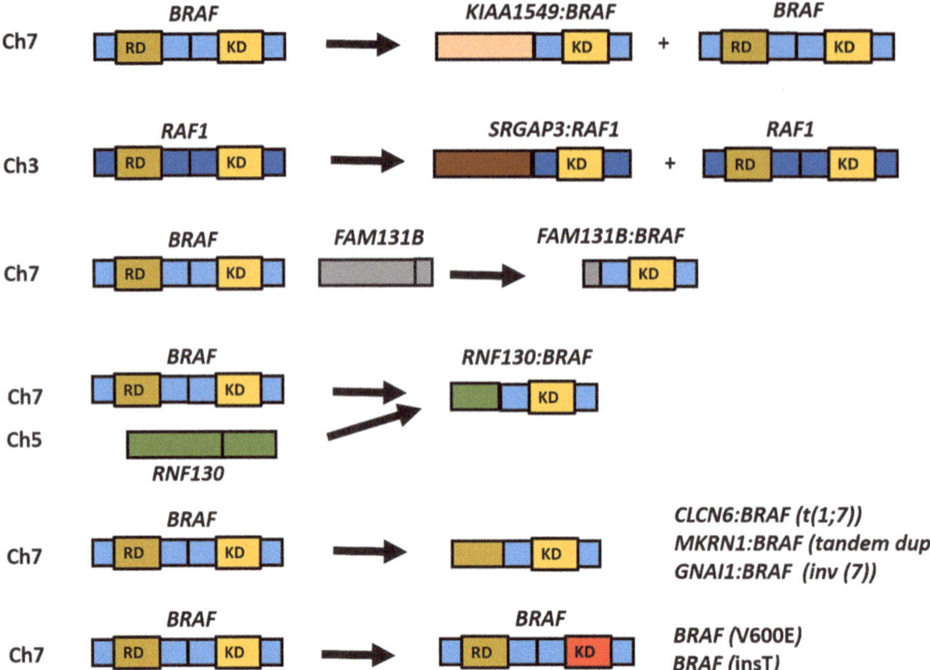

Fig. 4.6. Spectrum of BRAF alterations in pilocytic astrocytoma/circumscribed gliomas. Although tandem duplications involving the *BRAF* kinase domain (KD), excluding the regulatory domain (RD) and leading to a *KIAA1549:BRAF* fusion are the most frequent alterations associated with pilocytic astrocytoma in specific, alternative alterations occur in a small proportion of cases. These include an interstitial deletion leading to *FAM131B:BRAF* fusion, fusion events involving alternative partners, as well as point mutations (e.g., *BRAF V600E*) and small activating insertions (insT). A similar rearrangement involving the related gene *RAF1*, also occurs on rare occasions.

pathways [40, 41]. Conversely, *BRAF* fusions are less frequent in PA arising in the cerebral hemispheres. However, a small subset of unclassifiable low-grade astrocytomas and neuroepithelial/glioneuronal tumors may also have it [47]. In addition, it appears that the frequency of *BRAF-KIAA1549* fusion varies by age, being less frequent in PA of adults [48].

The development of low-grade astrocytomas in patients with germline *NF1* loss and the high frequency of somatic *BRAF* alterations in sporadic circumscribed low-grade gliomas provide strong evidence that the MAPK/ERK signaling pathway is critical for the biology of these tumors. Other studies have shown rarer genetic alterations leading to activation of this pathway, including small *BRAF* insertions, *RAF1-SRGAP3* fusions (at 3p25), activating *RAS* mutations, and a *FAM131B-BRAF* fusion mediated by an interstitial deletion [45, 49, 50] (Fig. 4.6). Some of these rearrangements seem to be facilitated by sequence microhomology [51]. A recent whole genome/transcriptome sequencing study of PA identified single MAPK pathway activating alterations, predominantly through *BRAF-KIAA11549* fusions, but also novel *BRAF* fusion partners in very rare cases (i.e., *RNF130-BRAF*, *CLCN6-BRAF*, *MKRN1-BRAF*, and *GNAI1-BRAF*) [52]. Alterations in other genes not involving *BRAF* were also identified in a small subset of non-cerebellar PA (*NTRK2* rearrangements, as well as *FGFR1* and *PTPN11* mutations). Of interest, in this study every PA had a genetic alteration in the MAPK pathway, which was almost always exclusive (except for *PTPN11* mutations which occurred only in combination with *FGFR1* alterations) [52].

BRAF (V600E) mutation, reported in numerous cancer types, is less restricted to histopathology and has been reported to occur with variable frequency in many brain tumor subtypes [53–58], including PXA, gangliogliomas, desmoplastic infantile gangliogliomas, PA, diffuse gliomas and even in dysembryoplastic neuroepithelial tumors. However, the frequency of *BRAF* (V600E) mutation appears to be higher in PXA, occurring in over half of cases [57, 59, 60].

At the current time, the prognostic significance of *BRAF* alterations in low-grade gliomas remains unclear. Several studies have not found a significant association with outcome in patients with low-grade gliomas containing *BRAF* fusions [13, 47, 49]. In a study by Hawkins et al. focusing on a clinically relevant group of 70 pediatric low-grade astrocytoma patients (i.e., sporadic, subtotally resected tumors in non-cerebellar locations), the investigators found *BRAF-KIAA1549* fusions to be significantly associated with better clinical outcome [61]. Conversely, Horbinski et al. in a study of 198 cases, found on multivariate analysis midline location and *p16* deletion (but not *BRAF* rearrangement) as independent prognostic factors [62]. In a meta-analysis of *BRAF* alteration data encompassing approximately 700 pediatric low-grade astrocytomas, specific *BRAF-KIAA1549* fusion variants have independent prognostic implications in extra-cerebellar PA, but *BRAF* fusions in general were not independently associated with outcome (Jones D et al., unpublished data). RT-PCR and FISH based methods that are able to detect this fusion in formalin-fixed paraffin-embedded tissue have been developed [63], and have been increasing applied for clinical use.

Given the high frequency of somatic *BRAF* genetic alterations in circumscribed low-grade gliomas, the possibility of pharmacologic inhibition as a therapeutic strategy is very appealing. However, targeted therapeutics for BRAF must be taken with caution, since recent pharmacologic evidence suggests that inhibitors that are effective against BRAF (V600E) may have paradoxic pro-growth effects in tumors that are *BRAF* wild type or contain activating *BRAF* fusions [64].

Oncogene-Induced Senescence

Senescence, i.e., irreversible growth arrest, is a cellular phenomenon that may occur as a result of oncogene activation. Clinical observations have documented stabilization, or even regression, of a subset of PA. Furthermore, PA shares frequent alterations in the *BRAF* oncogene with another limited neoplastic proliferation, cutaneous melanocytic nevi, which are known to senesce. Recent studies [65, 66] have shown markers of senescence, including p16 and acidic senescence-associated β-galactosidase, in primary PA and low passage cultures. Furthermore, senescence was also induced after introduction of *BRAF* (V600E) in neural stem cells, and p16 loss in clinical samples was associated with worse clinical outcome [66].

PI3K/mTOR

PI3K/mTOR signaling has been implicated as a frequent molecular property of a variety of tumor types. This pathway is of great interest for targeted therapeutics, since pharmacologic inhibitors (i.e., rapamycin and its analogs) are widely available. mTOR exists as part of two multiprotein complexes: mTORC1 and mTORC2 (mTORC1 is composed of RAPTOR, mLST8 and GBL), and signaling through this complex leads to increased protein translation, cell growth, and survival. In mTORC2, mTOR interacts with RICTOR, mSin1, and Protor, activation leads to AKT activation (identified by phosphorylation at S473)/PKC signaling, and subsequently increased cell survival and regulation of cytoskeletal dynamics [67].

Of relevance to low-grade glioma, particularly pediatric, is studies demonstrating increased mTOR signaling in the context of *NF1* loss. These include mouse models of NF1-optic glioma [68] and unusual low-grade gliomas in NF1 patients characterized by increased cell size [69]. mTOR activation is also more frequent in rare PA that develop anaplasia [70], and regulates proliferation of murine stem cells containing activating *BRAF* fusions [46]. A recent study of 177 pediatric low-grade gliomas and PA showed significant mTOR activation (~60 % of cases) as measured by pS6 protein [71]. In addition, mTOR inhibition led to decreased cell growth of two pediatric cell lines in vitro. Of great clinical interest, mTOR inhibitors have pharmacologic efficacy in SEGA and other manifestations of tuberous sclerosis [72], a syndrome essentially defined at the molecular level by constitutive mTOR activation. PI3K/mTOR pathway activation is also a frequent feature of both adult and pediatric diffuse gliomas, through alterations in *PTEN*, *NF1* and genes encoding for receptor tyrosine kinases (e.g., *FGFR1*) [73].

Diffuse Gliomas

One of the earliest molecular alterations described in diffuse gliomas, with morphologic and prognostic relevance was the identification of 1p19q co-deletion, particularly in tumors with oligodendroglial morphology (Fig. 4.7). Subsequent studies highlighted a strong association between 1p19q co-deletion and therapeutic response, particularly in anaplastic oligodendroglioma [74]. This alteration may be identified by a variety of methods that work in formalin-fixed paraffin-embedded tissue, most commonly FISH [75], but also array based platforms, such as SNP arrays [76]. Although partial deletions involving chromosome arm 1p and/or 19q are not uncommon in gliomas with various histologies, it is whole arm 1p and 19q co-deletion that is most closely associated with oligodendroglial histology, which is mediated by an unbalanced (t1;19) translocation [77, 78]. Subsequent whole exome sequencing studies have identified recurrent mutations in *FUBP1* (Ch 1p) and *CIC* (Ch 19q) as likely tumor suppressor genes inactivated at these locations [79, 80].

Another remarkable subsequent discovery in the biology of diffuse gliomas was the identification of recurrent point mutations in genes encoding for the cytosolic metabolic enzyme *IDH1* (and less frequently *IDH2*) through exome sequencing efforts. Although initially identified in a subset of glioblastomas, it was subsequently noted that these mutations were highly prevalent (>80 %) in diffuse gliomas grade II and III, both astrocytomas and oligodendrogliomas as well as in secondary glioblastomas [81–83]. These IDH mutations occur almost always at the same site (Arg132 of IDH1 and analogous Arg172 site in IDH2) and result in a neoenzymatic function leading to increased 2-hydroxyglutarate (2HG) [84], which has numerous cellular effects including inhibition of histone and DNA demethylation and global epigenetic alterations (reviewed in [85, 86]). *IDH1/2* mutations appear to be early events in tumorigenesis, since they show similar prevalence in grade II astrocytomas and oligodendrogliomas, and may occur earlier than 1p19q loss and *TP53* mutations. Diagnostically, an antibody directed against the most frequent IDH1 mutant protein in gliomas (IDH1 R132H), is in clinical use and valuable in differentiating infiltrating gliomas from other tumors and non-neoplastic conditions (i.e., gliosis) [87, 88].

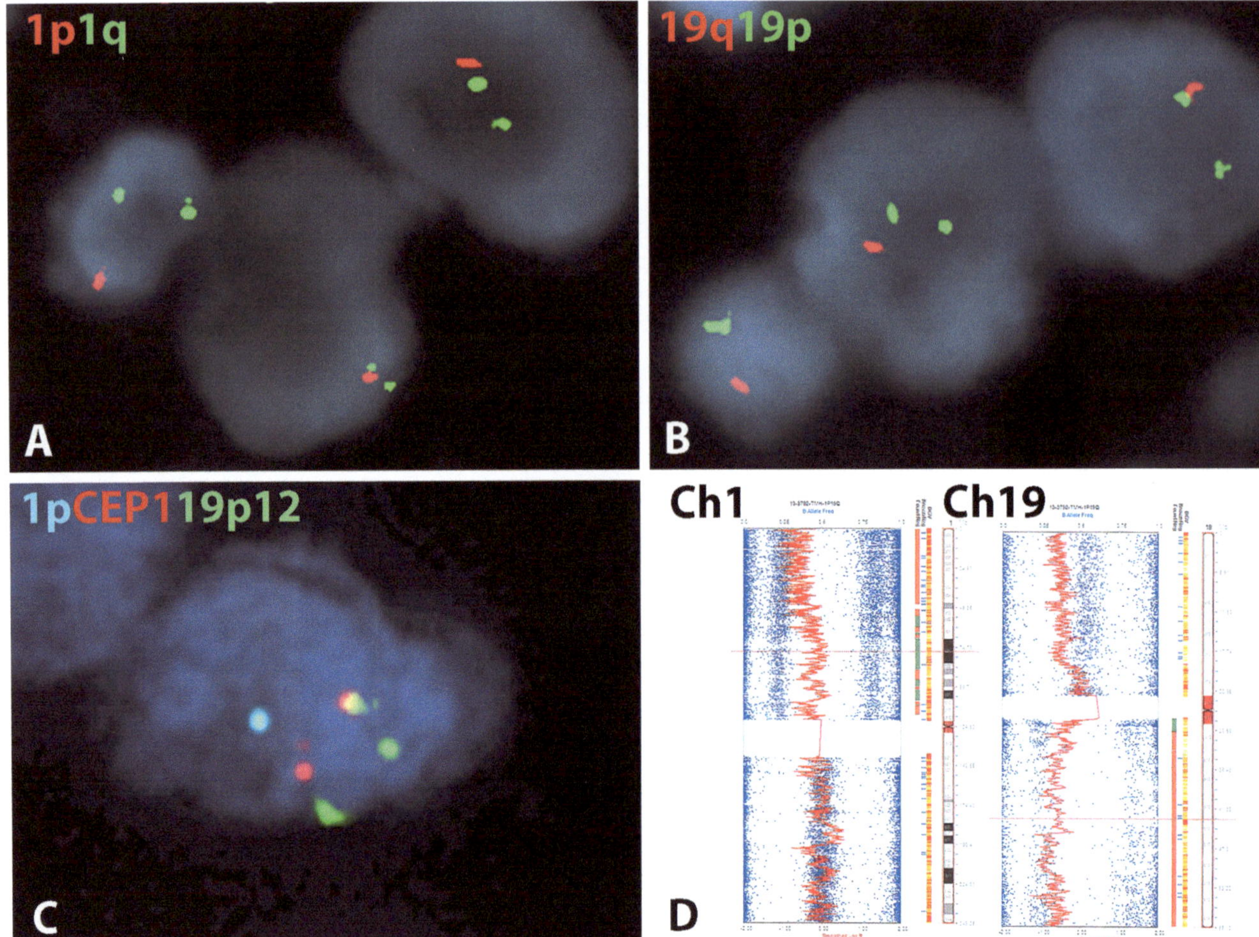

Fig. 4.7. Molecular genetic alterations in oligodendroglial neoplasms. The most characteristic molecular alteration in oligodendroglial tumors is combined deletions of 1p (**a**) and 19q (**b**) which is mediated by a t(1;19) translocation (**c**). The 1p19q co-deletion may also be recognized by array based methods (e.g., SNP platforms) in formalin-fixed tissue. As this case demonstrates, the classic co-deletion of oligodendroglioma involves the whole 1p and 19q chromosomal arms (**d**) (SNP figure courtesy of Christopher Gocke, MD).

Another molecular property of a subset of infiltrating astrocytomas is the presence of a telomerase independent mechanism of telomere maintenance known as the alternative lengthening of telomeres (ALT) (Fig. 4.8). Although present in a small subset of cancers of various types, this phenotype is enriched in DA (WHO grade II), anaplastic astrocytoma (WHO grade III), as well as secondary and pediatric glioblastoma (WHO grade IV). Subsequent studies found this phenotype to be strongly associated with mutations in the gene encoding the chromatin remodeling protein ATRX [89]. These mutations lead to ATRX protein loss and are strongly associated with *IDH* mutations [90–92], but are mutually exclusive with 1p19q co-deletion/*CIC*/*FUBP1* mutations [93].

All these recent studies highlighted an important role for telomere maintenance in the biology of diffuse gliomas, findings subsequently reinforced by the finding of mutations in the *TERT* promoter which leads to increased transcriptional activity [94]. Interestingly, among diffuse gliomas, *TERT* promoter mutations are more frequent in oligodendrogliomas and primary glioblastomas and mutually exclusive with *ATRX* mutations and the ALT phenotype. An expanding picture is now emerging with distinctive molecular signatures separating various low-grade glioma subtypes (Fig. 4.9).

Whole Genome Sequencing Studies of Pediatric Low-Grade Glioma

Whole genome/exome sequencing studies have also provided recent, important insights into the molecular genetics important for pediatric low-grade glioma development (Fig. 4.10). Zhang et al. in a whole genome sequencing study of 39 pediatric low-grade gliomas and glioneuronal tumors found very few genetic alterations, with 24 tumors (62 %) containing single relevant (non-silent) somatic alterations [73]. They found rearrangements of *MYB* and duplications of the gene segments of *FGFR1* encoding for the tyrosine kinase domain in approximately half of pediatric DA.

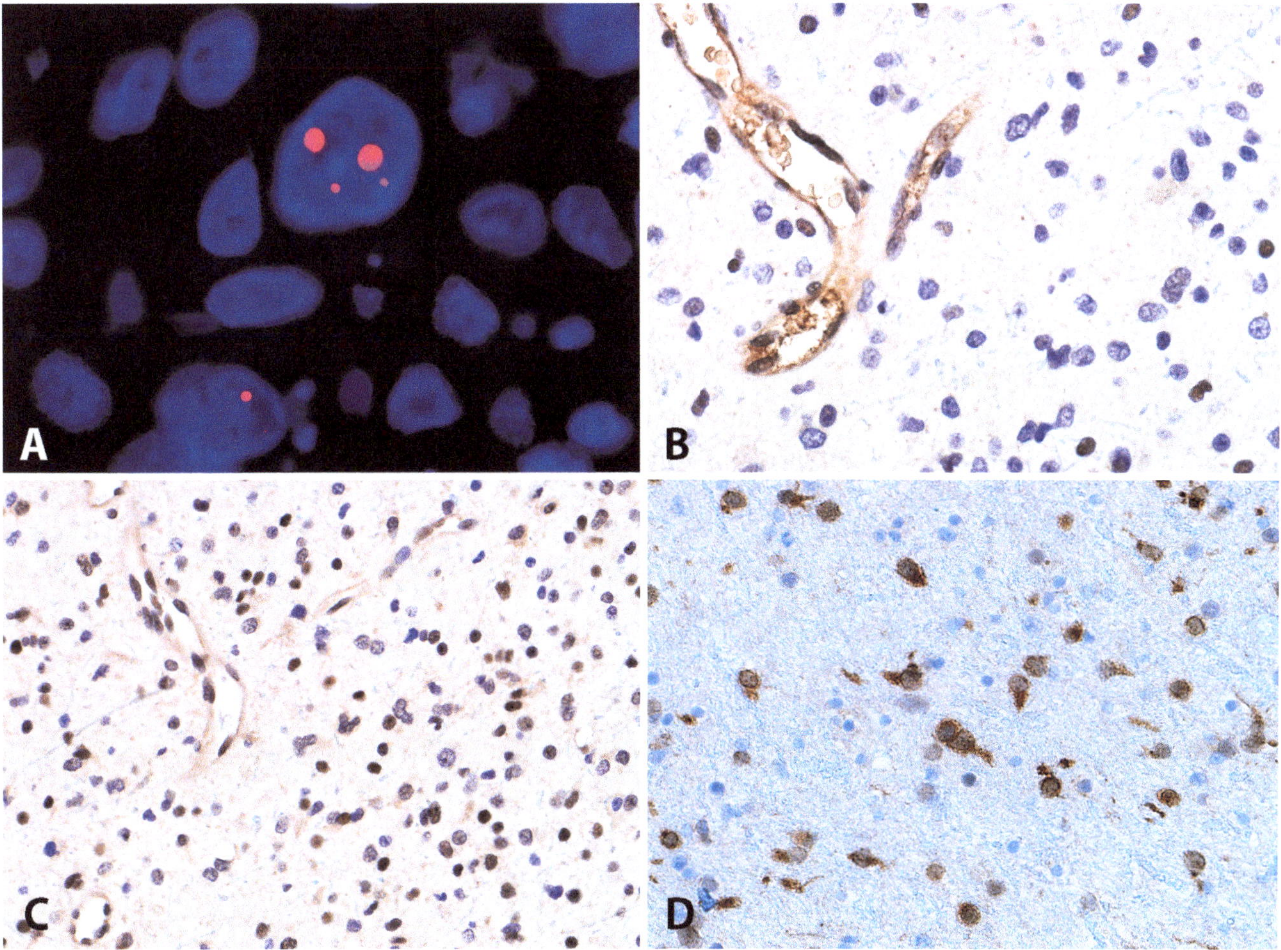

Fig. 4.8. Molecular features of adult diffuse astrocytomas. The alternative lengthening of telomeres (ALT) is a frequent phenotype identifiable in diffuse astrocytomas by telomere specific FISH, which demonstrates ultrabright signals (Courtesy of Christopher Heaphy, Ph.D.) (**a**). The ALT phenotype is frequently associated with *ATRX* mutations and protein loss in neoplastic cells (**b**). Conversely DAXX is usually preserved in most CNS tumors (**c**). IDH1 mutations are frequent in diffuse gliomas, and may be recognized by an antibody directed against the most frequent mutated protein product (R132H) (**d**).

Ramkissoon et al. studied 44 pediatric diffuse low-grade gliomas using high resolution copy number analysis and identified 8q13.1 alterations in 28 % of cases leading to *MYBL1* gain [95] (Fig. 4.11) The authors also found a similar alteration involving the related gene *MYB* in two angiocentric gliomas. These alterations frequently result in a duplication as well as truncation of a C-terminal regulatory domain.

In their study, Zhang et al. also identified various alterations in the small subset of the rarer pediatric oligodendroglial tumors [73]. For example, duplications of *FGFR* TK were present in 3 (of 5) pediatric oligodendrogoliomas and 4 (of 8) oligoastrocytomas. *FGFR1-TACC1* fusion, *NAV1-NTRK2* fusion, *FGFR1*:*p.N544K*, and *BRAF*:p.G503>EYSG were present in each of the two remaining oligoastrocytomas, and a *MYB-MAML2* fusion and adult oligodendroglioma alterations (*IDH1*, *CIC* mutations, 1p19q co-deletion) in one additional oligodendroglioma each. Prior studies have also found low frequencies of 1p19q co-deletion and IDH1 (R132H) in pediatric oligodendroglioma [22–24], and when present they tend to occur in older children (>15 years of age). Pending the study of additional cases, it therefore appears that there is genetic overlap between pediatric DA and oligodendrogliomas, unlike the morphologically similar tumors in adults.

Compound Genetic Alterations

Although initial studies suggested separation of different tumor types by molecular features, specifically by *BRAF-KIAA1549* fusion and *IDH1/2* mutations [96], subsequent studies have documented tumors with overlapping molecular alterations. For example, Badiali et al. found coexisting *IDH* mutations and *BRAF-KIAA1549* fusions in <10 % of 185 adult diffuse gliomas, particularly tumors with oligodendroglial morphology [97]. *BRAF* (7q34) gain was also even

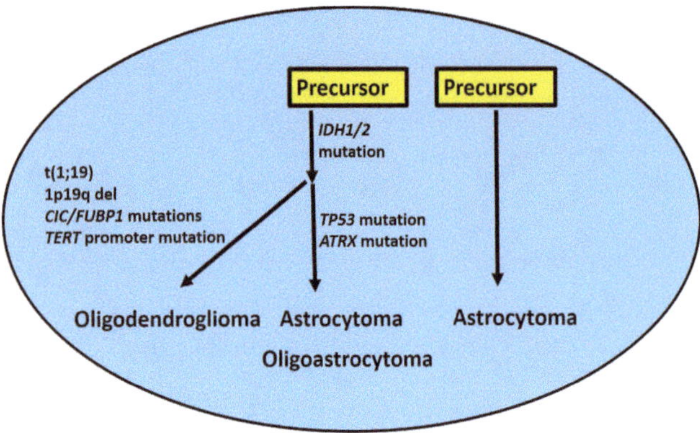

Fig. 4.9. Molecular pathogenesis of adult low-grade diffuse gliomas. Recent studies have also refined our classification of diffuse gliomas in adults. IDH mutations appear to be an early event, shared by oligodendroglial tumors and a subset of diffuse astrocytomas with a relatively better prognosis. Additional alterations (e.g., t(1;19)) are associated with the oligodendroglial subgroup, while ATRX alterations are associated with the astrocytic pathway. Other astrocytomas lack these alterations, and are associated with a worse prognosis. Often, they have molecular alterations more typical of primary glioblastoma. Oligoastrocytoma is an heterogeneous group, and may share molecular properties with oligodendrogliomas or astrocytomas.

more frequent in tumors with 1p19q loss (~40 %) in another study [98].

When focusing on activating alterations in the MAPK pathway, in most instances only a single alteration is encountered, particularly in PA. However, overlapping alterations (*BRAF-KIAA1549*, *BRAF* (V600E), NF1 syndrome) may also occur in a small proportion of cases [47, 49].

Epigenetics

One of the most important insights into the molecular biology of gliomas in the past several years is the presence of genetic mutations that lead to profound global alterations in the epigenetic landscape. For example, global methylation analysis of glioblastomas as part of the Cancer Genome Atlas (TCGA) led to the discovery of a CpG island methylator phenotype (CIMP) group of tumors that is strongly associated with *IDH1/2* mutations [99]. Interestingly, *IDH1* mutations are sufficient to induce this CIMP phenotype [100]. Subsequently, similar epigenetic alterations have been identified in lower grade tumors including oligodendrogliomas [101]. Mutations in genes encoding for chromatin remodelers (e.g., *ATRX/DAXX*) or components (*H3F3A*) transcription factors MYB or MYBL1. Many of these alterations particularly lead to MAPK and PI3K/mTOR pathway activation, an almost universal feature of these tumors.

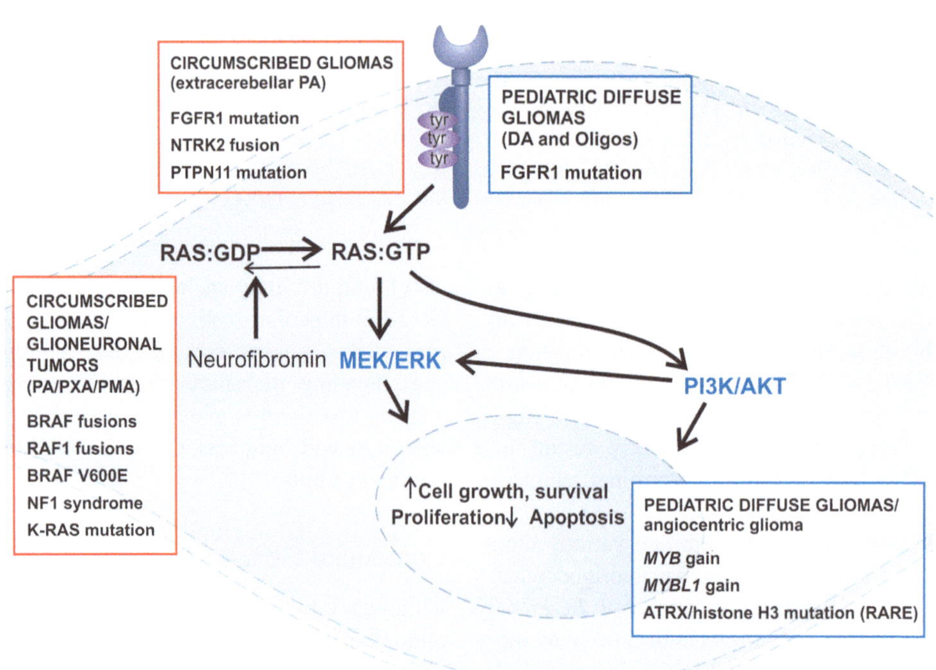

Fig. 4.10. Signaling pathways in pediatric low-grade gliomas. Recent genomic studies have clarified the molecular genetic alterations associated with pediatric low-grade gliomas and circumscribed gliomas, identifying alterations in BRAF, FGFR1 and

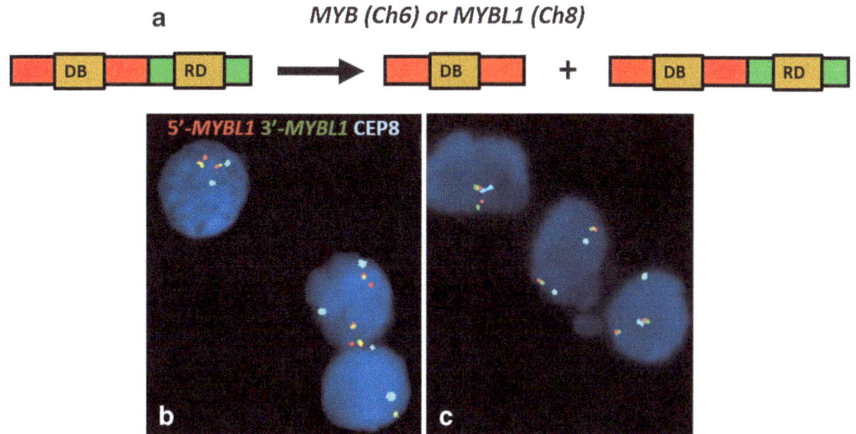

Fig. 4.11. Molecular alterations in *MYB* or *MYBL1* in pediatric diffuse gliomas. Diffuse gliomas in children, particularly astrocytic, and angiocentric gliomas have a relatively high frequency of MYB or MYBL1 rearrangements, often leading to a gain containing the DNA binding (DB) and activating domains, but lacking a C-terminal regulatory domain (RD) (**a**). FISH strategy identifies a pediatric glioma with *MYBL1* gain (three *red* copies) (**b**). Cells lacking *MYBL1* alteration for comparison (**c**) (FISH images courtesy of Azra Ligon, Ph.D.).

have also been identified in specific subsets of diffuse gliomas, particularly pediatric high-grade ones.

Epigenetic alterations, including dysregulation in microRNA levels [102] and DNA methylation [103] are also a recently recognized feature of PA, and may identify biologically and/or clinically relevant subsets that deserve further study. For example, the *AKAP12* tumor suppressor gene is underexpressed and methylated in DA and other infiltrating gliomas in contrast to PA [104].

Molecular Targeted Therapies

MAP Kinase Pathway: BRAF Duplication/BRAF V600E/MAPK/ERK Targeting Agents

Uncontrolled growth is a necessary step for the development of all cancers. In many cancers, a defect in the MAP Kinase Pathway has been demonstrated to regulate cell proliferation, mitosis, survival, and apoptosis. As a result of the relative high frequency of *BRAF* duplication/fusion mutations and activation of the MAP kinase pathway described among pediatric low-grade gliomas, including PA and PMA [39–41, 44, 47, 49, 61, 70, 105], there is considerable interest in targeted MAP kinase pathway inhibition as a potential therapy for these tumors (Fig. 4.12).

Sorafenib (Nexavar, Bayer and Onyx Pharmaceuticals) is an inhibitor of mutated BRAF including B-RAF and C-RAF (it has less potency against BRAF V600E). Sorafenib is approved the United States Food and Drug Administration (FDA) for the treatment of renal cell carcinoma and liver cancer. A recent phase II study of Sorafenib enrolled 11 patients with recurrent or progressive pediatric low-grade gliomas. Nine of 11 (82 %) patients enrolled had tumor progression at 3 months and thus the clinical trial was stopped early [106]. Furthermore, *KIAA1549-BRAF* fusions were identified among three of the nine patients with tumor progression, demonstrating a lack of activity among these patients. One patient with a ganglioglioma of the spinal cord completed six cycles with stable disease. Another patient with a PMA of the brainstem achieved a partial radiological response. The authors proposed that sorafenib may lead to ERK activation in both BRAF wild type and KIAA1549-BRAF mutant cell lines, and proposed that this paradoxical effect may be the mechanism by which Sorafenib promoted tumor growth in the patients with low-grade gliomas.

In general, BRAF V600E mutations are rare among pediatric low-grade astrocytomas, with the exception of being relatively common among PXA, gangliogliomas and a small subset of extra-cerebellar PA [57]. *Vemurafenib* (Plexxikon, Daiichi Sankyo) is a competitive inhibitor that is specific for the ATP binding domain of mutant BRAF V600E. As a result, it has activity against tumors with BRAF V600E, but not other mutant forms of BRAF [107, 108]. Following impressive, albeit transient, responses of recurrent melanoma to Vemurafenib [108], the United States Food and Drug Administration (FDA) approved Vemurafenib for the treatment of BRAF V600E mutation positive, inoperable or metastatic melanoma. A phase I clinical trial of Vemurafenib against BRAF V600E mutant pediatric low-grade gliomas is expected to be open in the near-term future. *Dabrafenib* (Tafinlar, GlaxoSmithKline) is another selective inhibitor of V600E-mutant BRAF and has been approved by the FDA for unresectable or metastatic melanoma. Recently, a phase I/II clinical trial of Dabrafenib has opened for pediatric brain tumors. *LGX818* (Novartis) is another selective BRAF V600E inhibitor that is undergoing clinical trials in adults,

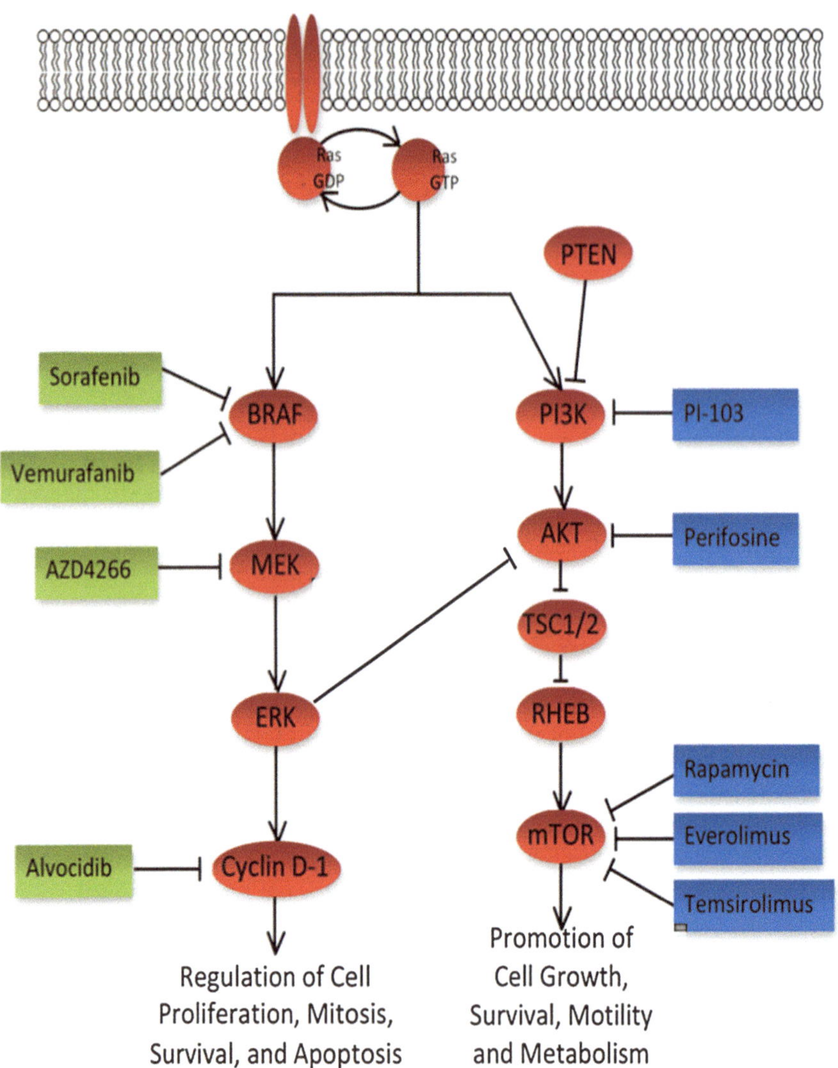

Fig. 4.12. Activated signal pathways and signal transduction inhibitors of potential clinical activity for pediatric low-grade glioma. Note that the agents listed below are just a few of the many new agents currently under development.

but there are no clinical trials of LGX818 for pediatric brain tumors at this time.

Selumetinib (AZD6244, AstraZeneca and Array BioPharma), a potent inhibitor of MEK, immediately downstream of BRAF, is an investigational therapy currently in clinical trials for non-small cell lung cancer and several other cancer types. AZD6244 is currently in phase I/II trials for pediatric low-grade astrocytomas through the Pediatric Brain Tumor Consortium.

Alvocidib (Flavopiridol, Sandofi) is a cyclin dependent kinase (CDK) inhibitor that has some activity against adult relapsed chronic lymphocytic leukemia, although it has not yet been approved by the FDA as treatment for cancer. Alvocidib has completed phase I trials in children which established the maximum tolerated dose, dose limiting toxicities were neutropenia and diarrhea. However, there are currently no ongoing studies of Alvocidib for pediatric brain tumors.

mTOR Pathway: PI3-K/AKT/mTOR Targeting Agents

The mTOR Pathway has been implicated as an important mechanism for tumor growth in many pediatric low-grade astrocytomas. Methylation of the PTEN promoter is associated with PI3-K activation and Akt phosphorylation in PLGAs [109]. Because of the clinical significance of PTEN promoter methylation and its effects on the PI3-K pathway, therapies that target tumors with PI3-K activation may be of clinical benefit in PLGAs. The mammalian target of rapamycin (mTOR) is downstream to the PI3-K and AKT and is therefore an ideal target for PLGAs with PTEN promoter methylation [110–115].

PI-103 is a dual inhibitor of PI3-K/mTOR and has activity in preclinical trials against malignant glioma cell lines. Unfortunately, because of its rapid in vivo metabolism, PI-103 is not being pursued further as an anticancer agent. Nonetheless, demonstration of dual PI3-K and mTOR inhibition suggests promise for this class of targeted agents. Currently, *SF-1126* (Semafore Pharmaceuticals) and *XL765* (Exelixis) are dual PI3-K/mTOR inhibitors that are currently in early phase trials in adults. New agents that are specific PI3-K inhibitors that are in early phase trials in adults include PX-866 (Oncothyreon) and XL147 (Exelixis). None of the PI3-K inhibitors have yet undergone phase clinical trials in children.

Akt, also, known as Protein Kinase-B, is a protein that is believed to play an important role in regulating development and growth of cancer cells. *Perifosine* (Keryx Biopharmaceuticals. Aeterna Zentaris) was the first drug that belongs to a class of agents known as "Akt-inhibitors." Perifosine has completed phase I testing in children with recurrent solid tumors [116]. However, results from the phase III trials of perifosine for recurrent colon cancer and myeloma were disappointing and it does not appear that there will be future studies of this agent. *GSK1120212* (GlaxoSmithKline) and *AZD5363* (Astex) are other Akt-inhibitors currently in early phase clinical trials in adults with recurrent cancer, but there are no clinical trials of these agents for children with brain tumors at this time. *MLN0128* (Millennium Pharmaceuticals) is a potent and selective small molecule active-site TORC1/2 kinase inhibitor that has demonstrated in vitro anticancer activity. MLN0128 is currently in early phase I, dose-finding clinical trials for adult malignancies.

SEGAs, found nearly exclusively among children with tuberous sclerosis, essentially always have activation of the AKT/mTOR pathway due to germline mutations in the *TSC1* or *TSC2* genes. Clinical trials have demonstrated that the mTOR inhibitors, *Sirolimus* (Pfizer) and *Everolimus* (Novartis Pharmaceuticals) have demonstrated activity against SEGAs [72, 117]. As of result of these studies, Everolimus has been approved by the FDA for the treatment of SEGAs not amenable to surgical resection. In addition, mTOR signaling may have a role in the biology of pediatric low-grade gliomas, especially among children with NF1 [118]. A report of a phase I/II study of Sirolimus and Erlotinib (Genentech) examined 16 patients with recurrent pediatric low-grade astrocytomas [119]. Of the seven children with NF1 in this clinical trial, all patients had either stable disease or tumor responses. Kieran and colleagues recently reported 23 patients with low-grade gliomas (median age: 9 years; range, 3–17 years) who were treated with single agent Everolimus after tumor progression following prior treatment with a carboplatin-containing chemotherapy regimen. Four of 23 patients had a partial response (>50 % decrease in tumor size) and 13 additional patients had stable disease. Therapy was generally well tolerated; two patients discontinued therapy due to mouth sores ($n=1$) and withdrawal of consent ($n=1$) [120].

As described above, recent advances in the understanding of PLGA biology suggest that pharmacologic targeting of these pathways will yield new therapies for PLGAs in the near- to intermediate-term future. However, multiple interactions and feedback loops exist between the MAP Kinase Pathway and the mTOR pathway which may explain the lack of clinical effect of single agent BRAF targeting. However, combination therapies with multiple signal transduction inhibitors or signal transduction inhibitors targeting of both the MAP kinase and mTOR pathways and conventional cytotoxic agents may yield antitumor activity [121, 122].

IDH1/2 Mutation Inhibition

Specific mutations in the isocitrate dehydrogenase genes IDH1 and IDH2 (IDH1/2) are often found in several adult brain tumors including low-grade (WHO grade II) diffuse gliomas, oligodendrogliomas, and nearly all cases of secondary glioblastomas which develop from lower grade gliomas [83, 123–125]. IDH1/2 mutations are also found in approximately 15 % of adults with acute myelogenous leukemia [126]. IDH1/2 mutations are rarely found in pediatric gliomas, with the exception being that IDH1 mutations are often found among children older than 14 years old with high-grade gliomas [4]. Although there is some conflicting data, reports of adults with low-grade gliomas whose tumors had an IDH1 and IDH2 mutations had longer survival [83, 127–129].

Investigators are examining strategies to inhibit mutant IDH1 activity and slow growth of IDH1-mutant gliomas [130, 131]. As one example, glutaminase is necessary for generation of α-KG from glutamine. Inhibition of glutaminase by either siRNA or the small molecule inhibitor, bis-2-(5-phenylacetamido-1,2,4-thiadiazol-2-yl)ethyl sulfide (BPTES) slowed growth of glioblastoma cells expressing mutant IDH1 compared with those expressing wild-type IDH1 [132]. AG-221 (Agios Pharmaceuticals) is an IDH2 inhibitor that is currently in early clinical trials for adults with IDH2 mutant-acute myelogenous leukemia. However, despite recognized potential for therapeutic strategies of IDH1 and IDH2 inhibitors, there are as yet no clinical trials of IDH1 or IDH2 inhibitors against low-grade gliomas.

References

1. Louis DN, Ohgaki H, Wiestler OD, Cavenee WK. WHO classification of tumours of the central nervous system. Lyon: IARC Press; 2007.
2. Cheng Y, Pang JC, Ng HK, Ding M, Zhang SF, Zheng J, et al. Pilocytic astrocytomas do not show most of the genetic changes commonly seen in diffuse astrocytomas. Histopathology. 2000;37(5):437–44. Epub 2000/12/19.
3. Buccoliero AM, Castiglione F, Rossi Degl'innocenti D, Gheri CF, Genitori L, Taddei GL. IDH1 mutation in pediatric gliomas: has it a diagnostic and prognostic value? Fetal Pediatr Pathol. 2012;31(5):278–82.
4. Pollack IF, Hamilton RL, Sobol RW, Nikiforova MN, Lyons-Weiler MA, LaFramboise WA, et al. IDH1 mutations are common in malignant gliomas arising in adolescents: a report from

the Children's Oncology Group. Childs Nerv Syst. 2011;27(1):87–94. Epub 2010/08/21.
5. Paugh BS, Qu C, Jones C, Liu Z, Adamowicz-Brice M, Zhang J, et al. Integrated molecular genetic profiling of pediatric high-grade gliomas reveals key differences with the adult disease. J Clin Oncol. 2010;28(18):3061–8. Epub 2010/05/19.
6. Giannini C, Scheithauer BW, Burger PC, Christensen MR, Wollan PC, Sebo TJ, et al. Cellular proliferation in pilocytic and diffuse astrocytomas. J Neuropathol Exp Neurol. 1999;58(1):46–53. Epub 1999/02/12.
7. Tibbetts KM, Emnett RJ, Gao F, Perry A, Gutmann DH, Leonard JR. Histopathologic predictors of pilocytic astrocytoma event-free survival. Acta Neuropathol. 2009;117(6):657–65. Epub 2009/03/10.
8. Bowers DC, Gargan L, Kapur P, Reisch JS, Mulne AF, Shapiro KN, et al. Study of the MIB-1 labeling index as a predictor of tumor progression in pilocytic astrocytomas in children and adolescents. J Clin Oncol. 2003;21(15):2968–73. Epub 2003/07/30.
9. Dirven CM, Koudstaal J, Mooij JJ, Molenaar WM. The proliferative potential of the pilocytic astrocytoma: the relation between MIB-1 labeling and clinical and neuro-radiological follow-up. J Neurooncol. 1998;37(1):9–16. Epub 1998/04/03.
10. Fisher BJ, Naumova E, Leighton CC, Naumov GN, Kerklviet N, Fortin D, et al. Ki-67: a prognostic factor for low-grade glioma? Int J Radiat Oncol Biol Phys. 2002;52(4):996–1001. Epub 2002/04/18.
11. Rodriguez FJ, Scheithauer BW, Burger PC, Jenkins S, Giannini C. Anaplasia in pilocytic astrocytoma predicts aggressive behavior. Am J Surg Pathol. 2010;34(2):147–60. Epub 2010/01/12.
12. Tihan T, Fisher PG, Kepner JL, Godfraind C, McComb RD, Goldthwaite PT, et al. Pediatric astrocytomas with monomorphous pilomyxoid features and a less favorable outcome. J Neuropathol Exp Neurol. 1999;58(10):1061–8. Epub 1999/10/09.
13. Colin C, Padovani L, Chappe C, Mercurio S, Scavarda D, Loundou A, et al. Outcome analysis of childhood pilocytic astrocytomas: a retrospective study of 148 cases at a single institution. Neuropathol Appl Neurobiol. 2012;39(6):693–705.
14. Johnson MW, Eberhart CG, Perry A, Tihan T, Cohen KJ, Rosenblum MK, et al. Spectrum of pilomyxoid astrocytomas: intermediate pilomyxoid tumors. Am J Surg Pathol. 2010;34(12):1783–91. Epub 2010/11/26.
15. Lopes MB, Altermatt HJ, Scheithauer BW, Shepherd CW, VandenBerg SR. Immunohistochemical characterization of subependymal giant cell astrocytomas. Acta Neuropathol. 1996;91(4):368–75. Epub 1996/01/01.
16. Reifenberger G, Kaulich K, Wiestler OD, Blumcke I. Expression of the CD34 antigen in pleomorphic xanthoastrocytomas. Acta Neuropathol. 2003;105(4):358–64. Epub 2003/03/08.
17. Giannini C, Scheithauer BW, Burger PC, Brat DJ, Wollan PC, Lach B, et al. Pleomorphic xanthoastrocytoma: what do we really know about it? Cancer. 1999;85(9):2033–45. Epub 1999/05/01.
18. Lellouch-Tubiana A, Boddaert N, Bourgeois M, Fohlen M, Jouvet A, Delalande O, et al. Angiocentric neuroepithelial tumor (ANET): a new epilepsy-related clinicopathological entity with distinctive MRI. Brain Pathol. 2005;15(4):281–6. Epub 2006/01/05.
19. Wang M, Tihan T, Rojiani AM, Bodhireddy SR, Prayson RA, Iacuone JJ, et al. Monomorphous angiocentric glioma: a distinctive epileptogenic neoplasm with features of infiltrating astrocytoma and ependymoma. J Neuropathol Exp Neurol. 2005;64(10):875–81. Epub 2005/10/11.
20. Jones DT, Mulholland SA, Pearson DM, Malley DS, Openshaw SW, Lambert SR, et al. Adult grade II diffuse astrocytomas are genetically distinct from and more aggressive than their paediatric counterparts. Acta Neuropathol. 2011;121(6):753–61. Epub 2011/02/18.
21. Ballester LY, Wang Z, Shandilya S, Miettinen M, Burger PC, Eberhart CG, et al. Morphologic characteristics and immunohistochemical profile of diffuse intrinsic pontine glioma. Am J Surg Pathol. 2013;37:1357–64.
22. Kreiger PA, Okada Y, Simon S, Rorke LB, Louis DN, Golden JA. Losses of chromosomes 1p and 19q are rare in pediatric oligodendrogliomas. Acta Neuropathol. 2005;109(4):387–92. Epub 2005/03/02.
23. Raghavan R, Balani J, Perry A, Margraf L, Vono MB, Cai DX, et al. Pediatric oligodendrogliomas: a study of molecular alterations on 1p and 19q using fluorescence in situ hybridization. J Neuropathol Exp Neurol. 2003;62(5):530–7. Epub 2003/05/29.
24. Rodriguez FJ, Burger PC, McDonald W, Nigro J, Lin D, Feuerstein B, et al. Clinicopathologic features of pediatric oligodendrogliomas with classic histology. J Neuropathol Exp Neurol. 2014;38(8):1058–70.
25. Agamanolis DP, Katsetos CD, Klonk CJ, Bartkowski HM, Ganapathy S, Staugaitis SM, et al. An unusual form of superficially disseminated glioma in children: report of 3 cases. J Child Neurol. 2012;27(6):727–33. Epub 2012/05/19.
26. Perilongo G, Gardiman M, Bisaglia L, Rigobello L, Calderone M, Battistella A, et al. Spinal low-grade neoplasms with extensive leptomeningeal dissemination in children. Childs Nerv Syst. 2002;18(9–10):505–12. Epub 2002/10/17.
27. Rodriguez FJ, Perry A, Rosenblum MK, Krawitz S, Cohen KJ, Lin D, et al. Disseminated oligodendroglial-like leptomeningeal tumor of childhood: a distinctive clinicopathologic entity. Acta Neuropathol. 2012;124(5):627–41. Epub 2012/09/04.
28. Schniederjan MJ, Alghamdi S, Castellano-Sanchez A, Mazewski C, Brahma B, Brat DJ, et al. Diffuse leptomeningeal neuroepithelial tumor: 9 pediatric cases with chromosome 1p/19q deletion status and IDH1 (R132H) immunohistochemistry. Am J Surg Pathol. 2013;37(5):763–71. Epub 2013/04/17.
29. Gupta K, Harreld JH, Sabin ND, Qaddoumi I, Kurian K, Ellison DW. Massively calcified low-grade glioma—a rare and distinctive entity. Neuropathol Appl Neurobiol. 2014;40(2):221–4.
30. Sharma MK, Mansur DB, Reifenberger G, Perry A, Leonard JR, Aldape KD, et al. Distinct genetic signatures among pilocytic astrocytomas relate to their brain region origin. Cancer Res. 2007;67(3):890–900. Epub 2007/02/07.
31. Sharma MK, Watson MA, Lyman M, Perry A, Aldape KD, Deak F, et al. Matrilin-2 expression distinguishes clinically relevant subsets of pilocytic astrocytoma. Neurology. 2006;66(1):127–30. Epub 2006/01/13.
32. Rodriguez FJ, Giannini C, Asmann YW, Sharma MK, Perry A, Tibbetts KM, et al. Gene expression profiling of NF-1-associated and sporadic pilocytic astrocytoma identifies aldehyde dehydrogenase 1 family member L1 (ALDH1L1) as an underexpressed candidate biomarker in aggressive subtypes. J Neuropathol Exp Neurol. 2008;67(12):1194–204. Epub 2008/11/20.

33. Wong KK, Chang YM, Tsang YT, Perlaky L, Su J, Adesina A, et al. Expression analysis of juvenile pilocytic astrocytomas by oligonucleotide microarray reveals two potential subgroups. Cancer Res. 2005;65(1):76–84. Epub 2005/01/25.
34. Gorovets D, Kannan K, Shen R, Kastenhuber ER, Islamdoust N, Campos C, et al. IDH mutation and neuroglial developmental features define clinically distinct subclasses of lower grade diffuse astrocytic glioma. Clin Cancer Res. 2012;18(9):2490–501. Epub 2012/03/15.
35. Dahlback HS, Gorunova L, Brandal P, Scheie D, Helseth E, Meling TR, et al. Genomic aberrations in diffuse low-grade gliomas. Genes Chromosomes Cancer. 2011;50(6):409–20. Epub 2011/03/18.
36. Kluwe L, Hagel C, Tatagiba M, Thomas S, Stavrou D, Ostertag H, et al. Loss of NF1 alleles distinguish sporadic from NF1-associated pilocytic astrocytomas. J Neuropathol Exp Neurol. 2001;60(9):917–20. Epub 2001/09/15.
37. Kleihues P, Schauble B, zur Hausen A, Esteve J, Ohgaki H. Tumors associated with p53 germline mutations: a synopsis of 91 families. Am J Pathol. 1997;150(1):1–13.
38. Jenkins RB, Xiao Y, Sicotte H, Decker PA, Kollmeyer TM, Hansen HM, et al. A low-frequency variant at 8q24.21 is strongly associated with risk of oligodendroglial tumors and astrocytomas with IDH1 or IDH2 mutation. Nat Genet. 2012;44(10):1122–5.
39. Bar EE, Lin A, Tihan T, Burger PC, Eberhart CG. Frequent gains at chromosome 7q34 involving BRAF in pilocytic astrocytoma. J Neuropathol Exp Neurol. 2008;67(9):878–87. Epub 2008/08/22.
40. Forshew T, Tatevossian RG, Lawson AR, Ma J, Neale G, Ogunkolade BW, et al. Activation of the ERK/MAPK pathway: a signature genetic defect in posterior fossa pilocytic astrocytomas. J Pathol. 2009;218(2):172–81. Epub 2009/04/18.
41. Jacob K, Albrecht S, Sollier C, Faury D, Sader E, Montpetit A, et al. Duplication of 7q34 is specific to juvenile pilocytic astrocytomas and a hallmark of cerebellar and optic pathway tumours. Br J Cancer. 2009;101(4):722–33. Epub 2009/07/16.
42. Jones DT, Kocialkowski S, Liu L, Pearson DM, Backlund LM, Ichimura K, et al. Tandem duplication producing a novel oncogenic BRAF fusion gene defines the majority of pilocytic astrocytomas. Cancer Res. 2008;68(21):8673–7. Epub 2008/11/01.
43. Pfister S, Janzarik WG, Remke M, Ernst A, Werft W, Becker N, et al. BRAF gene duplication constitutes a mechanism of MAPK pathway activation in low-grade astrocytomas. J Clin Invest. 2008;118(5):1739–49. Epub 2008/04/10.
44. Sievert AJ, Jackson EM, Gai X, Hakonarson H, Judkins AR, Resnick AC, et al. Duplication of 7q34 in pediatric low-grade astrocytomas detected by high-density single-nucleotide polymorphism-based genotype arrays results in a novel BRAF fusion gene. Brain Pathol. 2009;19(3):449–58. Epub 2008/11/20.
45. Yu J, Deshmukh H, Gutmann RJ, Emnett RJ, Rodriguez FJ, Watson MA, et al. Alterations of BRAF and HIPK2 loci predominate in sporadic pilocytic astrocytoma. Neurology. 2009;73(19):1526–31. Epub 2009/10/02.
46. Kaul A, Chen YH, Emnett RJ, Dahiya S, Gutmann DH. Pediatric glioma-associated KIAA1549:BRAF expression regulates neuroglial cell growth in a cell type-specific and mTOR-dependent manner. Genes Dev. 2012;26(23):2561–6. Epub 2012/11/16.
47. Lin A, Rodriguez FJ, Karajannis MA, Williams SC, Legault G, Zagzag D, et al. BRAF alterations in primary glial and glioneuronal neoplasms of the central nervous system with identification of 2 novel KIAA1549:BRAF fusion variants. J Neuropathol Exp Neurol. 2012;71(1):66–72. Epub 2011/12/14.
48. Hasselblatt M, Riesmeier B, Lechtape B, Brentrup A, Stummer W, Albert FK, et al. BRAF-KIAA1549 fusion transcripts are less frequent in pilocytic astrocytomas diagnosed in adults. Neuropathol Appl Neurobiol. 2011;37(7):803–6. Epub 2011/06/24.
49. Cin H, Meyer C, Herr R, Janzarik WG, Lambert S, Jones DT, et al. Oncogenic FAM131B-BRAF fusion resulting from 7q34 deletion comprises an alternative mechanism of MAPK pathway activation in pilocytic astrocytoma. Acta Neuropathol. 2011;121(6):763–74. Epub 2011/03/23.
50. Jones DT, Kocialkowski S, Liu L, Pearson DM, Ichimura K, Collins VP. Oncogenic RAF1 rearrangement and a novel BRAF mutation as alternatives to KIAA1549:BRAF fusion in activating the MAPK pathway in pilocytic astrocytoma. Oncogene. 2009;28(20):2119–23. Epub 2009/04/14.
51. Lawson AR, Hindley GF, Forshew T, Tatevossian RG, Jamie GA, Kelly GP, et al. RAF gene fusion breakpoints in pediatric brain tumors are characterized by significant enrichment of sequence microhomology. Genome Res. 2011;21(4):505–14. Epub 2011/03/12.
52. Jones DT, Hutter B, Jager N, Korshunov A, Kool M, Warnatz HJ, et al. Recurrent somatic alterations of FGFR1 and NTRK2 in pilocytic astrocytoma. Nat Genet. 2013;45(8):927–32. Epub 2013/07/03.
53. Chappe C, Padovani L, Scavarda D, Forest F, Nanni-Metellus I, Loundou A, et al. Dysembryoplastic neuroepithelial tumors share with pleomorphic xanthoastrocytomas and gangliogliomas BRAF(V600E) mutation and expression. Brain Pathol. 2013;23(5):574–83. Epub 2013/02/28.
54. Dougherty MJ, Santi M, Brose MS, Ma C, Resnick AC, Sievert AJ, et al. Activating mutations in BRAF characterize a spectrum of pediatric low-grade gliomas. Neuro Oncol. 2010;12(7):621–30. Epub 2010/02/17.
55. Ida C, Vrana J, Rodriguez FJ, Jentoft M, Caron A, Jenkins S, et al. Immunohistochemistry is highly sensitive and specific for detection of BRAF V600E mutation in pleomorphic xanthoastrocytoma. Acta Neuropathol Comm. 2013;1:20.
56. Koelsche C, Wohrer A, Jeibmann A, Schittenhelm J, Schindler G, Preusser M, et al. Mutant BRAF V600E protein in ganglioglioma is predominantly expressed by neuronal tumor cells. Acta Neuropathol. 2013;125(6):891–900. Epub 2013/02/26.
57. Schindler G, Capper D, Meyer J, Janzarik W, Omran H, Herold-Mende C, et al. Analysis of BRAF V600E mutation in 1,320 nervous system tumors reveals high mutation frequencies in pleomorphic xanthoastrocytoma, ganglioglioma and extra-cerebellar pilocytic astrocytoma. Acta Neuropathol. 2011;121(3):397–405. Epub 2011/01/29.
58. Koelsche C, Sahm F, Paulus W, Mittelbronn M, Giangaspero F, Antonelli M, et al. BRAF V600E expression and distribution in desmoplastic infantile astrocytoma/ganglioglioma. Neuropathol Appl Neurobiol. 2014;40(3):337–44.
59. Bettegowda C, Agrawal N, Jiao Y, Wang Y, Wood LD, Rodriguez FJ, et al. Exomic sequencing of four rare central nervous system tumor types. Oncotarget. 2013;4(4):572–83. Epub 2013/04/18.

60. Dias-Santagata D, Lam Q, Vernovsky K, Vena N, Lennerz JK, Borger DR, et al. BRAF V600E mutations are common in pleomorphic xanthoastrocytoma: diagnostic and therapeutic implications. PLoS One. 2011;6(3):e17948. Epub 2011/04/12.
61. Hawkins C, Walker E, Mohamed N, Zhang C, Jacob K, Shirinian M, et al. BRAF-KIAA1549 fusion predicts better clinical outcome in pediatric low-grade astrocytoma. Clin Cancer Res. 2011;17(14):4790–8. Epub 2011/05/26.
62. Horbinski C, Nikiforova MN, Hagenkord JM, Hamilton RL, Pollack IF. Interplay among BRAF, p16, p53, and MIB1 in pediatric low-grade gliomas. Neuro Oncol. 2012;14(6):777–89. Epub 2012/04/12.
63. Tian Y, Rich BE, Vena N, Craig JM, Macconaill LE, Rajaram V, et al. Detection of KIAA1549-BRAF fusion transcripts in formalin-fixed paraffin-embedded pediatric low-grade gliomas. J Mol Diagn. 2011;13(6):669–77. Epub 2011/09/03.
64. Sievert AJ, Lang SS, Boucher KL, Madsen PJ, Slaunwhite E, Choudhari N, et al. Paradoxical activation and RAF inhibitor resistance of BRAF protein kinase fusions characterizing pediatric astrocytomas. Proc Natl Acad Sci U S A. 2013;110(15):5957–62. Epub 2013/03/28.
65. Jacob K, Quang-Khuong DA, Jones DT, Witt H, Lambert S, Albrecht S, et al. Genetic aberrations leading to MAPK pathway activation mediate oncogene-induced senescence in sporadic pilocytic astrocytomas. Clin Cancer Res. 2011;17(14):4650–60. Epub 2011/05/26.
66. Raabe EH, Lim KS, Kim JM, Meeker A, Mao XG, Nikkhah G, et al. BRAF activation induces transformation and then senescence in human neural stem cells: a pilocytic astrocytoma model. Clin Cancer Res. 2011;17(11):3590–9. Epub 2011/06/04.
67. Guertin DA, Sabatini DM. The pharmacology of mTOR inhibition. Sci Signal. 2009;2(67):e24. Epub 2009/04/23.
68. Banerjee S, Crouse NR, Emnett RJ, Gianino SM, Gutmann DH. Neurofibromatosis-1 regulates mTOR-mediated astrocyte growth and glioma formation in a TSC/Rheb-independent manner. Proc Natl Acad Sci U S A. 2011;108(38):15996–6001. Epub 2011/09/08.
69. Jentoft M, Giannini C, Cen L, Scheithauer BW, Hoesley B, Sarkaria JN, et al. Phenotypic variations in NF1-associated low grade astrocytomas: possible role for increased mTOR activation in a subset. Int J Clin Exp Pathol. 2010;4(1):43–57. Epub 2011/01/14.
70. Rodriguez EF, Scheithauer BW, Giannini C, Rynearson A, Cen L, Hoesley B, et al. PI3K/AKT pathway alterations are associated with clinically aggressive and histologically anaplastic subsets of pilocytic astrocytoma. Acta Neuropathol. 2011;121(3):407–20. Epub 2010/11/30.
71. Hütt-Cabezas M, Karajannis MA, Zagzag D, Shah S, Horkayne-Szakaly I, Rushing EJ, et al. Activation of mTORC1/mTORC2 signaling in pediatric low-grade glioma and pilocytic astrocytoma reveals mTOR as a therapeutic target. Neuro Oncol. 2013;15(12):1604–14.
72. Franz DN, Belousova E, Sparagana S, Bebin EM, Frost M, Kuperman R, et al. Efficacy and safety of everolimus for subependymal giant cell astrocytomas associated with tuberous sclerosis complex (EXIST-1): a multicentre, randomised, placebo-controlled phase 3 trial. Lancet. 2013;381(9861):125–32. Epub 2012/11/20.
73. Zhang J, Wu G, Miller CP, Tatevossian RG, Dalton JD, Tang B, et al. Whole-genome sequencing identifies genetic alterations in pediatric low-grade gliomas. Nat Genet. 2013;45:602–12.
74. Cairncross JG, Ueki K, Zlatescu MC, Lisle DK, Finkelstein DM, Hammond RR, et al. Specific genetic predictors of chemotherapeutic response and survival in patients with anaplastic oligodendrogliomas. J Natl Cancer Inst. 1998;90(19):1473–9. Epub 1998/10/17.
75. Jenkins RB, Curran W, Scott CB, Cairncross G. Pilot evaluation of 1p and 19q deletions in anaplastic oligodendrogliomas collected by a national cooperative cancer treatment group. Am J Clin Oncol. 2001;24(5):506–8. Epub 2001/10/05.
76. Harada S, Henderson LB, Eshleman JR, Gocke CD, Burger P, Griffin CA, et al. Genomic changes in gliomas detected using single nucleotide polymorphism array in formalin-fixed, paraffin-embedded tissue: superior results compared with microsatellite analysis. J Mol Diagn. 2011;13(5):541–8. Epub 2011/07/06.
77. Griffin CA, Burger P, Morsberger L, Yonescu R, Swierczynski S, Weingart JD, et al. Identification of der(1;19)(q10;p10) in five oligodendrogliomas suggests mechanism of concurrent 1p and 19q loss. J Neuropathol Exp Neurol. 2006;65(10):988–94. Epub 2006/10/06.
78. Jenkins RB, Blair H, Ballman KV, Giannini C, Arusell RM, Law M, et al. A t(1;19)(q10;p10) mediates the combined deletions of 1p and 19q and predicts a better prognosis of patients with oligodendroglioma. Cancer Res. 2006;66(20):9852–61. Epub 2006/10/19.
79. Bettegowda C, Agrawal N, Jiao Y, Sausen M, Wood LD, Hruban RH, et al. Mutations in CIC and FUBP1 contribute to human oligodendroglioma. Science. 2011;333(6048):1453–5. Epub 2011/08/06.
80. Yip S, Butterfield YS, Morozova O, Chittaranjan S, Blough MD, An J, et al. Concurrent CIC mutations, IDH mutations, and 1p/19q loss distinguish oligodendrogliomas from other cancers. J Pathol. 2012;226(1):7–16. Epub 2011/11/11.
81. Hartmann C, Meyer J, Balss J, Capper D, Mueller W, Christians A, et al. Type and frequency of IDH1 and IDH2 mutations are related to astrocytic and oligodendroglial differentiation and age: a study of 1,010 diffuse gliomas. Acta Neuropathol. 2009;118(4):469–74. Epub 2009/06/26.
82. Watanabe T, Nobusawa S, Kleihues P, Ohgaki H. IDH1 mutations are early events in the development of astrocytomas and oligodendrogliomas. Am J Pathol. 2009;174(4):1149–53. Epub 2009/02/28.
83. Yan H, Parsons DW, Jin G, McLendon R, Rasheed BA, Yuan W, et al. IDH1 and IDH2 mutations in gliomas. N Engl J Med. 2009;360(8):765–73. Epub 2009/02/21.
84. Dang L, White DW, Gross S, Bennett BD, Bittinger MA, Driggers EM, et al. Cancer-associated IDH1 mutations produce 2-hydroxyglutarate. Nature. 2009;462(7274):739–44. Epub 2009/11/26.
85. Horbinski C. What do we know about IDH1/2 mutations so far, and how do we use it? Acta Neuropathol. 2013;125(5):621–36. Epub 2013/03/21.
86. Yang H, Ye D, Guan KL, Xiong Y. IDH1 and IDH2 mutations in tumorigenesis: mechanistic insights and clinical perspec-

tives. Clin Cancer Res. 2012;18(20):5562–71. Epub 2012/10/17.

87. Camelo-Piragua S, Jansen M, Ganguly A, Kim JC, Cosper AK, Dias-Santagata D, et al. A sensitive and specific diagnostic panel to distinguish diffuse astrocytoma from astrocytosis: chromosome 7 gain with mutant isocitrate dehydrogenase 1 and p53. J Neuropathol Exp Neurol. 2011;70(2):110–5. Epub 2011/02/24.
88. Capper D, Weissert S, Balss J, Habel A, Meyer J, Jager D, et al. Characterization of R132H mutation-specific IDH1 antibody binding in brain tumors. Brain Pathol. 2010;20(1):245–54. Epub 2009/11/12.
89. Heaphy CM, de Wilde RF, Jiao Y, Klein AP, Edil BH, Shi C, et al. Altered telomeres in tumors with ATRX and DAXX mutations. Science. 2011;333(6041):425. Epub 2011/07/02.
90. Kannan K, Inagaki A, Silber J, Gorovets D, Zhang J, Kastenhuber ER, et al. Whole-exome sequencing identifies ATRX mutation as a key molecular determinant in lower-grade glioma. Oncotarget. 2012;3(10):1194–203. Epub 2012/10/30.
91. Liu XY, Gerges N, Korshunov A, Sabha N, Khuong-Quang DA, Fontebasso AM, et al. Frequent ATRX mutations and loss of expression in adult diffuse astrocytic tumors carrying IDH1/IDH2 and TP53 mutations. Acta Neuropathol. 2012;124(5):615–25. Epub 2012/08/14.
92. Nguyen DN, Heaphy CM, de Wilde RF, Orr BA, Odia Y, Eberhart CG, et al. Molecular and morphologic correlates of the alternative lengthening of telomeres phenotype in high-grade astrocytomas. Brain Pathol. 2013;23(3):237–43. Epub 2012/08/30.
93. Jiao Y, Killela PJ, Reitman ZJ, Rasheed AB, Heaphy CM, de Wilde RF, et al. Frequent ATRX, CIC, FUBP1 and IDH1 mutations refine the classification of malignant gliomas. Oncotarget. 2012;3(7):709–22. Epub 2012/08/08.
94. Killela PJ, Reitman ZJ, Jiao Y, Bettegowda C, Agrawal N, Diaz Jr LA, et al. TERT promoter mutations occur frequently in gliomas and a subset of tumors derived from cells with low rates of self-renewal. Proc Natl Acad Sci U S A. 2013;110(15):6021–6. Epub 2013/03/27.
95. Ramkissoon LA, Horowitz PM, Craig JM, Ramkissoon SH, Rich BE, Schumacher SE, et al. Genomic analysis of diffuse pediatric low-grade gliomas identifies recurrent oncogenic truncating rearrangements in the transcription factor MYBL1. Proc Natl Acad Sci U S A. 2013;110(20):8188–93. Epub 2013/05/02.
96. Korshunov A, Meyer J, Capper D, Christians A, Remke M, Witt H, et al. Combined molecular analysis of BRAF and IDH1 distinguishes pilocytic astrocytoma from diffuse astrocytoma. Acta Neuropathol. 2009;118(3):401–5. Epub 2009/06/23.
97. Badiali M, Gleize V, Paris S, Moi L, Elhouadani S, Arcella A, et al. KIAA1549-BRAF fusions and IDH mutations can coexist in diffuse gliomas of adults. Brain Pathol. 2012;22(6):841–7. Epub 2012/05/18.
98. Kim YH, Nonoguchi N, Paulus W, Brokinkel B, Keyvani K, Sure U, et al. Frequent BRAF gain in low-grade diffuse gliomas with 1p/19q loss. Brain Pathol. 2012;22(6):834–40. Epub 2012/05/10.
99. Noushmehr H, Weisenberger DJ, Diefes K, Phillips HS, Pujara K, Berman BP, et al. Identification of a CpG island methylator phenotype that defines a distinct subgroup of glioma. Cancer Cell. 2010;17(5):510–22. Epub 2010/04/20.
100. Turcan S, Rohle D, Goenka A, Walsh LA, Fang F, Yilmaz E, et al. IDH1 mutation is sufficient to establish the glioma hypermethylator phenotype. Nature. 2012;483(7390):479–83. Epub 2012/02/22.
101. Mur P, Mollejo M, Ruano Y, de Lope AR, Fiano C, Garcia JF, et al. Codeletion of 1p and 19q determines distinct gene methylation and expression profiles in IDH-mutated oligodendroglial tumors. Acta Neuropathol. 2013;126(2):277–89. Epub 2013/05/22.
102. Ho CY, Bar E, Giannini C, Marchionni L, Karajannis MA, Zagzag D, et al. MicroRNA profiling in pediatric pilocytic astrocytoma reveals biologically relevant targets, including PBX3, NFIB, and METAP2. Neuro Oncol. 2013;15(1):69–82. Epub 2012/11/20.
103. Lambert SR, Witt H, Hovestadt V, Zucknick M, Kool M, Pearson DM, et al. Differential expression and methylation of brain developmental genes define location-specific subsets of pilocytic astrocytoma. Acta Neuropathol. 2013;126(2):291–301. Epub 2013/05/11.
104. Goeppert B, Schmidt CR, Geiselhart L, Dutruel C, Capper D, Renner M, et al. Differential expression of the tumor suppressor A-kinase anchor protein 12 in human diffuse and pilocytic astrocytomas is regulated by promoter methylation. J Neuropathol Exp Neurol. 2013;72(10):933–41. Epub 2013/09/18.
105. Tatevossian RG, Lawson ARJ, Forshew T, Hindley GFL, Ellison DW, Sheer D. MAPK pathway activation and the origins of pediatric low-grade astrocytomas. J Cell Physiol. 2010;222(3):509–14.
106. Karajannis M, Fisher M, Milla S, Cohen K, Legault G, Wisoff J, et al. Phase II study of sorafenib in children with recurrent/progressive low-grade astrocytomas. Neuro Oncol. 2013;15:32–3.
107. Shahabi V, Whitney G, Hamid O, Schmidt H, Chasalow S, Alaparthy S, et al. Assessment of association between BRAF-V600E mutation status in melanomas and clinical response to ipilimumab. Cancer Immunol Immunother. 2012;61(5):733–7.
108. Chapman PB, Hauschild A, Robert C, Haanen JB, Ascierto P, Larkin J, et al. Improved survival with vemurafenib in melanoma with BRAF V600E mutation. N Engl J Med. 2011;364(26): 2507–16.
109. Wiencke JK, Zheng S, Jelluma N, Tihan T, Vandenberg S, Tamguney T, et al. Methylation of the PTEN promoter defines low-grade gliomas and secondary glioblastoma. Neuro Oncol. 2007;9(3):271–9.
110. Neshat MS, Mellinghoff IK, Tran C, Stiles B, Thomas G, Petersen R, et al. Enhanced sensitivity of PTEN-deficient tumors to inhibition of FRAP/mTOR. Proc Natl Acad Sci U S A. 2001;98(18):10314–9.
111. Xu G, Zhang W, Bertram P, Zheng XF, McLeod H. Pharmacogenomic profiling of the PI3K/PTEN-AKT-mTOR pathway in common human tumors. Int J Oncol. 2004;24(4):893–900.
112. Choe G, Horvath S, Cloughesy TF, Crosby K, Seligson D, Palotie A, et al. Analysis of the phosphatidylinositol 3′-kinase

signaling pathway in glioblastoma patients in vivo. Cancer Res. 2003;63(11):2742–6.
113. Gera JF, Mellinghoff IK, Shi Y, Rettig MB, Tran C, Hsu JH, et al. AKT activity determines sensitivity to mammalian target of rapamycin (mTOR) inhibitors by regulating cyclin D1 and c-myc expression. J Biol Chem. 2004;279(4):2737–46.
114. Noh WC, Mondesire WH, Peng J, Jian W, Zhang H, Dong J, et al. Determinants of rapamycin sensitivity in breast cancer cells. Clin Cancer Res. 2004;10(3):1013–23.
115. Meric-Bernstam F, Gonzalez-Angulo AM. Targeting the mTOR signaling network for cancer therapy. J Clin Oncol. 2009;27(13): 2278–87.
116. Becher OJ, Trippett T, Gilheeney S, Khakoo Y, Lyden D, Haque S, et al. Phase I study of perifosine (AKT inhibitor) for recurrent pediatric solid tumors. Neuro Oncol. 2010;12(6):II42.
117. Franz DN, Leonard J, Tudor C, Chuck G, Care M, Sethuraman G, et al. Rapamycin causes regression of astrocytomas in tuberous sclerosis complex. Ann Neurol. 2006;59(3):490–8.
118. Dasgupta B, Yi Y, Chen DY, Weber JD, Gutmann DH. Proteomic analysis reveals hyperactivation of the mammalian target of rapamycin pathway in neurofibromatosis 1-associated human and mouse brain tumors. Cancer Res. 2005;65(7):2755–60. Epub 2005/04/05.
119. Packer RJ, Yalon M, Rood BR, Chao M, Miller MM, McCowage G, et al. Phase I/II study of Tarceva/Rapamcin for recurrent pediatric low-grade gliomas (LGG). Neuro Oncol. 2010;12(6):ii20.
120. Kieran MYX, Macy M, Geyer R, Cohen K, MacDonald T, Allen J, Boklan J, Smith A, Nazemi K, Gore L, Trippett T, DiRenzo J, Narendran A, Perentesis J, Prabhu S, Pinches N, Robison N, Manley P, Chi S. A prospective multi-institutional phase II study of everolimus (Rad001), an mTOR Inhibitor, in pediatric patients with recurrent or progressive low-grade glioma. Pediatric Blood & Cancer, SIOP 2013 Scientific Programme. 2013;60(S3):O-0068.
121. Cd B. PI3K and MEK inhibitor combinations: examining the evidence in selected tumor types. Cancer Chemother Pharmacol. 2013;71:1395–409.
122. Jokinen E, Laurila N, Koivunen J. Alternative dosing of dual PI3K and MEK inhibition in cancer therapy. BMC Cancer. 2012;12:612.
123. Juratli T, Kirsch M, Robel K, Soucek S, Geiger K, Kummer R, et al. IDH mutations as an early and consistent marker in low-grade astrocytomas WHO grade II and their consecutive secondary high-grade gliomas. J Neurooncol. 2012;108(3):403–10.
124. Kloosterhof NK, Bralten LBC, Dubbink HJ, French PJ, van den Bent MJ. Isocitrate dehydrogenase-1 mutations: a fundamentally new understanding of diffuse glioma? Lancet Oncol. 2011;12(1): 83–91.
125. Parsons DW, Jones S, Zhang X, Lin JC-H, Leary RJ, Angenendt P, et al. An integrated genomic analysis of human glioblastoma multiforme. Science. 2008;321(5897):1807–12.
126. Paschka P, Schlenk RF, Gaidzik VI, Habdank M, Krönke J, Bullinger L, et al. IDH1 and IDH2 mutations are frequent genetic alterations in acute myeloid leukemia and confer adverse prognosis in cytogenetically normal acute myeloid leukemia with NPM1 mutation without FLT3 internal tandem duplication. J Clin Oncol. 2010;28(22):3636–43.
127. Hartmann C, Hentschel B, Tatagiba M, Schramm J, Schnell O, Seidel C, et al. Molecular markers in low-grade gliomas: predictive or prognostic? Clin Cancer Res. 2011;17(13): 4588–99.
128. Houillier C, Wang X, Kaloshi G, Mokhtari K, Guillevin R, Laffaire J, et al. IDH1 or IDH2 mutations predict longer survival and response to temozolomide in low-grade gliomas. Neurology. 2010;75(17):1560–6.
129. Ahmadi R, Stockhammer F, Becker N, Hohlen K, Misch M, Christians A, et al. No prognostic value of IDH1 mutations in a series of 100 WHO grade II astrocytomas. J Neurooncol. 2012;109(1):15–22.
130. Rohle D, Popovici-Muller J, Palaskas N, Turcan S, Grommes C, Campos C, et al. An Inhibitor of mutant IDH1 delays growth and promotes differentiation of glioma cells. Science. 2013;340(6132): 626–30.
131. Popovici-Muller J, Saunders JO, Salituro FG, Travins JM, Yan S, Zhao F, et al. Discovery of the first potent inhibitors of mutant IDH1 that lower tumor 2-HG in vivo. ACS Med Chem Lett. 2012;3(10):850–5.
132. Seltzer MJ, Bennett BD, Joshi AD, Gao P, Thomas AG, Ferraris DV, et al. Inhibition of glutaminase preferentially slows growth of glioma cells with mutant IDH1. Cancer Res. 2010;70(22): 8981–7.

5
Ependymoma

Till Milde, Andrey Korshunov, Olaf Witt,
Stefan M. Pfister, and Hendrik Witt

Ependymomas constitute about 10 % of pediatric brain tumors, with an annual incidence of 0.3/100,000 children. Median age at diagnosis is 6 years and the male to female ratio is 1.2/1. Ependymomas are thought to arise from radial glia cells in the subventricular zone of the brain [1], and 2/3 of all ependymomas are located in the fourth ventricle [2]. Thus, clinical symptoms are often caused by obstruction of the ventricular system, and patients frequently present with headache, nausea, and vomiting. In addition, cerebellar ataxia or weakness of the abducens nerve can be present. Other common tumor locations include the supratentorial ventricular system, brain stem, and spinal canal.

Ependymomas pose a major challenge in pediatric oncology due to their large clinical and biological heterogeneity, as well as their limited sensitivity towards classical chemotherapy. The treatment of ependymomas therefore has rested largely on surgery and radiation therapy, with limited treatment options for patients with recurrent disease. In recent years, however, significant progress has been made in our understanding of the tumor genetics and biology of ependymoma. Based on molecular genetic information, it has become clear that histologically indistinguishable tumors can differ fundamentally in terms of disease biology. Although most of this new knowledge has yet to be translated successfully into clinical practice, the coming years promise to become a period of progress by incorporating disease biology into diagnostic and therapeutic algorithms. It is expected that further insights into tumor biology continue to be gained by rapidly evolving experimental technologies, such as next-generation sequencing and epigenetic profiling (DNA methylation, histone modifications, miRNA profiling), as well as improved preclinical models. We anticipate that these advances will improve risk stratification of newly diagnosed patients and allow for the development of novel, risk-adapted treatment protocols. Furthermore, the incorporation of molecular targeted therapies holds promise for future therapies that are less toxic and/or more effective than current standard approaches.

The following chapter will therefore attempt to summarize our current body of knowledge about the molecular genetics and biology of ependymomas, its application to clinically relevant risk stratification of patients, and the opportunities for developing novel molecular targeted therapies.

Histopathology

Macroscopically, ependymomas appear as well-circumscribed tumors. Histological features typically seen in ependymomas include perivascular pseudorosettes composed of glial tumor cells that are radially arranged around blood vessels, and true ependymal rosettes of tumor cells that form a central lumen. Perivascular pseudorosettes occur in the great majority of these neoplasms, whereas true ependymal rosettes are only present in a minority of tumors. Notably, these features can be found in ependymomas across all molecular subtypes. Regressive changes include areas of myxoid degeneration and calcifications. The current World Health Organization (WHO) classification [3] recognizes two histological grades of ependymomas: grade II ("classic" ependymoma) and III (anaplastic ependymoma).

The following histopathological variants of *WHO grade II ependymomas* can be distinguished [3]: (1) *Cellular ependymoma* shows conspicuous cellularity without a significant increase in mitotic activity. (2) *Papillary ependymoma* shows well-formed papillae in which tumor vessels are covered by a layer of tumor cells. (3) *Clear cell ependymoma* displays an oligodendroglia-like appearance with a perinuclear halo. These tumors appear to be preferentially located in the cerebral hemispheres and frequently progress to high-grade ependymomas. (4) Tanycytic ependymoma consists of cells which are arranged in the fascicles with variable width and cell density. These tumors are more frequent in the spinal cord. In addition, rare ependymoma variants including lipomatous ependymoma, giant cell ependymoma, melanotic ependymoma, signet ring cell ependymomas, and

M.A. Karajannis and D. Zagzag (eds.), *Molecular Pathology of Nervous System Tumors: Biological Stratification and Targeted Therapies*, Molecular Pathology Library 8,
DOI 10.1007/978-1-4939-1830-0_5,

ovarian ependymoma have been described. Occasional non-palisading tumor necrosis may be observed, and is compatible with ependymoma WHO grade II. Immunohistochemistry of GFAP is usually applied for routine diagnostics of ependymal tumors, together with the EMA antibody that typically reveals dot-like immunostaining with a predominant localization along the luminal surface of ependymal rosettes.

Anaplastic ependymomas (WHO grade III) tend to remain as well-demarcated lesions, but are sometimes frankly invasive. Occasionally, extraventricular location with extensive infiltration of white matter can be noted. Microscopically, these tumors include highly cellular and poorly differentiated areas with rare pseudorosettes, brisk mitotic activity and frequent microvascular proliferation and necroses with palisading cells. However, histological classification of ependymomas into WHO grades II and III can be challenging, and even experienced neuropathologists commonly differ in their grading [4].

Cytogenetics and Molecular Genetics

Although our knowledge of tumorigenesis, biology, and progression of ependymoma has advanced significantly during the past 10 years, we are still in the early stages of translating this knowledge into clinical research and practice. Several candidate oncogenes and tumor suppressor genes have emerged as potential therapeutic targets and a novel molecular staging system was recently proposed with the potential to improve future stratification of ependymoma patients in clinical studies [5].

Germline mutations of the tumor suppressor gene *NF2* on chromosome 22q are associated with a variety of central nervous system (CNS) tumors, including ependymomas, schwannomas, and meningiomas. In sporadic ependymoma, however, *NF2* mutations appear to be restricted to a subset of spinal ependymomas in adult patients [6].

Early cytogenetic and comparative genomic hybridization studies provided the first evidence that ependymoma represents a biologically heterogeneous group of diseases [7, 8]. These initial studies, however, were limited by low genomic resolution, limited numbers of tumor samples from different CNS locations, and lack of detailed clinical and patient outcome data. In contrast, more recent studies using larger sample sizes and at higher resolutions have identified genetic signatures that could readily distinguish ependymomas arising in different anatomic localizations [1].

The most frequent genetic abnormalities in primary pediatric ependymoma involve gains of chromosome 1q, 5, 7, 9, 11, 18, and 20 and of losses chromosome 1p, 3, 6q, 6, 9p, 13q, 17, and 22. Several groups reported chromosome gain at 1q with an incidence of approximately 25 % to be the most frequently detected aberration in childhood ependymoma. Notably, gain of chromosome 1q has also been identified as the most consistent biomarker being associated with poor outcome and fossa posterior location in independent studies [6, 7]. These findings suggest that chromosome 1q may host candidate genes involved in ependymoma tumorigenesis and/or progression. Potential driver oncogenes located on chromosome 1q, especially within the hotspot region 1q21–32, include *DUSP12* (1q23.3), *S100A10* (1q21), *CHI3LI* (1q32.1), *TPR*, *SHC1*, *JTB*, and *HSPA6* (1q32) [9].

Loss of chromosome 22, especially complete or partial monosomy of chromosome 22, was reported as one of the most common aberrations in sporadic ependymomas. Aside from *NF2*, reduced expression of other candidate genes contained in the minimally deleted region at chromosome 22q has been observed, including *SULTA4*, a gene widely expressed in several compartments of the human brain, as well as *CBX7*, *G22P1*, and *MCM5*, which may be involved in cellular DNA repair and/or replication [8, 10].

Another recurrent finding in pediatric intracranial ependymoma is loss of chromosome 6q, which has been linked to an increased risk of recurrence. In particular, deletion of chromosome 6q23 has been associated with poor progression-free survival. Several genes located within this region were found to be downregulated in tumors with a heterozygous deletion, including *SASH1*, *TCP1*, *ADM1*, and *CDK11* [9].

Recently, chromosome 9q33–34 was identified as one of the most frequently gained regions (up to 36 % of patients), mainly occurring in posterior fossa tumors arising in children. The prognostic value of 9q gain remains controversial, since one study showed an association with increased risk of relapse, whereas a more recent one found this aberration to define a lower-risk group [5, 11]. Since different markers were used to identify 9q gains in these studies, one likely explanation for these differing results is that the precise genomic location is of major importance. Nevertheless, the biological relevance of this genomic region is supported by the fact that it harbors two oncogenes, namely *NOTCH1* and *TNC* which had previously been linked to brain tumorigenesis [11]. The *TNC* gene was shown to be upregulated in infant ependymomas, and overexpression was associated with a short time to relapse and poor prognosis [11, 12]. In addition, Notch pathway members, including receptors (Notch1 and Notch2), ligands (JAG1, DLL1, and DLL2), and downstream targets (HES1, HEY2, and MYC), were observed to be consistently overexpressed in ependymoma [11, 13]. The first hint towards involvement of Notch signaling came from a report by Taylor et al., in which activation of Notch signaling was observed in both supratentorial and spinal ependymomas [1].

Homozygous deletion of *CDKN2A/p16*$^{\mathrm{INK4a}}$ has repeatedly been detected in supratentorial ependymomas [1, 7, 14]. *CDKN2A/p16*$^{\mathrm{INK4a}}$, a tumor suppressor gene located at 9p21.3, regulates neural stem cell (NSC) proliferation, and its deletion has been shown to rapidly expand progenitor cell numbers in developing neural tissue.

Although we were able to demonstrate stepwise accumulation of genetic aberrations during disease progression for the first time in a case with anaplastic ependymoma [15], much work remains to be done to define the molecular changes that underlie disease recurrence and progression in ependymoma.

Gene Expression Profiling

A decade ago, the first studies were published to reveal distinct gene expression patterns separating subgroups of ependymoma [8]. Supporting this initial finding, a comprehensive picture of tumor heterogeneity associated with disease localization has emerged on a transcriptional and cytogenetic levels [1, 13, 16–18]. Recently, two distinct variants of posterior fossa ependymomas were identified by gene expression profiling, defined as Group A (Group 1 in [16]) and Group B (Group 2 in [16]) [18]. Group A tumors were associated with very poor outcomes, recurred at significantly higher rates, and developed metastases in more than 80 % of cases. Patients diagnosed with this disease variant were younger on average and their tumors tended to be located laterally within the posterior fossa. Approximately half of Group A patients developed a relapse of their disease, which notably was independent of the extent of surgical resection. From the genomic point of view, it was somewhat surprising to find that the genomes of these aggressive Group A tumors were without large cytogenetic alterations. This variant of ependymomas, however, comprised activation of classic cancer-related signaling pathways, such as EGFR, PDGF, RAS, ECM, VEGF, MAPK, and integrins. Strikingly, Group B ependymomas showed a highly disparate molecular profile, featuring large chromosomal aberrations, partially affecting whole p- or q-arms of a chromosome or the entire chromosome. Transcriptome profiling of Group B ependymomas showed highly specific overexpression of genes involved in ciliogenesis and microtubule assembly, as well as mitochondrial metabolism.

The existence of two biologically distinct variants of posterior fossa ependymomas was confirmed in a subsequent study [16]. Wani and colleagues observed overexpression of genes associated with mesenchyme in Group 1 tumors, as well as an association with younger age and reduced recurrence-free survival, similar to the findings by Witt and colleagues in Group A ependymomas [18]. Comparable to Group B tumors [18], Group 2 tumors were associated with an excellent prognosis, tended to occur in adolescent children and young adults, and did not express genes associated with altered gene ontology terms in their transcriptomes [16]. In addition, Wani et al. were able to define and validate a 10-gene signature to reliably classify posterior fossa ependymomas into the two groups. This gene signature, which can be obtained from small amounts of routine formalin-fixed, paraffin-embedded tissue, is of major interest as a clinically feasible approach for patient stratification in future clinical trials.

Another study by Johnson and colleagues performed a gene expression analysis of 83 ependymomas, including both supra- and infratentorial locations [17]. They were able to identify nine molecular subgroups in total, although their clinical relevance was uncertain, as detailed patient information and outcome data was unavailable [17]. The following molecular subgroups related to localization were described: four supratentorial subgroups (A–D), two subgroups of posterior fossa ependymomas including some spinal tumors (E, F), and three subgroups consisting of tumors of posterior fossa localization only (G, H, I) [17]. Integrating these findings of two variants of posterior fossa tumors, the distribution would be as follows: one variant corresponds to Group A by Witt et al., Group 1 by Wani et al., and Cluster G, H, and I by Johnson et al.; the other variant corresponds to Group B by Witt et al., Group 2 by Wani et al., and Cluster E and F by Johnson et al. (Fig. 5.1).

In conclusion, several independent studies have confirmed the presence of at least two, genetically and biologically, different variants of posterior fossa ependymoma. At present, the standard treatment for patients with posterior fossa ependymomas remains maximal safe surgical resection followed by adjuvant radiation therapy. The role of additional adjuvant chemotherapy is being investigated in an ongoing phase III clinical trial by the Children's Oncology Group (COG), ACNS0831, which includes planned post hoc molecular subgroup analysis. Future studies will be needed to investigate experimental, intensified treatment regimens in prospectively selected high-risk patients.

Subgroup-specific preclinical models are being developed [17, 19] and are expected to help inform the rational selection of novel therapies for testing in future clinical trials.

Prognostic Stratification

The two most widely accepted factors used for patient stratification are extent of resection, metastatic status, and WHO grading. WHO grading, as an important, independent prognostic marker has been described early on [20], and has recently been confirmed by a large meta-analysis investigating 2408 ependymoma patients [21], whereas other studies have suggested that tumor grading is highly dependent upon the experience of individual neuropathologists [22, 23]. Regarding molecular markers, deletion of *CDKN2A* along with 1q gain was identified as the strongest indicator of poor prognosis in a cohort of 292 intracranial ependymomas [5]. The same study was able to identify reliable cytogenetic markers for standard, intermediate, and high-risk ependymoma, comprising the first molecular staging system for ependymoma that could be validated in a completely non-overlapping patient cohort [5]. This cytogenetic risk stratification model for intracranial ependymoma comprises three cytogenetic subgroups. Group 1 is associated with standard risk, with tumors displaying large aberrations of chromosomes

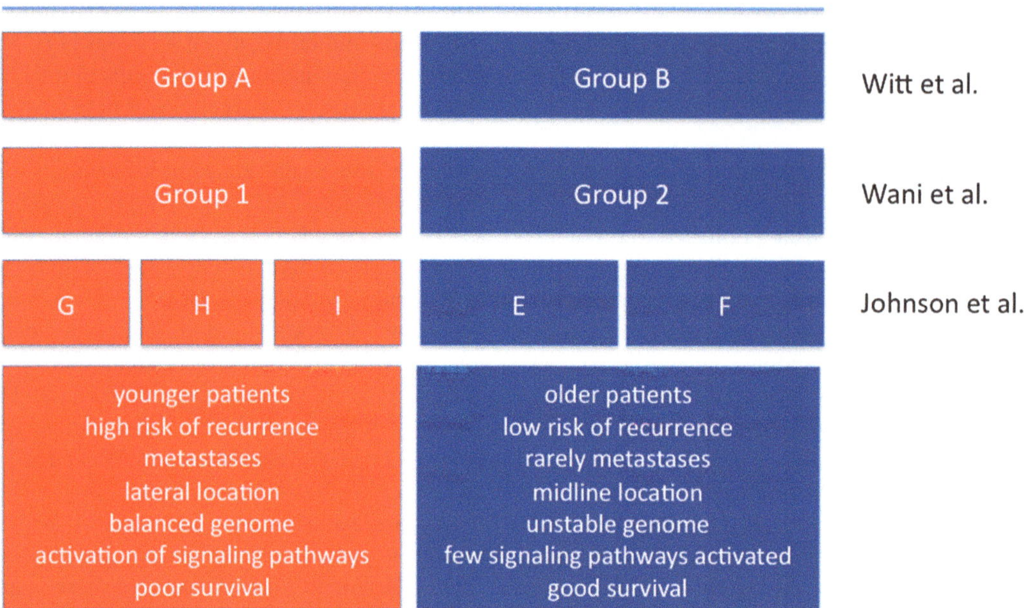

FIG. 5.1. Molecular subgroups of posterior fossa ependymoma, as described by Witt et al., Wani et al., and Johnson et al. Group A, Group 1, and clusters G, H, and I describe to same biological subgroup (*red*), as do Group B, Group 2, and clusters E and F (*blue*). Both subgroups differ significantly in their molecular and clinical variables.

6, 9, 15, and 18. Group 2 is associated with intermediate risk, and tumors show a balanced genome. Group 3 is associated with high risk, and defined by 1q gain and/or homozygous deletion of CDKN2A/B [5]. Gain of 1q25 as a negative prognostic marker has since been confirmed in three independent clinical cohorts (CCLG/SIOP, BBSFOP, and SIOP) [24]. A separate study confirmed gain of 1q as a negative prognostic marker in posterior fossa ependymoma [25].

In conclusion, copy number gain of chromosome 1q is the most widely published negative prognostic molecular marker and applies to both supra- and infratentorial ependymoma [5, 7, 18, 24–28].

Other prognostic markers that are based on immunohistochemistry, rather than cytogenetics, have also been identified. Tenascin C is an extracellular matrix protein and has been shown to be a negative prognostic marker in ependymoma [11, 12, 18]. The NSC marker Nestin is a negative prognostic marker identifying ependymoma with poor prognosis especially in WHO II tumors [29], possibly indicating a less favorable, undifferentiated phenotype. Conversely, expression of neurofilament light polypeptide 70 (encoded by *NEFL*) is a positive predictive marker in supratentorial ependymoma [30] and may indicate a more favorable, differentiated phenotype. The immunohistochemical markers LAMA2 and NELL2 delineate the two molecular subgroups in posterior fossa ependymoma described above: Group A tumors (with poor prognosis) are characterized by the pattern LAMA2 positive and NELL2 negative, and Group B tumors (with more favorable prognosis) by the pattern LAMA2 negative and NELL2 positive [18]. The delineation of two molecular subgroups by the expression of LAMA2 and NELL2, and their prognostic values, have since been confirmed in a separate study [16].

Finally, miRNAs associated with prognosis have been described in ependymoma: let-7d, miR-596, and miR-367 are associated with poor survival, and miR-203 is an independent predictor for time to relapse [31].

Molecular Signaling Pathways

Identification of molecular signaling pathways that can be targeted for therapeutic purposes will be crucial for the rational development of novel drug-based treatments. It is important to note that thorough characterization of molecular subgroups and establishment of faithful subgroup-specific models will be needed for successful preclinical testing. It has become evident that different molecular subgroups of posterior fossa ependymoma show distinct activation of molecular signaling pathways (Fig. 5.2): Group A shows activation of epidermal growth factor receptor (EGFR), platelet-derived growth factor (PDGF), vascular endothelial growth factor (VEGF), and mitogen-activated protein kinase (MAPK) among others [18]. Group B shows less activation of classic oncogenic signaling pathways; gene expression profiles, however, indicate activation of ciliogenesis, microtubule assembly and mitochondrial metabolism [18]. These promising findings display novel treatment opportunities in a

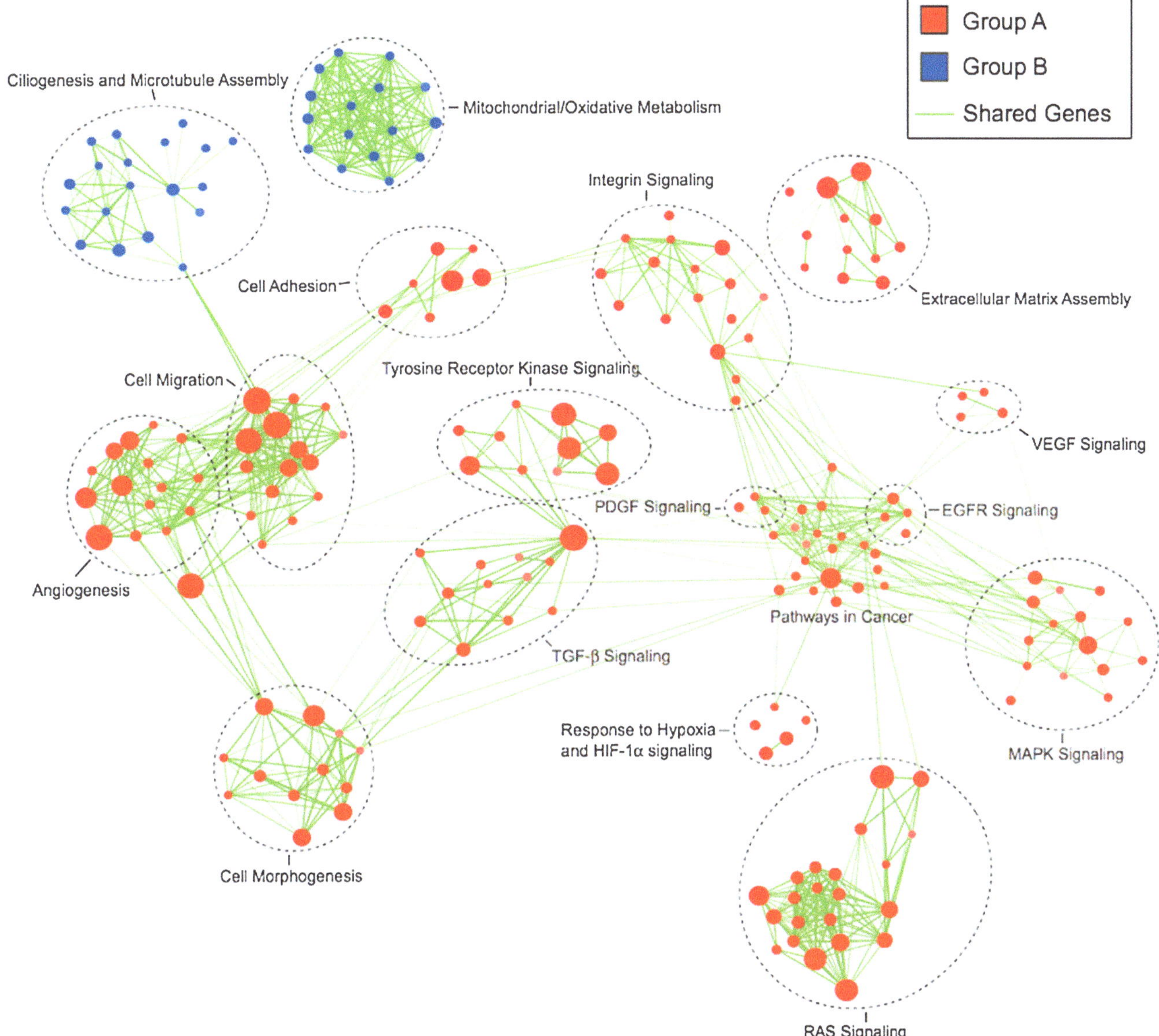

Fig. 5.2. Group A (*red*) and Group B (*blue*) posterior fossa ependymomas show distinct activation of signaling pathways and biological functions. The map was created by geneset enrichment analysis of transcriptomes of the two molecular subgroups of posterior fossa ependymomas, using Cytoscape and Enrichment Map (Adapted from Witt H, Mack SC, Ryzhova M, Bender S, Sill M, Isserlin R, et al. Delineation of two clinically and molecularly distinct subgroups of posterior fossa ependymoma. Cancer Cell. 2011;20:143-57, with permission).

fashion of subgroup-specific targeted therapies. A large number of therapeutic drugs inhibiting these molecular pathways (e.g. MAPK-, EGFR-, PDGF-, VEGF- and integrin-inhibitors) are already approved for other cancers and/or in various stages of clinical development, including those for pediatric patients. Carefully designed clinical studies will be needed to assess the potential of these agents to complement current standard therapies (surgery, radiotherapy) and/or other investigational therapies, such as chemotherapy. Of note, an integrated in vivo high-throughput drug screen using the preclinical supratentorial subgroup D-specific model [19] recently showed that the most active compounds against ependymoma which showed the least toxicity on NSCs were 5-FU and bortezomib, a proteasome inhibitor [19].

Other signaling pathways implicated in ependymoma biology are the Notch pathway, p53 and ERBB (EGFR and ERBB2/3/4), among others. Notch activation is associated with ependymoma progression [11], and inhibition of the Notch pathway using gamma-secretase inhibitors reduces neurosphere formation in vitro [11]. Aberrant expression of p53 was identified as an unfavorable prognostic marker in ependymoma, whereas its regulator MDM2 did not show an association with prognosis [12, 32]. The molecular mechanism of p53 pathway dysregulation in ependymoma is not yet understood. Despite frequent p53 overexpression in ependymoma, known mechanisms such as *TP53* mutation or promoter hypermethylation, MDM2 overexpression, P14[ARF] promoter hypermethylation or increased PAX5 expression are not observed in ependymoma. Furthermore, some studies implied the RTK1 family of proteins including EGFR, ERBB2, ERBB3, and ERBB4, in ependymoma biology, promoting growth, motility, and survival of ependymoma cells, whereas ERBB2 overexpression may potentiate radial glia proliferation [14]. In two studies, EGFR expression was found to be associated with an increased risk of disease recurrence [7, 12].

Molecular Targeted Therapies

Radical surgical resection, whenever feasible, remains the mainstay of ependymoma treatment and may be sufficient in a subset of patients with supratentorial ependymomas [33]. Because of high rates of local recurrence without additional therapy, adjuvant involved-field radiation therapy is generally employed in current standard treatment protocols. Nevertheless, local or distant disease recurrence is common, including for approximately half of all patients with posterior fossa ependymoma. In case of metastatic dissemination at diagnosis, craniospinal radiation therapy is typically used. The role of chemotherapy in the treatment of ependymoma is not well established, and response rates to single agent or combination chemotherapy in recurrent ependymoma are disappointing [34]. It has been shown, however, that chemotherapy can be effectively used to delay the beginning of radiotherapy in very young children, without compromising their prognosis [35]. Recent and ongoing clinical trials are examining the role of neoadjuvant chemotherapy in unresectable or disseminated disease, as well as in the adjuvant setting post radiation therapy for high-risk patients [36]. Due to the generally limited efficacy of classical chemotherapy in disseminated and recurrent ependymoma, however, novel therapies are urgently needed.

Based on the discovery of molecular signaling pathways relevant to ependymoma biology, several targeted therapy approaches are currently in development, including chromatin-modifying drugs. Early phase clinical trials are currently investigating compounds targeting Notch, EGFR, HDACs, and ERBB among others, as single agents or in combination with chemotherapy, in children with ependymoma.

Targeting the Notch pathway in a phase I clinical trial by using the gamma-secretase inhibitor MK-0752 showed that the MK-0752 is well tolerated in children, and response was seen in one ependymoma and one glioblastoma patient [37]. Promising preclinical data on EGFR inhibitors in ependymoma show success alone or in combination with phosphoinositide 3-kinase inhibitors [38, 39]. In vitro, ependymoma cells are sensitive to HDAC inhibitor (HDACi) treatment, which induced differentiation in subgroup C ependymoma cells [40] and increased apoptosis in others [41]. As a result, HDACis, such as vorinostat (suberoylanilide hydroxamic acid, SAHA), are being investigated in recent and ongoing clinical studies including patients with ependymoma [42, 43].

For both traditional chemotherapy and targeted agents, however, sufficient drug penetration into CNS tumor tissue and efficient target inhibition in vivo represent formidable challenges for successful translation of preclinical discoveries into effective clinical therapy. For example, a recent clinical and molecular biology study using the EGFR/ERBB2 inhibitor lapatinib in children with refractory brain tumors revealed that the drug failed to achieve meaningful concentration in the tumor tissues and, as a result, failed to inhibit the molecular targets [44].

Recently, two studies highlighted genetic and epigenetic alterations as therapeutic targets of different subtypes of ependymoma.

Posterior fossa ependymoma harbor nonrecurrent somatic mutations in a cohort of 47 tumors using whole-exome and whole-genome sequencing technologies [45]. Notably, a very low mutation rate was found in these tumors regardless of subgroups, with an average of only five somatic mutations per tumor (4.6 and 5.6 somatic mutations in Group A and Group B ependymomas, respectively). In contrast, DNA methylation patterns were highly dissimilar between both subtypes. When comparing only PF ependymoma subtypes, Group A ependymomas display a much higher proportion of methylated CpG-islands within the promoter regions as compared to Group B ependymomas. Based on this distinct pattern of epigenetic alteration, Group A tumors show a CpG-island methylator phenotype (CIMP). Additionally, Group A/CIMP-positive tumors show a greater extent of epigenetic silencing of targets of the polycomb repressive complex 2, including downregulation of differentiation genes through histone H3-lysine 27 (H3K27) trimethylation. To investigate if epigenetic agents can be used as potential novel treatment option for Group A tumors, in vitro and in vivo tests were performed. The preclinical treatment approaches using either 5-aza-2′-deoxycytidine, 3-deazaneplanocin A, or GSK343 (a selective inhibitor of the H3K27 methyltransferase EZH2) have shown very good response of cells and mice bearing Group A tumors. These results are promising treatment strategies targeting DNA CpG methylation, PRC2/EZH2, and/or histone deacetylases of this chemotherapy-resistant disease.

Another study, using whole-genome sequencing and/or RNA sequencing of 77 ependymomas, identified a novel gene fusion affecting *RELA* and *C11orf95* [46]. In line with findings of the study by Mack and colleagues, no recurrent somatic mutations were detected in posterior fossa ependymomas, including Group A and Group B. Notably, among supratentorial ependymomas Parker and colleagues discovered a frequent translocation within a region of chromosome 11q, which is possibly caused by chromotripsis (a recently discovered phenomenon of genomic rearrangement arising during a single genome-shattering event) and resulted in a *C11orf95-RELA* gene fusion in about 70 % of cases. RELA is a downstream target of the NF-κB signaling pathway, acting as a transcription factor and regulating several biological actions of cell maintenance. Importantly, a genetically engineered mouse model was successfully developed based of the *C11orf95-RELA* gene fusion. NSC from a Ink4a/Arf-null background were transduced with the retroviruses carrying the *C11orf95-RELA* fusion. These transgenic NSCs were then implanted into the cerebrum and developed supratentorial ependymomas within a few days. Hence, this model delivers excellent opportunities for preclinical drug testing in vivo of a supratentorial subtype of ependymomas.

Summary

As has been shown, genomic and gene expression profiling in ependymomas not only identifies biologically distinct subgroups but also allows for the stratification of patients into clinically meaningful prognostic subgroups. As demonstrated by the delineation of Group A and B posterior fossa ependymomas, the tight association between molecular profile and clinical behavior is of high practical relevance for the individual patient. One simple consequence of the identification of a Group A vs. Group B tumor for the patient is the new possibility of truly risk-adapted adjuvant treatment of previously equally treated tumors. Thus, the identification of the molecular profile adds considerable additional information to the classical histopathological analysis, enabling better informed clinical decisions.

The first steps toward better tumor diagnostics and disease stratification have been completed on the molecular level, now the key to successful translation into the clinic lies in (1) faithful preclinical models, (2) appropriate patient selection, and (3) careful consideration of pharmacological issues in brain tumors.

The strong heterogeneity of the tumor biology between different ependymoma subgroups, such as Group A and B, implies that the therapeutic treatment of each subgroup needs to be addressed individually. As has been shown in subgroup specific mouse models, new drugs can be validated and "old" drugs rediscovered for a very specific subset of ependymomas. Thorough characterization of preclinical models and their molecular subgroup therefore has to be a prerequisite for preclinical studies in order to yield results that can be translated into the clinic. Accordingly, the appropriate patient selection is of paramount importance for the success of future clinical trials. Not only do the trial design and therapy need to be tailored to the molecular ependymoma subgroups, but individual patients' molecular subgroup and targets will need to be confirmed reliably and in real-time. Future clinical studies should therefore include thorough molecular characterization of the tumor to be treated. Finally, pharmacological issues such as clinically achievable concentrations of the drug of interest, as well as the blood brain barrier (BBB) need to be taken into account for clinical trial design, and confirmation of successful target inhibition in the tumor tissue itself would be highly desirable as part of trials exploring novel, molecular targeted drugs.

The advent of high-throughput molecular analyses such as whole genome sequencing or genome-wide methylome analysis at affordable prices will undoubtedly allow for rapid and comprehensive molecular characterization of individual patients' tumors not only for research, but also in routine clinical practice. The patients will benefit from these insights if we can succeed in the translation of the molecular knowledge into novel and more effective individual treatment strategies.

References

1. Taylor MD, Poppleton H, Fuller C, Su X, Liu Y, Jensen P, et al. Radial glia cells are candidate stem cells of ependymoma. Cancer Cell. 2005;8:323–35.
2. McGuire CS, Sainani KL, Fisher PG. Both location and age predict survival in ependymoma: a SEER study. Pediatr Blood Cancer. 2009;52:65–9.
3. Louis D, Ohgaki H, Wiestler O, Cavenee W, Burger P, Jouvet A, et al. The 2007 WHO classification of tumours of the central nervous system. Acta Neuropathol. 2007;114:97–109.
4. Ellison DW, Kocak M, Figarella-Branger D, Felice G, Catherine G, Pietsch T, et al. Histopathological grading of pediatric ependymoma: reproducibility and clinical relevance in European trial cohorts. J Negat Results Biomed. 2011;10:7.
5. Korshunov A, Witt H, Hielscher T, Benner A, Remke M, Ryzhova M, et al. Molecular staging of intracranial ependymoma in children and adults. J Clin Oncol. 2010;28(19):3182–90.
6. Mack SC, Taylor MD. The genetic and epigenetic basis of ependymoma. Childs Nerv Syst. 2009;25:1195–201.
7. Mendrzyk F, Korshunov A, Benner A, Toedt G, Pfister S, Radlwimmer B, et al. Identification of gains on 1q and epidermal growth factor receptor overexpression as independent prognostic markers in intracranial ependymoma. Clin Cancer Res. 2006;12:2070–9.
8. Korshunov A, Neben K, Wrobel G, Tews B, Benner A, Hahn M, et al. Gene expression patterns in ependymomas correlate with tumor location, grade, and patient age. Am J Pathol. 2003;163: 1721–7.
9. Kilday JP, Rahman R, Dyer S, Ridley L, Lowe J, Coyle B, et al. Pediatric ependymoma: biological perspectives. Mol Cancer Res. 2009;7:765–86.
10. Suarez-Merino B, Hubank M, Revesz T, Harkness W, Hayward R, Thompson D, et al. Microarray analysis of pediatric ependymoma identifies a cluster of 112 candidate genes including four transcripts at 22q12.1-q13.3. Neuro Oncol. 2005;7:20–31.
11. Puget S, Grill J, Valent A, Bieche I, Dantas-Barbosa C, Kauffmann A, et al. Candidate genes on chromosome 9q33-34 involved in the progression of childhood ependymomas. J Clin Oncol. 2009;27:1884–92.
12. Korshunov A, Golanov A, Timirgaz V. Immunohistochemical markers for intracranial ependymoma recurrence. An analysis of 88 cases. J Neurol Sci. 2000;177:72–82.

13. Modena P, Lualdi E, Facchinetti F, Veltman J, Reid JF, Minardi S, et al. Identification of tumor-specific molecular signatures in intracranial ependymoma and association with clinical characteristics. J Clin Oncol. 2006;24:5223–33.
14. Poppleton H, Gilbertson RJ. Stem cells of ependymoma. Br J Cancer. 2007;96:6–10.
15. Milde T, Pfister S, Korshunov A, Deubzer H, Oehme I, Ernst A, et al. Stepwise accumulation of distinct genomic aberrations in a patient with progressively metastasizing ependymoma. Genes Chromosomes Cancer. 2009;48(3):229–38.
16. Wani K, Armstrong TS, Vera-Bolanos E, Raghunathan A, Ellison D, Gilbertson R, et al. A prognostic gene expression signature in infratentorial ependymoma. Acta Neuropathol. 2012;123(5):727–38.
17. Johnson RA, Wright KD, Poppleton H, Mohankumar KM, Finkelstein D, Pounds SB, et al. Cross-species genomics matches driver mutations and cell compartments to model ependymoma. Nature. 2010;466:632–6.
18. Witt H, Mack SC, Ryzhova M, Bender S, Sill M, Isserlin R, et al. Delineation of two clinically and molecularly distinct subgroups of posterior fossa ependymoma. Cancer Cell. 2011;20: 143–57.
19. Atkinson JM, Shelat AA, Carcaboso AM, Kranenburg TA, Arnold LA, Boulos N, et al. An integrated in vitro and in vivo high-throughput screen identifies treatment leads for ependymoma. Cancer Cell. 2011;20:384–99.
20. Korshunov A, Golanov A, Sycheva R, Timirgaz V. The histologic grade is a main prognostic factor for patients with intracranial ependymomas treated in the microneurosurgical era: an analysis of 258 patients. Cancer. 2004;100:1230–7.
21. Rodriguez D, Cheung MC, Housri N, Quinones-Hinojosa A, Camphausen K, Koniaris LG. Outcomes of malignant CNS ependymomas: an examination of 2408 cases through the Surveillance, Epidemiology, and End Results (SEER) database (1973–2005). J Surg Res. 2009;156:340–51.
22. Messahel B, Ashley S, Saran F, Ellison D, Ironside J, Phipps K, et al. Relapsed intracranial ependymoma in children in the UK: patterns of relapse, survival and therapeutic outcome. Eur J Cancer. 2009;45:1815–23.
23. Tihan T, Zhou T, Holmes E, Burger PC, Ozuysal S, Rushing EJ. The prognostic value of histological grading of posterior fossa ependymomas in children: a Children's Oncology Group study and a review of prognostic factors. Mod Pathol. 2008;21: 165–77.
24. Kilday JP, Mitra B, Domerg C, Ward J, Andreiuolo F, Osteso-Ibanez T, et al. Copy number gain of 1q25 predicts poor progression-free survival for pediatric intracranial ependymomas and enables patient risk stratification: a prospective European clinical trial cohort analysis on behalf of the Children's Cancer Leukaemia Group (CCLG), Societe Francaise d'Oncologie Pediatrique (SFOP), and International Society for Pediatric Oncology (SIOP). Clin Cancer Res. 2012;18:2001–11.
25. Godfraind C, Kaczmarska JM, Kocak M, Dalton J, Wright KD, Sanford RA, et al. Distinct disease-risk groups in pediatric supratentorial and posterior fossa ependymomas. Acta Neuropathol. 2012;124:247–57.
26. Carter M, Nicholson J, Ross F, Crolla J, Allibone R, Balaji V, et al. Genetic abnormalities detected in ependymomas by comparative genomic hybridisation. Br J Cancer. 2002;86:929–39.
27. Dyer S, Prebble E, Davison V, Davies P, Ramani P, Ellison D, et al. Genomic imbalances in pediatric intracranial ependymomas define clinically relevant groups. Am J Pathol. 2002;161:2133–41.
28. Grill J, Avet-Loiseau H, Lellouch-Tubiana A, Sevenet N, Terrier-Lacombe MJ, Venuat AM, et al. Comparative genomic hybridization detects specific cytogenetic abnormalities in pediatric ependymomas and choroid plexus papillomas. Cancer Genet Cytogenet. 2002;136:121–5.
29. Milde T, Hielscher T, Witt H, Kool M, Mack SC, Deubzer HE, et al. Nestin expression identifies ependymoma patients with poor outcome. Brain Pathol. 2012;22(6):848–60.
30. Andreiuolo F, Puget S, Peyre M, Dantas-Barbosa C, Boddaert N, Philippe C, et al. Neuronal differentiation distinguishes supratentorial and infratentorial childhood ependymomas. Neuro Oncol. 2010;12:1126–34.
31. Costa FF, Bischof JM, Vanin EF, Lulla RR, Wang M, Sredni ST, et al. Identification of microRNAs as potential prognostic markers in ependymoma. PLoS One. 2011;6:e25114.
32. Korshunov A, Golanov A, Timirgaz V. p14ARF protein (FL-132) immunoreactivity in intracranial ependymomas and its prognostic significance: an analysis of 103 cases. Acta Neuropathol. 2001;102:271–7.
33. Venkatramani R, Rosenberg S, Indramohan G, Jeng M, Jubran R. An exploratory epidemiological study of Langerhans cell histiocytosis. Pediatr Blood Cancer. 2012;59:1324–6.
34. Bouffet E, Tabori U, Huang A, Bartels U. Ependymoma: lessons from the past, prospects for the future. Childs Nerv Syst. 2009;25:1383–4; author reply 5.
35. Grundy RG, Wilne SA, Weston CL, Robinson K, Lashford LS, Ironside J, et al. Primary postoperative chemotherapy without radiotherapy for intracranial ependymoma in children: the UKCCSG/SIOP prospective study. Lancet Oncol. 2007;8: 696–705.
36. Gajjar A, Packer RJ, Foreman NK, Cohen K, Haas-Kogan D, Merchant TE, et al. Children's Oncology Group's 2013 blueprint for research: central nervous system tumors. Pediatr Blood Cancer. 2013;60:1022–6.
37. Fouladi M, Stewart CF, Olson J, Wagner LM, Onar-Thomas A, Kocak M, et al. Phase I trial of MK-0752 in children with refractory CNS malignancies: a pediatric brain tumor consortium study. J Clin Oncol. 2011;29:3529–34.
38. Guan S, Shen R, Lafortune T, Tiao N, Houghton P, Yung WK, et al. Establishment and characterization of clinically relevant models of ependymoma: a true challenge for targeted therapy. Neuro Oncol. 2011;13:748–58.
39. Servidei T, Meco D, Trivieri N, Patriarca V, Vellone VG, Zannoni GF, et al. Effects of epidermal growth factor receptor blockade on ependymoma stem cells in vitro and in orthotopic mouse models. Int J Cancer. 2012;131:E791–803.
40. Milde T, Kleber S, Korshunov A, Witt H, Hielscher T, Koch P, et al. A novel human high-risk ependymoma stem cell model reveals the differentiation-inducing potential of the histone deacetylase inhibitor Vorinostat. Acta Neuropathol. 2012; 122:637–50.
41. Rahman R, Osteso-Ibanez T, Hirst RA, Levesley J, Kilday JP, Quinn S, et al. Histone deacetylase inhibition attenuates cell growth with associated telomerase inhibition in high-grade childhood brain tumor cells. Mol Cancer Ther. 2010;9:2568–81.
42. Witt O, Milde T, Deubzer HE, Oehme I, Witt R, Kulozik A, et al. Phase I/II intra-patient dose escalation study of vorinostat

in children with relapsed solid tumor, lymphoma or leukemia. Klin Padiatr. 2012;224:398–403.
43. Hummel TR, Wagner L, Ahern C, Fouladi M, Reid JM, McGovern RM, et al. A pediatric phase 1 trial of vorinostat and temozolomide in relapsed or refractory primary brain or spinal cord tumors: a Children's Oncology Group phase 1 consortium study. Pediatr Blood Cancer. 2013;60:1452–7.
44. Fouladi M, Stewart CF, Blaney SM, Onar-Thomas A, Schaiquevich P, Packer RJ, et al. A molecular biology and phase II trial of lapatinib in children with refractory CNS malignancies: a pediatric brain tumor consortium study. J Neurooncol. 2013;114:173–9.
45. Mack SM, Witt H, Piro R, Gu L, Zuyderduyn S, Stütz AM, et al. Epigenomic alterations define lethal CIMP-positive ependymomas of infancy. Nature. 2014;506:445–50.
46. Parker M, Mohankumar KM, Punchihewa C, Weinlich R, Dalton JD, Li Y, et al. C11orf95-RELA fusions drive oncogenic NF-κB signalling in ependymoma. Nature. 2014;506:451–5.

6 Adult High-Grade (Diffuse) Glioma

Katharine McNeill, Kenneth Aldape, and Howard A. Fine

The central brain tumor registry of the United States (CBTRUS) estimates that there will be about 70,000 primary CNS tumor diagnosed in 2013. Of these, about 20 % will be malignant gliomas [1]. Glioblastomas (WHO grade IV, formerly termed glioblastoma multiforme or GBM) are the most common malignant primary brain tumors, with an incidence of about 3–4 per 100,000 [2]. Peak incidence for malignant glioma is in the fifth or sixth decade of life, and there is a slight male preponderance (1.1–1.3:1) [2]. Incidence and median age of diagnosis by histology is summarized in Table 6.1.

While traditionally high-grade "malignant" gliomas (grades III and IV) are distinguished from low-grade gliomas (grades I and II), this distinction does not correspond with the known biology of these tumors and is therefore probably outdated. Grade I gliomas are usually circumscribed, with a very low propensity for malignant transformation, and, while not the subject of this chapter, occur predominantly in children and have a molecular pathogenesis that is unrelated to diffuse glioma. In contrast, the diffusely infiltrating gliomas (grades II–IV) are prone to tumor recurrence and progression to higher grades, and their clinical behavior is malignant to varying degrees. As an added complexity, while the histologic diagnosis of glioblastoma (grade IV) is relatively straightforward, the histopathologic distinction of grade II from grade III glioma is ill-defined and subject to considerable inter-observer variability. In addition, the molecular genetics of grade II and III gliomas largely overlap, arguing that these are best considered within a spectrum of a single disease entity. Median survival varies with histologic diagnosis, and ranges from 5 to 7 years for diffuse (grade II) astrocytoma, 3–5 years for anaplastic astrocytoma [3] to 15–16 months for glioblastoma [4]. One-, 2-, 5-, and 10-year survival by histologic diagnosis are summarized in Table 6.2. There is some evidence that average survival times are improving modestly. Median survival for patients with glioblastoma treated in a large randomized trial that defined our current standard of care was 15 months [4], while outcomes in patients treated on clinical trials in the 5 years after that study was published was 20 months [5]. Apart from a possible element of patient selection bias, reasons may include improved treatments at the time of disease recurrence or an improvement in the standard of clinical and supportive patient care over time.

Standard treatment of glioblastoma includes maximal safe resection, involved field radiation, and concomitant and adjuvant temozolomide. Large retrospective studies have shown that patients who receive a more extensive resection, defined as 78–98 % of contrast enhancing tumor, have improved survival compared to patients who receive a subtotal resection or biopsy [6, 7], so extensive resection is warranted when feasible. The benefit from radiotherapy was defined by randomized trials, which showed a significant improvement in outcomes with radiotherapy compared to chemotherapy alone or best conventional care [8, 9]. A series of randomized studies established the standard dosing and fractionation of 60 Gy in 30 daily fractions [10–17].

A large randomized study defined the role of adjuvant chemotherapy with temozolomide, and found that patients who received concomitant and adjuvant temozolomide had a significant improvement in median survival compared to patients treated with radiation alone (12.1 vs. 14.6 months) [4] The proportion of patients surviving 5-years after diagnosis was five times higher in the temozolomide group (9.8 % vs. 1.9 %) [18]. This "Stupp protocol" has become the standard of care for initial management of glioblastoma. More recently, non-randomized data suggest that bevacizumab may improve outcomes after disease recurrence, with median progression-free survival of 4–6 months and median overall survival of 8–9 months [19, 20], which compared favorably to historical controls [21, 22].

Prospective, randomized trial data defining the utility of these modalities in anaplastic gliomas (WHO grade III) is lacking. These tumors are more heterogeneous in terms of

M.A. Karajannis and D. Zagzag (eds.), *Molecular Pathology of Nervous System Tumors: Biological Stratification and Targeted Therapies*, Molecular Pathology Library 8, DOI 10.1007/978-1-4939-1830-0_6, © Springer Science+Business Media New York 2015

TABLE 6.1. CBTRUS estimates of the number and age-adjusted incidence rates of malignant glial tumors, 2005–2009.

Histology	*N*	% of all tumors	Median age	Rate (95 % CI)
Glioblastoma	49,088	15.8	64	3.19 (3.16–3.22)
Anaplastic astrocytoma	5,374	1.7	54	0.36 (0.35–0.37)
Anaplastic oligodendroglioma	1,687	0.5	49	0.11 (0.11–0.12)
Glioma, malignant, NOS	6,574	2.1	40	0.45 (0.44–0.46)

From Dolecek TA, Propp JM, Stroup NE, Kruchko C: CBTRUS statistical report: primary brain and central nervous system tumors diagnosed in the United States in 2005-2009. *Neuro Oncol* 2012, 14 Suppl 5:v1-49, with permission

TABLE 6.2. CBTRUS estimates of 1-, 2-, 5-, and 10-year relative survival rates, 1995–2009.

Histology	1-year	2-years	5-years	10-year
Glioblastoma (%)	35.7	13.6	4.7	2.3
Anaplastic astrocytoma (%)	60.1	41.5	25.9	17.6
Anaplastic oligodendroglioma (%)	81.0	66.9	49.4	34.2
Glioma, malignant, NOS	61.9 %	50.4 %	43.3	38.3 %

From Dolecek TA, Propp JM, Stroup NE, Kruchko C: CBTRUS statistical report: primary brain and central nervous system tumors diagnosed in the United States in 2005-2009. *Neuro Oncol* 2012, 14 Suppl 5:v1-49, with permission

their behavior, genetics, and response to therapy compared to glioblastomas, so the most appropriate up-front treatment has not been established, and may vary depending on the histologic and genetic subtype. Early clinical trials that defined the benefit from radiotherapy included patients with grade III tumors, and based on those data it is generally accepted that radiotherapy improves outcomes in anaplastic glioma, although the number of patients with grade III tumors on those trials was too small to allow a statistically robust subgroup analysis [8, 9]. Most physicians treat patients with anaplastic astrocytoma with radiation and temozolomide per the Stupp protocol [23], and there are retrospective data that suggests a benefit of chemoradiotherapy over radiotherapy alone in patients whose tumors do not harbor a 1p/19q co-deletion [24]. Recent data indicate that in anaplastic oligodendrogliomas, addition of chemotherapy to radiotherapy also benefits patients with non-co-deleted, isocitrate dehydrogenase 1 (IDH1) mutant tumors [25]. The benefit of adjuvant temozolomide, however, has not been confirmed in prospective trials [23, 25–27]. The prospective data that do exist used a more toxic regimen of procarbazine, lomustine, and vincristine, so whether patients with anaplastic tumors benefit from adjuvant temozolomide is still an open question, and large randomized trials in patients with co-deleted [28] and non-co-deleted tumors [29] are ongoing. In order to circumvent the risk of radiation-induced neurocognitive deficits, there is a growing interest in treating selected patients with chemosensitive tumors (e.g., those with 1p/19q co-deletion) with chemotherapy alone based on retrospective [24] and prospective [30] data suggesting outcomes similar to radiation alone.

After more than three decades of clinical trials, it is clear that there is significant heterogeneity in the biology and behavior of these tumors and their response to treatment. A better understanding of the histopathologic, genetic, and epigenetic changes that underlie tumor biology will allow for more tailored treatment of these heterogeneous tumors, and this will be the subject of the rest of this review.

Histopathology

Diffuse gliomas are infiltrative glial tumors characterized by increased cellularity, nuclear atypia, and mitotic activity. They are subclassified according to their cellular morphology as either astrocytic, oligodendroglial, or mixed gliomas.

Astrocytomas are composed of cells with elongated or irregular hyperchromatic nuclei and scant cytoplasm. Cell processes form a loose fibrillary matrix and glial fibrillary acidic protein (GFAP) staining highlights both the cytoplasm and cell processes. Proliferative index, as measured by Ki-67 or MIB-1, is generally between 5 and 10 % but is highly variable. Oligodendrogliomas also exhibit GFAP immunoreactivity, but morphologically the cells have rounded hyperchromatic nuclei, perinuclear halos, and few cellular processes. They have a characteristic branching capillary pattern and focal microcalcifications are common (Fig. 6.1). Oligoastrocytomas display features intermediate between astrocytoma and oligodendroglioma. While a biphasic distribution where distinct areas display astrocytic or oligodendroglial differentiation has been described in the literature, this is extremely rare and when found is of uncertain clinical significance. Most commonly mixed oligoastrocytomas represent an indeterminate diffuse variant where the two phenotypes are intermingled [2]. Recent data suggest that from a biologic perspective, mixed oligoastrocytoma is not a distinct entity and as a category is likely composed of a mix of tumors with "oligodendroglioma" biology (e.g., 1p/19q co-deletion) together with tumors with "astrocytoma" biology (e.g., TP53 mutation). These considerations

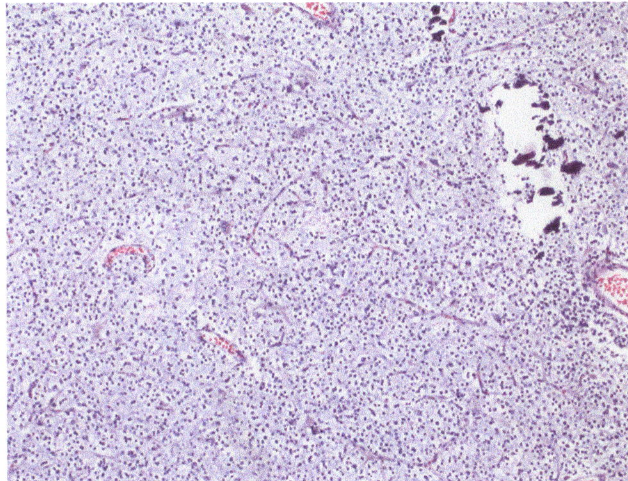

Fig. 6.1. Oligodendroglioma, with characteristic rounded hyperchromatic nuclei, perinuclear halos, and branching capillary pattern.

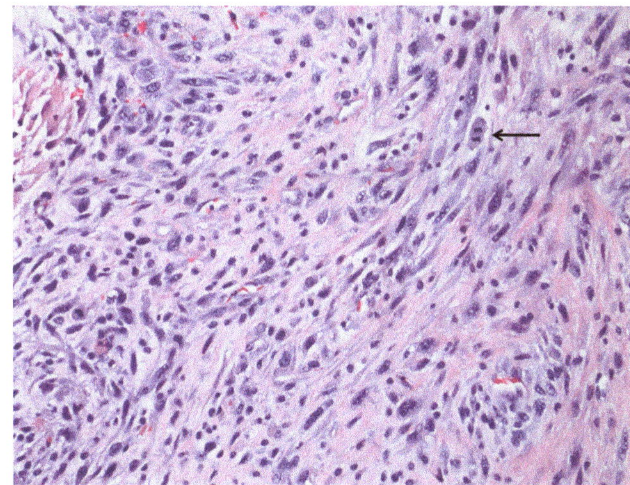

Fig. 6.3. Gliosarcoma, with bundles of elongated spindle cells.

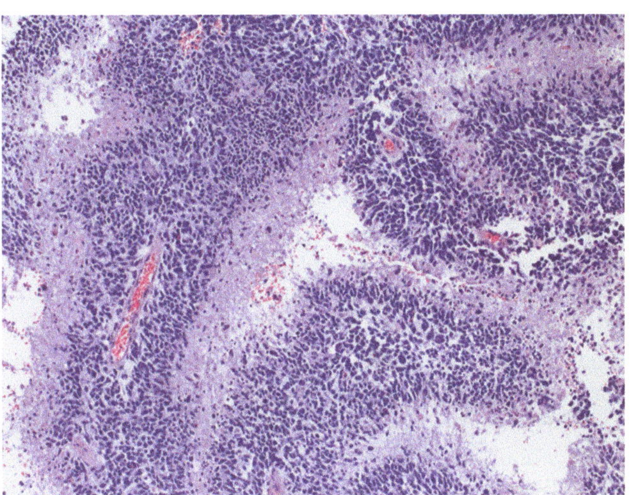

Fig. 6.2. Glioblastoma, with pseudopalisading necrosis.

highlight an important concept likely to be introduced into future classification systems of glioma, where key molecular markers are to be used as an important adjunct to conventional histopathologic analysis.

In addition to the features described above, glioblastomas are defined by the presence of microvascular proliferation and/or necrosis (Fig. 6.2). The cells are poorly differentiated and pleomorphic, and regional heterogeneity is common. Several variants have been described, including small cell glioblastoma, glioblastoma with an oligodendroglioma component, giant cell glioblastoma, and gliosarcoma [2].

Small cell glioblastoma is characterized by a monomorphic population of densely packed small, round cells with a high nuclear:cytoplasmic ratio and modest atypia. Proliferative activity is high, and GFAP immunoreactivity can be minimal. Their outcome is similar to standard GBMs [31]. Glioblastomas with an oligodendroglial component contain foci that resemble oligodendroglioma. The presence of areas with both astrocytic differentiation and necrosis differentiates them from anaplastic oligoastrocytomas. Giant cell glioblastomas have numerous multinucleated giant cells along with smaller fusiform cells. There is some data to suggest that the prognosis of glioblastomas with an oligodendroglial component and giant cell glioblastomas may be better compared to standard glioblastomas [32–34]. Gliosarcomas have a mixture of cells with gliomatous and sarcomatous differentiation, either in distinct geographic areas or intermixed. The gliomatous areas show typical features of glioblastoma. Sarcomatous areas often resemble fibrosarcoma, with bundles of spindle cells, but can also show mesenchymal differentiation with cartilaginous, osteoid, myomatous, or lipomatous features. These areas are GFAP negative [2] (Fig. 6.3). The prognosis of gliosarcoma is similar to standard glioblastoma [35].

Cytogenetics and Molecular Genetics

1p/19q Co-deletion

Loss of heterozygosity (LOH) of 1p and 19q is a common event in oligodendroglial tumors, occurring in 80–90 % of low-grade oligodendrogliomas and 50–70 % of anaplastic oligodendrogliomas [36]. However, since the distinction of oligodendroglioma from astrocytic tumors is subject to interobserver variability, the rate of 1p/19q co-deletion relative to histologic diagnosis is only approximate. Several groups have reported that it is mutually exclusive from genetic changes common to astrocytic tumors, including TP53 mutations [37, 38], EGFR amplification [38, 39], and LOH 10q [39, 40]. It is associated with oligodendroglial morphology [41] and is felt to be a reliable diagnostic biomarker of the oligodendroglial phenotype [37, 42]. Tumors with 1p/19q co-deletion often exhibit several other genetic and epigenetic changes including IDH mutations [43, 44], methylguanine methyltransferase (MGMT) promoter methylation [44], CpG island methylator phenotype (G-CIMP) [45], and a proneural gene expression profile [46, 47], which will be discussed in greater detail below.

Recent work has identified candidate tumor suppressor genes on 1p and 19q. Mutations in the homolog of the *Drosophila capicua* gene (CIC) on 19q13.2 are present in 50–80 % of 1p/19q co-deleted oligodendrogliomas [48–50]. CIC is a downstream transcriptional repressor of receptor tyrosine kinase (RTK) pathways, including EGFR, Ras, Raf, and MAP kinases [48]. The exact mechanism of tumor pathogenesis remains unclear [42]. Mutations in the far-upstream element (FUSE) binding protein 1 (FUBP1) on 1p31.1 are seen in about 20 % of oligodendrogliomas [48, 50]. FUBP1 binds to the FUSE of Myc, a well-known oncogene [51] and negatively regulates Myc expression [52]. Although these are theoretically attractive genes for being involved in the pathogenesis of oligodendrogliomas, no definitive mechanism has yet been identified.

Chromosome 10 Deletion

LOH of chromosome 10 is the most frequent genetic alteration in GBM, and occurs in 60–80 % of cases [53, 54]. Loss of the entire chromosome is common, but partial deletions in three common regions have been described, suggesting that several tumor suppressor genes may exist in chromosome 10 [2, 55]. LOH 10q occurs in both primary and secondary glioblastomas at similar frequencies [53] while LOH 10p is generally seen in primary glioblastomas [56]. One established tumor suppressor in this region is the PTEN (phosphatase and tensin homology) gene on 10q23.3 [57]. PTEN is a phosphatase which inhibits PIP3 signaling, and thereby downregulates the activity of AKT and mTOR and inhibits cell proliferation [58]. It is mutated in 15–40 % of glioblastomas [59, 60] most often in primary glioblastomas [53, 61].

Chromosome 7 Amplification

The most frequent amplification event in glioblastoma is amplification of 7p12 in the region of the EGFR gene [62]. Like PTEN mutation and LOH 10q, EGFR amplification is common in primary glioblastoma, where it occurs in about 40 % of cases [53, 63]. EGFR amplification is significantly less frequent in secondary glioblastoma [63]. About 50–60 % of tumors with EGFR amplification also express a truncated variant of the receptor, EGFR variant III (EGFRvIII), which is constitutively active and ligand-independent [64, 65]. EGFR amplification and EGFRvIII mutation have been associated with an increased proliferation rate, increased invasiveness, resistance to cytotoxic therapy, and worse patient outcomes [66–68]. When other clinical and genetic variables and known prognostic factors are considered in a multivariant analysis, however, it is less clear that EGFR amplification and particularly the EGFRvIII mutation turn out to be independent prognostic factors. The EGFR signaling pathway will be discussed in further detail below.

IDH1 and IDH2

Mutations in isocitrate dehydrogenase-1 and -2 (IDH1 and -2) were first identified as important driver mutations in a subset of glioblastomas by Parsons et al. in 2008 [69]. IDH catalyzes the oxidative carboxylation of isocitrate to α-ketoglutarate (α-KG) within the citric acid cycle. The IDH family of genes code for enzymes that catalyze the NADP/NAD-dependent oxidative decarboxylation of isocitrate to alpha-ketoglutarate, with subsequent NADPH/NADH release [5]. These enzymes are found both in the cytoplasm (IDH1), and in the mitochondria (IDH2 and IDH3). IDH mutations are present in 50–75 % of anaplastic tumors and 75–85 % secondary glioblastomas, but are uncommon in primary glioblastomas, occurring in about 5 % [43, 44, 69–71]. IDH mutations frequently occur in association with other mutations common to secondary glioblastomas, such as TP53 mutations, 1p/19q co-deletions, and methylated MGMT promoter, and are inversely associated with alterations in PTEN, EGFR, and LOH 10, which are common to primary glioblastomas [70, 72, 73].

IDH1 mutations are point mutations at position 395 (G395A) of the IDH1 gene (codon 132 of the IDH1 binding site), most commonly with replacement of arginine with histidine (IDH1-R132H) [69], which accounts for >90 % of IDH1 mutations [43, 69, 71]. IDH2 mutations are less common, accounting for only 4–5 % of IDH mutations, and appear largely in the setting of 1p/19q co-deleted tumors [43, 71] IDH2 are also point mutations at a homologous codon (172) within the binding site [42]. Collective data suggest that IDH mutation is a very early lesion in the pathogenesis of lower grade (grade II–III) diffuse glioma. Co-deletion of 1p/19q is almost invariably observed in the setting of an IDH mutation. Interestingly, IDH-mutated but non-1p/19q-co-deleted tumors are nearly always TP53-mutated, suggesting that either co-deletion or TP53 mutation occur after IDH mutation and either of these aberrations is required for most cases of glioma pathogenesis. There is a mutant-specific commercially available antibody to the IDH1-R132H protein which is a reliable diagnostic biomarker [74]. From a practical and clinical perspective, this immunohistochemical test has several diagnostic uses, which include mutation detection and distinction of diffuse glioma from entities not associated with IDH mutation (for example circumscribed glioma and ependymoma). In addition, in the setting of a differential diagnosis of diffuse glioma versus reactive conditions (astrogliosis, treatment effects), R132H-specific immunohistochemistry can be very useful when positive. It is important to remember that absence of staining/mutation is not always helpful, since not all diffuse gliomas are IDH-mutated.

The pathogenesis of IDH mutations is still under active investigation. The mutation causes reduced enzymatic activity in the conversion of isocitrate to α-KG [75], but since the remaining allele produces functional enzyme it is likely that it is a gain of function which is pathogenic [76]. The mutated enzyme has been shown to catalyze the reduction of α-KG to 2-hydroxyglutarate (2-HG), and 2-HG levels are elevated in IDH1 mutated tumors, suggesting that 2-HG is an oncometabolite [77]. This is supported by the fact that patients with inborn errors of metabolism leading to accumulation of 2-HG in the brain have an elevated risk of brain tumors [78]. 2-HG is a competitive inhibitor of α-KG-dependent dioxygenases including histone demethylases and the TET family of hydroxylases [79], which are involved in DNA methylation [80]. Recent data shows that IDH mutation causes DNA hypermethylation over serial passages and is sufficient to establish the G-CIMP hypermethylated phenotype [81]. Mutations in IDH genes are not specific to gliomas, and have been described in other neoplasms, including acute myelogenous leukemia (AML) and cartilaginous neoplasms, among others. IDH mutations in these tumors, unlike gliomas, have not been shown to have a more favorable outcome.

The absence or presence of IDH mutation in diffuse gliomas largely accounts for the prior designation of primary and secondary pathways to glioblastoma, respectively. Lower grade diffuse gliomas (grade II–III) are largely IDH mutant, while grade IV gliomas (glioblastomas) are largely IDH wild type. However, a subset of grade II–III gliomas are IDH wild type and likely represent a precursor lesion to glioblastoma. In addition, while IDH-mutant glioblastomas are rare in the setting of a new glioma diagnosis, they likely represent malignant progression from a previously undiagnosed lower grade IDH-mutant glioma. Although indistinguishable histologically, many distinctions exist between IDH-mutant and IDH wild-type diffuse gliomas in terms of methylation pattern, DNA copy number aberrations, gene expression profiles, and somatic mutational profiles. Future progress in the classification and management of diffuse gliomas will likely benefit by treating IDH-mutant and IDH wild-type tumors as separate clinico-pathological entities.

ATRX

Alpha Thalassemia/Mental Retardation Syndrome X-Linked (ATRX) is a component of the SWI/SNF complex of chromatin remodeling proteins and is involved in gene regulation. Jiao et al. have recently described mutations in ATRX in gliomas, occurring in more than one third of astrocytomas (71 %, grades II and III), 57 % of secondary glioblastomas, and 68 % of mixed oligoastrocytomas. The frequency in primary glioblastoma and oligodendroglioma was much lower (4 % and 14 %, respectively). ATRX mutation was almost always seen in the presence of a TP53 mutation (94 %) and IDH mutations (99 %) in adult gliomas [82].

Epigenetics and Gene Expression Profiling

MGMT

O^6-MGMT is a DNA repair protein on 10q26 that removes alkyl groups from the O^6 position of guanine, thereby counteracting the activity of alkylating agents such as temozolomide and nitrosoureas [83]. It can be epigenetically silenced via methylation of 5′-CpG islands within the transcription factor binding sites [84]. MGMT is methylated in about 40 % of primary glioblastomas, 70 % of secondary glioblastomas, and 50 % of anaplastic astrocytomas [85, 86]. MGMT methylation is strongly associated with 1p/19q co-deletion [87, 88] and IDH mutations [44, 86]. MGMT methylation is predictive of response to temozolomide [89] and nitrosoureas [90], consistent with their mechanism of action. There is emerging evidence, however, that MGMT methylation is also an independent prognostic marker and associated with improved outcome in patients treated with radiotherapy alone [30, 72, 91], suggesting that this epigenetic change is associated with biological effects beyond DNA alkylator damage repair [92]. MGMT methylation is also associated with the G-CIMP hypermethylated phenotype [45] and it is possible that these genetic and global epigenetic changes underlie the prognostic effect of MGMT methylation. That said, whether MGMT methylation has the same prognostic significance in patients with IDH-mutant tumors as has been shown in patient cohorts with largely IDH wild-type glioblastomas, is not entirely clear.

Glioma-CpG-Island Methylator Phenotype (G-CIMP)

Noushmehr et al. have identified a subgroup of glioblastomas characterized by a distinct pattern of hypermethylation of CpG islands in a subset of glioma-specific genes, including genes involved in cell adhesion, regulation of transcription, metabolic processes, and nucleic acid synthesis [93]. This glioma-CpG-island methylator phenotype (G-CIMP) leads to transcriptional silencing of specific genes via methylation of promoter regions. It is associated with younger age, the "proneural" gene expression profile, a high frequency of IDH1 and TP53 mutations, and a low frequency of PTEN, NF1, and EGFR mutations. As outlined above, there is evidence to suggest that IDH mutations are sufficient to cause this glioma-specific methylation phenotype.

Gene Expression Subtypes

The Cancer Genome Atlas (TCGA) has identified four gene expression subtypes within glioblastoma including proneural, neural, classical, and mesenchymal subtypes [94]. The frequency of copy number alterations and mutations by subtype in this cohort are described in Tables 6.3 and 6.4.

Table 6.3. Copy number alterations in glioblastoma subtypes in TCGA samples.

	Proneural (%)	Neural (%)	Classical (%)	Mesenchymal (%)	Gene(s) in ROI
Low and high level amplified events					
7p11.2	54	96	100	95	EGFR
7q21.2	46	96	92	89	CDK6
7q31.2	54	92	86	91	MET
7q34	52	92	86	91	
High level amplification events					
7p11.2	17	67	95	29	EGFR
4q12	35	13	5	9	PDGFRA
Homozygous and hemizygous deletion events					
17q11.2	6	17	5	38	NF1
10q23	69	96	100	87	PTEN
9p21.3	56	71	95	67	CDKN2A/ CDKN2B
13q14	52	46	16	53	RB1
Homozygous deletion events					
9p21.3	41	54	92	53	CDKN2A/ CDKN2B

From Verhaak RG, Hoadley KA, Purdom E, Wang V, Qi Y, Wilkerson MD, Miller CR, Ding L, Golub T, Mesirov JP et al.: Integrated genomic analysis identifies clinically relevant subtypes of glioblastoma characterized by abnormalities in PDGFRA, IDH1, EGFR, and NF1. *Cancer Cell* 2010, 17(1):98-110, with permission

Table 6.4. Distribution of mutated genes in glioblastoma subtypes.

Gene	Proneural (%)	Neural (%)	Classical (%)	Mesenchymal (%)
TP53	54	21	0	32
PTEN	16	21	23	32
NF1	5	16	5	37
EGFR	16	26	32	5
IDH1	30	5	0	0
PIK3R1	19	11	5	0
RB1	3	5	0	13
ERBB2	5	16	5	3
EGFRvIII	3	0	23	3
PIK3CA	8	5	5	3
PDGFRA	11	0	0	0

From Verhaak RG, Hoadley KA, Purdom E, Wang V, Qi Y, Wilkerson MD, Miller CR, Ding L, Golub T, Mesirov JP et al.: Integrated genomic analysis identifies clinically relevant subtypes of glioblastoma characterized by abnormalities in PDGFRA, IDH1, EGFR, and NF1. *Cancer Cell* 2010, 17(1):98-110, with permission

The proneural subtype has an oligodendroglial signature, and is characterized by alterations in PDGFRA and IDH1 as well as TP53 mutations. Copy number changes that are common in classic glioblastoma, such as chromosome 7 amplification and chromosome 10 loss, are significantly less frequent in the proneural subtype. Oligodendrocytic development genes, including PDGFRA, NKX2-2, and Olig-2, are highly expressed. Patients with proneural tumors are younger and have a better prognosis, and secondary glioblastomas are more common in this subtype. It is important to realize that the improved prognosis observed by the proneural subclass is likely due to its inclusion of IDH-mutant tumors, which represent a subset of this transcriptomal class.

The neural subtype is associated with both oligodendrocytic and astrocytic gene signatures, and is also characterized by expression of neuronal markers, including NEFL, GABRA1, SYT1, and SLC12A5. Its expression patterns are most similar to normal brain.

The Classical subtype has an astrocytic signature, and is characterized by chromosome 7 amplification and chromosome 10 loss, EGFR amplification and EGFRvIII mutation, and increased expression of Notch and Sonic hedgehog (SHH) signaling pathway constituents. TP53 mutations are not seen in this subtype.

The mesenchymal subtype has a cultured astroglial signature, and microglial markers such as CD68, PTPRC, and TNF are highly expressed. NF1 mutations and PTEN loss are common in this subtype. Phenotypically, these tumors have more abundant necrosis, perhaps related to high expression of genes in the tumor necrosis factor (TNF) and NF-κB pathways. Both mesenchymal (CHI3L1, MET) and astrocytic markers (CD44, MERTK) are expressed.

While the TCGA classification is the most widely cited, it is important to realize that the TCGA classification system for gene expression analysis has not been validated using an unsupervised analysis from an independent data set. However, examination of additional analyses in the literature would suggest that, with some variation in nomenclature, the mesenchymal and proneural subtypes appear to be reproducibly identified in gene expression datasets [95, 96]. In addition, while the mesenchymal subtype is generally restricted to IDH wild-type glioblastoma, the proneural subtype is observed in diffuse gliomas of all three WHO grades. In addition, IDH-mutated gliomas are almost invariably proneural, but a subset of IDH wild-type tumors can also cluster in the proneural class.

Prognostic Stratification

Traditionally, prognostic stratification for malignant gliomas has been based on clinical and histologic features of the tumors. Regressive partitioning analysis has identified age, histologic grade, performance status, and extent of resection as important prognostic factors [97]. Outcomes stratified by these variables are markedly different, and vary from 5 months in the worst prognostic group to almost 60 months in the best prognostic group [97]. The significance of these prognostic markers has been born out in multiple studies [3, 6, 7, 21, 98–100], and they continue to be the foundation for estimating prognosis.

There is evidence that several of the genetic and molecular features of these tumors discussed above have prognostic significance, and they are increasingly being incorporated into prognostic schema. It has long been recognized, for instance, that 1p/19q loss is associated with a better response to chemotherapy [101, 102] and radiotherapy [25], as well as with longer survival [25, 27, 101]. As discussed above, there is also evidence that MGMT methylation is both a predictive [89, 90] and prognostic [30, 72, 91] biomarker. Both tests are now commercially available, and are routinely used as part of the diagnostic evaluation of these tumors.

More recently IDH1 and 2 mutations have emerged as another important prognostic factor. Several groups have established that gliomas with IDH mutations have a relatively favorable prognosis [43, 69], and that IDH mutations are more prognostic than grade [73, 103] As outlined above, current evidence suggests that IDH status defines two biologically and clinically distinct types of diffuse glioma, and IDH-mutant tumors are less aggressive than IDH wild-type gliomas when matched for histological grade. In contrast, EGFR overexpression is associated with worse prognosis and therapeutic resistance [104, 105]. Although TP53 mutations have emerged as a useful diagnostic biomarker given their higher incidence in secondary glioblastoma compared to primary glioblastoma [63], they do not appear to have prognostic significance in glioblastoma [106].

Molecular Signaling Pathways

The PI3K kinase pathway is altered in the majority of glioblastomas through a variety of mechanisms. Activating mutations or amplifications of multiple RTKs which activate this pathway, including EGFR, Her2, PDGFRα, or MET have been described [107]. PI3K is activated by RTKs and leads to increased cell proliferation and survival via activation of multiple downstream effectors including Akt and mTOR [58, 108]. Activating mutations of the pathway components Ras, PI3K, and Akt are often identified [107]. Inactivating mutations or deletions of NF1, a negative regulator of Ras, or PTEN, a negative regulator of PI3K, are also common [53, 107, 109]. Constituents in this pathway and the frequency of alterations in glioblastoma are summarized in Fig. 6.4a.

TCGA identified alterations in the TP53 tumor suppressor pathway in 87 % of glioblastomas [107]. Disruption of this pathway leads to clonal expansion and genetic instability, as outlined above [110, 111]. Alterations in this pathway can occur via inactivating mutations or deletions in TP53 itself, or amplification of negative regulators of TP53, MDM2, and MDM4. These two events are generally mutually exclusive [107, 112]. Homozygous deletion of the CDKN2A gene, which leads to loss of $p14^{ARF}$, an inhibitor of MDM2, also leads to functional loss of p53 activity [113]. A summary of this pathway and frequency of alterations in glioblastoma is provided in Fig. 6.4b.

The Rb pathway is altered in 78 % of glioblastomas [107]. Rb is a tumor suppressor that controls cell cycle progression from G1 to S phase [113]. Alterations in this pathway are most often due to deletions or mutations of Rb, amplification of its negative regulator CDK4, or deletions of $p16^{INK4a}$ or CDKN2B, which are in turn inhibitors of CDK4 [113]. Of note, $p16^{INK4a}$ is also translated from the CDKN2A gene, underscoring the connectedness of the TP53 and Rb pathways [114]. This pathway is summarized in Fig. 6.4c.

There has been increasing interest in stem-like cell (GSCs) signaling pathways in recent years. GSCs are characterized by their ability for self-renewal, their ability to differentiate into multiple lineages, and their tumorgenicity [115, 116]. GSCs have been identified as an important cause of treatment resistance in malignant gliomas [117, 118]. Two main stem cell signaling pathways that have inconsistently been implicated in GSC biology are the Notch pathway and the SHH pathway. Jagged and Delta-like ligands bind to Notch, which leads to γ-secretase-mediated cleavage of the intracellular domain of the Notch receptor [119]. Notch-IC then translocates to the nucleus where it functions as a transcriptional activator of several physiologic processes, including angiogenesis, specification of cell fate, and regulation of differentiation [119, 120]. SHH binds to the patched homolog receptor, and thereby releases the membrane protein Smoothened homolog, resulting in the activation of Gli proteins [121]. Gli proteins are transcription factors that modulate several target genes including MYC and CCND1 [121]. Different studies have implicated one, both or neither of these pathways in GSC biology. It is therefore likely that these pathways have variable activities and roles in different GSC lines from different tumors. These two pathways are summarized in Fig. 6.5.

Finally, it has long been recognized that gliomas are highly angiogenic tumors, so angiogenic signaling pathways represent a major area of glioma research. The vascular endothelial growth factor (VEGF) signaling pathway is pivotal to the development of tumor-associated blood vessels [120]. VEGF is secreted by tumor cells and binds to the VEGF receptor (VEGFR) on tumor-associated endothelium. This stimulates a signaling cascade through the PI3K/Ras/MAPK pathway, leading to endothelial cell proliferation and migration [120, 122]. Other pro-angiogenic factors and their receptors can stimulate these pathways, including platelet-derived growth factor (PDGF), fibroblast growth factor 2 (FGF-2), hypoxia-inducible factor 1-alpha (HIF-1α), hepatocyte growth factor (HGF), and angiopoetin-1 and -2, via their receptors PDGFR, FGFR, Met, and Tie2 and may be important causes of resistance to VEGF targeted therapy [120, 123, 124]. These pathways are summarized in Fig. 6.5.

Molecular Targeted Therapies

The elucidation of these important signaling pathways in malignant glioma has stimulated extensive research in the use of molecular targeted therapies. The most successful of the targeted therapies to date is bevacizumab, a humanized

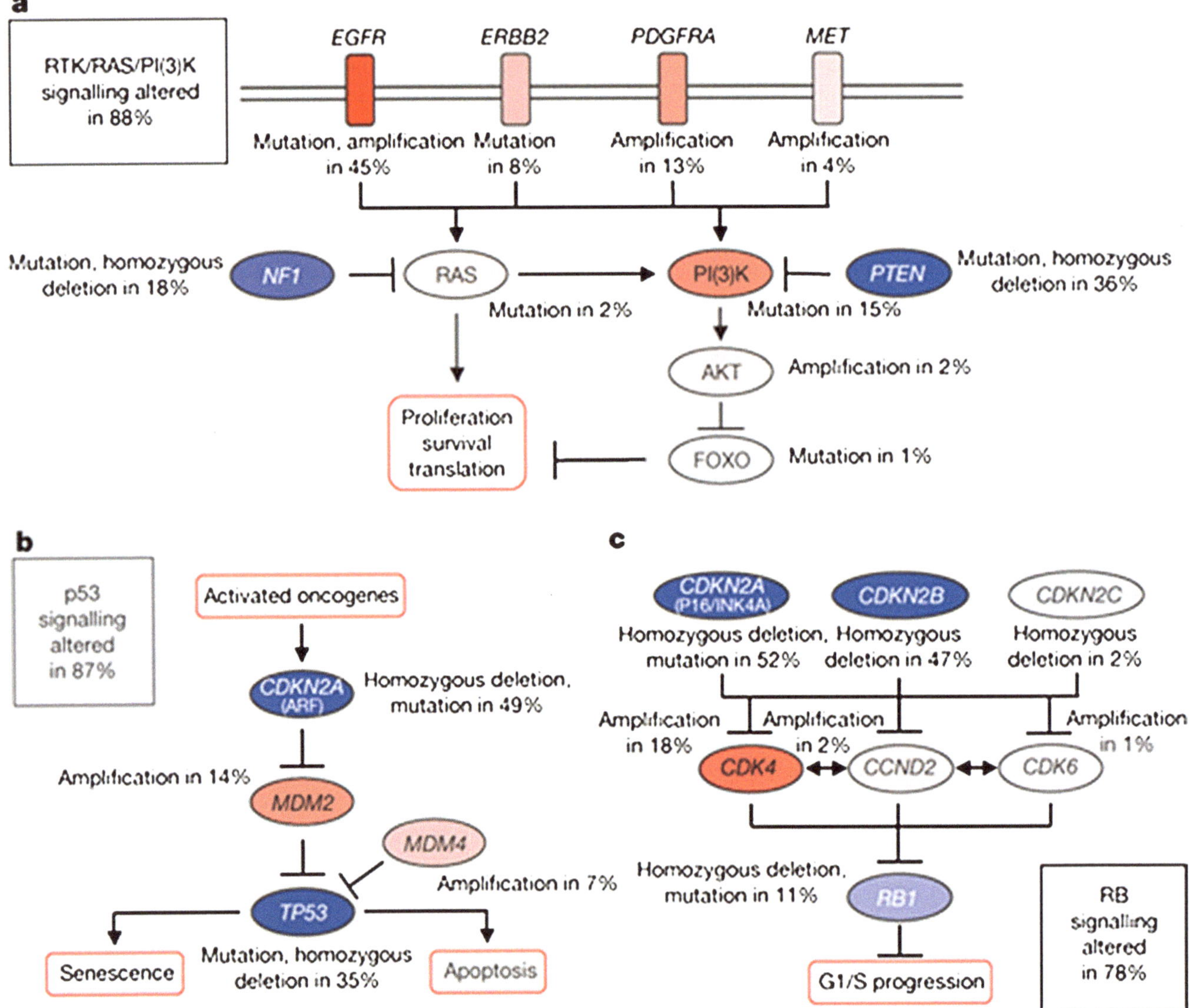

Fig. 6.4 Common signaling pathway alterations in glioblastoma (From Comprehensive genomic characterization defines human glioblastoma genes and core pathways. *Nature* 2008, 455(7216):1061-1068, with permission)

monoclonal antibody against VEGF-A ligand, which was approved by the FDA in 2009 for the treatment of recurrent glioblastoma [125]. Treatment with bevacizumab in phase II trials resulted in radiographic responses in 28–57 % of patients, median progression-free survival of 4–6 months, and median overall survival of 8–10 months [19, 20, 126], which compared favorably to historical controls [21, 22].

Two recent phase III trials examined the utility of bevacizumab added to chemoradiation as initial therapy for newly diagnosed glioblastoma. They showed an improvement in progression-free survival, but not overall survival, compared to controls, many of whom received bevacizumab at recurrence [127–129]. These data suggest that bevacizumab is not indicated as part of initial therapy. It should be noted that overall survival in both arms of these two trials was 16–17 months, which was a modest improvement compared to the 14.6 months seen in earlier phase III studies with radiation and temozolomide alone [4].

The success of bevacizumab has spurred interest in other VEGF targeted therapies, including decoy receptors, pan-VEGFR tyrosine kinase inhibitors (TKIs), multitargeted TKIs, integrin inhibitors, protein kinase C-β inhibitors, and inhibitors of other pro-angiogenic pathways. Although some have shown modest antitumor activity [130, 131], many have proven ineffective alone [132–135], or in combination with other targeted agents [136, 137], and none has proven more efficacious than bevacizumab to date. Ongoing clinical trials are exploring the activity of anti-angiogenic agents in combination with other targeted agents [138, 139], and in combination with bevacizumab [140]. Anti-angiogenic agents tested in clinical trials are summarized in Table 6.5.

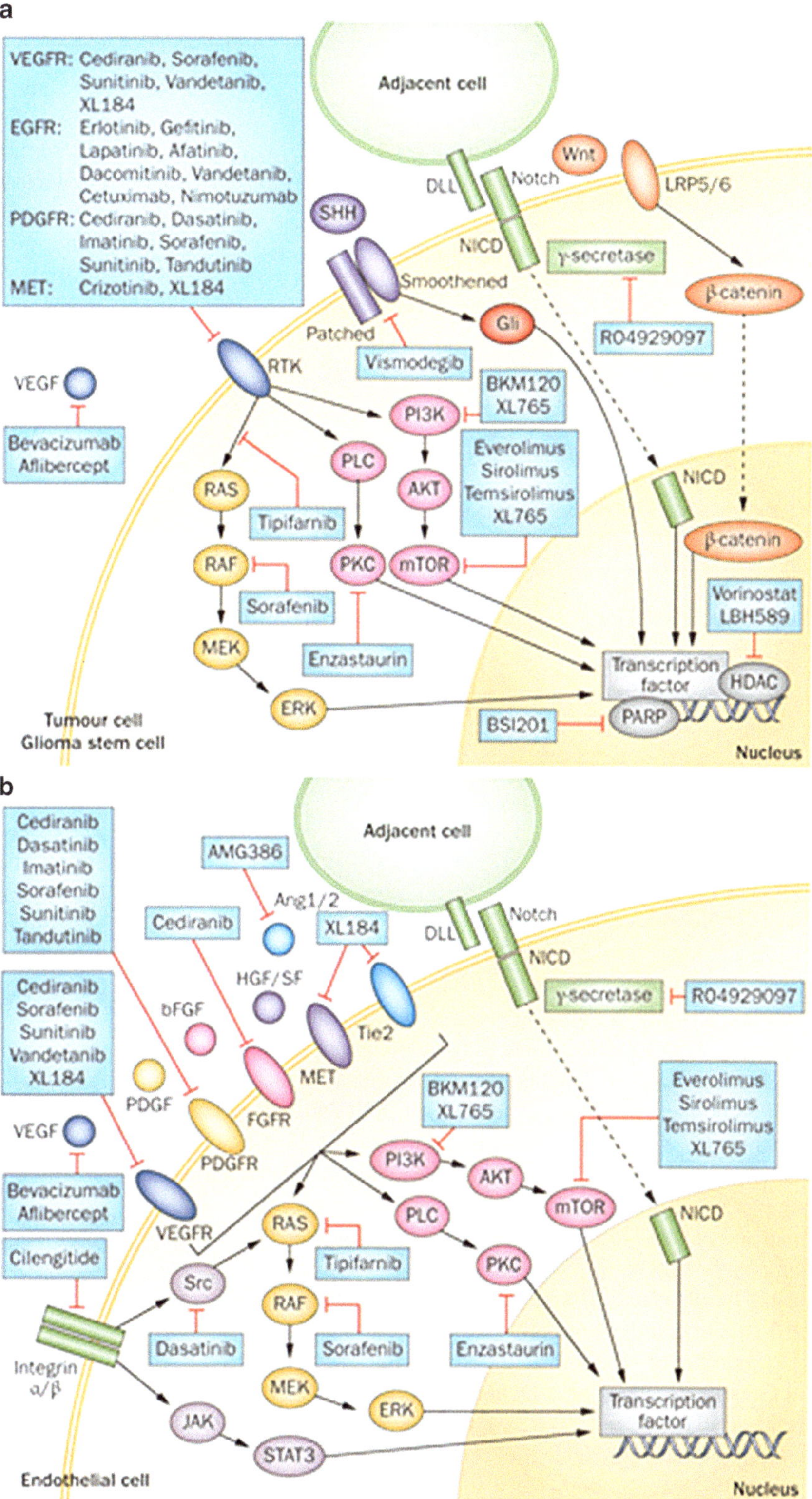

FIG. 6.5 Cell signaling pathways in malignant glioma cells (**a**) and tumor-associated endothelial cells (**b**), and agents under investigation to target these pathways (From Tanaka S, Louis DN, Curry WT, Batchelor TT, Dietrich J: Diagnostic and therapeutic avenues for glioblastoma: no longer a dead end? *Nat Rev Clin Oncol* 2013, 10(1):14-26, with permission)

Another major area of interest is EGFR targeted therapy. Although EGFR alterations are common in glioblastoma, first generation EGFR TKIs including erlotinib and gefitinib, as well as cetuximab, a monoclonal antibody against EGFR, had limited activity [141–147]. This may be due to amplification of multiple RTKs within tumors, which maintain downstream signaling in the setting of EGFR inhibition [148–151]. Vandetanib, an EGFR and VEGFR-2 inhibitor, and lapatanib, a HER-1 and HER-2 inhibitor also had limited activity [132, 152, 153]. A second generation of

Table 6.5. Anti-angiogenic agents under investigation.

Agent	Target	References
Bevacizumab	VEGF-A	[19, 20, 126]
Aflibercept	VEGF-A, VEGF-B, PlGF	[135]
Cediranib	VEGFR-1,2,3, PDGFR-α,β, FGFR-1, c-Kit	[130, 161]
Sorafenib	VEGFR-2,3, PDGFR-α,β, BRAF, c-Kit, Ras	[136, 137, 162–164]
Sunitinib	VEGFR-2, PDGFR-β, c-Kit, RET, Flt3	[134, 165, 166]
Vandetanib	VEGFR-2, EGFR, RET	[132, 152]
Cabozantinib	VEGFR-2, Met, RET, c-Kit, Flt3, Tie-2	[133]
Cilengitide	αvβ3, αvβ5 integrins	[131, 167]
Enzastaurin	PKC-β, Akt	[168, 169]
AMG386	Ang-1, Ang-2	[170, 171]

Table 6.6. Molecular targeted agents under investigation.

Agent	Target	References
Temsirolimus	mTOR	[172, 173]
Everolimus	mTOR	[174–176]
BKM-120	PI3K	[177–179]
XL-765	PI3K, mTOR	[180]
Sorafenib	VEGFR-2,3, PDGFR-α,β, BRAF, c-Kit, Ras	[136, 137, 162–164]
Imatinib	PDGFR-α,β, c-Kit, Bcr-Abl	[181–183]
Tandutinib	PDGFR-α,β, c-Kit, Flt3	[184, 185]
Dasatinib	PDGFR-α,β, Src, Bcr-Abl, c-Kit, EphA2	[186–190]
PD-0332991	CDK4, CDK6	[191]
RO492097	γ-secretase	[192–195]
Vismodegib	Smoothened homolog	[196]

EGFR TKIs which cause irreversible target inhibition are currently being studied, and may prove more beneficial [154–157]. Several immunotherapy approaches targeting EGFRvIII have also been evaluated. An EGFRvIII peptide vaccine, CDX-110, was evaluated in a phase II trial in patients with newly diagnosed glioblastoma, and showed a significant improvement in overall survival compared to a matched cohort [158]. A phase III trial in newly diagnosed patients is ongoing [159]. A phase I/II trial is also ongoing using T-cells genetically modified to express an anti-EGFRvIII chimeric antigen receptor [160].

A number of other molecular targets have been explored in the past decade. These include inhibitors of other RTKs such as PDGFR and MET, and inhibitors of downstream signaling molecules such as mTOR, PI3K, RAS, RAF, Src, and PKC. Recently there has also been interest in targeting signaling pathways specifically involved in stem cell biology, such as γ-secretase inhibitors, which are involved in Notch signaling, and SHH signaling inhibitors. A schematic of these pathways, and drugs under investigation to target these pathways, is provided in Fig. 6.5. Current clinical trials investigating these agents are summarized in Table 6.6.

Conclusion

The last decade has seen an explosion in our knowledge of the genetic and molecular biology of high-grade gliomas. New data support the great biological heterogeneity that underlies what was previously thought to represent just a few tumor types affirming the heterogeneity of observed clinical endpoints such as response to specific treatments and overall survival. The discovery of discrete mutational events in subsets of high-grade gliomas yield hopes of targeted therapies directed at those genetic and epigenetic aberrations, as well as more rationale clinical trials selected for subgroups of patients enriched for tumors most likely to respond to a particular targeted therapy. Nevertheless, the heterogeneity of genomic and epigenomic profiles from multiple gliomas, as well as the relatively disappointing results of targeted treatments to date, raises the realistic possibility that the future of targeted treatment will not be matching a drug against its specific mutated gene, but rather the need for a more complete understanding of the complexity of the gene regulatory network hardwired into each of those tumors as defined by their specific mutational and epigenetic profiles. Understanding this network may then allow us to identify points of network vulnerability for which future targeted therapies may be developed. Thus, although our understanding of the biology and molecular signatures of diffuse glioma has increased, the pace of clinical improvements for this disease has unfortunately lagged behind and much work to successfully match tumor-specific alterations with specific and efficacious therapeutics is yet to be done.

References

1. Dolecek TA, Propp JM, Stroup NE, Kruchko C. CBTRUS statistical report: primary brain and central nervous system tumors diagnosed in the United States in 2005-2009. Neuro Oncol. 2012;14 Suppl 5:v1–49.
2. Louis DN, Ohgaki H, Wiestler OD, Cavenee WK. WHO classification of tumours of the central nervous system. 4th ed. Lyon: International Agency for Research on Cancer (IARC); 2007.
3. Scott CB, Scarantino C, Urtasun R, Movsas B, Jones CU, Simpson JR, Fischbach AJ, Curran Jr WJ. Validation and predictive power of Radiation Therapy Oncology Group (RTOG) recursive partitioning analysis classes for malignant glioma patients: a report using RTOG 90-06. Int J Radiat Oncol Biol Phys. 1998;40(1):51–5.
4. Stupp R, Mason WP, van den Bent MJ, Weller M, Fisher B, Taphoorn MJ, Belanger K, Brandes AA, Marosi C, Bogdahn U, et al. Radiotherapy plus concomitant and adjuvant temozolomide for glioblastoma. N Engl J Med. 2005;352(10):987–96.
5. Grossman SA, Ye X, Piantadosi S, Desideri S, Nabors LB, Rosenfeld M, Fisher J. Survival of patients with newly diagnosed glioblastoma treated with radiation and temozolomide in research studies in the United States. Clin Cancer Res. 2010;16(8):2443–9.

6. Lacroix M, Abi-Said D, Fourney DR, Gokaslan ZL, Shi W, DeMonte F, Lang FF, McCutcheon IE, Hassenbusch SJ, Holland E, et al. A multivariate analysis of 416 patients with glioblastoma multiforme: prognosis, extent of resection, and survival. J Neurosurg. 2001;95(2):190–8.
7. Sanai N, Polley MY, McDermott MW, Parsa AT, Berger MS. An extent of resection threshold for newly diagnosed glioblastomas. J Neurosurg. 2011;115(1):3–8.
8. Walker MD, Green SB, Byar DP, Alexander Jr E, Batzdorf U, Brooks WH, Hunt WE, MacCarty CS, Mahaley Jr MS, Mealey Jr J, et al. Randomized comparisons of radiotherapy and nitrosoureas for the treatment of malignant glioma after surgery. N Engl J Med. 1980;303(23):1323–9.
9. Walker MD, Alexander Jr E, Hunt WE, MacCarty CS, Mahaley Jr MS, Mealey Jr J, Norrell HA, Owens G, Ransohoff J, Wilson CB, et al. Evaluation of BCNU and/or radiotherapy in the treatment of anaplastic gliomas. A cooperative clinical trial. J Neurosurg. 1978;49(3):333–43.
10. Chang CH, Horton J, Schoenfeld D, Salazer O, Perez-Tamayo R, Kramer S, Weinstein A, Nelson JS, Tsukada Y. Comparison of postoperative radiotherapy and combined postoperative radiotherapy and chemotherapy in the multidisciplinary management of malignant gliomas. A joint Radiation Therapy Oncology Group and Eastern Cooperative Oncology Group study. Cancer. 1983;52(6):997–1007.
11. Bleehen NM, Stenning SP. A Medical Research Council trial of two radiotherapy doses in the treatment of grades 3 and 4 astrocytoma. The Medical Research Council Brain Tumour Working Party. Br J Cancer. 1991;64(4):769–74.
12. Walker MD, Strike TA, Sheline GE. An analysis of dose-effect relationship in the radiotherapy of malignant gliomas. Int J Radiat Oncol Biol Phys. 1979;5(10):1725–31.
13. Kristiansen K, Hagen S, Kollevold T, Torvik A, Holme I, Nesbakken R, Hatlevoll R, Lindgren M, Brun A, Lindgren S, et al. Combined modality therapy of operated astrocytomas grade III and IV. Confirmation of the value of postoperative irradiation and lack of potentiation of bleomycin on survival time: a prospective multicenter trial of the Scandinavian Glioblastoma Study Group. Cancer. 1981;47(4):649–52.
14. Shapiro WR, Green SB, Burger PC, Mahaley Jr MS, Selker RG, VanGilder JC, Robertson JT, Ransohoff J, Mealey Jr J, Strike TA, et al. Randomized trial of three chemotherapy regimens and two radiotherapy regimens and two radiotherapy regimens in postoperative treatment of malignant glioma. Brain Tumor Cooperative Group Trial 8001. J Neurosurg. 1989;71(1):1–9.
15. Coughlin C, Scott C, Langer C, Coia L, Curran W, Rubin P. Phase II, two-arm RTOG trial (94-11) of bischloroethylnitrosourea plus accelerated hyperfractionated radiotherapy (64.0 or 70.4 Gy) based on tumor volume (>20 or < or = 20 cm(2), respectively) in the treatment of newly-diagnosed radiosurgery-ineligible glioblastoma multiforme patients. Int J Radiat Oncol Biol Phys. 2000;48(5):1351–8.
16. Deutsch M, Green SB, Strike TA, Burger PC, Robertson JT, Selker RG, Shapiro WR, Mealey Jr J, Ransohoff II J, Paoletti P, et al. Results of a randomized trial comparing BCNU plus radiotherapy, streptozotocin plus radiotherapy, BCNU plus hyperfractionated radiotherapy, and BCNU following misonidazole plus radiotherapy in the postoperative treatment of malignant glioma. Int J Radiat Oncol Biol Phys. 1989;16(6):1389–96.
17. Werner-Wasik M, Scott CB, Nelson DF, Gaspar LE, Murray KJ, Fischbach JA, Nelson JS, Weinstein AS, Curran Jr WJ. Final report of a phase I/II trial of hyperfractionated and accelerated hyperfractionated radiation therapy with carmustine for adults with supratentorial malignant gliomas. Radiation Therapy Oncology Group Study 83-02. Cancer. 1996;77(8):1535–43.
18. Stupp R, Hegi ME, Mason WP, van den Bent MJ, Taphoorn MJ, Janzer RC, Ludwin SK, Allgeier A, Fisher B, Belanger K, et al. Effects of radiotherapy with concomitant and adjuvant temozolomide versus radiotherapy alone on survival in glioblastoma in a randomised phase III study: 5-year analysis of the EORTC-NCIC trial. Lancet Oncol. 2009;10(5):459–66.
19. Friedman HS, Prados MD, Wen PY, Mikkelsen T, Schiff D, Abrey LE, Yung WK, Paleologos N, Nicholas MK, Jensen R, et al. Bevacizumab alone and in combination with irinotecan in recurrent glioblastoma. J Clin Oncol. 2009;27(28):4733–40.
20. Kreisl TN, Kim L, Moore K, Duic P, Royce C, Stroud I, Garren N, Mackey M, Butman JA, Camphausen K, et al. Phase II trial of single-agent bevacizumab followed by bevacizumab plus irinotecan at tumor progression in recurrent glioblastoma. J Clin Oncol. 2009;27(5):740–5.
21. Wong ET, Hess KR, Gleason MJ, Jaeckle KA, Kyritsis AP, Prados MD, Levin VA, Yung WK. Outcomes and prognostic factors in recurrent glioma patients enrolled onto phase II clinical trials. J Clin Oncol. 1999;17(8):2572–8.
22. Lamborn KR, Yung WK, Chang SM, Wen PY, Cloughesy TF, DeAngelis LM, Robins HI, Lieberman FS, Fine HA, Fink KL, et al. Progression-free survival: an important end point in evaluating therapy for recurrent high-grade gliomas. Neuro Oncol. 2008;10(2):162–70.
23. DeAngelis LM. Anaplastic glioma: how to prognosticate outcome and choose a treatment strategy. [corrected]. J Clin Oncol. 2009;27(35):5861–2.
24. Lassman AB, Iwamoto FM, Cloughesy TF, Aldape KD, Rivera AL, Eichler AF, Louis DN, Paleologos NA, Fisher BJ, Ashby LS, et al. International retrospective study of over 1000 adults with anaplastic oligodendroglial tumors. Neuro Oncol. 2011;13(6):649–59.
25. Cairncross G, Berkey B, Shaw E, Jenkins R, Scheithauer B, Brachman D, Buckner J, Fink K, Souhami L, Laperierre N, et al. Phase III trial of chemotherapy plus radiotherapy compared with radiotherapy alone for pure and mixed anaplastic oligodendroglioma: Intergroup Radiation Therapy Oncology Group Trial 9402. J Clin Oncol. 2006;24(18):2707–14.
26. Medical Research Council Brain Tumor Working Party. Randomized trial of procarbazine, lomustine, and vincristine in the adjuvant treatment of high-grade astrocytoma: a Medical Research Council trial. J Clin Oncol. 2001;19(2):509–18.
27. van den Bent MJ, Carpentier AF, Brandes AA, Sanson M, Taphoorn MJ, Bernsen HJ, Frenay M, Tijssen CC, Grisold W, Sipos L, et al. Adjuvant procarbazine, lomustine, and vincristine improves progression-free survival but not overall survival in newly diagnosed anaplastic oligodendrogliomas and oligoastrocytomas: a randomized European Organisation for Research and Treatment of Cancer phase III trial. J Clin Oncol. 2006;24(18):2715–22.
28. http://clinicaltrials.gov/ct2/results?term=NCT00887146

29. http://clinicaltrials.gov/ct2/results?term=NCT00626990
30. Wick W, Hartmann C, Engel C, Stoffels M, Felsberg J, Stockhammer F, Sabel MC, Koeppen S, Ketter R, Meyermann R, et al. NOA-04 randomized phase III trial of sequential radiochemotherapy of anaplastic glioma with procarbazine, lomustine, and vincristine or temozolomide. J Clin Oncol. 2009;27(35):5874–80.
31. Perry A, Aldape KD, George DH, Burger PC. Small cell astrocytoma: an aggressive variant that is clinicopathologically and genetically distinct from anaplastic oligodendroglioma. Cancer. 2004;101(10):2318–26.
32. He J, Mokhtari K, Sanson M, Marie Y, Kujas M, Huguet S, Leuraud P, Capelle L, Delattre JY, Poirier J, et al. Glioblastomas with an oligodendroglial component: a pathological and molecular study. J Neuropathol Exp Neurol. 2001;60(9):863–71.
33. Homma T, Fukushima T, Vaccarella S, Yonekawa Y, Di Patre PL, Franceschi S, Ohgaki H. Correlation among pathology, genotype, and patient outcomes in glioblastoma. J Neuropathol Exp Neurol. 2006;65(9):846–54.
34. Shinojima N, Kochi M, Hamada J, Nakamura H, Yano S, Makino K, Tsuiki H, Tada K, Kuratsu J, Ishimaru Y, et al. The influence of sex and the presence of giant cells on postoperative long-term survival in adult patients with supratentorial glioblastoma multiforme. J Neurosurg. 2004;101(2):219–26.
35. Galanis E, Buckner JC, Dinapoli RP, Scheithauer BW, Jenkins RB, Wang CH, O'Fallon JR, Farr Jr G. Clinical outcome of gliosarcoma compared with glioblastoma multiforme: North Central Cancer Treatment Group results. J Neurosurg. 1998;89(3):425–30.
36. Reifenberger G, Louis DN. Oligodendroglioma: toward molecular definitions in diagnostic neuro-oncology. J Neuropathol Exp Neurol. 2003;62(2):111–26.
37. Aldape K, Burger PC, Perry A. Clinicopathologic aspects of 1p/19q loss and the diagnosis of oligodendroglioma. Arch Pathol Lab Med. 2007;131(2):242–51.
38. Ino Y, Betensky RA, Zlatescu MC, Sasaki H, Macdonald DR, Stemmer-Rachamimov AO, Ramsay DA, Cairncross JG, Louis DN. Molecular subtypes of anaplastic oligodendroglioma: implications for patient management at diagnosis. Clin Cancer Res. 2001;7(4):839–45.
39. Hoang-Xuan K, He J, Huguet S, Mokhtari K, Marie Y, Kujas M, Leuraud P, Capelle L, Delattre JY, Poirier J, et al. Molecular heterogeneity of oligodendrogliomas suggests alternative pathways in tumor progression. Neurology. 2001;57(7):1278–81.
40. Sasaki H, Zlatescu MC, Betensky RA, Ino Y, Cairncross JG, Louis DN. PTEN is a target of chromosome 10q loss in anaplastic oligodendrogliomas and PTEN alterations are associated with poor prognosis. Am J Pathol. 2001;159(1):359–67.
41. Scheie D, Cvancarova M, Mork S, Skullerud K, Andresen PA, Benestad I, Helseth E, Meling T, Beiske K. Can morphology predict 1p/19q loss in oligodendroglial tumours? Histopathology. 2008;53(5):578–87.
42. Olar A, Aldape KD. Biomarkers classification and therapeutic decision-making for malignant gliomas. Curr Treat Options Oncol. 2012;13(4):417–36.
43. Yan H, Parsons DW, Jin G, McLendon R, Rasheed BA, Yuan W, Kos I, Batinic-Haberle I, Jones S, Riggins GJ, et al. IDH1 and IDH2 mutations in gliomas. N Engl J Med. 2009;360(8):765–73.
44. Sanson M, Marie Y, Paris S, Idbaih A, Laffaire J, Ducray F, El Hallani S, Boisselier B, Mokhtari K, Hoang-Xuan K, et al. Isocitrate dehydrogenase 1 codon 132 mutation is an important prognostic biomarker in gliomas. J Clin Oncol. 2009;27(25):4150–4.
45. van den Bent MJ, Gravendeel LA, Gorlia T, Kros JM, Lapre L, Wesseling P, Teepen JL, Idbaih A, Sanson M, Smitt PA, et al. A hypermethylated phenotype is a better predictor of survival than MGMT methylation in anaplastic oligodendroglial brain tumors: a report from EORTC study 26951. Clin Cancer Res. 2011;17(22):7148–55.
46. Ducray F, Idbaih A, de Reynies A, Bieche I, Thillet J, Mokhtari K, Lair S, Marie Y, Paris S, Vidaud M, et al. Anaplastic oligodendrogliomas with 1p19q codeletion have a proneural gene expression profile. Mol Cancer. 2008;7:41.
47. Cooper LA, Gutman DA, Long Q, Johnson BA, Cholleti SR, Kurc T, Saltz JH, Brat DJ, Moreno CS. The proneural molecular signature is enriched in oligodendrogliomas and predicts improved survival among diffuse gliomas. PLoS One. 2010;5(9):e12548.
48. Bettegowda C, Agrawal N, Jiao Y, Sausen M, Wood LD, Hruban RH, Rodriguez FJ, Cahill DP, McLendon R, Riggins G, et al. Mutations in CIC and FUBP1 contribute to human oligodendroglioma. Science. 2011;333(6048):1453–5.
49. Yip S, Butterfield YS, Morozova O, Chittaranjan S, Blough MD, An J, Birol I, Chesnelong C, Chiu R, Chuah E, et al. Concurrent CIC mutations, IDH mutations, and 1p/19q loss distinguish oligodendrogliomas from other cancers. J Pathol. 2012;226(1):7–16.
50. Sahm F, Koelsche C, Meyer J, Pusch S, Lindenberg K, Mueller W, Herold-Mende C, von Deimling A, Hartmann C. CIC and FUBP1 mutations in oligodendrogliomas, oligoastrocytomas and astrocytomas. Acta Neuropathol. 2012;123(6):853–60.
51. Duncan R, Bazar L, Michelotti G, Tomonaga T, Krutzsch H, Avigan M, Levens D. A sequence-specific, single-strand binding protein activates the far upstream element of c-myc and defines a new DNA-binding motif. Genes Dev. 1994;8(4):465–80.
52. Hsiao HH, Nath A, Lin CY, Folta-Stogniew EJ, Rhoades E, Braddock DT. Quantitative characterization of the interactions among c-myc transcriptional regulators FUSE, FBP, and FIR. Biochemistry. 2010;49(22):4620–34.
53. Ohgaki H, Dessen P, Jourde B, Horstmann S, Nishikawa T, Di Patre PL, Burkhard C, Schuler D, Probst-Hensch NM, Maiorka PC, et al. Genetic pathways to glioblastoma: a population-based study. Cancer Res. 2004;64(19):6892–9.
54. Ohgaki H, Schauble B, zur Hausen A, Von Ammon K, Kleihues P. Genetic alterations associated with the evolution and progression of astrocytic brain tumours. Virchows Arch. 1995;427(2):113–8.
55. Rasheed BK, McLendon RE, Friedman HS, Friedman AH, Fuchs HE, Bigner DD, Bigner SH. Chromosome 10 deletion mapping in human gliomas: a common deletion region in 10q25. Oncogene. 1995;10(11):2243–6.
56. Fujisawa H, Reis RM, Nakamura M, Colella S, Yonekawa Y, Kleihues P, Ohgaki H. Loss of heterozygosity on chromosome 10 is more extensive in primary (de novo) than in secondary glioblastomas. Lab Invest. 2000;80(1):65–72.
57. Li J, Yen C, Liaw D, Podsypanina K, Bose S, Wang SI, Puc J, Miliaresis C, Rodgers L, McCombie R, et al. PTEN, a putative

protein tyrosine phosphatase gene mutated in human brain, breast, and prostate cancer. Science. 1997;275(5308):1943–7.
58. Choe G, Horvath S, Cloughesy TF, Crosby K, Seligson D, Palotie A, Inge L, Smith BL, Sawyers CL, Mischel PS. Analysis of the phosphatidylinositol 3′-kinase signaling pathway in glioblastoma patients in vivo. Cancer Res. 2003;63(11):2742–6.
59. Duerr EM, Rollbrocker B, Hayashi Y, Peters N, Meyer-Puttlitz B, Louis DN, Schramm J, Wiestler OD, Parsons R, Eng C, et al. PTEN mutations in gliomas and glioneuronal tumors. Oncogene. 1998;16(17):2259–64.
60. Knobbe CB, Merlo A, Reifenberger G. Pten signaling in gliomas. Neuro Oncol. 2002;4(3):196–211.
61. Tohma Y, Gratas C, Biernat W, Peraud A, Fukuda M, Yonekawa Y, Kleihues P, Ohgaki H. PTEN (MMAC1) mutations are frequent in primary glioblastomas (de novo) but not in secondary glioblastomas. J Neuropathol Exp Neurol. 1998;57(7):684–9.
62. Fuller GN, Bigner SH. Amplified cellular oncogenes in neoplasms of the human central nervous system. Mutat Res. 1992;276(3):299–306.
63. Ohgaki H, Kleihues P. Genetic pathways to primary and secondary glioblastoma. Am J Pathol. 2007;170(5):1445–53.
64. Gan HK, Kaye AH, Luwor RB. The EGFRvIII variant in glioblastoma multiforme. J Clin Neurosci. 2009;16(6):748–54.
65. Prigent SA, Nagane M, Lin H, Huvar I, Boss GR, Feramisco JR, Cavenee WK, Huang HS. Enhanced tumorigenic behavior of glioblastoma cells expressing a truncated epidermal growth factor receptor is mediated through the Ras-Shc-Grb2 pathway. J Biol Chem. 1996;271(41):25639–45.
66. Nishikawa R, Ji XD, Harmon RC, Lazar CS, Gill GN, Cavenee WK, Huang HJ. A mutant epidermal growth factor receptor common in human glioma confers enhanced tumorigenicity. Proc Natl Acad Sci U S A. 1994;91(16):7727–31.
67. Schlegel J, Merdes A, Stumm G, Albert FK, Forsting M, Hynes N, Kiessling M. Amplification of the epidermal-growth-factor-receptor gene correlates with different growth behaviour in human glioblastoma. Int J Cancer. 1994;56(1):72–7.
68. Hurtt MR, Moossy J, Donovan-Peluso M, Locker J. Amplification of epidermal growth factor receptor gene in gliomas: histopathology and prognosis. J Neuropathol Exp Neurol. 1992;51(1):84–90.
69. Parsons DW, Jones S, Zhang X, Lin JC, Leary RJ, Angenendt P, Mankoo P, Carter H, Siu IM, Gallia GL, et al. An integrated genomic analysis of human glioblastoma multiforme. Science. 2008;321(5897):1807–12.
70. Watanabe T, Nobusawa S, Kleihues P, Ohgaki H. IDH1 mutations are early events in the development of astrocytomas and oligodendrogliomas. Am J Pathol. 2009;174(4):1149–53.
71. Hartmann C, Meyer J, Balss J, Capper D, Mueller W, Christians A, Felsberg J, Wolter M, Mawrin C, Wick W, et al. Type and frequency of IDH1 and IDH2 mutations are related to astrocytic and oligodendroglial differentiation and age: a study of 1,010 diffuse gliomas. Acta Neuropathol. 2009;118(4):469–74.
72. van den Bent MJ, Dubbink HJ, Marie Y, Brandes AA, Taphoorn MJ, Wesseling P, Frenay M, Tijssen CC, Lacombe D, Idbaih A, et al. IDH1 and IDH2 mutations are prognostic but not predictive for outcome in anaplastic oligodendroglial tumors: a report of the European Organization for Research and Treatment of Cancer Brain Tumor Group. Clin Cancer Res. 2010;16(5):1597–604.
73. Metellus P, Coulibaly B, Colin C, de Paula AM, Vasiljevic A, Taieb D, Barlier A, Boisselier B, Mokhtari K, Wang XW, et al. Absence of IDH mutation identifies a novel radiologic and molecular subtype of WHO grade II gliomas with dismal prognosis. Acta Neuropathol. 2010;120(6):719–29.
74. Horbinski C, Kofler J, Kelly LM, Murdoch GH, Nikiforova MN. Diagnostic use of IDH1/2 mutation analysis in routine clinical testing of formalin-fixed, paraffin-embedded glioma tissues. J Neuropathol Exp Neurol. 2009;68(12):1319–25.
75. Zhao S, Lin Y, Xu W, Jiang W, Zha Z, Wang P, Yu W, Li Z, Gong L, Peng Y, et al. Glioma-derived mutations in IDH1 dominantly inhibit IDH1 catalytic activity and induce HIF-1alpha. Science. 2009;324(5924):261–5.
76. Ichimura K. Molecular pathogenesis of IDH mutations in gliomas. Brain Tumor Pathol. 2012;29(3):131–9.
77. Dang L, White DW, Gross S, Bennett BD, Bittinger MA, Driggers EM, Fantin VR, Jang HG, Jin S, Keenan MC, et al. Cancer-associated IDH1 mutations produce 2-hydroxyglutarate. Nature. 2009;462(7274):739–44.
78. Aghili M, Zahedi F, Rafiee E. Hydroxyglutaric aciduria and malignant brain tumor: a case report and literature review. J Neurooncol. 2009;91(2):233–6.
79. Xu W, Yang H, Liu Y, Yang Y, Wang P, Kim SH, Ito S, Yang C, Xiao MT, Liu LX, et al. Oncometabolite 2-hydroxyglutarate is a competitive inhibitor of alpha-ketoglutarate-dependent dioxygenases. Cancer Cell. 2011;19(1):17–30.
80. Guo JU, Su Y, Zhong C, Ming GL, Song H. Hydroxylation of 5-methylcytosine by TET1 promotes active DNA demethylation in the adult brain. Cell. 2011;145(3):423–34.
81. Turcan S, Rohle D, Goenka A, Walsh LA, Fang F, Yilmaz E, Campos C, Fabius AW, Lu C, Ward PS, et al. IDH1 mutation is sufficient to establish the glioma hypermethylator phenotype. Nature. 2012;483(7390):479–83.
82. Jiao Y, Killela PJ, Reitman ZJ, Rasheed AB, Heaphy CM, de Wilde RF, Rodriguez FJ, Rosemberg S, Oba-Shinjo SM, Nagahashi Marie SK, et al. Frequent ATRX, CIC, FUBP1 and IDH1 mutations refine the classification of malignant gliomas. Oncotarget. 2012;3(7):709–22.
83. Gerson SL. MGMT: its role in cancer aetiology and cancer therapeutics. Nat Rev Cancer. 2004;4(4):296–307.
84. Riemenschneider MJ, Hegi ME, Reifenberger G. MGMT promoter methylation in malignant gliomas. Target Oncol. 2010;5(3):161–5.
85. Weller M, Stupp R, Reifenberger G, Brandes AA, van den Bent MJ, Wick W, Hegi ME. MGMT promoter methylation in malignant gliomas: ready for personalized medicine? Nat Rev Neurol. 2010;6(1):39–51.
86. Mellai M, Monzeglio O, Piazzi A, Caldera V, Annovazzi L, Cassoni P, Valente G, Cordera S, Mocellini C, Schiffer D. MGMT promoter hypermethylation and its associations with genetic alterations in a series of 350 brain tumors. J Neurooncol. 2012;107(3):617–31.
87. van den Bent MJ, Dubbink HJ, Sanson M, van der Lee-Haarloo CR, Hegi M, Jeuken JW, Ibdaih A, Brandes AA, Taphoorn MJ, Frenay M, et al. MGMT promoter methylation is prognostic

but not predictive for outcome to adjuvant PCV chemotherapy in anaplastic oligodendroglial tumors: a report from EORTC Brain Tumor Group Study 26951. J Clin Oncol. 2009;27(35):5881–6.

88. Mollemann M, Wolter M, Felsberg J, Collins VP, Reifenberger G. Frequent promoter hypermethylation and low expression of the MGMT gene in oligodendroglial tumors. Int J Cancer. 2005;113(3):379–85.
89. Hegi ME, Diserens AC, Gorlia T, Hamou MF, de Tribolet N, Weller M, Kros JM, Hainfellner JA, Mason W, Mariani L, et al. MGMT gene silencing and benefit from temozolomide in glioblastoma. N Engl J Med. 2005;352(10):997–1003.
90. Esteller M, Garcia-Foncillas J, Andion E, Goodman SN, Hidalgo OF, Vanaclocha V, Baylin SB, Herman JG. Inactivation of the DNA-repair gene MGMT and the clinical response of gliomas to alkylating agents. N Engl J Med. 2000;343(19):1350–4.
91. Rivera AL, Pelloski CE, Gilbert MR, Colman H, De La Cruz C, Sulman EP, Bekele BN, Aldape KD. MGMT promoter methylation is predictive of response to radiotherapy and prognostic in the absence of adjuvant alkylating chemotherapy for glioblastoma. Neuro Oncol. 2010;12(2):116–21.
92. Olson RA, Brastianos PK, Palma DA. Prognostic and predictive value of epigenetic silencing of MGMT in patients with high grade gliomas: a systematic review and meta-analysis. J Neurooncol. 2011;105(2):325–35.
93. Noushmehr H, Weisenberger DJ, Diefes K, Phillips HS, Pujara K, Berman BP, Pan F, Pelloski CE, Sulman EP, Bhat KP, et al. Identification of a CpG island methylator phenotype that defines a distinct subgroup of glioma. Cancer Cell. 2010;17(5):510–22.
94. Verhaak RG, Hoadley KA, Purdom E, Wang V, Qi Y, Wilkerson MD, Miller CR, Ding L, Golub T, Mesirov JP, et al. Integrated genomic analysis identifies clinically relevant subtypes of glioblastoma characterized by abnormalities in PDGFRA, IDH1, EGFR, and NF1. Cancer Cell. 2010;17(1):98–110.
95. Li A, Walling J, Ahn S, Kotliarov Y, Su Q, Quezado M, Oberholtzer JC, Park J, Zenklusen JC, Fine HA. Unsupervised analysis of transcriptomic profiles reveals six glioma subtypes. Cancer Res. 2009;69(5):2091–9.
96. Shen R, Mo Q, Schultz N, Seshan VE, Olshen AB, Huse J, Ladanyi M, Sander C. Integrative subtype discovery in glioblastoma using iCluster. PLoS One. 2012;7(4):e35236.
97. Curran Jr WJ, Scott CB, Horton J, Nelson JS, Weinstein AS, Fischbach AJ, Chang CH, Rotman M, Asbell SO, Krisch RE, et al. Recursive partitioning analysis of prognostic factors in three Radiation Therapy Oncology Group malignant glioma trials. J Natl Cancer Inst. 1993;85(9):704–10.
98. Siker ML, Wang M, Porter K, Nelson DF, Curran WJ, Michalski JM, Souhami L, Chakravarti A, Yung WK, Delrowe J, et al. Age as an independent prognostic factor in patients with glioblastoma: a Radiation Therapy Oncology Group and American College of Surgeons National Cancer Data Base comparison. J Neurooncol. 2011;104(1):351–6.
99. Stummer W, Reulen HJ, Meinel T, Pichlmeier U, Schumacher W, Tonn JC, Rohde V, Oppel F, Turowski B, Woiciechowsky C, et al. Extent of resection and survival in glioblastoma multiforme: identification of and adjustment for bias. Neurosurgery. 2008;62(3):564–76; discussion 564–76.
100. Buckner JC. Factors influencing survival in high-grade gliomas. Semin Oncol. 2003;30(6 Suppl 19):10–4.
101. Kaloshi G, Benouaich-Amiel A, Diakite F, Taillibert S, Lejeune J, Laigle-Donadey F, Renard MA, Iraqi W, Idbaih A, Paris S, et al. Temozolomide for low-grade gliomas: predictive impact of 1p/19q loss on response and outcome. Neurology. 2007;68(21):1831–6.
102. Cairncross JG, Ueki K, Zlatescu MC, Lisle DK, Finkelstein DM, Hammond RR, Silver JS, Stark PC, Macdonald DR, Ino Y, et al. Specific genetic predictors of chemotherapeutic response and survival in patients with anaplastic oligodendrogliomas. J Natl Cancer Inst. 1998;90(19):1473–9.
103. Hartmann C, Hentschel B, Wick W, Capper D, Felsberg J, Simon M, Westphal M, Schackert G, Meyermann R, Pietsch T, et al. Patients with IDH1 wild type anaplastic astrocytomas exhibit worse prognosis than IDH1-mutated glioblastomas, and IDH1 mutation status accounts for the unfavorable prognostic effect of higher age: implications for classification of gliomas. Acta Neuropathol. 2010;120(6):707–18.
104. Salomon DS, Brandt R, Ciardiello F, Normanno N. Epidermal growth factor-related peptides and their receptors in human malignancies. Crit Rev Oncol Hematol. 1995;19(3):183–232.
105. Holbro T, Civenni G, Hynes NE. The ErbB receptors and their role in cancer progression. Exp Cell Res. 2003;284(1):99–110.
106. Bleeker FE, Molenaar RJ, Leenstra S. Recent advances in the molecular understanding of glioblastoma. J Neurooncol. 2012;108(1):11–27.
107. Comprehensive genomic characterization defines human glioblastoma genes and core pathways. Nature. 2008;455(7216):1061–8.
108. Li B, Yuan M, Kim IA, Chang CM, Bernhard EJ, Shu HK. Mutant epidermal growth factor receptor displays increased signaling through the phosphatidylinositol-3 kinase/AKT pathway and promotes radioresistance in cells of astrocytic origin. Oncogene. 2004;23(26):4594–602.
109. Liu W, James CD, Frederick L, Alderete BE, Jenkins RB. PTEN/MMAC1 mutations and EGFR amplification in glioblastomas. Cancer Res. 1997;57(23):5254–7.
110. Sidransky D, Mikkelsen T, Schwechheimer K, Rosenblum ML, Cavanee W, Vogelstein B. Clonal expansion of p53 mutant cells is associated with brain tumour progression. Nature. 1992;355(6363):846–7.
111. Bogler O, Huang HJ, Cavenee WK. Loss of wild-type p53 bestows a growth advantage on primary cortical astrocytes and facilitates their in vitro transformation. Cancer Res. 1995;55(13):2746–51.
112. Reifenberger G, Liu L, Ichimura K, Schmidt EE, Collins VP. Amplification and overexpression of the MDM2 gene in a subset of human malignant gliomas without p53 mutations. Cancer Res. 1993;53(12):2736–9.
113. Ohgaki H, Kleihues P. Genetic alterations and signaling pathways in the evolution of gliomas. Cancer Sci. 2009;100(12):2235–41.
114. Stott FJ, Bates S, James MC, McConnell BB, Starborg M, Brookes S, Palmero I, Ryan K, Hara E, Vousden KH, et al. The alternative product from the human CDKN2A locus, p14(ARF), participates in a regulatory feedback loop with p53 and MDM2. EMBO J. 1998;17(17):5001–14.

115. Dietrich J, Imitola J, Kesari S. Mechanisms of disease: the role of stem cells in the biology and treatment of gliomas. Nat Clin Pract Oncol. 2008;5(7):393–404.
116. Singh SK, Hawkins C, Clarke ID, Squire JA, Bayani J, Hide T, Henkelman RM, Cusimano MD, Dirks PB. Identification of human brain tumour initiating cells. Nature. 2004;432(7015): 396–401.
117. Bao S, Wu Q, McLendon RE, Hao Y, Shi Q, Hjelmeland AB, Dewhirst MW, Bigner DD, Rich JN. Glioma stem cells promote radioresistance by preferential activation of the DNA damage response. Nature. 2006;444(7120):756–60.
118. Dean M, Fojo T, Bates S. Tumour stem cells and drug resistance. Nat Rev Cancer. 2005;5(4):275–84.
119. Shih Ie M, Wang TL. Notch signaling, gamma-secretase inhibitors, and cancer therapy. Cancer Res. 2007;67(5):1879–82.
120. Kerbel RS. Tumor angiogenesis. N Engl J Med. 2008;358(19): 2039–49.
121. Dietrich J, Diamond EL, Kesari S. Glioma stem cell signaling: therapeutic opportunities and challenges. Expert Rev Anticancer Ther. 2010;10(5):709–22.
122. Gomez-Manzano C, Fueyo J, Jiang H, Glass TL, Lee HY, Hu M, Liu JL, Jasti SL, Liu TJ, Conrad CA, et al. Mechanisms underlying PTEN regulation of vascular endothelial growth factor and angiogenesis. Ann Neurol. 2003;53(1):109–17.
123. Norden AD, Drappatz J, Wen PY. Antiangiogenic therapies for high-grade glioma. Nat Rev Neurol. 2009;5(11):610–20.
124. Jain RK, di Tomaso E, Duda DG, Loeffler JS, Sorensen AG, Batchelor TT. Angiogenesis in brain tumours. Nat Rev Neurosci. 2007;8(8):610–22.
125. Cohen MH, Shen YL, Keegan P, Pazdur R. FDA drug approval summary: bevacizumab (Avastin) as treatment of recurrent glioblastoma multiforme. Oncologist. 2009;14(11):1131–8.
126. Vredenburgh JJ, Desjardins A, Herndon II JE, Marcello J, Reardon DA, Quinn JA, Rich JN, Sathornsumetee S, Gururangan S, Sampson J, et al. Bevacizumab plus irinotecan in recurrent glioblastoma multiforme. J Clin Oncol. 2007;25(30):4722–9.
127. Chinot OL, Wick W, Mason W, Henriksson R, Saran F, Nishikawa R, Carpentier AF, Hoang-Xuan K, Kavan P, Cernea D, et al. Bevacizumab plus radiotherapy-temozolomide for newly diagnosed glioblastoma. N Engl J Med. 2014;370(8):709–22.
128. Gilbert MR, Dignam JJ, Armstrong TS, Wefel JS, Blumenthal DT, Vogelbaum MA, Colman H, Chakravarti A, Pugh S, Won M, et al. A randomized trial of bevacizumab for newly diagnosed glioblastoma. N Engl J Med. 2014;370(8):699–708.
129. Weller M, Yung WK. Angiogenesis inhibition for glioblastoma at the edge: beyond AVAGlio and RTOG 0825. Neuro Oncol. 2013;15(8):971.
130. Batchelor TT, Duda DG, di Tomaso E, Ancukiewicz M, Plotkin SR, Gerstner E, Eichler AF, Drappatz J, Hochberg FH, Benner T, et al. Phase II study of cediranib, an oral pan-vascular endothelial growth factor receptor tyrosine kinase inhibitor, in patients with recurrent glioblastoma. J Clin Oncol. 2010;28(17):2817–23.
131. Reardon DA, Fink KL, Mikkelsen T, Cloughesy TF, O'Neill A, Plotkin S, Glantz M, Ravin P, Raizer JJ, Rich KM, et al. Randomized phase II study of cilengitide, an integrin-targeting arginine-glycine-aspartic acid peptide, in recurrent glioblastoma multiforme. J Clin Oncol. 2008;26(34):5610–7.
132. Kreisl TN, McNeill KA, Sul J, Iwamoto FM, Shih J, Fine HA. A phase I/II trial of vandetanib for patients with recurrent malignant glioma. Neuro Oncol. 2012;14(12):1519–26.
133. Wen PY. American Society of Clinical Oncology 2010: report of selected studies from the CNS tumors section. Expert Rev Anticancer Ther. 2010;10(9):1367–9.
134. Kreisl TN, Smith P, Sul J, Salgado C, Iwamoto FM, Shih JH, Fine HA. Continuous daily sunitinib for recurrent glioblastoma. J Neurooncol. 2013;111(1):41–8.
135. de Groot JF, Lamborn KR, Chang SM, Gilbert MR, Cloughesy TF, Aldape K, Yao J, Jackson EF, Lieberman F, Robins HI, et al. Phase II study of aflibercept in recurrent malignant glioma: a North American Brain Tumor Consortium study. J Clin Oncol. 2011;29(19):2689–95.
136. Lee EQ, Kuhn J, Lamborn KR, Abrey L, DeAngelis LM, Lieberman F, Robins HI, Chang SM, Yung WK, Drappatz J, et al. Phase I/II study of sorafenib in combination with temsirolimus for recurrent glioblastoma or gliosarcoma: North American Brain Tumor Consortium study 05-02. Neuro Oncol. 2012;14(12):1511–8.
137. Peereboom DM, Ahluwalia MS, Ye X, Supko JG, Hilderbrand SL, Phuphanich S, Nabors LB, Rosenfeld MR, Mikkelsen T, Grossman SA. NABTT 0502: a phase II and pharmacokinetic study of erlotinib and sorafenib for patients with progressive or recurrent glioblastoma multiforme. Neuro Oncol. 2013;15(4):490–6.
138. http://clinicaltrials.gov/ct2/show/NCT00720356
139. http://clinicaltrials.gov/ct2/show/NCT00329719
140. http://clinicaltrials.gov/ct2/show/NCT01609790. 2013.
141. Rich JN, Reardon DA, Peery T, Dowell JM, Quinn JA, Penne KL, Wikstrand CJ, Van Duyn LB, Dancey JE, McLendon RE, et al. Phase II trial of gefitinib in recurrent glioblastoma. J Clin Oncol. 2004;22(1):133–42.
142. van den Bent MJ, Brandes AA, Rampling R, Kouwenhoven MC, Kros JM, Carpentier AF, Clement PM, Frenay M, Campone M, Baurain JF, et al. Randomized phase II trial of erlotinib versus temozolomide or carmustine in recurrent glioblastoma: EORTC brain tumor group study 26034. J Clin Oncol. 2009;27(8):1268–74.
143. Raizer JJ, Abrey LE, Lassman AB, Chang SM, Lamborn KR, Kuhn JG, Yung WK, Gilbert MR, Aldape KA, Wen PY, et al. A phase II trial of erlotinib in patients with recurrent malignant gliomas and nonprogressive glioblastoma multiforme postradiation therapy. Neuro Oncol. 2010;12(1):95–103.
144. Yung WK, Vredenburgh JJ, Cloughesy TF, Nghiemphu P, Klencke B, Gilbert MR, Reardon DA, Prados MD. Safety and efficacy of erlotinib in first-relapse glioblastoma: a phase II open-label study. Neuro Oncol. 2010;12(10):1061–70.
145. Brown PD, Krishnan S, Sarkaria JN, Wu W, Jaeckle KA, Uhm JH, Geoffroy FJ, Arusell R, Kitange G, Jenkins RB, et al. Phase I/II trial of erlotinib and temozolomide with radiation therapy in the treatment of newly diagnosed glioblastoma multiforme: North Central Cancer Treatment Group Study N0177. J Clin Oncol. 2008;26(34):5603–9.
146. Lassman AB, Rossi MR, Raizer JJ, Abrey LE, Lieberman FS, Grefe CN, Lamborn K, Pao W, Shih AH, Kuhn JG, et al. Molecular study of malignant gliomas treated with epidermal growth factor receptor inhibitors: tissue analysis from North American Brain Tumor Consortium Trials 01-03 and 00-01. Clin Cancer Res. 2005;11(21):7841–50.

147. Neyns B, Sadones J, Joosens E, Bouttens F, Verbeke L, Baurain JF, D'Hondt L, Strauven T, Chaskis C, In't Veld P, et al. Stratified phase II trial of cetuximab in patients with recurrent high-grade glioma. Ann Oncol. 2009;20(9):1596–603.
148. Snuderl M, Fazlollahi L, Le LP, Nitta M, Zhelyazkova BH, Davidson CJ, Akhavanfard S, Cahill DP, Aldape KD, Betensky RA, et al. Mosaic amplification of multiple receptor tyrosine kinase genes in glioblastoma. Cancer Cell. 2011;20(6):810–7.
149. Stommel JM, Kimmelman AC, Ying H, Nabioullin R, Ponugoti AH, Wiedemeyer R, Stegh AH, Bradner JE, Ligon KL, Brennan C, et al. Coactivation of receptor tyrosine kinases affects the response of tumor cells to targeted therapies. Science. 2007;318(5848):287–90.
150. Szerlip NJ, Pedraza A, Chakravarty D, Azim M, McGuire J, Fang Y, Ozawa T, Holland EC, Huse JT, Jhanwar S, et al. Intratumoral heterogeneity of receptor tyrosine kinases EGFR and PDGFRA amplification in glioblastoma defines subpopulations with distinct growth factor response. Proc Natl Acad Sci U S A. 2012;109(8):3041–6.
151. Hegi ME, Diserens AC, Bady P, Kamoshima Y, Kouwenhoven MC, Delorenzi M, Lambiv WL, Hamou MF, Matter MS, Koch A, et al. Pathway analysis of glioblastoma tissue after preoperative treatment with the EGFR tyrosine kinase inhibitor gefitinib—a phase II trial. Mol Cancer Ther. 2011;10(6):1102–12.
152. Drappatz J, Norden AD, Wong ET, Doherty LM, Lafrankie DC, Ciampa A, Kesari S, Sceppa C, Gerard M, Phan P, et al. Phase I study of vandetanib with radiotherapy and temozolomide for newly diagnosed glioblastoma. Int J Radiat Oncol Biol Phys. 2010;78(1):85–90.
153. Thiessen B, Stewart C, Tsao M, Kamel-Reid S, Schaiquevich P, Mason W, Easaw J, Belanger K, Forsyth P, McIntosh L, et al. A phase I/II trial of GW572016 (lapatinib) in recurrent glioblastoma multiforme: clinical outcomes, pharmacokinetics and molecular correlation. Cancer Chemother Pharmacol. 2010;65(2):353–61.
154. http://clinicaltrials.gov/ct2/show/NCT00977431
155. http://clinicaltrials.gov/ct2/show/NCT00727506
156. http://clinicaltrials.gov/ct2/show/NCT01520870
157. http://clinicaltrials.gov/ct2/show/NCT00753246
158. Sampson JH, Heimberger AB, Archer GE, Aldape KD, Friedman AH, Friedman HS, Gilbert MR, Herndon II JE, McLendon RE, Mitchell DA, et al. Immunologic escape after prolonged progression-free survival with epidermal growth factor receptor variant III peptide vaccination in patients with newly diagnosed glioblastoma. J Clin Oncol. 2010;28(31):4722–9.
159. http://clinicaltrials.gov/ct2/show/NCT01480479
160. http://clinicaltrials.gov/ct2/show/NCT01454596
161. Batchelor TT, Mulholland P, Neyns B, Nabors LB, Campone M, Wick A, Mason W, Mikkelsen T, Phuphanich S, Ashby LS, et al. Phase III randomized trial comparing the efficacy of cediranib as monotherapy, and in combination with lomustine, versus lomustine alone in patients with recurrent glioblastoma. J Clin Oncol. 2013;31(26):3212–8.
162. Reardon DA, Vredenburgh JJ, Desjardins A, Peters K, Gururangan S, Sampson JH, Marcello J, Herndon II JE, McLendon RE, Janney D, et al. Effect of CYP3A-inducing anti-epileptics on sorafenib exposure: results of a phase II study of sorafenib plus daily temozolomide in adults with recurrent glioblastoma. J Neurooncol. 2011;101(1):57–66.
163. Hainsworth JD, Ervin T, Friedman E, Priego V, Murphy PB, Clark BL, Lamar RE. Concurrent radiotherapy and temozolomide followed by temozolomide and sorafenib in the first-line treatment of patients with glioblastoma multiforme. Cancer. 2010;116(15):3663–9.
164. Galanis E, Anderson SK, Lafky JM, Uhm JH, Giannini C, Kumar SK, Kimlinger TK, Northfelt DW, Flynn PJ, Jaeckle KA, et al. Phase II study of bevacizumab in combination with sorafenib in recurrent glioblastoma (N0776): a north central cancer treatment group trial. Clin Cancer Res. 2013;19(17):4816–23.
165. Pan E, Yu D, Yue B, Potthast L, Chowdhary S, Smith P, Chamberlain M. A prospective phase II single-institution trial of sunitinib for recurrent malignant glioma. J Neurooncol. 2012;110(1):111–8.
166. Neyns B, Sadones J, Chaskis C, Dujardin M, Everaert H, Lv S, Duerinck J, Tynninen O, Nupponen N, Michotte A, et al. Phase II study of sunitinib malate in patients with recurrent high-grade glioma. J Neurooncol. 2011;103(3):491–501.
167. Stupp R, Hegi ME, Neyns B, Goldbrunner R, Schlegel U, Clement PM, Grabenbauer GG, Ochsenbein AF, Simon M, Dietrich PY, et al. Phase I/IIa study of cilengitide and temozolomide with concomitant radiotherapy followed by cilengitide and temozolomide maintenance therapy in patients with newly diagnosed glioblastoma. J Clin Oncol. 2010;28(16):2712–8.
168. Kreisl TN, Kotliarova S, Butman JA, Albert PS, Kim L, Musib L, Thornton D, Fine HA. A phase I/II trial of enzastaurin in patients with recurrent high-grade gliomas. Neuro Oncol. 2010;12(2):181–9.
169. Wick W, Puduvalli VK, Chamberlain MC, van den Bent MJ, Carpentier AF, Cher LM, Mason W, Weller M, Hong S, Musib L, et al. Phase III study of enzastaurin compared with lomustine in the treatment of recurrent intracranial glioblastoma. J Clin Oncol. 2010;28(7):1168–74.
170. http://clinicaltrials.gov/ct2/show/NCT01609790
171. http://clinicaltrials.gov/ct2/show/NCT01290263
172. Galanis E, Buckner JC, Maurer MJ, Kreisberg JI, Ballman K, Boni J, Peralba JM, Jenkins RB, Dakhil SR, Morton RF, et al. Phase II trial of temsirolimus (CCI-779) in recurrent glioblastoma multiforme: a North Central Cancer Treatment Group Study. J Clin Oncol. 2005;23(23):5294–304.
173. Chang SM, Wen P, Cloughesy T, Greenberg H, Schiff D, Conrad C, Fink K, Robins HI, De Angelis L, Raizer J, et al. Phase II study of CCI-779 in patients with recurrent glioblastoma multiforme. Invest New Drugs. 2005;23(4):357–61.
174. Kreisl TN, Lassman AB, Mischel PS, Rosen N, Scher HI, Teruya-Feldstein J, Shaffer D, Lis E, Abrey LE. A pilot study of everolimus and gefitinib in the treatment of recurrent glioblastoma (GBM). J Neurooncol. 2009;92(1):99–105.
175. Chinnaiyan P, Won M, Wen PY, Rojiani AM, Wendland M, Dipetrillo TA, Corn BW, Mehta MP. RTOG 0913: a phase 1 study of daily everolimus (RAD001) in combination with radiation therapy and temozolomide in patients with newly diagnosed glioblastoma. Int J Radiat Oncol Biol Phys. 2013;86(5):880–4.

176. http://clinicaltrials.gov/ct2/show/NCT01062399
177. http://clinicaltrials.gov/ct2/show/NCT01339052
178. http://clinicaltrials.gov/ct2/show/NCT01349660
179. http://clinicaltrials.gov/ct2/show/NCT01473901
180. http://clinicaltrials.gov/ct2/show/NCT00704080
181. Wen PY, Yung WK, Lamborn KR, Dahia PL, Wang Y, Peng B, Abrey LE, Raizer J, Cloughesy TF, Fink K, et al. Phase I/II study of imatinib mesylate for recurrent malignant gliomas: North American Brain Tumor Consortium Study 99-08. Clin Cancer Res. 2006;12(16):4899–907.
182. Reardon DA, Dresemann G, Taillibert S, Campone M, van den Bent M, Clement P, Blomquist E, Gordower L, Schultz H, Raizer J, et al. Multicentre phase II studies evaluating imatinib plus hydroxyurea in patients with progressive glioblastoma. Br J Cancer. 2009;101(12):1995–2004.
183. Dresemann G, Weller M, Rosenthal MA, Wedding U, Wagner W, Engel E, Heinrich B, Mayer-Steinacker R, Karup-Hansen A, Fluge O, et al. Imatinib in combination with hydroxyurea versus hydroxyurea alone as oral therapy in patients with progressive pretreated glioblastoma resistant to standard dose temozolomide. J Neurooncol. 2010;96(3):393–402.
184. http://clinicaltrials.gov/ct2/show/NCT00667394
185. http://clinicaltrials.gov/ct2/show/NCT00379080
186. Franceschi E, Stupp R, van den Bent MJ, van Herpen C, Laigle Donadey F, Gorlia T, Hegi M, Lhermitte B, Strauss LC, Allgeier A, et al. EORTC 26083 phase I/II trial of dasatinib in combination with CCNU in patients with recurrent glioblastoma. Neuro Oncol. 2012;14(12):1503–10.
187. Reardon DA, Vredenburgh JJ, Desjardins A, Peters KB, Sathornsumetee S, Threatt S, Sampson JH, Herndon II JE, Coan A, McSherry F, et al. Phase 1 trial of dasatinib plus erlotinib in adults with recurrent malignant glioma. J Neurooncol. 2012;108(3):499–506.
188. http://clinicaltrials.gov/ct2/show/NCT00892177
189. http://clinicaltrials.gov/ct2/show/NCT00895960
190. http://clinicaltrials.gov/ct2/show/NCT00869401
191. http://clinicaltrials.gov/ct2/show/NCT01227434
192. http://clinicaltrials.gov/ct2/show/NCT01269411
193. http://clinicaltrials.gov/ct2/show/NCT01119599
194. http://clinicaltrials.gov/ct2/show/NCT01189240
195. http://clinicaltrials.gov/ct2/show/NCT01122901
196. http://clinicaltrials.gov/ct2/show/NCT00980343

7 Pediatric High-Grade Gliomas and DIPG

Oren J. Becher, Kelly L. Barton, Kyle G. Halvorson, and Roger McLendon

The central nervous system (CNS) is the second most common location for tumorigenesis in children with the majority of tumors being benign. Pediatric high-grade gliomas (pHGGs) only account for approximately 8–12 % of all childhood CNS tumors but are a leading cause of mortality in children [1, 2]. pHGG histologies include anaplastic astrocytomas (World Health Organization or WHO grade III), anaplastic oligodendrogliomas (WHO grade III), and glioblastomas/gliosarcomas (WHO grade IV). pHGGs can arise anywhere in the CNS and those that arise in the brainstem are also called diffuse intrinsic pontine glioma or DIPG. Unfortunately, little therapeutic progress has been made over the last few decades, and clinical outcomes for these patients remain dismal. To date the only effective modality is focal radiation, which provides only temporary tumor control in most patients. One of the reasons for this lack of clinical progress has been our limited understanding of the molecular genetics and tumor biology of pHGGs. Very recently, next generation sequencing studies have led to the discovery of a fundamentally novel class of genetic alterations, implicating epigenetic reprogramming as a central component of pHGG pathogenesis and opening potential avenues for new, biology-based treatment approaches.

Additional key insights from recent genomic studies of pHGG include the appreciation of molecular genetic heterogeneity not only between patients, but also within the tumor tissue of the same patients, distinct biological differences compared to adult high-grade gliomas, and the recognition of differences in tumorigenesis based on age and tumor location within the CNS. Clearly, these insights will need to be taken into account in developing novel therapeutic strategies that will hopefully lead to improved outcomes of patients afflicted with these highly aggressive and lethal tumors. In this chapter, we will briefly describe the histopathology, cytogenetic, molecular genetic and epigenetic alterations, as well as gene expression profiling of pHGGs. We will also discuss key signaling pathways pertinent to the advancement of molecular targeted therapies in pHGGs. Lastly, we will review current clinical trials of molecular targeted therapies for pHGGs and emerging future avenues of clinical investigation.

Histopathology

High-grade gliomas consist of the gliomas graded by the World Health Organization as Grades III and IV. As such, the following tumors fall into this group: anaplastic astrocytoma, glioblastoma multiforme (GBM), anaplastic oligodendroglioma, and anaplastic oligo-astrocytoma. While not a strictly histogenetic type, anaplastic glioma has been assigned to those cases that do not clearly fall into either anaplastic astrocytoma or anaplastic oligodendroglioma due to small sample size, therapeutic effect, or some other histologic artifact that renders specific classification difficult.

High-grade gliomas of all types share common features of high mitotic activity, vascular endothelial proliferation and, quite commonly, focal necrosis. Oligodendrogliomas share features with the myelinating cells of the CNS, the oligodendrocytes. These include round, regular nuclei and clear cytoplasm that ring the nuclei producing a fried-egg appearance. Anaplastic oligodendrogliomas exhibit dense hypercellularity, frequent mitotic figures, vascular endothelial proliferation, and foci of necrosis. These foci may or may not be ringed by cells tightly surrounding the focus, defined as pseudopalisading necrosis (Fig. 7.1).

Anaplastic astrocytomas differ from anaplastic oligodendrogliomas by having hyperchromatic nuclei that are often elongated, irregular, or smudged. Mitotic figures may not be common, but can be found by immunohistochemical markers of proliferation such as the MIB-1 index. While the tumor cells are not as densely packed as in the oligodendroglioma, they are nonetheless, obviously more hypercellular than the white matter by a factor of three- to tenfold. Vascular changes are frequent in anaplastic astrocytoma, but the defining element of vascular proliferation as found in the Grade IV

M.A. Karajannis and D. Zagzag (eds.), *Molecular Pathology of Nervous System Tumors: Biological Stratification and Targeted Therapies*, Molecular Pathology Library 8,
DOI 10.1007/978-1-4939-1830-0_7, © Springer Science+Business Media New York 2015

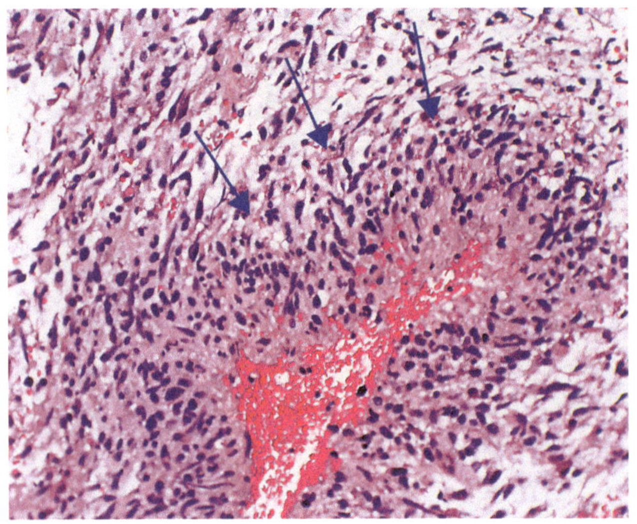

Fig. 7.1 Pediatric glioblastoma exhibiting pseudopalisading necrosis. Hematoxylin and eosin staining of a Grade IV GBM (40× magnification). *Arrows* point to pseudopalisading necrosis

glioblastoma, is debated. While most brain tumor neuropathologists agree that endothelial duplication circumferentially ringing the vessel is a feature of glioblastomas, it is unclear where glomeruloid vessels and vascular garlands or loops of vessels fall in astrocytoma grading. Among astrocytic tumors, foci of necrosis are reserved for glioblastomas.

Glioblastoma multiforme, the most malignant and most common of the high-grade gliomas, is an astrocytic neoplasm that has been found to most commonly arise de novo without a preceding history of glioma, with only 5 % of glioblastomas occurring as a result of progression from a lower grade astrocytoma. Both de novo and progressive GBMs exhibit nuclear pleomorphism, mitotic activity, vascular proliferation, and/or necrosis. While densely cellular in some foci of the tumor, there is commonly an infiltrative component that can be found distant from the central mass. This infiltrative capability currently makes GBMs impossible to cure by surgery or local–regional radiation therapy.

Epigenetics

With the advent of next generation sequencing, our understanding of the genetic alterations in pHGGs has been turned upside down. This technological advance has led to the discovery of heterozygous K27M or G34R/V mutations in the tail of histone 3.3 or K27M mutations in the tail of histone 3.1 and loss of function mutations in the chromatin remodelers ATRX (α-thalassaemia/mental retardation syndrome X-linked) and DAXX (death-domain associated protein) in pHGGs (Fig. 7.2; [3, 4]). As a brief review, the fundamental repeating unit of chromatin is the nucleosome, which consists of approximately 147 bp of superhelical DNA wrapped around the radial surface of an octamer of highly conserved core histone proteins (two copies of each H2A, H2B, H3, and H4). Histone proteins are subject to a wide array of covalent modifications that occur primarily at amino (N^-) and carboxy (C^-) termini. The tail regions of core histones contain flexible and highly basic amino acid sequences that are highly conserved and serve as substrates for several post-translational modifications such as acetylation, methylation, ADP-ribosylation, ubiquitylation, and phosphorylation. These modifications impact gene transcription, DNA replication, and chromatin assembly. The histone code states that distinct patterns of histone modifications act in concert with DNA methylation, noncoding RNAs, and transcription factors to generate "histone-epigenetic codes" that are read by effector proteins [5]. Lastly, another level of complexity is histone variants (e.g., H3.3 vs. H3.1), which are relevant to pHGGs. Although the difference between H3.3 and H3.1 is only four amino acids, H3.1 (also called canonical core H3) is only incorporated into nucleosomes during the S-phase of the cell cycle while H3.3 incorporation into nucleosomes is cell-cycle independent. Furthermore, ATRX and DAXX are both H3.3 chaperones and together they facilitate the deposition and remodeling of H3.3 containing nucleosomes [6].

The initial two manuscripts describing these mutations noted, in the brainstem there are K27M mutations in either H3.3 or H3.1 in up to 80 % of DIPGs, while the G34R/V mutations are found only in H3.3 and were primarily found in pHGGs located in the cerebral cortex. In addition, G34R/V mutations co-occur with loss of function ATRX or DAXX mutations and are associated with the ALT (alternative lengthening of telomeres) phenotype [3, 4, 7, 8]. In a follow-up paper, Sturm and colleagues [9] pursue an integrative approach based on epigenetic, copy number, expression, and genetic analyses on over 200 adult and pediatric GBMs to identify six distinct DNA methylation clusters which were labeled as "IDH," "K27," "G34," "receptor tyrosine kinase (RTK) I (platelet-derived growth factor receptor A or PDGFR-A)," "mesenchymal," and "RTK II (Classic)." A key finding of this analysis was that H3F3A K27 and H3F3A G34 mutations were exclusively distributed to the K27 and G34 clusters, respectively, and these were mutually exclusive of the isocitrate dehydrogenase (IDH1) mutations. The RTK I (PDGFR-A) group had a high frequency of PDGFR-A amplification and the RTK II Classic group had a very high frequency of whole chromosome seven gain, whole chromosome ten loss, frequent deletion of cyclin-dependent kinase inhibitor 2a (CDKN2A), and amplification of epidermal growth factor receptor (EGFR). This RTK II Classic subgroup is completely devoid of pediatric patients. Remarkably, the clusters are associated with patient age, with K27M patients being the youngest (median age 10.5; range 5–23) and G34 patients being the second youngest (median age 18 years; range 9–42). The RTK I "PDGFR-A" cluster (median age 36 years, range 8–74 years) and the IDH cluster (median age 40 years, range 13–71 years) mostly comprised young

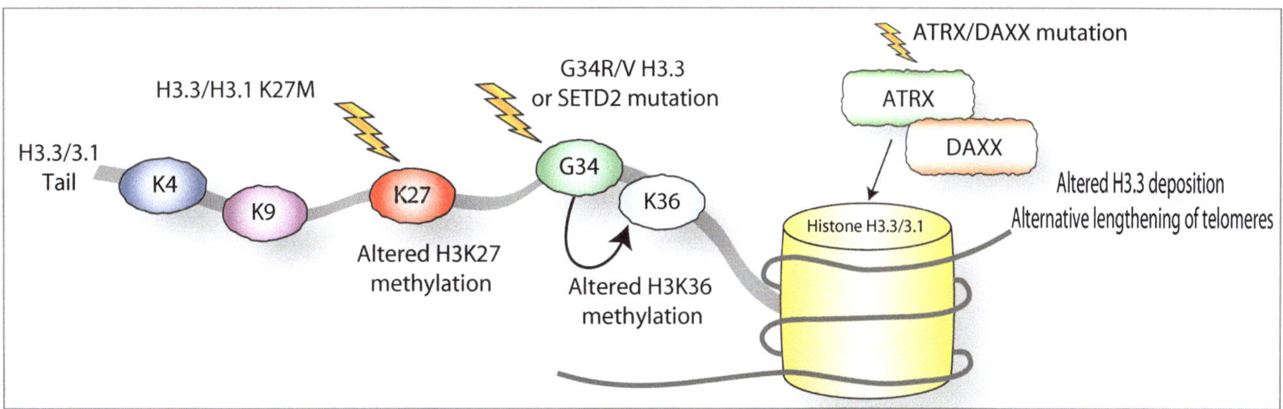

Fig. 7.2 Epigenetic alterations associated with pediatric high-grade gliomagenesis. This schematic of the H3.3/H3.1 tail illustrates the three types of epigenetic mutations seen in pHGG: (1) K27M mutations which impact H3K27 methylation, (2) G34R/V or SETD2 mutations, both of which impact H3K36 methylation, and (3) ATRX/DAXX mutations which likely impact H3.3 deposition and alternative lengthening of telomeres

adults, while the oldest cluster, the RTK II "Classic" cluster, comprised older adults (median age 58, range 36–81 years). The other remarkable finding was that the epigenetic GBM subgroups showed region-specific predilection within the CNS whereby the K27-mutant tumors were predominantly seen in midline locations such as the thalamus, pons, and the spinal cord while the tumors in the other five subgroups almost exclusively arose in the cerebral hemispheres. This remarkable observation clearly suggests that the mechanism of gliomagenesis is distinct in different regions of the CNS. Lastly, these subgroups also correlated with survival with the K27 subgroup having the shortest survival, the IDH subgroup with the longest survival, and the other subgroups in between. Interestingly, both the IDH and H3F3A mutations co-occur with p53 mutations, suggesting that p53 mutations do not have independent prognostic significance [9].

How histone mutations contribute to pHGG pathogenesis is subject to current investigations, but Lewis and colleagues recently reported an initial glimpse into the mechanism. They reported that the K27M H3.3/H3.1 mutations inhibit polycomb repressive complex 2 (PRC2), the enzyme complex that adds methyl groups to H3 lysine 27. Under normal circumstances, this histone mark is repressive, and inhibition of PRC2 results in global loss of H3 lysine 27 trimethylation. The mechanism of the G34R/V histone mutations is less well understood, but results in a local decrease in H3 lysine 36 trimethylation [10]. In addition to the epigenetic mutations described above, pHGGs recently have also been reported to harbor loss of function mutations in SETD2, an H3K36 trimethyltransferase. Perhaps not surprisingly, SET2D mutations were mutually exclusive with H3F3A mutations, but they did overlap with IDH1 mutations [11]. High-grade gliomas with SET2D mutations were found exclusively in tumors arising in the cerebral hemispheres, reinforcing the notion that H3K36 is important for gliomagenesis in the cerebral hemispheres, while H3K27 is central in the etiology of tumors arising in midline structures of the CNS. Lastly, while IDH mutations are primarily found in adult gliomas, adolescents 13 years old and older can also harbor activating mutations in IDH1 in amino acid 132 [12, 13]. These IDH1 mutations have also been reported to impact histone marks, but through a completely different mechanism [14].

Cytogenetics

Several studies have investigated the spectrum of copy number aberrations in pHGGs [15–22]. Copy number changes in pHGGs are best subdivided between broad chromosomal gains and losses and focal gains and losses. Broad low-amplitude gains of chromosome 1q were identified as well as broad losses of 10q, 13q, and 14q. Focal gains have been reported in PDGFR-A, cyclin D1-3 (CCND1-3), cyclin-dependent kinase 4 (CDK4), cyclin-dependent kinase 6 (CDK6), MYC, v-myc avian myelocytomatosis viral oncogene neuroblastoma-derived homolog (MYCN), EGFR, V-Erb-A Avian Erythroblastic Leukemia Viral Oncogene Homolog-Like 4 (ERBB4), MET, hepatocyte growth factor (HGF), insulin-like growth factor-1 receptor (IGF1R), insulin-like growth factor 2 (IGF2), platelet-derived growth factor B (PDGFB), Neuregulin 1 (NRG1), phosphatidylinositol-4,5-bisphosphate 3-kinase, catalytic subunit alpha (PIK3CA), PIK3C2B, PIK3C2G, PIK3R5, Kirsten rat sarcoma viral oncogene homolog (KRAS), v-akt murine thymoma viral oncogene homolog 1 (AKT1), AKT3, S6K1, and murine double minute 4 (MDM4). The most common homozygous focal loss was at CDKN2A/CDKN2B. Other homozygous focal losses included the following genes: CDKN2C, neurofibromin-1 (NF1), PTEN

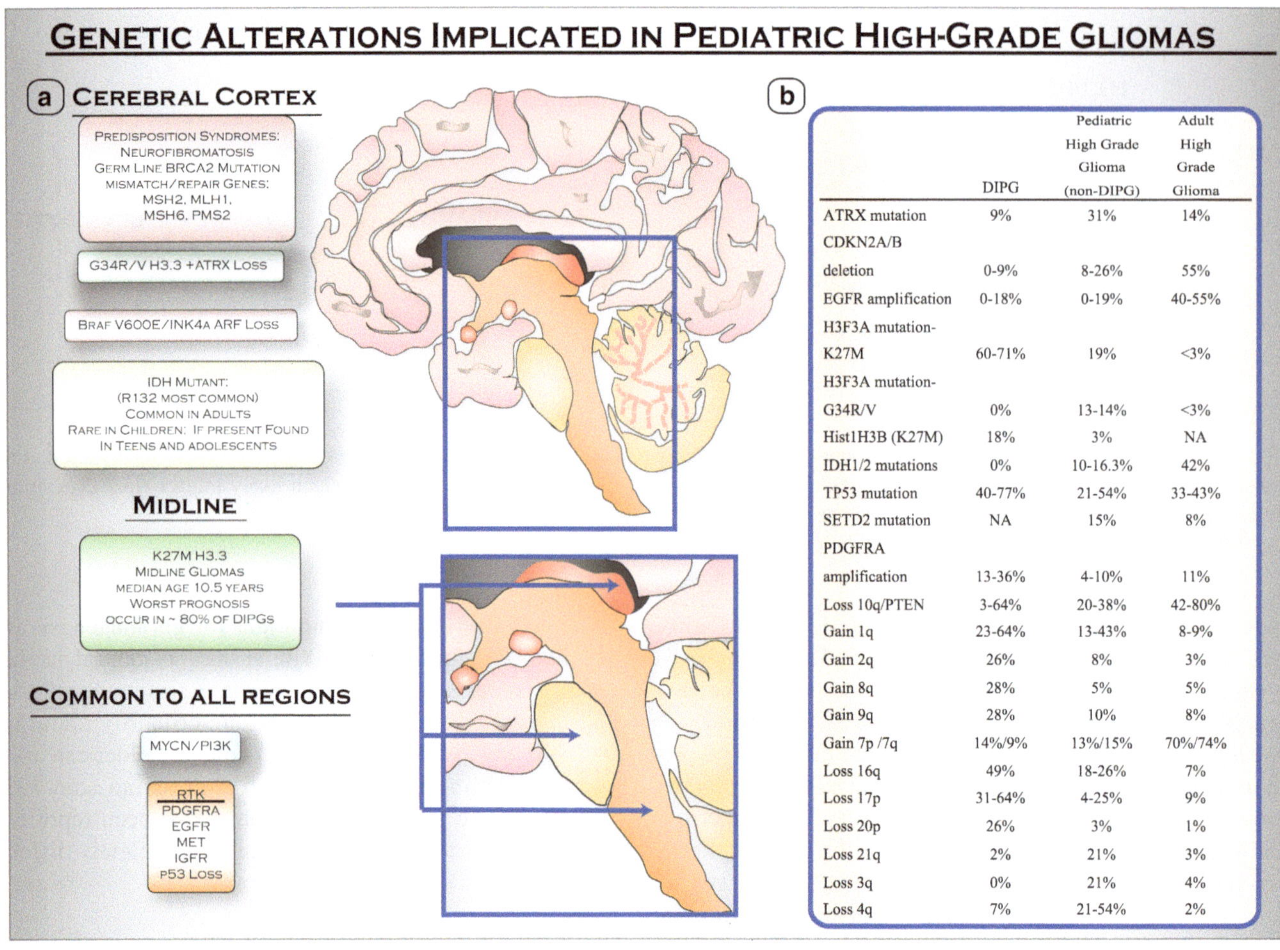

	DIPG	Pediatric High Grade Glioma (non-DIPG)	Adult High Grade Glioma
ATRX mutation	9%	31%	14%
CDKN2A/B deletion	0-9%	8-26%	55%
EGFR amplification	0-18%	0-19%	40-55%
H3F3A mutation-K27M	60-71%	19%	<3%
H3F3A mutation-G34R/V	0%	13-14%	<3%
Hist1H3B (K27M)	18%	3%	NA
IDH1/2 mutations	0%	10-16.3%	42%
TP53 mutation	40-77%	21-54%	33-43%
SETD2 mutation	NA	15%	8%
PDGFRA amplification	13-36%	4-10%	11%
Loss 10q/PTEN	3-64%	20-38%	42-80%
Gain 1q	23-64%	13-43%	8-9%
Gain 2q	26%	8%	3%
Gain 8q	28%	5%	5%
Gain 9q	28%	10%	8%
Gain 7p /7q	14%/9%	13%/15%	70%/74%
Loss 16q	49%	18-26%	7%
Loss 17p	31-64%	4-25%	9%
Loss 20p	26%	3%	1%
Loss 21q	2%	21%	3%
Loss 3q	0%	21%	4%
Loss 4q	7%	21-54%	2%

Fig. 7.3 Genetic alterations implicated in pHGGs. Genetic alterations vary by location and age. (**a**) Genetic alterations observed in pHGGs located in the cerebral cortex, or in midline areas of the CNS, or common to all pHGGs. Arrows pointing to midline areas from top to bottom: thalamus, pons, and spinal cord. (**b**) Distinct molecular genetics of DIPG as compared to pHGGs (non-DIPG) and adult high-grade gliomas. Table is adapted from: Kristin M Schroeder, Christine M Hoeman, and Oren J Becher, Children are not just little adults: recent advances in understanding of diffuse intrinsic pontine glioma biology, *Pediatric Research*, 2014 [57]

(phosphatase and tensin homolog), retinoblastoma (RB1), TP53, TP73, and protein tyrosine phosphatase receptor type D (PTPRD). Interestingly, copy number alterations are also age- and region specific. PDGFR-A is the most common amplified receptor tyrosine kinase (RTK) in pHGGs while EGFR amplification is the most common amplified RTK in adult high-grade glioma. Gains of chromosomes 2q, 8q, and 9q and losses of 16q, 17p, and 20p were significantly more frequent in DIPG than in non-brainstem pHGGs. Furthermore, focal deletions of CDKN2A are extremely rare in DIPGs and are found in 26 % of non-brainstem pHGGs [23]. Lastly, Barrow et al. described homozygous loss of ADAM3A in 16 % of pHGGs, although the function of this gene and how its loss contributes to pediatric gliomagenesis is not known [17]. Figure 7.3 includes a summary figure of the genetic alterations in pHGGs, as well as a table, which lists the genetic alterations in DIPG, non-brainstem pHGG, and adult HGG.

Gene Expression

Gene expression profiling, a method to analyze the mRNA expression of all genes in the tumor, is another useful technique to study the complex biology of cancer. In fact, mRNA analysis of a select number of genes is used to make clinical decisions in some types of breast cancer. In pHGGs, unsupervised hierarchical clustering identified three main tumor subgroups: HC1/proliferative, HC2/proneural, and HC3/mesenchymal [15]. Gene ontology analysis across the groups revealed that HC1 is most associated with cell-cycle genes; HC2 is most associated with neuronal differentiation, while HC3 is most associated with extracellular matrix–receptor interactions and cell adhesion. Interestingly, HC1 is most associated with amplifications targeting the PDGFR signaling cascade, which ties together PDGF signaling with cell growth. If one were to compare the expression profiling of pHGGs to adult high-grade gliomas, PDGFR-A mRNA is significantly overexpressed in pHGGs relative to adult high-grade gliomas while EGFR mRNA is significantly repressed in pHGGs relative to adult high-grade gliomas. With regard to the HC3/mesenchymal group, immune response genes were also enriched and more specifically associated with microglia/macrophages and monocytes [24]. Lastly, using principal component analysis (PCA), two independent groups noted that the expression profiling of DIPGs consists of a distinct cluster separate from non-brainstem gliomas, reinforcing the notion of region-specific differences in pediatric CNS gliomagenesis [23, 25].

Prognostic Stratification

Until recently, the concept that HGGs comprise several, biologically distinct diseases associated with age and location was not fully appreciated. As a consequence, current research efforts center on developing a better understanding of tumor biology and accordingly, devise appropriate classification schemes. Similar to the increased stratification of leukemias in children, molecular stratification of pHGG will continue to become increasingly refined, in parallel with advances in our understanding of disease biology. The ongoing challenge is how to best incorporate new molecular prognostic factors with well-established prognostic factors, such as extent of resection and tumor grade [2]. For over a decade, p53 overexpression has been recognized as a poor prognostic factor in pHGGs. Most importantly, this association was found to be independent of age, histologic features, the extent of resection, or tumor location [26]. Overexpression of p53 as determined by immunohistochemistry, however, is an imperfect proxy for oncogenic p53 mutations, and taken in context with our current knowledge of the molecular genetics of HGG, a clearer picture emerges. For example, as previously mentioned in the epigenetics section of this chapter, IDH mutations frequently co-occur with p53 mutations, and these tumors currently have the best prognosis. However, p53 mutations also overlap with K27M mutations, which appear to have the worst prognosis. According to retrospective studies, K27M is a poor prognostic factor in pediatric GBM, although it is unclear whether this is due to a different biology versus the midline location of these tumors, which limits surgical options [9, 27]. Within the K27M subgroup, DIPGs have the worst prognosis, with a median survival time of 9–12 months and greater than 90 % of children dying within 2 years [28]. Lastly, PTEN mutations or loss of PTEN expression by IHC have been reported to be significantly associated with decreased survival in pHGGs, but this has so far only been reported in small cohorts and will require further validation [29, 30].

Molecular Signaling Pathways

Three pathways that are most implicated in pHGG pathogenesis are the p53, retinoblastoma protein (Rb), and RTK/Ras/phosphoinositide 3-kinase (PI3K) signaling pathways. These pathways are dysregulated in both pediatric and adult high-grade gliomas, and the importance of these three pathways in adult gliomagenesis was recently underscored by the mutual exclusivity of alterations affecting these pathways [31]. Evolving knowledge of precisely how these pathways contribute to tumor initiation and growth is expected to lead to better-informed molecular targeted therapeutic approaches. With regard to activation of the RTK/Ras/PI3K pathway, 80 % of pHGGs activate this pathway through amplification of RTKs, and/or activating mutations in PI3K, and/or loss of PTEN either through deletion or promoter methylation [32]. Below is a brief summary of the key molecular signaling pathways.

RTK/Ras/PI3K Pathway

The axis of PI3K signaling in cancer begins with engagement of growth factors by RTKs such as PDGFR, MET, EGFR, and IGF-1R (Fig. 7.4). PI3K, a lipid kinase, is then recruited to plasma membrane-anchored receptors, is activated, and phosphorylates PIP2 to generate PIP3. Through its pleckstrin homology (PH) domain, the nodal kinase AKT (also known as PKB) binds to PIP3, where it is activated by two phosphorylation events, and triggers a complex cascade of signals that regulate growth, proliferation, survival, and motility. The lipid phosphatase, PTEN, antagonizes this process by dephosphorylating PIP3 to inhibit activation of AKT. PI3K is activated downstream of numerous RTKs that directly, or through adaptor proteins, bind and activate PI3K. PI3K activity is thus carefully regulated by growth factor–receptor interactions. In fact, the vast majority of PI3K remains inactive in the cytoplasm, removed from its plasma membrane-associated substrates, and only a small percentage of PI3K becomes activated upon growth factor stimulation. Therefore, even slight modulations in receptor activity can lead to manyfold increases in PI3K activity [33].

In addition to copy number alterations, pHGGs can also harbor additional alterations in the RTK/Ras/PI3K pathways through somatic mutations or alternative splicing. The most commonly mutated RTK in pHGGs is PDGFR-A where mutations in the extracellular domain as well as in the tyrosine kinase domain have been described in approximately 10 % of these tumors [3, 25, 34]. By contrast, the most commonly mutated RTK in adult high-grade glioma is EGFR. EGFRvIII (an EGFR lacking exons 2–7 resulting in ligand-independent signaling) is an alternatively spliced EGFR variant found in 19 % of adult HGGs, but has also been reported in 17 % of pHGGs [31,

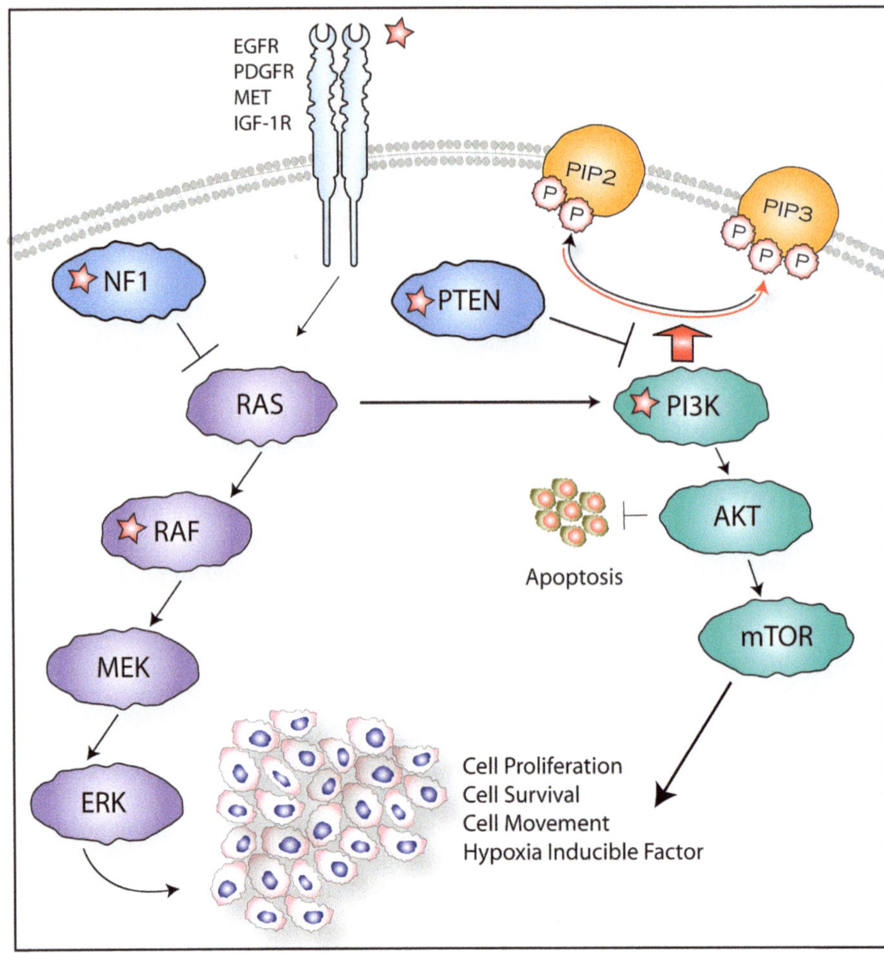

Fig. 7.4 RTK/Ras/PI3K pathway. Growth factors such as EGF, PDGF, HGF, and IGF2 engage with their respective RTKs leading to PI3K activation. PI3K activation phosphorylates PIP2 to generate PIP3. AKT binds to PIP3, becomes activated, and triggers a complex cascade of signals that regulate growth, proliferation, survival, and motility. PTEN, a naturally occurring antagonist of this pathway, dephosphorylates PIP3 inhibiting activation of AKT. Growth factors and RTK interactions also regulate cell proliferation and survival through activation of Ras followed by sequential activation of Raf, Mek, and Erk. Starred (*asterisk*) factors mutated in RTK/Ras/PI3K pathway are prevalent in pHGGs

35]. Downstream of RTKs, activating mutations in PIK3CA have been described in a subset of pHGGs both inside and outside of the brainstem [36, 37]. While activating Ras mutations have rarely been described in pHGGs (G12V Kras reported by Schiffman et al. [16]), loss of function NF1 (neurofibromatosis type 1 which negatively regulates the Ras pathway) mutations has been identified in a subset of pHGGs outside of the brainstem [3]. Furthermore, activating V600E Braf mutations have also been described in pHGGs [11, 16, 38, 39]. V600E Braf mutations can also be found in low-grade gliomas, but usually in isolation, suggesting that cooperating mutations (such as CDKN2A) may be required for a high-grade phenotype in V600E Braf mutant tumors [16].

RB Pathway

The retinoblastoma protein (RB) is a tumor suppressor protein and key regulator of cell-cycle control. The RB pathway consists of five families of proteins: CDKN (e.g., Ink4a), D-type cyclins, D-cyclin-dependent protein kinases (cdk4, cdk6), RB-family of pocket proteins (RB, p107, p130), and the E2F-family of transcription factors. Each Ink4-protein (p16Ink4a, p15Ink4b, and p18Ink4c) can bind to and inhibit the activity of cdk4 and cdk6. Each D-cyclin protein can associate with cdk4 or cdk6 to form the active kinase complex. Therefore, Ink4 proteins compete with the D-cyclins for cdk4/6 to prevent the formation of the active kinase complex [40]. Importantly, proteins in this pathway are com-

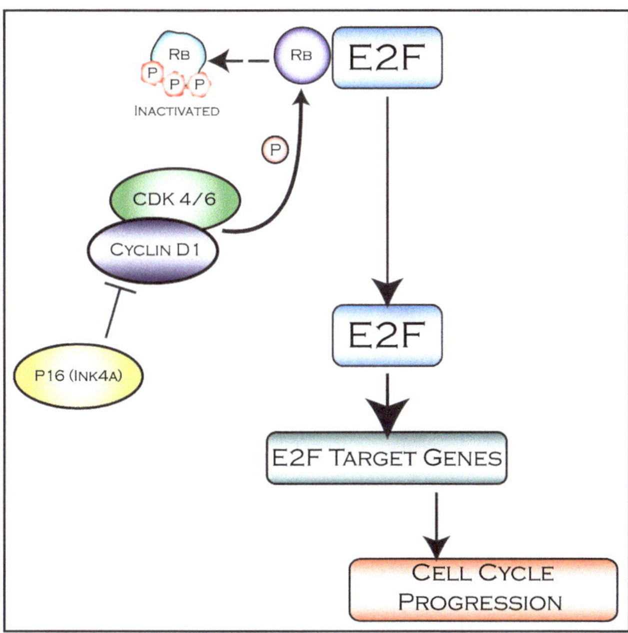

Fig. 7.5 RB pathway. The RB pathway is an important regulator of cell-cycle control. Cyclin D1 and cdk4/6 bind to form a complex that phosphorylates RB. In its active form RB is bound to E2F transcription factors. Hyperphosphorylation of RB renders it inactive and allows for the release of E2F transcription factors. E2F transcription factors activate E2F target genes, leading to initiation of S-phase and cell-cycle progression. CDKN (e.g., INK4a) is a tumor suppressor gene that inactivates the cyclin D1/cdk4/6 complex. Cdkn2a deletions and/or amplification of cdk4, cdk6, cyclin D1, D2, or D3 are common in pHGGs

monly altered in pHGGs, primarily through copy number aberrations: cdkn2a deletions and/or amplification of cdk4, cdk6, cyclin d1, d2, and d3 [15, 19, 23].

The RB pathway regulates cell proliferation as the proteins in this pathway are activated and/or inhibited by growth-promoting, as well as growth-suppressing signals (Fig. 7.5). During regulated cell proliferation, as cells respond to mitogenic signals and commit to cell-cycle entry the complex of D-cyclin/cdk4/6 is activated. The primary cellular targets of the D-cyclin/cdk4/6 complex are the RB-family of pocket proteins (henceforward referred to as RB), which inhibit transcription by directly inhibiting the activity of E2F. Hyperphosphorylation of RB by activated D-cyclin/cdk4/6 complexes renders RB inactive and in turn allows for the release of E2F transcription factors, leading to the activation of E2F target genes involved in cell-cycle progression [40]. Recently, a preclinical trial using genetically engineered mouse models identified a population of pHGG patients that may be sensitive to treatment with a highly selective cdk4/6 inhibitor [41]. Inhibition of cdk4/6 in murine high-grade gliomas harboring CDKN2A loss provided a significant survival benefit and holds promise for translation into clinical trials.

P53 Pathway

The p53 protein plays a key role in eliciting cellular responses to a variety of stress signals, such as DNA damage, hypoxia, and aberrant proliferative signals such as oncogene activation. Following cellular stresses, p53 is stabilized and binds to DNA as a tetramer, in a sequence-specific manner that results in the transcriptional regulation of genes involved in DNA repair, cell-cycle arrest, senescence, and apoptosis [42]. The critical role of this gene in tumor suppression in pHGG is clear as evidenced by the abundant, inactivating somatic mutations, which were recently reported in as many as 77 % of DIPGs [27]. Besides p53 mutations, other mechanisms to inactivate the p53 pathway include amplification of mouse double minute 2 homolog (MDM2) and MDM4. MDM2 is an important negative regulator of p53 working through two mechanisms: It is an E3 ubiquitin ligase that targets p53 for proteosomal degradation and it can also inhibit p53 transcriptional activation. MDM4 is a homolog of MDM2 and can also inhibit p53 transcriptional activity. In pHGGs, MDM2 is overexpressed but it is not amplified while MDM4 amplifications have been observed [15, 19, 43]. Interestingly, p53 mutations were reported to occur significantly more often in pediatric GBM relative to adult GBM [3]. This may be related to the fact that CDKN2A deletions are significantly more common in adult GBMs. CDKN2A encodes two transcripts: Ink4a (an endogenous cdk4/6 inhibitor discussed in the RB section) and alternative reading frame (ARF). ARF inhibits p53 degradation by sequestering MDM2 to the nucleolus and rendering it inactive. In summary, the p53 pathway is inactivated in the majority of pHGGs primarily through p53 mutations but also through MDM2 overexpression, MDM4 amplification, and CDKN2A loss, preventing the tumor cells from responding appropriately to cellular stresses.

Molecular Targeted Therapies

Despite recent advancements in our knowledge of key molecular alterations in pHGGs, this new depth of understanding has not translated into improved clinical therapies thus far. There have been numerous clinical trials with molecular targeted therapies for children with high-grade gliomas, but none have been demonstrated to significantly prolong survival. Most of the targeted therapy trials to date have focused on targeting RTKs (the upstream part of the RTK/Ras/PI3K pathway), and angiogenesis (VEGF or αv integrins). The lack of efficacy is likely due to activation of feedback loops, redundant activation of RTK pathways in glioma [44], intratumoral heterogeneity [15], and potentially inadequate drug delivery across the blood–brain barrier [45]. The following is not an exhaustive list of all targeted therapies that have been evaluated in pHGGs, but a brief description of some of the most relevant studies.

There have been multiple studies evaluating EGFR inhibitors (erlotinib, lapatinib, gefitinib) in pHGGs and none of them have demonstrated significant efficacy, even though the target has been demonstrated as present in a subset of pHGGs ([13, 45–49]. Other studies evaluating molecular targeted therapies in pHGGs include evaluation of inhibitors of PDGFR (imatinib), mTOR (temsirolimus), Ras (tipifarnib), VEGF (bevacizumab), αv integrin antagonist (cilengitide), Notch (MK-0752), and VEGFR2 (vandetanib) without success [47, 50–55]. Recently, a combination study of vandetanib and dasatinib (PDGFR inhibitor) was also reported with limited success [56]. Interestingly, the authors noted a 2 % cerebrospinal fluid to plasma exposure in two of the patients in the study, suggesting that inadequate drug delivery may explain the lack of response. Adequate drug delivery across the blood–brain barrier remains an obstacle in pHGG, and particularly in DIPG.

Future Directions

It is our hope that advances in our understanding of the genetic alterations of pHGGs will eventually translate into improved therapies. There is a great deal of excitement surrounding the discovery of highly specific histone mutations in pHGGs, and it remains to be seen how one can target such genetic alterations therapeutically. So far, there are two classes of epigenetic drugs that have been FDA approved for cancer: histone deacetylase (HDAC) inhibitors for cutaneous T-cell lymphoma and DNA methyltransferase (DNMT) inhibitors for myelodysplastic syndrome. In addition, there are numerous new classes of epigenetic drugs that have shown promise in preclinical trials and have recently entered clinical trials such as bromodomain inhibitors (a bromodomain is a protein domain that can bind an acetylated lysine) and enhancer of zeste 2 (EZH2) inhibitors. Furthermore, there are new therapeutic targets that are currently being evaluated in clinical trials for children with high-grade gliomas such as inhibitors of the enzyme poly (ADP-ribose) polymerase (PARP), inhibitors of telomerase (Imetelstat), and V600E Braf inhibitors. In summary, there are numerous new promising therapeutic targets in pHGGs, and the challenge is how to prioritize the translation of novel agents into clinical trials in children with high-grade gliomas and how to combine these novel agents synergistically. Undoubtedly, deeper insights into the biology of pHGGs will continue to emerge over the next years, opening new therapeutic avenues. The inter-patient heterogeneity of the genetic alterations in pHGGs implies that more personalized approaches may be needed, and a current V600E Braf inhibitor pediatric study with dabrafenib (ClinicalTrials.gov NCT01677741) is one example in the right direction, as only patients whose tumors harbor a V600E Braf mutation are allowed to enroll.

References

1. Fangusaro J. Pediatric high grade glioma: a review and update on tumor clinical characteristics and biology. Front Oncol. 2012;2:105.
2. Finlay JL, et al. Randomized phase III trial in childhood high-grade astrocytoma comparing vincristine, lomustine, and prednisone with the eight-drugs-in-1-day regimen. Childrens Cancer Group. J Clin Oncol. 1995;13(1):112–23.
3. Schwartzentruber J, et al. Driver mutations in histone H3.3 and chromatin remodelling genes in paediatric glioblastoma. Nature. 2012;482(7384):226–31.
4. Wu G, et al. Somatic histone H3 alterations in pediatric diffuse intrinsic pontine gliomas and non-brainstem glioblastomas. Nat Genet. 2012;44(3):251–3.
5. Maze I, Noh KM, Allis CD. Histone regulation in the CNS: basic principles of epigenetic plasticity. Neuropsychopharmacology. 2013;38(1):3–22.
6. Lewis PW, et al. Daxx is an H3.3-specific histone chaperone and cooperates with ATRX in replication-independent chromatin assembly at telomeres. Proc Natl Acad Sci U S A. 2010;107(32):14075–80.
7. Heaphy CM, et al. Altered telomeres in tumors with ATRX and DAXX mutations. Science. 2011;333(6041):425.
8. Nguyen DN, et al. Molecular and morphologic correlates of the alternative lengthening of telomeres phenotype in high-grade astrocytomas. Brain Pathol. 2013;23(3):237–43.
9. Sturm D, et al. Hotspot mutations in H3F3A and IDH1 define distinct epigenetic and biological subgroups of glioblastoma. Cancer Cell. 2012;22(4):425–37.
10. Lewis PW, et al. Inhibition of PRC2 activity by a gain-of-function H3 mutation found in pediatric glioblastoma. Science. 2013;340(6134):857–61.
11. Fontebasso AM, et al. Mutations in SETD2 and genes affecting histone H3K36 methylation target hemispheric high-grade gliomas. Acta Neuropathol. 2013;125(5):659–69.
12. Yan H, et al. IDH1 and IDH2 mutations in gliomas. N Engl J Med. 2009;360(8):765–73.
13. Pollack IF, et al. IDH1 mutations are common in malignant gliomas arising in adolescents: a report from the Children's Oncology Group. Childs Nerv Syst. 2011;27(1):87–94.
14. Losman JA, Kaelin Jr WG. What a difference a hydroxyl makes: mutant IDH, (R)-2-hydroxyglutarate, and cancer. Genes Dev. 2013;27(8):836–52.
15. Paugh BS, et al. Integrated molecular genetic profiling of pediatric high-grade gliomas reveals key differences with the adult disease. J Clin Oncol. 2010;28(18):3061–8.

16. Schiffman JD, et al. Oncogenic BRAF mutation with CDKN2A inactivation is characteristic of a subset of pediatric malignant astrocytomas. Cancer Res. 2010;70(2):512–9.
17. Barrow J, et al. Homozygous loss of ADAM3A revealed by genome-wide analysis of pediatric high-grade glioma and diffuse intrinsic pontine gliomas. Neuro Oncol. 2011;13(2):212–22.
18. Bax DA, et al. A distinct spectrum of copy number aberrations in pediatric high-grade gliomas. Clin Cancer Res. 2010;16(13):3368–77.
19. Warren KE, et al. Genomic aberrations in pediatric diffuse intrinsic pontine gliomas. Neuro Oncol. 2012;14(3):326–32.
20. Zarghooni M, et al. Whole-genome profiling of pediatric diffuse intrinsic pontine gliomas highlights platelet-derived growth factor receptor alpha and poly (ADP-ribose) polymerase as potential therapeutic targets. J Clin Oncol. 2010;28(8):1337–44.
21. Wong KK, et al. Genome-wide allelic imbalance analysis of pediatric gliomas by single nucleotide polymorphic allele array. Cancer Res. 2006;66(23):11172–8.
22. Phillips JJ, et al. PDGFRA amplification is common in pediatric and adult high-grade astrocytomas and identifies a poor prognostic group in IDH1 mutant glioblastoma. Brain Pathol. 2013;23(5):565–73.
23. Paugh BS, et al. Genome-wide analyses identify recurrent amplifications of receptor tyrosine kinases and cell-cycle regulatory genes in diffuse intrinsic pontine glioma. J Clin Oncol. 2011;29(30):3999–4006.
24. Engler JR, et al. Increased microglia/macrophage gene expression in a subset of adult and pediatric astrocytomas. PLoS One. 2012;7(8):e43339.
25. Puget S, et al. Mesenchymal transition and PDGFRA amplification/mutation are key distinct oncogenic events in pediatric diffuse intrinsic pontine gliomas. PLoS One. 2012;7(2):e30313.
26. Pollack IF, et al. Expression of p53 and prognosis in children with malignant gliomas. N Engl J Med. 2002;346(6):420–7.
27. Khuong-Quang DA, et al. K27M mutation in histone H3.3 defines clinically and biologically distinct subgroups of pediatric diffuse intrinsic pontine gliomas. Acta Neuropathol. 2012;124(3):439–47.
28. Freeman CR, Perilongo G. Chemotherapy for brain stem gliomas. Childs Nerv Syst. 1999;15(10):545–53.
29. Raffel C, et al. Analysis of oncogene and tumor suppressor gene alterations in pediatric malignant astrocytomas reveals reduced survival for patients with PTEN mutations. Clin Cancer Res. 1999;5(12):4085–90.
30. Thorarinsdottir HK, et al. Protein expression of platelet-derived growth factor receptor correlates with malignant histology and PTEN with survival in childhood gliomas. Clin Cancer Res. 2008;14(11):3386–94.
31. Brennan CW, et al. The somatic genomic landscape of glioblastoma. Cell. 2013;155(2):462–77.
32. Mueller S, et al. PTEN promoter methylation and activation of the PI3K/Akt/mTOR pathway in pediatric gliomas and influence on clinical outcome. Neuro Oncol. 2012;14(9):1146–52.
33. Yuan TL, Cantley LC. PI3K pathway alterations in cancer: variations on a theme. Oncogene. 2008;27(41):5497–510.
34. Paugh BS, et al. Novel oncogenic PDGFRA mutations in pediatric high-grade gliomas. Cancer Res. 2013;73(20):6219–29.
35. Bax DA, et al. EGFRvIII deletion mutations in pediatric high-grade glioma and response to targeted therapy in pediatric glioma cell lines. Clin Cancer Res. 2009;15(18):5753–61.
36. Gallia GL, et al. PIK3CA gene mutations in pediatric and adult glioblastoma multiforme. Mol Cancer Res. 2006;4(10):709–14.
37. Grill J, et al. Critical oncogenic mutations in newly diagnosed pediatric diffuse intrinsic pontine glioma. Pediatr Blood Cancer. 2012;58(4):489–91.
38. Bettegowda C, et al. Exomic sequencing of four rare central nervous system tumor types. Oncotarget. 2013;4(4):572–83.
39. Kleinschmidt-DeMasters BK, et al. Epithelioid GBMs show a high percentage of BRAF V600E mutation. Am J Surg Pathol. 2013;37(5):685–98.
40. Knudsen ES, Wang JY. Targeting the RB-pathway in cancer therapy. Clin Cancer Res. 2010;16(4):1094–9.
41. Barton KL, et al. PD-0332991, a CDK4/6 inhibitor, significantly prolongs survival in a genetically engineered mouse model of brainstem glioma. PLoS One. 2013;8(10):e77639.
42. Vazquez A, et al. The genetics of the p53 pathway, apoptosis and cancer therapy. Nat Rev Drug Discov. 2008;7(12):979–87.
43. Sung T, et al. Preferential inactivation of the p53 tumor suppressor pathway and lack of EGFR amplification distinguish de novo high grade pediatric astrocytomas from de novo adult astrocytomas. Brain Pathol. 2000;10(2):249–59.
44. Stommel JM, et al. Coactivation of receptor tyrosine kinases affects the response of tumor cells to targeted therapies. Science. 2007;318(5848):287–90.
45. Fouladi M, et al. A molecular biology and phase II trial of lapatinib in children with refractory CNS malignancies: a pediatric brain tumor consortium study. J Neurooncol. 2013;114(2):173–9.
46. Broniscer A, et al. Phase I and pharmacokinetic studies of erlotinib administered concurrently with radiotherapy for children, adolescents, and young adults with high-grade glioma. Clin Cancer Res. 2009;15(2):701–7.
47. Geoerger B, et al. Phase II trial of temsirolimus in children with high-grade glioma, neuroblastoma and rhabdomyosarcoma. Eur J Cancer. 2012;48(2):253–62.
48. Geoerger B, et al. Innovative therapies for children with cancer pediatric phase I study of erlotinib in brainstem glioma and relapsing/refractory brain tumors. Neuro Oncol. 2011;13(1):109–18.
49. Pollack IF, et al. A phase II study of gefitinib and irradiation in children with newly diagnosed brainstem gliomas: a report from the Pediatric Brain Tumor Consortium. Neuro Oncol. 2011;13(3):290–7.
50. Pollack IF, et al. Phase I trial of imatinib in children with newly diagnosed brainstem and recurrent malignant gliomas: a Pediatric Brain Tumor Consortium report. Neuro Oncol. 2007;9(2):145–60.
51. Broniscer A, et al. Phase I study of vandetanib during and after radiotherapy in children with diffuse intrinsic pontine glioma. J Clin Oncol. 2010;28(31):4762–8.

52. Fouladi M, et al. Phase I trial of MK-0752 in children with refractory CNS malignancies: a pediatric brain tumor consortium study. J Clin Oncol. 2011;29(26):3529–34.
53. Gururangan S, et al. Lack of efficacy of bevacizumab plus irinotecan in children with recurrent malignant glioma and diffuse brainstem glioma: a Pediatric Brain Tumor Consortium study. J Clin Oncol. 2010;28(18):3069–75.
54. Haas-Kogan DA, et al. Phase II trial of tipifarnib and radiation in children with newly diagnosed diffuse intrinsic pontine gliomas. Neuro Oncol. 2011;13(3):298–306.
55. MacDonald TJ, et al. Phase II study of cilengitide in the treatment of refractory or relapsed high-grade gliomas in children: a report from the Children's Oncology Group. Neuro Oncol. 2013;15(10):1438–44.
56. Broniscer A, et al. Phase I trial, pharmacokinetics, and pharmacodynamics of vandetanib and dasatinib in children with newly diagnosed diffuse intrinsic pontine glioma. Clin Cancer Res. 2013;19(11):3050–8.
57. Schroeder KM, Hoeman CM, Becher OJ. Children are not just little adults: recent advances in understanding of diffuse intrinsic pontine glioma biology. Pediatr Res. 2014;75(1–2):205–9.

8 Oligodendroglial Tumors

Stephen Yip and Jaishri Blakeley

Oligodendroglioma: An Infiltrating Glioma

The broad category of gliomas encompasses tumors comprised of neoplastic astrocytes and oligodendrocytes. Traditionally, these are classified based on morphologic pathology and clinical behavior. The most widely applied classification system was developed (and updated) by the World Health Organization (WHO) [1]. In this framework, gliomas are divided into astrocytomas, oligodendrogliomas (ODG), and mixed oligoastrocytomas (MOA) (Table 8.1). Oligodendroglial tumors are the least common of all gliomas, accounting for only 3–20 % of all glial tumors [2]. Of these, roughly 70 % are WHO grade II low-grade oligodendrogliomas (LGO) and 30 % are WHO grade III anaplastic oligodendrogliomas (AO) [3]. Given that ODG are a subtype of infiltrating glioma, they share many of the features common to this group of tumors, such as invasive growth often involving expansive regions of brain parenchyma, increasing aggressiveness with progression from low-grade to high-grade histology over time and ultimately, causing death, with the exception of small and localized tumors that are amenable to radical surgical resection. However, OGDs have several unique molecular genetic and clinical features that distinguish them from other infiltrating gliomas.

Specifically, ODG tend to be less diffuse than the other gliomas. Although there are certainly widely infiltrative ODG, these tumors are often confined to the superficial rather than deep portions of the cerebral hemispheres and in some cases, are relatively well demarcated, allowing for more radical surgical debulking compared to other infiltrative gliomas [4, 5] (Fig. 8.1). Another highly favorable property is the chemosensitivity of ODG, particularly those with 1p19q co-deletion. This was first noted more than 20 years ago when AO were shown to be responsive to cytotoxic chemotherapy [6]. These initial observations have matured into multiple randomized controlled clinical trials for AO that have had encouraging results relative to other diffuse or high-grade glioma subtypes [7, 8]. Unfortunately, despite these favorable properties, both LGO and AO remain almost always incurable and inevitably progress to an increasingly aggressive and treatment-resistant disease. This sobering reality is the major driver of the ongoing research into the unique features of ODG that is hoped to result in improved therapies and outcomes for patients with ODG.

Histopathology

ODG is characterized by tumor cells that morphologically and phenotypically resemble oligodendrocytes, which produce myelin that serves to optimize nerve transmission via the insulation of axons. This helps to facilitate saltatory transmission of action potential that greatly expedites nerve impulse speed. They are located within the white matter of the brain, an area that is rich in myelin due to the concentration of axons in this region. ODG display classical histological appearance marked by "back-to-back" tumor cells with regular, round hyperchromatic nuclei in association with clearing of the cytoplasm and close proximity to fine branching vasculature [1]. The former is whimsically referred to as "fried-egg appearance" and the latter as "chicken-wire vasculature." Nonetheless, these terms accurately describe the classical histological appearance of ODG (Fig. 8.2a). Note that perinuclear clearing is secondary to the "washing out" of cytoplasmic content by organic solvent during the process of formalin-fixed paraffin-embedded (FFPE) specimen preparation and is absent in frozen sections. ODG can also present with subpopulations of gliofibrillary oligodendrocytes and minigemistocytes. Other associated histological features include the frequent presence of microscopic calcospherites which often coalesce into grossly observable calcific deposits that lend themselves to stereotypical radio-dense appearance in computer tomography imaging (Fig. 8.2b).

M.A. Karajannis and D. Zagzag (eds.), *Molecular Pathology of Nervous System Tumors: Biological Stratification and Targeted Therapies*, Molecular Pathology Library 8,
DOI 10.1007/978-1-4939-1830-0_8, © Springer Science+Business Media New York 2015

Table 8.1. 2007 World Health Organization (WHO) classification of gliomas.

Grade I	Grade II	Grade III	Grade IV
Angiocentric glioma	Diffuse astrocytoma	Anaplastic astrocytoma	Glioblastoma
Pilocytic astrocytoma	Oligodendroglioma	Anaplastic oligodendroglioma	Giant cell glioblastoma
Subependymal giant cell astrocytoma (SEGA)	Oligoastrocytoma	Anaplastic oligoastrocytoma	Gliosarcoma
	Pilomyxoid astrocytoma		Small cell glioblastoma
	Pleomorphic xanthoastrocytoma		Glioblastoma with oligodendroglioma features

From WHO Classification of Tumours of the Central Nervous System (IARC WHO Classification of Tumours) (v. 1), 2007, with permission of the World Health Organization

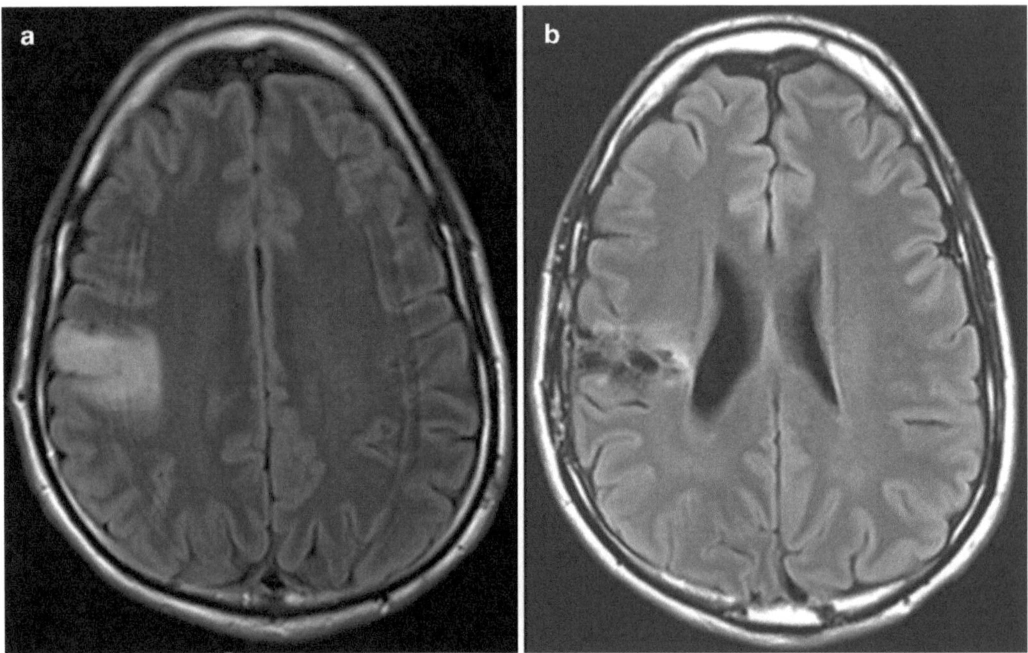

Fig. 8.1. Low-grade oligodendroglioma of the right frontal lobe as depicted in FLAIR brain MRI sequences before (**a**) and after (**b**) surgical resection. This is a classic presentation with the predominant involvement being in the cortical rather than deep regions.

Other histological features include foci of microcystic change and nuclear palisading, which historically was referred to as spongioblastic pattern usually associated with anaplastic ODG (WHO III) [9] (Fig. 8.2c). A feature shared by most ODG is the rather benign nuclear morphology which is frequently lost during malignant transformation to higher grade glioma. However, a focus with low-grade histological feature is sometimes present within glioblastoma suggestive of transformation. ODG tumor cells exhibit a strong physical affinity for non-neoplastic elements of the adjacent neuropil, a common characteristic shared with other infiltrating gliomas. These histological entities, including perineuronal and perivascular satellitoses, as well as subpial and intrafascicular spread, are collectively known as secondary structures of Scherer [10] (Fig. 8.2d).

Immunohistochemically, ODG tumor cells, especially those exhibiting classical morphology, are negative for glial fibrillary acidic protein (GFAP) expression. Morphological variants such as gliofibrillary oligodendrocytes and minigemistocytes display GFAP immunopositive cytoplasm and processes. Nonetheless, there is frequent background of GFAP reactivity due to the infiltrative nature of the tumor. Also, one must be cognizant of the reactive astrocytes admixed with tumor cells (Fig. 8.3a). Ki67 specific antibody highlights the proliferative fraction of the tumor. Immunoexpression of P53 is not very informative given *TP53* mutation is a rare event in ODG (Fig. 8.3b) [11]. The clinical introduction of IDH1 R132H mutant specific antibody (clone H-09) has dramatically altered the daily practice of neuropathology (Fig. 8.3c) [12]. Since a majority of WHO II/III infiltrating gliomas exhibit *IDH1* mutations, and R132H variant is the dominant form, the antibody is very useful in pinpointing tumor cells, even in small and challenging specimens.

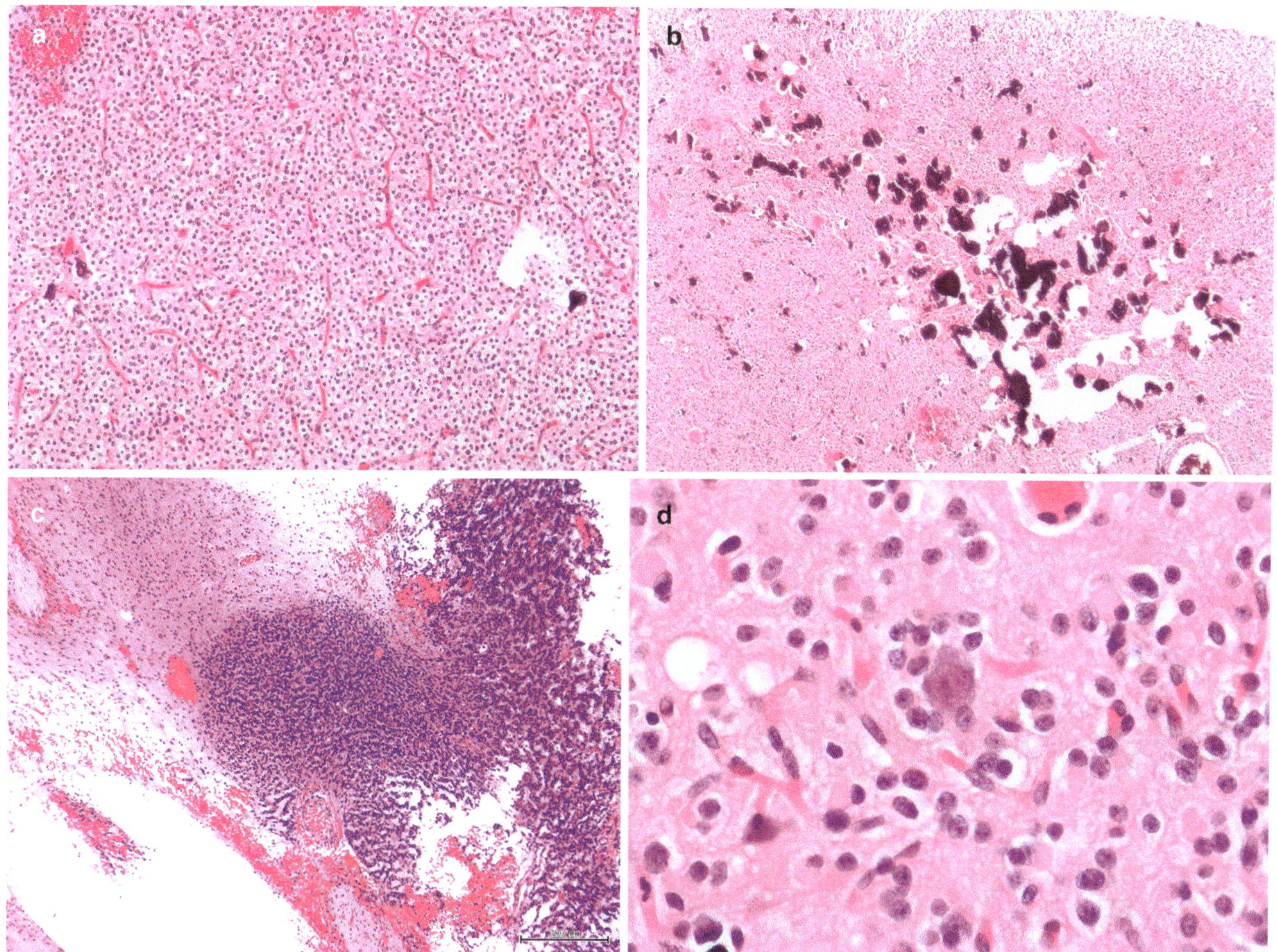

FIG. 8.2 (**a**) ODG displays classical appearance of perinuclear clearing and fine branching vasculatures, (**b**) frequent deposits of microcalcifications are common in ODG, (**c**) nuclear palisading is sometimes seen in ODG and especially associated with WHO III anaplastic ODG, (**d**) perineuronal satellitoses by ODG tumor cells is a feature shared with other infiltrating gliomas

As mentioned previously, the WHO grading scheme divides ODG with predominantly malignant oligodendroglial morphology into grades II and III, with the latter known as anaplastic oligodendroglioma (AO). The principal features of WHO III AO include predominance of hypercellular foci, worsening cytological pleomorphism, tumor necrosis, conspicuous microvascular proliferation, and significantly elevated mitotic activity. The latter two are particularly associated with aggressive behavior [13]. Presence of necrosis, even of the pseudopalisading variant, might not portend a worse prognosis as long as there is a predominance of tumor cells with classic ODG morphology [14]. Conversely, necrosis in tumors with mixed oligoastrocytic populations is associated with poor outcome.

Given the considerable subjectivity in the histological differentiation of WHO grade II and III oligodendroglial neoplasms, there is an even greater challenge in differentiating between pure ODG and mixed oligoastrocytomas (WHO grade II and III). Recently, this conundrum has extended further to clinical diagnosis of glioblastoma with oligodendroglioma component, or GBMO, vs. glioblastoma, or GBM—both of which are WHO grade IV malignant gliomas with poor prognosis. GBMO, when using strict diagnostic criteria, certainly presents distinctly from GBM under the microscope. Recent studies have also highlighted the uniqueness of the molecular underpinnings in GBMO [15]. It remains contentious whether GBMO is associated with a more favorable outcome compared to GBM, and this is exacerbated by the relatively loose definition of this entity along with the absence of agreed upon molecular biomarkers [16].

Inclusion of subjective histomorphological criteria presents significant problems in ensuring diagnostic uniformity among neuropathologists. This is especially problematic in accounting for the malignant oligodendroglial component in an infiltrating glioma and whether to diagnose a tumor as pure ODG or a mixed oligoastrocytoma. However, the most important issue arises from the vagaries of glioma cell morphology, which can lead to over-diagnosis of

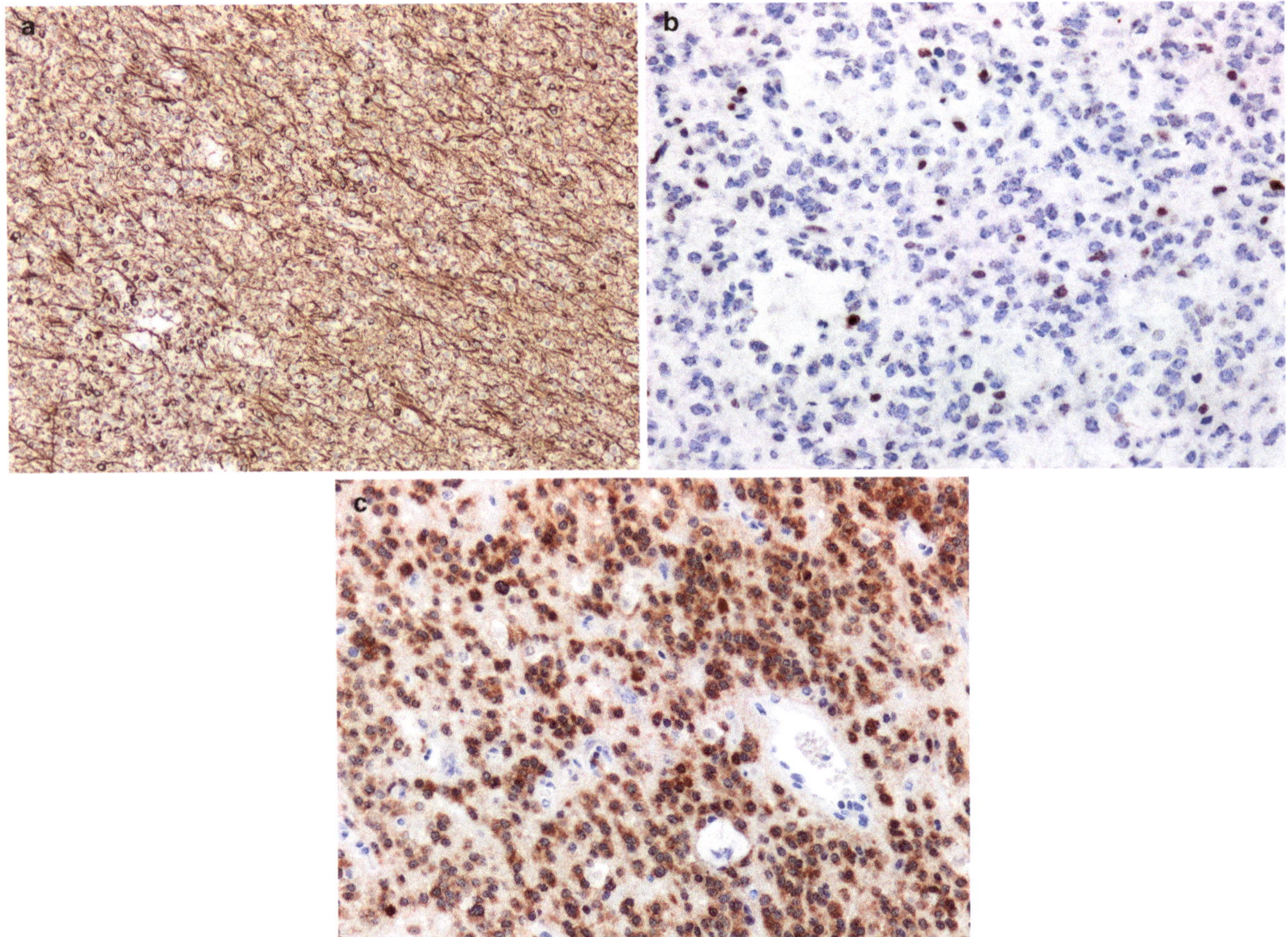

Fig. 8.3 (**a**) ODG is generally immunonegative for GFAP except for tumor cells with gliofibrillary oligodendrocytic and minigemistocytic morphology. There is strong background immunopositivity consistent with infiltrative nature of tumor cells, (**b**) ODG is typically negative for mutations in *TP53* and is reflected in "non-neoplastic" pattern of TP53 reactivity, (**c**) ODG tumor cells display strong cytoplasmic reactivity for IDH1 R132H mutant protein

oligodendroglial neoplasms, pure or mixed. Strong correlation between 1p19q co-deletions and the classical ODG morphology described above highlights association between underlying glioma genetics and histopathology [17]. This is an especially powerful finding given the survival benefits observed in 1p19q co-deleted WHO grade II and III oligodendroglial neoplasms [18, 19].

Clinical Behavior of Oligodendroglial Tumors

The clinical behavior of ODG is characterized by slow progression. LGO have a peak incidence commiserate with all low-grade gliomas, in the third decade of life. There is no clear gender or race distribution. The most common clinical presentation is seizures. Seizures, rather than focal neurologic deficits such as hemiplegia, are thought to be the presenting symptom due to the slow growth rate and infiltrative pattern of LGO, leading to brain irritation rather than to mass effect (source?). However, in some cases of AO where the tumor may grow more rapidly, patients may present with focal neurologic symptoms such as weakness, sensory alteration, vision change or personality change depending on the specific location of the tumor. Alternatively, patients with rapidly growing AO may present with more general symptoms of elevated intracranial pressure such as new and persistent headache or confusion. However, as above, new onset seizure is the most common presentation for ODG (50–90 % of patients) [2, 20].

The event of a first time seizure in an adult often leads to urgent medical evaluation including a computed tomography (CT) of the head or a magnetic resonance imaging (MRI) of the brain. Head CT will commonly show an area of hypodensity and in the case of more chronic tumors, may show punctate hyperdensities consistent with calcification or

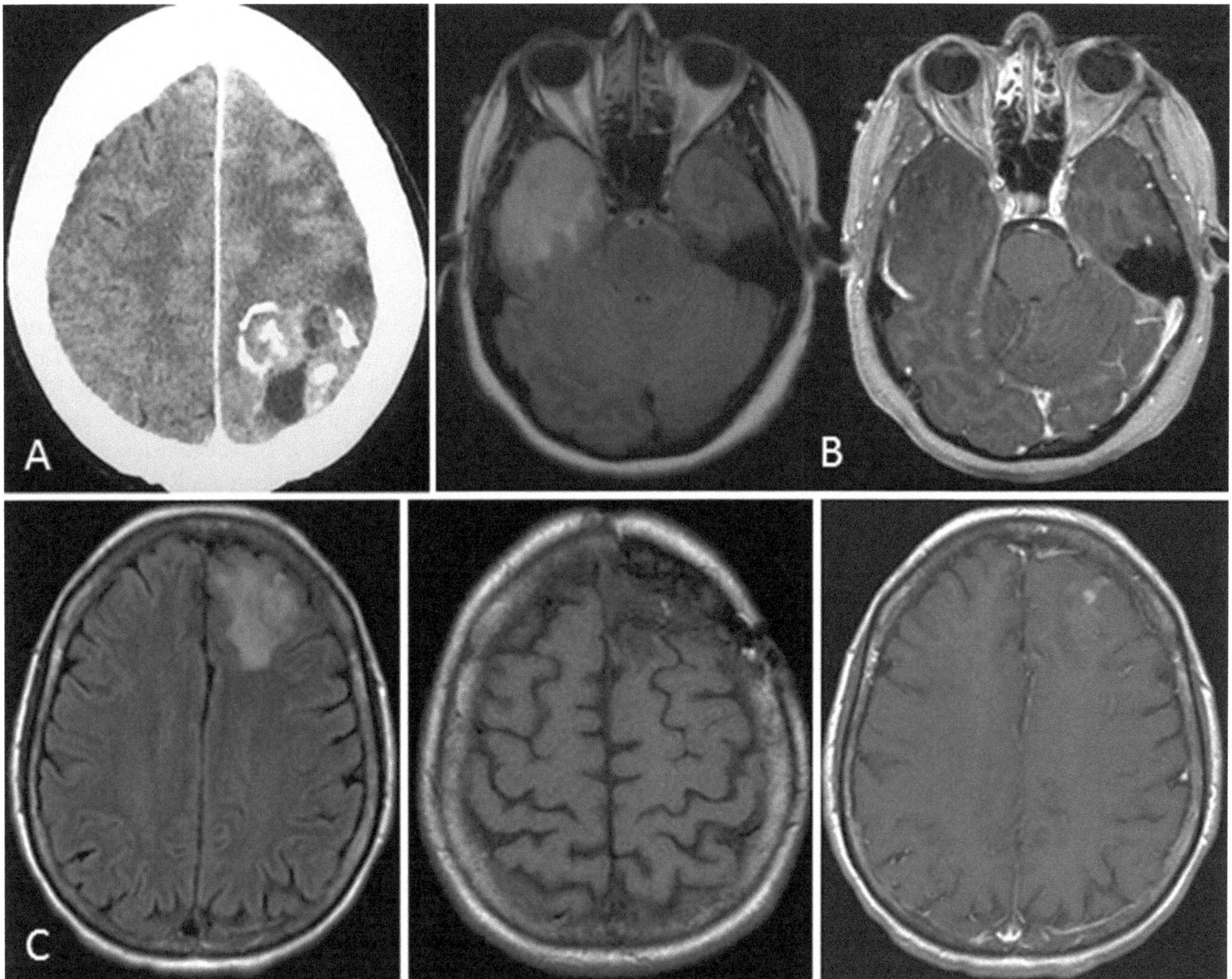

Fig. 8.4 Classic imaging features of ODG. (**a**) computed tomography scan showing hyperdensities consistent with calcification and possibly, microhemorrhages; magnetic resonance imaging (MRI) of AO with (**b**) FLAIR, (**c**) T1w, and (**d**) T1wGd sequences

microhemorrhages (Fig. 8.4a). The typical MRI features for a LGO include diffuse hyperintensity on T2-weighted or fluid attenuated inverse recovery (FLAIR) imaging sequences, a lack of gadolinium contrast enhancement, and normal diffusion weighted imaging (Fig. 8.4b). In comparison, the characteristic MRI features for AO include a mixed-intensity central core with diffuse surrounding signal hyperintensity on T2-weighted or FLAIR sequences and hypointensity on T1-weighted sequences, with some scattered hyperintensity due to calcification or microhemorrhage, as well as heterogeneous enhancement after administration of gadolinium [21–23] (Fig. 8.4c). Importantly, the presence of contrast enhancement does not uniformly predict a higher histological grade. In fact, in a recent study of MRI features of ODG, 28 % of AO did not have gadolinium (Gd) enhancement whereas 20 % of LGO did demonstrate Gd enhancement [24].

Functional MRI has recently been applied to ODG for the purpose of predicting grade as well as allele status (1p19q co-deletion vs. intact), since 1p19q status has been confirmed as both a prognostic and predictive marker [25, 26]. For example, perfusion-weighted imaging and proton MR spectroscopy added to standard anatomical imaging result in 72 % accuracy (83 % sensitivity and 65 % specificity) for distinguishing tumors with intact vs. co-deleted 1p/19q [25]. Although applying functional MRI and metabolic imaging remains experimental, interesting observations have been made that may offer insights into the molecular behavior of ODG subtypes in vivo. Specifically, when the metabolic radiolabelled tracers ^{201}Thallium (^{201}Tl) and ^{18F}fluorodeoxyglucose (^{18F}F-FDG) were assessed in patients with LGO, AO, and mixed oligoastrocytoma (with and without 1p19q co-deletion), 80 % of high-grade tumor had markers of elevated metabolism as might be expected [27].

Interestingly, LGO with 1p19q co-deletion also had an elevated metabolism profile compared to tumors without this molecular marker. In summary, the unique features of ODG tumors are increasingly being explored with specialized imaging techniques in the context of molecular discoveries, with the goal to better understand disease biology of these tumors and aid in the clinical management.

The time of disease progression for both LGO and AO is highly variable. Traditionally, factors such as age at diagnosis, degree of surgical resection, and tumor grade were considered the major predictors. Recently, based on data from the European Organization for Research and Treatment of Cancer (EORTC) study 26951 for AO [28], nine variables including adjuvant treatment received, age, tumor location (frontal or other), extent of resection, WHO performance status, the presence of endothelial abnormalities or necrosis, and finally, 1p/19q co-deletion and *IDH1* mutation status, were shown to be important prognostic factors. Based on these factors, they divided patients into low, intermediate, and high risk groups, with the best prognosis being associated with patients with age of diagnosis <40 years, a good performance status, tumor location in the frontal lobe, confirmed extensive resection without residual tumor on imaging, absence of endothelial abnormalities or necrosis, and 1p/19q co-deletion with *IDH1* mutation. For patients with AO who met all of these criteria, the median overall survival (OS) was 127 months (95 % CI: 95 months—not reached).

Treatment of Oligodendroglial Tumors

The first step in establishing a treatment plan for any patient with a suspected diagnosis of glioma is surgery. Surgery serves the role of both obtaining tissue to confirm the histology and molecular subtype and offering an opportunity for cytoreduction. Although the advanced imaging techniques discussed above may help in distinguishing tumor subtypes with increasing confidence, tissue is required for diagnostic confirmation. As discussed below, it is now widely accepted that initial molecular studies in any tumor suspected of being ODG should include analysis of 1p19q status. Studies such as *IDH1/2* status and *MGMT* promoter methylation are also commonly obtained at the time of initial diagnosis, as these allow for molecular subclassification and have impact on both overall prognosis and treatment decisions.

The first therapeutic intervention for all ODG is maximum safe surgical resection. There are a series of single center studies that all support the conclusion that gross total resection of the entire area of tumor involvement based on abnormal MRI signal is optimal as long as this can be accomplished safely without causing significant postoperative neurologic deficits [5, 29–31]. If significant tumor debulking is not feasible due to tumor location and risk for neurologic injury, the options are biopsy to confirm diagnosis, or if LGO is suspected, it may be reasonable to proceed with cautious surveillance in select patients until clinical or radiologic evidence of tumor progression. In widely infiltrative tumors where there is no clearly optimal location for diagnostic sampling, recent studies suggest that functional imaging techniques (diffusion tensor imaging, MR spectroscopy, perfusion imaging) may help determine the optimal location of tissue sampling [32, 33].

When the diagnosis of an AO is confirmed histologically, the next question to address is 1p19q status. For patients with 1p19q co-deleted AO, there is level one evidence in support of the use of procarbazine, carmustine (CCNU), vincristine (PCV) either before or after radiation therapy [7, 8]. This is based on two independent studies, EORTC 26951 and RTOG 9402, that had very similar conclusions despite slightly different designs. In EORTC 26951, patients with newly diagnosed AO were treated with RT alone vs. RT followed by up to six cycles of PCV [8]. At median 5-year follow-up, there was a significant difference in progression free survival (PFS), but not OS between the RT+PVC group and the RT alone group regardless of 1p19q status. However, at median 140 months follow-up, in patients with 1p19q co-deleted AO treated with RT+PCV median OS had not been reached vs. median OS of 9 years in patients treated with RT alone. In the RTOG 9402 trial, patients with AO were randomized to either four cycles of PCV followed by RT or RT alone. Similar to the EORTC study, there was no statistically significant difference in median OS at 5 years or at 12 years when all AO patients are analyzed in aggregate. However, at 12 year follow-up, the subpopulation of patients with 1p19q co-deleted AO treated with PCV+RT had a median OS of 14.7 vs. 7.3 months for those treated with RT alone [7] In contrast, there was no statistically significant difference in median OS for patients without 1p19q co-deletion treated with RT alone vs. RT+PCV. In summary, for patients with 1p19q co-deleted AO, there is strong evidence in support of a treatment paradigm that incorporates PCV and RT, however, there is no clear data to support a specific sequence (Table 8.2).

TABLE 8.2. Evidence for PCV chemotherapy for 1p19q co-deleted anaplastic oligodendrogliomas.

Study	Tumor grade	Treatment	Molecular subtype	mPFS (years)	mOS (years)
RTOG 9402 [7]	AO	PCV+RT	1p/19q co-deleted (*n*=59)	8.4	14.7
			All others (*n*=89)	1.2	2.6
		RT	1p/19q co-deleted (*n*=67)	2.9	7.3
			All others (*n*=76)	1.0	2.7
EORTC 26951 [8]	AO	PCV+RT	1p/19q co-deleted (*n*=43)	13.1	Not reached
			All others (*n*=114)	1.2	2.1
		RT	1p/19q co-deleted (*n*=37)	4.1	9.3
			All others (*n*=122)	0.73	1.8

Despite the compelling data using PCV, many neuro-oncologists advocate for consideration of RT and temozolomide (TMZ) as first line therapy for patients with newly diagnosed AO. This practice is based on the fact that as alkylator-based chemotherapies, PCV and TMZ have similar mechanisms of action and that PCV is much more toxic, resulting in only 42 % of the patients in RTOG 9402 and 30 % of the patients in EORTC 26951 receiving all prescribed chemotherapy [7, 8]. When the initial reports of these studies were published in 2006, the high rates of toxicity and lack of OS benefit led many neuro-oncologists to apply the regimen of RT + TMZ followed by six cycles of TMZ to AO based on the proven benefit of this regimen in glioblastoma [34–36]. However, despite evidence that TMZ does have activity in AO (newly diagnosed and recurrent), it remains to be proven that TMZ plus RT has similar efficacy to PCV plus RT in patients with newly diagnosed AO [37–41]. Ongoing studies that assess the benefit of RT + TMZ in patients with anaplastic gliomas segregated based on 1p19q status will help further clarify this issue. Specifically, the Chemoradiation and Adjuvant Temozolomide in Non-deleted anaplastic glial tumors (CATNON, NCT00626990) trial is addressing the question of whether adding TMZ to RT improves OS for non-deleted anaplastic gliomas. A concurrent study, a randomized trial of Chemoradiation vs. Radiation vs. Temozolomide in 1p/19q Co-deleted anaplastic gliomas (CODEL, NCT 00887146) was initially designed to assess the impact of RT alone, vs. RT + TMZ, vs. TMZ alone on OS in the setting of 1p19q co-deleted anaplastic gliomas. However, in the wake of the long-term results of the RTOG 9402 and EORTC 26951 studies, it was amended to include three comparator arms: RT + PCV, RT + TMZ and adjuvant TMZ, and TMZ alone. In summary, to date the only level 1 evidence to guide treatment recommendations is for the use of RT + PCV for patients with newly diagnosed 1p19q co-deleted AO, while there remains no agreed upon optimal therapy for non-deleted AO.

There is also no agreed upon optimal therapy for LGO. Even more so than for high-grade tumors, the extent of resection has been associated with better PFS and OS [42]. After maximal safe surgical resection, the treatment options include surveillance, RT, or for patients with 1p19q co-deletion, possibly chemotherapy. RT has been the traditional first line therapy for all low-grade gliomas, including LGO. However, data shows that there is no difference in OS between patients who received RT at the time of initial diagnosis or at the time of progression [43]. To help clarify which patients may benefit from early RT treatment, the definition of high and low risk groups for low-grade glioma has been proposed [44]. The high risk group is defined as having tumor dimension ≥6 cm and astrocytoma histology. Low risk gliomas were defined as tumor <6 cm with oligodendroglioma histology. Additional prognostic factors include 1p19q status, Mini Mental Status Examination score and extent of resection. Another unanswered question is whether there is benefit to adding chemotherapy to RT for LGO. RTOG 98-02 assessed the effect of RT + PCV vs. RT alone on OS. There was no statistically significant difference between the RT + PCV and RT groups, although there was an improvement for the combined therapy group in PFS (5-year PFS 63 % RT + PCV vs. 46 % RT) alone (HR, 0.6; 95 % CI, 0.41–0.86; $p = 0.06$; log-rank $p = 0.005$) [45]. The ongoing Eastern Oncology Group E3F05 study: Radiation Therapy with or without Temozolomide in Treating Patients With Low-Grade Glioma (NCT 00978458) is assessing the benefit of RT alone vs. RT + TMZ as first line therapy in patients with symptomatic or progressive low-grade gliomas. Finally, there remains the question about whether RT should be deferred for LGO with chemotherapy being offered as first line therapy. A series of studies have suggested that TMZ shows significant activity in patients with LGO, with the most robust effects seen in patients with 1p19q co-deletion, *IDH1* mutation status, and *MGMT* methylation [46–49].

Molecular Genetics of ODG: Predictive, Prognostic, and the Impact on Treatment Decisions

The discovery of associations between ODG histomorphology, 1p19q co-deletion, and clinical outcome resulting from slow and predictable natural history and chemosensitivity remains a landmark in modern neuro-oncology and pathology [50]. Initial observations of a favorable response to the PCV regimen have been extended to TMZ [48, 51]. Due to its strong association with chemoresponsiveness, molecular testing for 1p19q co-deletion, either via fluorescence in situ hybridization (FISH) or loss of heterozygosity (LOH) assays, in gliomas with oligodendroglial features on histology has become a standard diagnostic adjunct in modern neuro-oncology (Fig. 8.5) [52, 53]. The unique yet simple histology

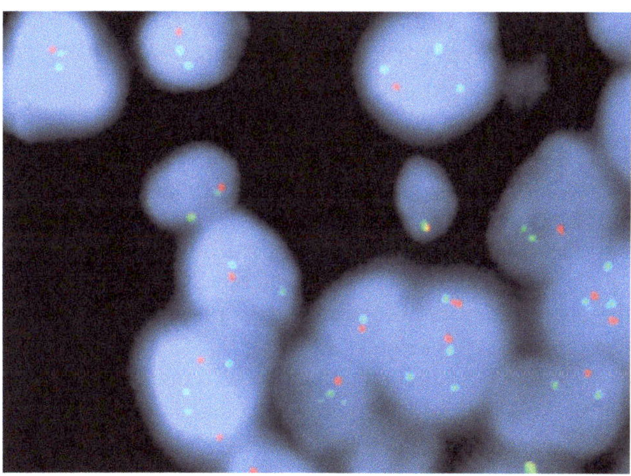

Fig. 8.5. 1p FISH shows individual ODG tumor cells contain relatively more 1q chromosomes (*green* probe) compared to 1p chromosomes (*red* probe) consistent with 1p deletion.

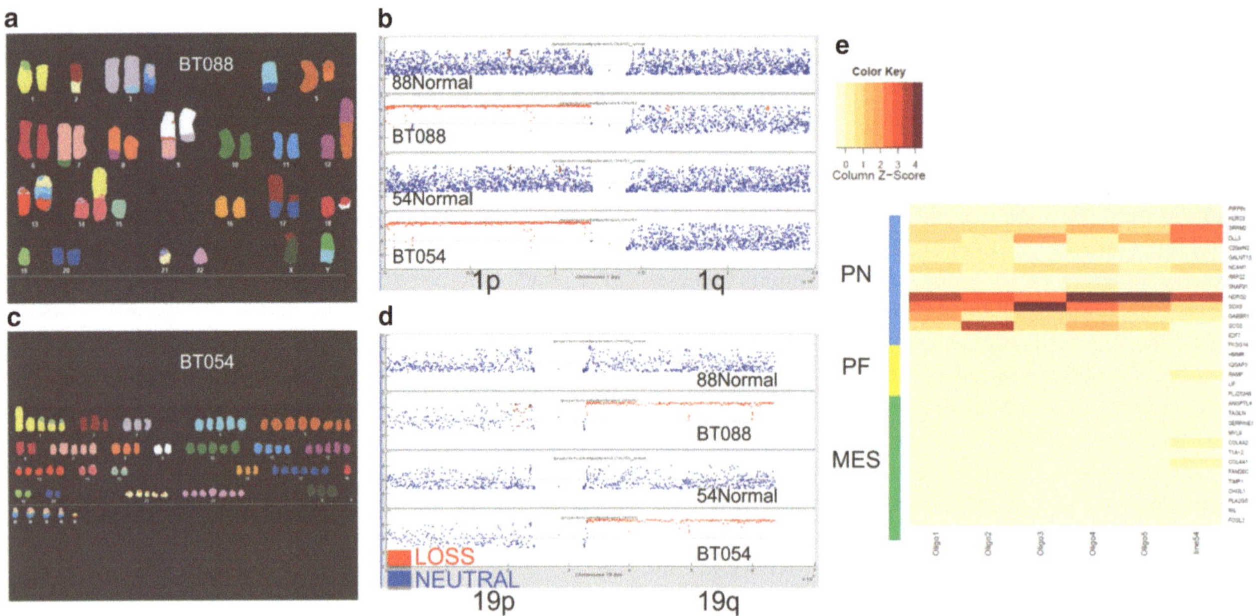

FIG. 8.6. Next generation sequencing of two 1p19q co-deleted brain tumor initiating cell lines derived from ODG patients (**a**, **c**) confirmed copy number losses of 1p and 19q (**b**, **d**) as well as proneural gene expression signature compatible with ODG (**e**).

of ODG also belies other distinctive molecular features that span the genomic, transcriptomic, and epigenomic realms, which will be explored in detail below [54–58]. A recent report highlighted how a genetic variant rs55705857 in 8q24.21 is associated with ODG development in a background of mutant *IDH1/2* [59]. This study suggests that germline variants may be important factors in acquiring OGD, and perhaps other gliomas as well.

Fundamentally, ODG is defined by 1p19q co-deletion, or more specifically, unbalanced translocations of chromosomes 1p and 19q [60, 61]. This essentially leads to loss of one copy each of 1p and 19q, resulting in loss of heterozygosity (LOH) affecting the regions of numerical loss. Moreover, 1p19q co-deleted anaplastic ODG that exhibits polysomy for chromosomes 1p and 19q has intermediate survival between 1p19q retained tumors and 1p19q co-deleted ODGs in a euploidy background [62, 63]. This suggests that accumulation of additional genetic aberrations, such as those regulating cell cycling and homologous recombination that contribute to the polysomy state, might contribute to earlier recurrence. An issue raised by these data is the importance of the specific assay used for determination of 1p19q status, since only FISH (and not LOH PCR) permits the enumeration of absolute numbers of chromosomes and determination of ploidy status.

In addition to 1p19q co-deletion as a unique biomarker of ODG chemoresponsiveness, early studies have identified somatic mutations in *TP53* as virtually restricted to astrocytomas and not occurring in ODG [11, 64]. Whole exome sequencing has confirmed this early finding in untreated ODG [65]. Another significant molecular feature of OGD is the strong association with mutations of *IDH1/2* [66]. In the same study, 99 of 107 WHO II/III pure ODG tumors showed 1p19q co-deletion or loss of heterozygosity of which 90 contain *IDH1* and three contain *IDH2* mutations [67]. In a review of published studies by Kloosterhof and colleagues, they found 76 % and 67 % *IDH1* and 4 % and 5 % *IDH2* mutations in LGO (WHO II) and AO (WHO III), respectively [68]. These percentages are similar to WHO II/III infiltrating astrocytomas and mixed oligoastrocytomas. Heterozygous neomorphic mutations in *IDH* genes result in the generation of the onco-metabolite 2-hydroxyglutarate or 2HG [69, 70]. 2HG has significant pleiotropic effects on the tumor epigenome, leading to aberrant histone regulation and development of the glioma hypermethylator phenotype [71–73]. This important discovery has generated leads for practical applications in improved diagnosis and treatment of *IDH* mutated gliomas [74–76]. Prior to the discovery of recurrent mutations in the *IDH* genes, the sole focus was on uncovering genetic candidates within the 1p and 19q LOH regions and particular effort on the former given its stronger association with the ODG phenotype and superior clinical performance [77]. Obvious candidates such as *NOTCH2*, located at 1p11 have been extensively investigated [78, 79]. Identification of recurrent somatic mutations in *CIC*, a gene that resides in chromosome 19q, is 69 % of ODG with 1p19q co-deletions and *IDH* gene mutation using next generation sequencing (NGS) [66, 80]. NGS excels at the unprecedented depth and breadth of profiling of the transcriptome, exome, and genome of cancer. NGS has refined many long-standing molecular findings of ODG at basepair resolution (Fig. 8.6). Data from subsequent studies have

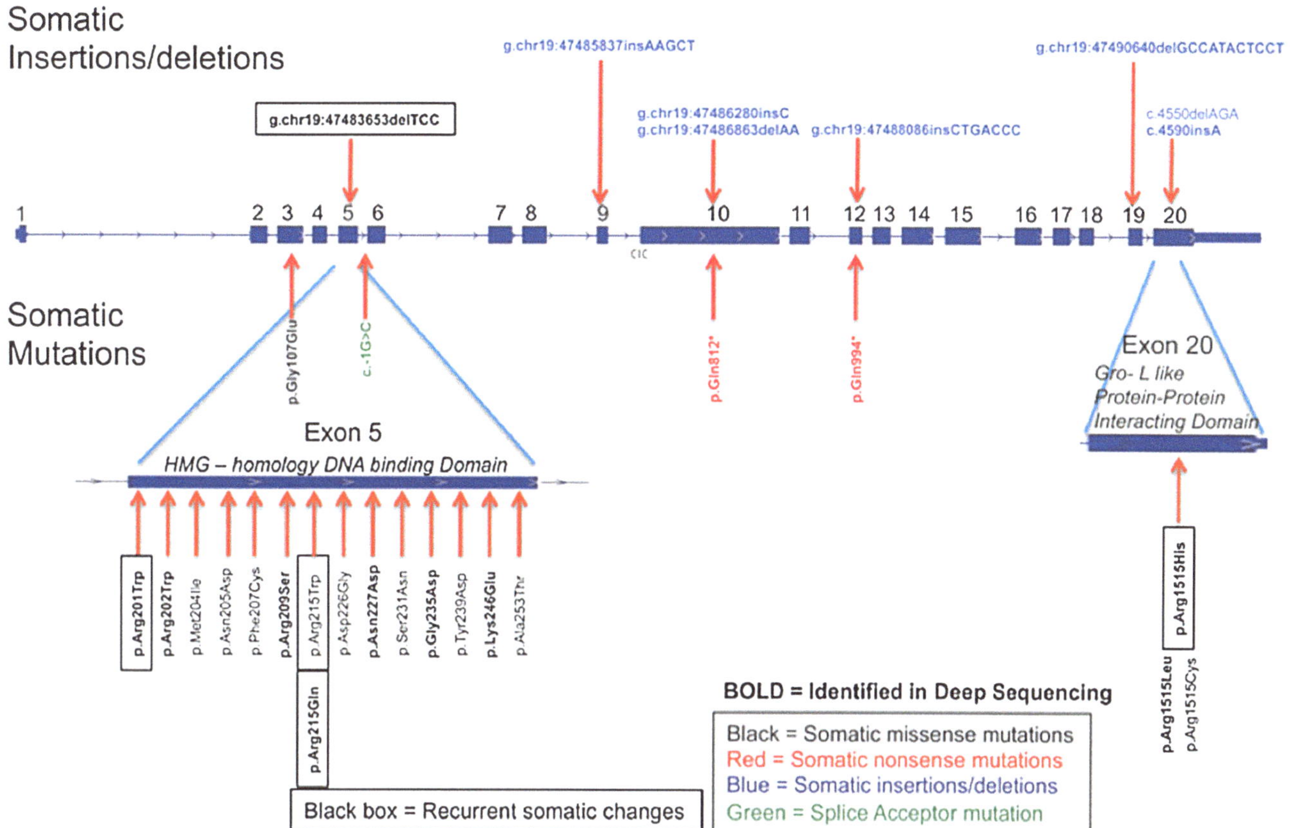

FIG. 8.7. Somatic mutations in the remaining allele of *CIC* in 19q are distributed across the gene but cluster in exons 5 and 20, which code for functionally crucial domains.

added to these initial findings [81, 82]. The *CIC* gene encodes the mammalian homolog of *Capicua*, a transcriptional repressor in *Drosophila* that is essential for inhibition of RAS/MAPK signaling [83–85]. There is a high level of cross-species homology of the *CIC* gene, especially in the functionally critical DNA-binding and protein-interacting domains. Somatic *CIC* mutations in oligodendrogliomas most commonly cluster in the HMG-homology DNA-binding domain in exon 5, and recurrent mutations affecting codons 201, 202, and 215 have been identified (Fig. 8.7). The second most common recurrent mutations are clustered within the exon 20 protein-interacting Gro-L homology domain. A slightly lesser number of *CIC* mutations are scattered throughout the gene. Strikingly, somatic *CIC* mutations are very strongly associated with 1p19q co-deleted and *IDH* mutated OGD, and only found in 2 % of astrocytomas not associated with 1p19q co-deletion. Importantly, the majority of the *CIC* mutations in this cohort are located outside of exons 5 and 20. This highlights potential selective pressure on the development of *CIC* mutations in ODG and also the functional significance of these domains. At this time, very little is known about the mechanistic role of CIC in brain tumor development, and hence the impetus to pursue ongoing impetus to pursue ongoing functional investigations into its role functional investigations into its role in the development of this tumor [86]. The close association of CIC mutations with *IDH* mutations in 1p19q co-deleted ODG suggests that both cooperate in tumorigenesis, which may require a pro-oncogenic environment facilitated by the presence of 2HG. However, it remains unclear whether *CIC* mutations represent loss-of-function or gain-of-function, and how they contribute mechanistically to the development of ODG. Somatic mutations in *FUBP1*, located in 1p, also appear to cluster in 1p19q co-deleted ODG [80, 81]. Inactivating mutations of *ATRX*, which code for a chromatin remodeler, are virtually exclusive to astrocytomas and mixed oligoastrocytomas and rarely found in ODG, whereas *CIC* and *FUBP1* mutations are preferentially associated with ODG and only discovered in 10 % of the former [82]. Therefore, ODG biology and clinical behavior are governed by the complex interactions of the presence and absence of unique genetic alterations. These emerging data highlight the need to develop a molecular classification for these tumors that goes beyond histology and accurately reflects entities with distinct biology and clinical behavior.

Gene Expression in OGD

ODG with 1p19q co-deletion exhibits a proneural gene expression signature that is associated with a more favorable prognosis [54, 57], in keeping with similar findings in glioblastoma [87]. One of the differentially expressed genes dependent on 1p19q status, *α-internexin* [88], can be easily interrogated with economical, automated immunohistochemical (IHC) testing in lieu of molecular genetic testing. Another example of a biomarker associated with clinical tumor behavior that can be assessed by IHC is EGFR protein expression in ODG [89].

Epigenetics of ODG

In addition to somatic DNA aberrations, the epigenome of brain tumors, including OGD, has emerged as a key driver of tumor biology, as illustrated by the broad epigenetic consequences of *IDH* mutations. LOH can be mediated genetically via the acquisition of mutations in the remaining allele or epigenetic silencing of regulatory regions of a gene in the remaining allele [90]. Therefore, epigenetic modification of genes located within 1p and 19q, such as *CIC* and *FUBP1*, could perhaps provide for an alternative mechanism of gene silencing. Transcriptome studies of 1p19q co-deleted ODG have confirmed the selective down-regulation of *SLC9A1* gene expression in the absence of somatic mutation. This gene, located in chr1p36.1, codes for a sodium/hydrogen exchanger essential for the maintenance of intracellular pH [91]. Attenutation of *SLC9A1* gene expression in 1p loss tumors is a result of promoter hypermethylation and reversible upon the introduction of 5-azacytidine. Aberrant expression of this protein results in significantly reduced intracellular pH which affects acid load recovery in ODG that may partly explain the biological and phenotypic difference between ODG and other infiltrating gliomas. Hypermethylation of the *MGMT* promoter is associated with improved outcome in glioblastoma patients receiving concurrent TMZ and ionizing irradiation [92]. However, in AO a hypermethylated phenotype is a stronger predictor of survival than selective *MGMT* methylation [93, 94]. This so-called G-CIMP (glioma—CpG island methylator phenotype) signature is tightly associated with IDH-mutant low-grade gliomas with proneural gene expression signature [95]. Therefore, one can start to appreciate the interconnectivity between the genomic, transcriptomic, and epigenomic spaces of ODG and the significance of an integrative approach to studying this tumor.

Future Directions

Evolving concepts of ODG molecular pathology are directly impacting the way this tumor is managed clinically. Traditional reliance on subjective descriptive terminology is slowly being replaced by objective molecular findings, with a significantly stronger association with outcome and response to specific targeted therapeutics [96, 97]. Introduction of advanced diagnostic platforms in routine laboratory workflow has provided the opportunity to profile large cohorts of ODG at an unprecedented depth and breadth. Both the Ion Torrent PGM and Illumina MiSeq sequencing platforms accommodate deep amplicon sequencing suitable for DNA extracted from formalin-fixed paraffin-embedded (FFPE) tissues [98]. Since FFPE is the common currency of pathology labs, the ability to extract potentially informative genetic material for multiplex deep-sequencing assays from archival samples will dramatically alter the landscape of genetic-clinical outcome correlative studies by increasing the number of eligible study cases (Fig. 8.8) [98, 99]. Similarly, introduction of the Nanostring nCounter platform that can perform multiplex gene expression analysis of FFPE-derived mRNA has opened up limitless research opportunities as illustrated in several recent publications [100, 101]. A custom designed codeset was able to distinguish between ODG and other brain tumors (Fig. 8.9).

Infiltrating glioma is an ideal disease model that lends itself to deeper interrogation of spatial and temporal heterogeneity of cancer. Given the diverse histology of tumor cells within GBM, the discovery of substantial underlying genomic heterogeneity is perhaps not surprising. For example, a recent landmark study has demonstrated mosaic amplification of growth factor genes in GBM [102]. This raises the fundamental question whether tumors with more homogeneous and regular histology, such as ODG, also exhibit underlying genomic heterogeneity. One of the authors (SY) has embarked on a study to address this question via deep sequencing and gene expression profiling of F-DOPA-PET-guided biopsy specimens of WHO II/III infiltrating gliomas including ODG. Tumor from a patient may yield several spatially unique tissue samples based on F-DOPA signatures—these are subjected to NGS to reveal allelic frequencies of mutations and to enumerate expression of selected genes. Clinical follow-up and repeated metabolic imaging permits for the association of metabolic signatures, genomic and transcriptomic profiles, and location of disease recurrence to generate a "radio-metabolo-genomic" signature of glioma recurrence. This epitomizes the emerging concept of "integrative diagnostics" which amalgamate traditional and functional imaging with pathology and advanced molecular diagnostics. This may not only direct the use of currently available therapies, but lead to

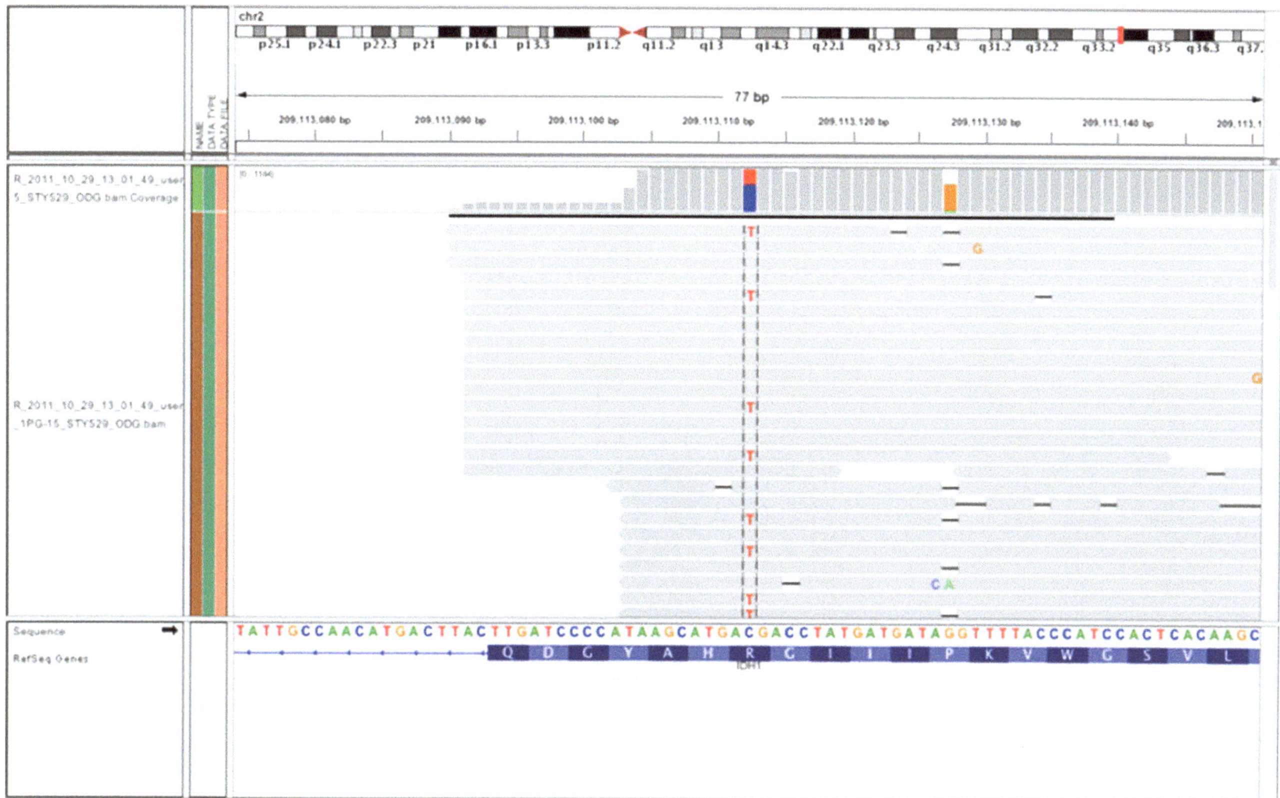

Fig. 8.8. Deep amplicon sequencing of 10 ng of FFPE DNA from an ODG using the AmpliSeq cancer panel on the Ion Torrent PGM sequencing platform reveals heterozygous mutation leading to R132H change in *IDH1*.

the identification of new targetable nodes and therefore, the development of new therapies.

Such scientifically driven advances are desperately needed, as although the last 5–10 years have been full of great discovery for ODG tumors, they remain an enigmatic entity and a cure is still out of reach today. However, there is promise for further advancement in the near future. Historical observation of good clinical behavior was supplemented by discovery of strong association with 1p19q co-deletions, that later transcended into unique gene expression and epigenetic features of ODG. NGS has allowed for unbiased and genome-wide interrogation of ODG which resulted in the discoveries of *CIC* and *FUBP1* mutations. However, these are unlikely to be the sole molecular drivers and not all mutations can be readily converted to therapeutic targets. Hence, ongoing investigation into the wide range of genetic and epigenetic components in addition to a permissive metabolic milieu permitted by *IDH* mutations, for example, is required. Ongoing efforts by the TCGA low-grade glioma consortium will significantly augment our knowledge of this enigmatic tumor. Fortunately, the field is well versed in the practice of clinical-translational research allowing close collaboration between laboratory and clinical scientists that will yield the next treatment breakthrough.

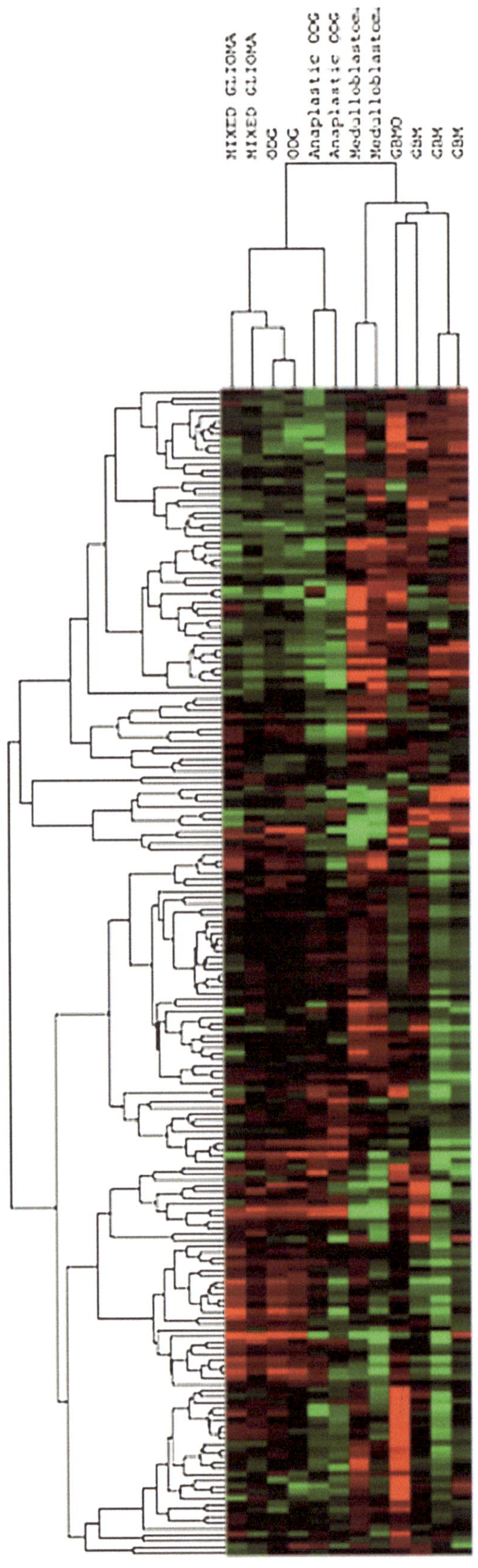

FIG. 8.9. Unsupervised hierarchical clustering of gene expression data generated from 250 ng mRNA extracted from FFPE blocks of various brain tumors show distinctive clustering pattern.

References

1. Louis DN, Ohgaki H, Wiestler OD, Cavenee WK, editors. WHO classification of tumours of the central nervous system. Lyon: IARC; 2007.
2. van den Bent MJ. Anaplastic oligodendroglioma and oligoastrocytoma. Neurol Clin. 2007;25:1089–109, ix–x.
3. CBTRUS: statistical report: primary brain tumors in the United States, 1998-2002. Central Brain Tumor Registry of the United States; 2005. Available at http://www.cbtrus.org/reports//2005-2006/2006report.pdf. Accessed 24 March 2008.
4. Jenkinson MD, du Plessis DG, Smith TS, et al. Histological growth patterns and genotype in oligodendroglial tumours: correlation with MRI features. Brain. 2006;129:1884–91.
5. Laws ER, Parney IF, Huang W, et al. Survival following surgery and prognostic factors for recently diagnosed malignant glioma: data from the Glioma Outcomes Project. J Neurosurg. 2003;99:467–73.
6. Cairncross JG, Macdonald DR. Successful chemotherapy for recurrent malignant oligodendroglioma. Ann Neurol. 1988;23: 360–4.
7. Cairncross G, Wang M, Shaw E, Jenkins R, Brachman D, Buckner J, Fink K, Souhami L, Laperriere N, Curran W, Mehta M. Phase III trial of chemoradiotherapy for anaplastic oligodendroglioma: long-term results of RTOG 9402. J Clin Oncol. 2013;31(3):337–43.
8. van den Bent MJ, Brandes AA, Taphoorn MJ, Kros JM, Kouwenhoven MC, Delattre JY, Bernsen HJ, Frenay M, Tijssen CC, Grisold W, Sipos L, Enting RH, French PJ, Dinjens WN, Vecht CJ, Allgeier A, Lacombe D, Gorlia T, Hoang-Xuan K. Adjuvant procarbazine, lomustine, and vincristine chemotherapy in newly diagnosed anaplastic oligodendroglioma: long-term follow-up of EORTC brain tumor group study 26951. J Clin Oncol. 2013;31(3):344–50.
9. Wippold II FJ, Lammle M, Anatelli F, et al. Neuropathology for the neuroradiologist: palisades and pseudopalisades. AJNR Am J Neuroradiol. 2006;27:2037–41.
10. Scherer HJ. Structural development in glioma. Am J Cancer. 1938;34:333–51.
11. Ueki K, Nishikawa R, Nakazato Y, et al. Correlation of histology and molecular genetic analysis of 1p, 19q, 10q, TP53, EGFR, CDK4, and CDKN2A in 91 astrocytic and oligodendroglial tumors. Clin Cancer Res. 2002;8:196–201.
12. Capper D, Zentgraf H, Balss J, et al. Monoclonal antibody specific for IDH1 R132H mutation. Acta Neuropathol. 2009;118:599–601.
13. Giannini C, Scheithauer BW, Weaver AL, et al. Oligodendrogliomas: reproducibility and prognostic value of histologic diagnosis and grading. J Neuropathol Exp Neurol. 2001;60:248–62.
14. Miller CR, Dunham CP, Scheithauer BW, et al. Significance of necrosis in grading of oligodendroglial neoplasms: a clinicopathologic and genetic study of newly diagnosed high-grade gliomas. J Clin Oncol. 2006;24:5419–26.
15. Appin CL, Gao J, Chisolm C, et al. Glioblastoma with oligodendroglioma component (GBM-O): molecular genetic and clinical characteristics. Brain Pathol. 2013;23:454–61.
16. Hegi ME, Janzer RC, Lambiv WL, et al. Presence of an oligodendroglioma-like component in newly diagnosed glioblastoma identifies a pathogenetically heterogeneous subgroup and lacks prognostic value: central pathology review of the EORTC_26981/NCIC_CE.3 trial. Acta Neuropathol. 2012;123:841–52.
17. McDonald JM, See SJ, Tremont IW, et al. The prognostic impact of histology and 1p/19q status in anaplastic oligodendroglial tumors. Cancer. 2005;104:1468–77.
18. Mason W, Louis DN, Cairncross JG. Chemosensitive gliomas in adults: which ones and why? J Clin Oncol. 1997;15:3423–6.
19. Cairncross JG, Ueki K, Zlatescu MC, et al. Specific genetic predictors of chemotherapeutic response and survival in patients with anaplastic oligodendrogliomas. J Natl Cancer Inst. 1998;90:1473–9.
20. Daumas-Duport C, Varlet P, Tucker ML, et al. Oligodendrogliomas. Part I: patterns of growth, histological diagnosis, clinical and imaging correlations: a study of 153 cases. J Neurooncol. 1997;34:37–59.
21. Jenkinson MD, du Plessis DG, Smith TS, et al. Histological growth patterns and genotype in oligodendroglial tumours: correlation with MRI features. Brain. 2006;129:1884–91.
22. Kondziolka D, Bernstein M, Resch L, et al. Significance of hemorrhage into brain tumors: clinicopathological study. J Neurosurg. 1987;67:852–7.
23. Liwnicz BH, Wu SZ, Tew Jr JM. The relationship between the capillary structure and hemorrhage in gliomas. J Neurosurg. 1987;66:536–41.
24. Khalid L, Carone M, Dumrongpisutikul N, Intrapiromkul J, Bonekamp D, Barker PB, Yousem DM. Imaging characteristics of oligodendrogliomas that predict grade. AJNR Am J Neuroradiol. 2012;33(5):852–7.
25. Chawla S, Krejza J, Vossough A, Zhang Y, Kapoor GS, Wang S, O'Rourke DM, Melhem ER, Poptani H. Differentiation between oligodendroglioma genotypes using dynamic susceptibility contrast perfusion-weighted imaging and proton MR spectroscopy. AJNR Am J Neuroradiol. 2013;34(8):1542–9.
26. Jia Z, Geng D, Liu Y, Chen X, Zhang J. Low-grade and anaplastic oligodendrogliomas: differences in tumour microvascular permeability evaluated with dynamic contrast-enhanced magnetic resonance imaging. J Clin Neurosci. 2013;20(8):1110–3.
27. Walker C, du Plessis DG, Fildes D, et al. Correlation of molecular genetics with molecular and morphological imaging in gliomas with an oligodendroglial component. Clin Cancer Res. 2004;10:7182–91.
28. Gorlia T, Delattre JY, Brandes AA, Kros JM, Taphoorn MJ, Kouwenhoven MC, Bernsen HJ, Frénay M, Tijssen CC, Lacombe D, van den Bent MJ. New clinical, pathological and molecular prognostic models and calculators in patients with locally diagnosed anaplastic oligodendroglioma or oligoastrocytoma. A prognostic factor analysis of European Organisation for Research and Treatment of Cancer Brain Tumour Group Study 26951. Eur J Cancer. 2013;49(16):3477–85.
29. McGirt MJ, Chaichana KL, Attenello FJ, Weingart JD, Than K, Burger PC, Olivi A, Brem H, Quinoñes-Hinojosa A. Extent of surgical resection is independently associated with survival in patients with hemispheric infiltrating low-grade gliomas. Neurosurgery. 2008;63(4):700–7.
30. McGirt MJ, Mukherjee D, Chaichana KL, Than KD, Weingart JD, Quinones-Hinojosa A. Association of surgically acquired motor and language deficits on overall survival after resection of glioblastoma multiforme. Neurosurgery. 2009;65(3):463–9, discussion 469–70.
31. Tsitlakidis A, Foroglou N, Venetis CA, Patsalas I, Hatzisotiriou A, Selviaridis P. Biopsy versus resection in the management of

malignant gliomas: a systematic review and meta-analysis. J Neurosurg. 2010;112(5):1020–32.
32. Pamir MN, Özduman K, Yıldız E, Sav A, Dinçer A. Intraoperative magnetic resonance spectroscopy for identification of residual tumor during low-grade glioma surgery: clinical article. J Neurosurg. 2013;118(6):1191–8.
33. Sahin N, Melhem ER, Wang S, Krejza J, Poptani H, Chawla S, Verma G. Advanced MR imaging techniques in the evaluation of nonenhancing gliomas: perfusion-weighted imaging compared with proton magnetic resonance spectroscopy and tumor grade. Neuroradiol J. 2013;26(5):531–41.
34. Panageas KS, Iwamoto FM, Cloughesy TF, Aldape KD, Rivera AL, Eichler AF, Louis DN, Paleologos NA, Fisher BJ, Ashby LS, Cairncross JG, Roldán Urgoiti GB, Wen PY, Ligon KL, Schiff D, Robins HI, Rocque BG, Chamberlain MC, Mason WP, Weaver SA, Green RM, Kamar FG, Abrey LE, Deangelis LM, Jhanwar SC, Rosenblum MK, Lassman AB. Initial treatment patterns over time for anaplastic oligodendroglial tumors. Neuro Oncol. 2012;14(6):761–7.
35. Abrey LE, Louis DN, Paleologos N, Lassman AB, Raizer JJ, Mason W, Finlay J, MacDonald DR, DeAngelis LM, Cairncross JG, Oligodendroglioma Study Group. Survey of treatment recommendations for anaplastic oligodendroglioma. Neuro Oncol. 2007;9(3):314–8.
36. Stupp R, Mason WP, van den Bent MJ, Weller M, Fisher B, Taphoorn MJ, Belanger K, Brandes AA, Marosi C, Bogdahn U, Curschmann J, Janzer RC, Ludwin SK, Gorlia T, Allgeier A, Lacombe D, Cairncross JG, Eisenhauer E, Mirimanoff RO, European Organisation for Research and Treatment of Cancer Brain Tumor and Radiotherapy Groups, National Cancer Institute of Canada Clinical Trials Group. Radiotherapy plus concomitant and adjuvant temozolomide for glioblastoma. N Engl J Med. 2005;352(10):987–96.
37. Chinot OL, Honore S, Dufour H, Barrie M, Figarella-Branger D, Muracciole X, Braguer D, Martin PM, Grisoli F. Safety and efficacy of temozolomide in patients with recurrent anaplastic oligodendrogliomas after standard radiotherapy and chemotherapy. J Clin Oncol. 2001;19(9):2449–55.
38. Taliansky-Aronov A, Bokstein F, Lavon I, Siegal T. Temozolomide treatment for newly diagnosed anaplastic oligodendrogliomas: a clinical efficacy trial. J Neurooncol. 2006;79(2):153–7.
39. Wick W, Hartmann C, Engel C, Stoffels M, Felsberg J, Stockhammer F, Sabel MC, Koeppen S, Ketter R, Meyermann R, Rapp M, Meisner C, Kortmann RD, Pietsch T, Wiestler OD, Ernemann U, Bamberg M, Reifenberger G, von Deimling A, Weller M. NOA-04 randomized phase III trial of sequential radiochemotherapy of anaplastic glioma with procarbazine, lomustine, and vincristine or temozolomide. J Clin Oncol. 2009;27(35):5874–80.
40. Vogelbaum MA, Berkey B, Peereboom D, Macdonald D, Giannini C, Suh JH, Jenkins R, Herman J, Brown P, Blumenthal DT, Biggs C, Schultz C, Mehta M. Phase II trial of preirradiation and concurrent temozolomide in patients with newly diagnosed anaplastic oligodendrogliomas and mixed anaplastic oligoastrocytomas: RTOG BR0131. Neuro Oncol. 2009;11(2):167–75.
41. Lassman AB, Iwamoto FM, Cloughesy TF, Aldape KD, Rivera AL, Eichler AF, Louis DN, Paleologos NA, Fisher BJ, Ashby LS, Cairncross JG, Roldán GB, Wen PY, Ligon KL, Schiff D, Robins HI, Rocque BG, Chamberlain MC, Mason WP, Weaver SA, Green RM, Kamar FG, Abrey LE, DeAngelis LM, Jhanwar SC, Rosenblum MK, Panageas KS. International retrospective study of over 1000 adults with anaplastic oligodendroglial tumors. Neuro Oncol. 2011;13(6):649–59.
42. Youland RS, Brown PD, Giannini C, Parney IF, Uhm JH, Laack NN. Adult low-grade glioma: 19-year experience at a single institution. Am J Clin Oncol. 2013;36(6):612–9.
43. van den Bent MJ, Afra D, de Witte O, Ben Hassel M, Schraub S, Hoang-Xuan K, Malmström PO, Collette L, Piérart M, Mirimanoff R, Karim AB, EORTC Radiotherapy and Brain Tumor Groups and the UK Medical Research Council. Long-term efficacy of early versus delayed radiotherapy for low-grade astrocytoma and oligodendroglioma in adults: the EORTC 22845 randomised trial. Lancet. 2005;366(9490):985–90.
44. Daniels TB, Brown PD, Felten SJ, Wu W, Buckner JC, Arusell RM, Curran WJ, Abrams RA, Schiff D, Shaw EG. Validation of EORTC prognostic factors for adults with low-grade glioma: a report using intergroup 86-72-51. Int J Radiat Oncol Biol Phys. 2011;81(1):218–24.
45. Shaw EG, Wang M, Coons SW, Brachman DG, Buckner JC, Stelzer KJ, Barger GR, Brown PD, Gilbert MR, Mehta MP. Randomized trial of radiation therapy plus procarbazine, lomustine, and vincristine chemotherapy for supratentorial adult low-grade glioma: initial results of RTOG 9802. J Clin Oncol. 2012;30(25):3065–70.
46. Hoang-Xuan K, Capelle L, Kujas M, Taillibert S, Duffau H, Lejeune J, Polivka M, Crinière E, Marie Y, Mokhtari K, Carpentier AF, Laigle F, Simon JM, Cornu P, Broët P, Sanson M, Delattre JY. Temozolomide as initial treatment for adults with low-grade oligodendrogliomas or oligoastrocytomas and correlation with chromosome 1p deletions. J Clin Oncol. 2004;22(15):3133–8.
47. Levin N, Lavon I, Zelikovitsh B, Fuchs D, Bokstein F, Fellig Y, Siegal T. Progressive low-grade oligodendrogliomas: response to temozolomide and correlation between genetic profile and O6-methylguanine DNA methyltransferase protein expression. Cancer. 2006;106(8):1759–65.
48. Brandes AA, Tosoni A, Cavallo G, Reni M, Franceschi E, Bonaldi L, Bertorelle R, Gardiman M, Ghimenton C, Iuzzolino P, Pession A, Blatt V, Ermani M, GICNO. Correlations between O6-methylguanine DNA methyltransferase promoter methylation status, 1p and 19q deletions, and response to temozolomide in anaplastic and recurrent oligodendroglioma: a prospective GICNO study. J Clin Oncol. 2006;24(29):4746–53.
49. Kaloshi G, Benouaich-Amiel A, Diakite F, Taillibert S, Lejeune J, Laigle-Donadey F, Renard MA, Iraqi W, Idbaih A, Paris S, Capelle L, Duffau H, Cornu P, Simon JM, Mokhtari K, Polivka M, Omuro A, Carpentier A, Sanson M, Delattre JY, Hoang-Xuan K. Temozolomide for low-grade gliomas: predictive impact of 1p/19q loss on response and outcome. Neurology. 2007;68(21):1831–6.
50. Louis DN, Holland EC, Cairncross JG. Glioma classification: a molecular reappraisal. Am J Pathol. 2001;159:779–86.
51. Kouwenhoven MC, Kros JM, French PJ, et al. 1p/19q loss within oligodendroglioma is predictive for response to first

line temozolomide but not to salvage treatment. Eur J Cancer. 2006;42:2499–503.

52. Yip S, Iafrate AJ, Louis DN. Molecular diagnostic testing in malignant gliomas: a practical update on predictive markers. J Neuropathol Exp Neurol. 2008;67:1–15.
53. Jansen M, Yip S, Louis DN. Molecular pathology in adult gliomas: diagnostic, prognostic, and predictive markers. Lancet Neurol. 2010;9:717–26.
54. Ducray F, Idbaih A, de Reynies A, et al. Anaplastic oligodendrogliomas with 1p19q codeletion have a proneural gene expression profile. Mol Cancer. 2008;7:41.
55. Gravendeel LA, Kloosterhof NK, Bralten LB, et al. Segregation of non-p.R132H mutations in IDH1 in distinct molecular subtypes of glioma. Hum Mutat. 2010;31:E1186–99.
56. van den Bent MJ, Dubbink HJ, Marie Y, et al. IDH1 and IDH2 mutations are prognostic but not predictive for outcome in anaplastic oligodendroglial tumors: a report of the European Organization for Research and Treatment of Cancer Brain Tumor Group. Clin Cancer Res. 2010;16:1597–604.
57. Cooper LA, Gutman DA, Long Q, et al. The proneural molecular signature is enriched in oligodendrogliomas and predicts improved survival among diffuse gliomas. PLoS One. 2010;5:e12548.
58. Huse JT, Phillips HS, Brennan CW. Molecular subclassification of diffuse gliomas: seeing order in the chaos. Glia. 2011;59:1190–9.
59. Jenkins RB, Xiao Y, Sicotte H, et al. A low-frequency variant at 8q24.21 is strongly associated with risk of oligodendroglial tumors and astrocytomas with IDH1 or IDH2 mutation. Nat Genet. 2012;44:1122–5.
60. Jenkins RB, Blair H, Ballman KV, et al. A t(1;19)(q10;p10) mediates the combined deletions of 1p and 19q and predicts a better prognosis of patients with oligodendroglioma. Cancer Res. 2006;66:9852–61.
61. Griffin CA, Burger P, Morsberger L, et al. Identification of der(1;19)(q10;p10) in five oligodendrogliomas suggests mechanism of concurrent 1p and 19q loss. J Neuropathol Exp Neurol. 2006;65:988–94.
62. Snuderl M, Eichler AF, Ligon KL, et al. Polysomy for chromosomes 1 and 19 predicts earlier recurrence in anaplastic oligodendrogliomas with concurrent 1p/19q loss. Clin Cancer Res. 2009;15:6430–7.
63. Wiens AL, Cheng L, Bertsch EC, et al. Polysomy of chromosomes 1 and/or 19 is common and associated with less favorable clinical outcome in oligodendrogliomas: fluorescent in situ hybridization analysis of 84 consecutive cases. J Neuropathol Exp Neurol. 2012;71:618–24.
64. Okamoto Y, Di Patre PL, Burkhard C, et al. Population-based study on incidence, survival rates, and genetic alterations of low-grade diffuse astrocytomas and oligodendrogliomas. Acta Neuropathol. 2004;108:49–56.
65. Yip S, Butterfield YS, Morozova O, Chittaranjan S, Blough MD, An J, Birol I, Chesnelong C, Chiu R, Chuah E, Corbett R, Docking R, Firme M, Hirst M, Jackman S, Karsan A, Li H, Louis DN, Maslova A, Moore R, Moradian A, Mungall KL, Perizzolo M, Qian J, Roldan G, Smith EE, Tamura-Wells J, Thiessen N, Varhol R, Weiss S, Wu W, Young S, Zhao Y, Mungall AJ, Jones SJ, Morin GB, Chan JA, Cairncross JG, Marra MA. Concurrent CIC mutations, IDH mutations, and 1p/19q loss distinguish oligodendrogliomas from other cancers. J Pathol. 2012;226(1):7–16.
66. Balss J, Meyer J, Mueller W, et al. Analysis of the IDH1 codon 132 mutation in brain tumors. Acta Neuropathol. 2008;116: 597–602.
67. Yip S, Butterfield YS, Morozova O, Chittaranjan S, Blough MD, An J, Birol I, Chesnelong C, Chiu R, Chuah E, Corbett R, Docking R, Firme M, Hirst M, Jackman S, Karsan A, Li H, Louis DN, Maslova A, Moore R, Moradian A, Mungall KL, Perizzolo M, Qian J, Roldan G, Smith EE, Tamura-Wells J, Thiessen N, Varhol R, Weiss S, Wu W, Young S, Zhao Y, Mungall AJ, Jones SJ, Morin GB, Chan JA, Cairncross JG, Marra MA. Concurrent CIC mutations, IDH mutations, and 1p/19q loss distinguish oligodendrogliomas from other cancers. J Pathol. 2012;226(1):7–16.
68. Kloosterhof NK, Bralten LB, Dubbink HJ, et al. Isocitrate dehydrogenase-1 mutations: a fundamentally new understanding of diffuse glioma? Lancet Oncol. 2010;12:83–91.
69. Dang L, White DW, Gross S, et al. Cancer-associated IDH1 mutations produce 2-hydroxyglutarate. Nature. 2010;465:966.
70. Cairns RA, Mak TW. Oncogenic isocitrate dehydrogenase mutations: mechanisms, models, and clinical opportunities. Cancer Discov. 2013;3:730–41.
71. Lu C, Ward PS, Kapoor GS, et al. IDH mutation impairs histone demethylation and results in a block to cell differentiation. Nature. 2012;483:474–8.
72. Figueroa ME, Abdel-Wahab O, Lu C, et al. Leukemic IDH1 and IDH2 mutations result in a hypermethylation phenotype, disrupt TET2 function, and impair hematopoietic differentiation. Cancer Cell. 2010;18:553–67.
73. Turcan S, Rohle D, Goenka A, et al. IDH1 mutation is sufficient to establish the glioma hypermethylator phenotype. Nature. 2012;483:479–83.
74. Andronesi OC, Kim GS, Gerstner E, et al. Detection of 2-hydroxyglutarate in IDH-mutated glioma patients by in vivo spectral-editing and 2D correlation magnetic resonance spectroscopy. Sci Transl Med. 2012;4:116ra114.
75. Sahm F, Capper D, Pusch S, et al. Detection of 2-hydroxyglutarate in formalin-fixed paraffin-embedded glioma specimens by gas chromatography/mass spectrometry. Brain Pathol. 2012;22:26–31.
76. Rohle D, Popovici-Muller J, Palaskas N, et al. An inhibitor of mutant IDH1 delays growth and promotes differentiation of glioma cells. Science. 2013;340:626–30.
77. Bralten LB, Nouwens S, Kockx C, et al. Absence of common somatic alterations in genes on 1p and 19q in oligodendrogliomas. PLoS One. 2011;6:e22000.
78. Boulay JL, Miserez AR, Zweifel C, et al. Loss of NOTCH2 positively predicts survival in subgroups of human glial brain tumors. PLoS One. 2007;2:e576.
79. Benetkiewicz M, Idbaih A, Cousin PY, et al. NOTCH2 is neither rearranged nor mutated in t(1;19) positive oligodendrogliomas. PLoS One. 2009;4:e4107.
80. Bettegowda C, Agrawal N, Jiao Y, et al. Mutations in CIC and FUBP1 contribute to human oligodendroglioma. Science. 2011;333:1453–5.
81. Sahm F, Koelsche C, Meyer J, et al. CIC and FUBP1 mutations in oligodendrogliomas, oligoastrocytomas and astrocytomas. Acta Neuropathol. 2012;123:853–60.

82. Jiao Y, Killela PJ, Reitman ZJ, et al. Frequent ATRX, CIC, FUBP1 and IDH1 mutations refine the classification of malignant gliomas. Oncotarget. 2012;3:709–22.
83. Jimenez G, Guichet A, Ephrussi A, et al. Relief of gene repression by torso RTK signaling: role of capicua in Drosophila terminal and dorsoventral patterning. Genes Dev. 2000;14:224–31.
84. Goff DJ, Nilson LA, Morisato D. Establishment of dorsal-ventral polarity of the Drosophila egg requires capicua action in ovarian follicle cells. Development. 2001;128:4553–62.
85. Tseng AS, Tapon N, Kanda H, et al. Capicua regulates cell proliferation downstream of the receptor tyrosine kinase/ras signaling pathway. Curr Biol. 2007;17:728–33.
86. Klink B, Miletic H, Stieber D, et al. A novel, diffusely infiltrative xenograft model of human anaplastic oligodendroglioma with mutations in FUBP1, CIC, and IDH1. PLoS One. 2013;8:e59773.
87. Phillips HS, Kharbanda S, Chen R, et al. Molecular subclasses of high-grade glioma predict prognosis, delineate a pattern of disease progression, and resemble stages in neurogenesis. Cancer Cell. 2006;9:157–73.
88. Ducray F, Criniere E, Idbaih A, et al. alpha-Internexin expression identifies 1p19q codeleted gliomas. Neurology. 2009;72:156–61.
89. Horbinski C, Hobbs J, Cieply K, et al. EGFR expression stratifies oligodendroglioma behavior. Am J Pathol. 2011;179: 1638–44.
90. Jones PA, Laird PW. Cancer epigenetics comes of age. Nat Genet. 1999;21:163–7.
91. Blough MD, Al-Najjar M, Chesnelong C, et al. DNA hypermethylation and 1p Loss silence NHE-1 in oligodendroglioma. Ann Neurol. 2012;71:845–9.
92. Hegi ME, Diserens AC, Gorlia T, et al. MGMT gene silencing and benefit from temozolomide in glioblastoma. N Engl J Med. 2005;352:997–1003.
93. van den Bent MJ, Dubbink HJ, Sanson M, et al. MGMT promoter methylation is prognostic but not predictive for outcome to adjuvant PCV chemotherapy in anaplastic oligodendroglial tumors: a report from EORTC Brain Tumor Group Study 26951. J Clin Oncol. 2009;27:5881–6.
94. van den Bent MJ, Gravendeel LA, Gorlia T, et al. A hypermethylated phenotype is a better predictor of survival than MGMT methylation in anaplastic oligodendroglial brain tumors: a report from EORTC study 26951. Clin Cancer Res. 2011;17:7148–55.
95. Noushmehr H, Weisenberger DJ, Diefes K, et al. Identification of a CpG island methylator phenotype that defines a distinct subgroup of glioma. Cancer Cell. 2010;17:510–22.
96. Louis DN. The next step in brain tumor classification: "let us now praise famous men"… or molecules? Acta Neuropathol. 2012;124:761–2.
97. Riemenschneider MJ, Louis DN, Weller M, et al. Refined brain tumor diagnostics and stratified therapies: the requirement for a multidisciplinary approach. Acta Neuropathol. 2013;126:21–37.
98. Yang MM, Singhal A, Rassekh SR, et al. Possible differentiation of cerebral glioblastoma into pleomorphic xanthoastrocytoma: an unusual case in an infant. J Neurosurg Pediatr. 2012;9:517–23.
99. Bashashati A, Ha G, Tone A, et al. Distinct evolutionary trajectories of primary high-grade serous ovarian cancers revealed through spatial mutational profiling. J Pathol. 2013;231:21–34.
100. Payton JE, Grieselhuber NR, Chang LW, et al. High throughput digital quantification of mRNA abundance in primary human acute myeloid leukemia samples. J Clin Invest. 2009;119:1714–26.
101. Northcott PA, Shih DJ, Remke M, et al. Rapid, reliable, and reproducible molecular sub-grouping of clinical medulloblastoma samples. Acta Neuropathol. 2012;123:615–26.
102. Snuderl M, Fazlollahi L, Le LP, et al. Mosaic amplification of multiple receptor tyrosine kinase genes in glioblastoma. Cancer Cell. 2011;20:810–7.

9 Medulloblastoma and CNS Primitive Neuroectodermal Tumors

David T.W. Jones, Andrey Korshunov, Stefan M. Pfister, Michael D. Taylor, and Paul A. Northcott

Medulloblastoma

Medulloblastoma is a malignant (WHO Grade IV) small round blue cell tumor of the cerebellum that constitutes one of the most common malignant brain tumors in children [1]. The disease has a peak age of onset of ~7–8 years, but is also diagnosed in young infants and well into adulthood. Males are more commonly affected than females, with a male:female ratio of ~1.5:1. Current treatment strategies for medulloblastoma include a combination of surgical resection, craniospinal radiation (in children older than 3 years), and cytotoxic chemotherapy. Five-year overall survival rates for standard-risk patients (i.e., patients older than 3 years with less than 1.5 cm^2 residual disease and no evidence of metastasis) are in the range of 70–80 %. In contrast, patients currently stratified as high-risk, including those that are less than 3 years old, patients with greater than 1.5 cm^2 residual disease, and/or those with metastatic dissemination, typically have inferior outcomes. Patients that are effectively cured of their disease currently face significant challenges and treatment-related sequelae, including pronounced developmental, neurological, and psychosocial deficits.

The WHO currently recognizes five distinct histological subtypes of medulloblastoma: classic, desmoplastic, medulloblastoma with extensive nodularity (MBEN), large cell, and anaplastic (Fig. 9.1) [1]. The classic medulloblastoma subtype accounts for the majority of cases, followed by the desmoplastic subtype, collectively accounting for ~80 % of cases, and the other subtypes comprising the remainder. Numerous studies have demonstrated improved survival rates for desmoplastic/nodular medulloblastoma, which is contrasted by an inferior prognosis usually encountered with large cell/anaplastic disease [2–7]. Varying degrees of desmoplasia, anaplasia, and intratumoral heterogeneity can make the diagnosis of these histological subtypes difficult and subjective, confounding consistency in diagnoses.

Understanding the molecular biology underlying medulloblastoma is currently an area of intense interest among the pediatric neuro-oncology community. It is anticipated that knowledge gained from genomic and biological studies will translate to more accurate and consistent diagnoses, improved risk-stratification schemes, and the development and implementation of molecularly targeted therapies that are more effective and less toxic.

Molecular Genetics of Medulloblastoma: A Historical Perspective

Recurrent cytogenetic aberrations have been observed in medulloblastoma specimens for several decades [8]. The presence of an isochromosome 17q (i[17]q), essentially resulting in the net loss of one copy of the chromosome 17 p-arm and a net gain of one copy of the q-arm, is a signature event in medulloblastoma, found in up to 50 % of patient samples (Fig. 9.2a). Other chromosomal abnormalities that are commonly encountered include gains of chromosomes 1q and 7 and losses of chromosomes 6, 8p, 9q, 10q, 11, 16q, and X.

High-level amplification of the *MYC* proto-oncogene in the form of double-minute chromosomes has been observed for more than two decades, reported to occur in 5–10 % of patients (Fig. 9.2b). Historically, amplification of *MYC* has been recognized as a marker of poor patient outcome, often occurring in patients with a particularly aggressive form of the disease [3, 9–16].

Rare familial tumor syndromes, namely Gorlin and Turcot Syndromes, have provided considerable insight into the genetics underlying specific subsets of medulloblastoma patients [17]. Gorlin Syndrome (also referred to as Nevoid Basal Cell Carcinoma Syndrome, NBCCS) is an autosomal dominant disorder that results in abnormal facial and skeletal phenotypes, with affected individuals prone to the

M.A. Karajannis and D. Zagzag (eds.), *Molecular Pathology of Nervous System Tumors: Biological Stratification and Targeted Therapies*, Molecular Pathology Library 8,
DOI 10.1007/978-1-4939-1830-0_9,

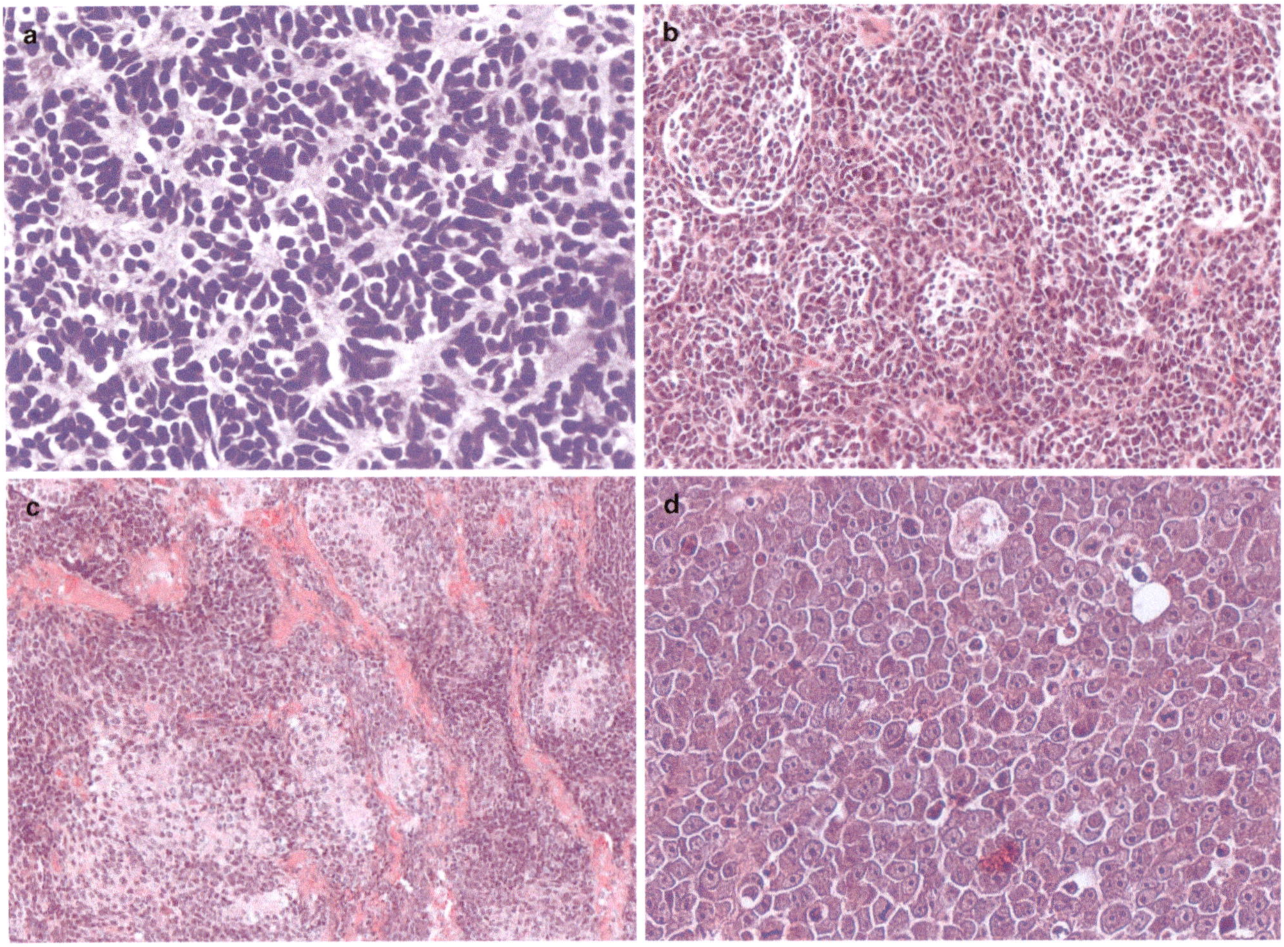

Fig. 9.1. Histological subtypes of medulloblastoma. (**a**) Classic histology; (**b**) desmoplastic histology; (**c**) medulloblastoma with extensive nodularity (MBEN); (**d**) large cell/anaplastic (LC/A) histology.

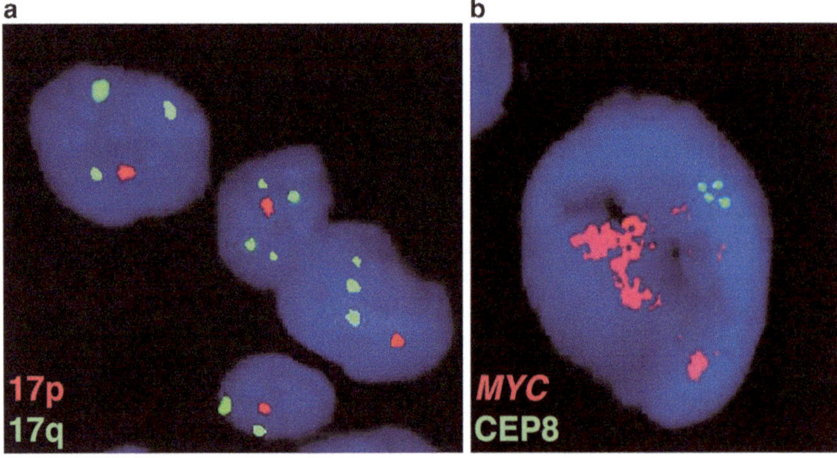

Fig. 9.2. Historical cytogenetic aberrations of medulloblastoma. (**a**) Interphase FISH performed on a medulloblastoma sample exhibiting copy number imbalance on chromosome 17, characterized by deletion of 17p and duplication of 17q (i[17]q). (**b**) A medulloblastoma sample with high-level amplification of the *MYC* proto-oncogene on chromosome 8q24 as demonstrated by FISH.

development of numerous basal cell carcinomas and predisposed to medulloblastoma. Germline loss-of-function mutations in the *PTCH1* tumor suppressor gene on chromosome 9q are responsible for this disorder [18–20]. PTCH1 is a negative regulator of the Sonic Hedgehog (SHH) signal transduction pathway, an important developmental signaling cascade. As will be discussed in detail below, aberrant activation of the SHH pathway is found in ~25–30 % of all

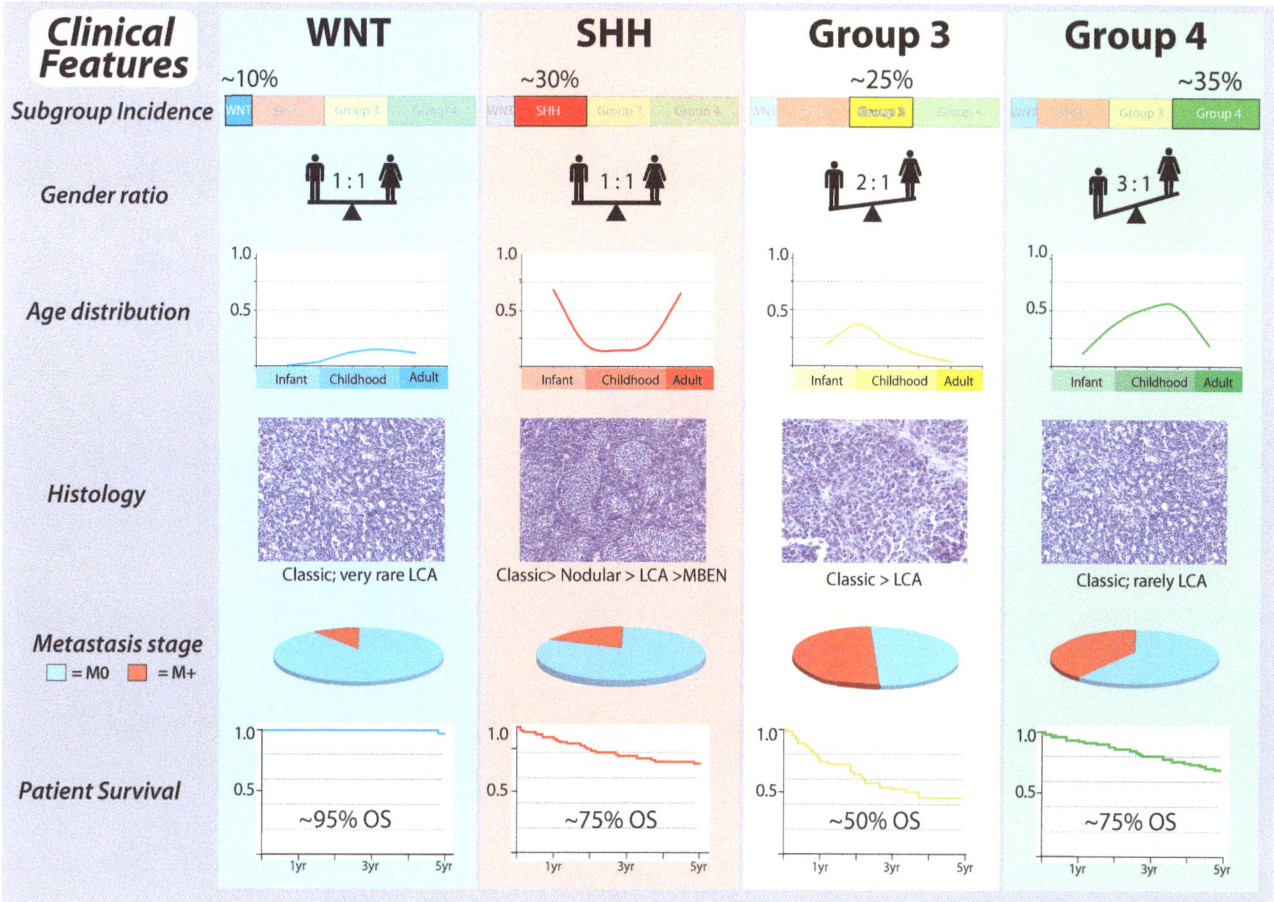

FIG. 9.3. Clinical features of medulloblastoma subgroups. General summary of the clinical characteristics intrinsic to the core molecular subgroups of medulloblastoma. *LCA* large cell and anaplastic, *MBEN* medulloblastoma with extensive nodularity, *OS* overall survival.

medulloblastoma patients and is perhaps the most well characterized molecular pathway involved in medulloblastoma development.

Turcot Syndrome is also an autosomal dominant condition; attributed to germline mutations in either *APC* or the DNA mismatch repair genes *MLH1* or *PMS2*. Affected individuals are predisposed to either medulloblastoma (linked with *APC* mutation) or glioblastoma multiforme (linked with *MLH1* or *PMS2* mutations) [21]. The APC protein functions to control the activity of β-Catenin, the central molecule of the Wingless (WNT) signaling pathway. Activation of WNT signaling is observed in ~10–15 % of medulloblastomas, a distinct subset of patients with a highly favorable outcome, as will be discussed in detail below.

Molecular Subgroups of Medulloblastoma: Discovery and Initial Characterization

The Molecular Subgroup Concept

Clinical outcome of patients with medulloblastoma can be highly variable, irrespective of parameters routinely used in the clinic to predict patient risk (i.e., patient age, extent of resection, and metastatic stage). This is often exemplified by the very disparate therapeutic responses observed among patients with histologically identical disease. Furthermore, survival patterns reported for different age groups of medulloblastoma patients have strongly suggested underlying biological differences that must account for the distinct age of onset and therapeutic response of these patient subgroups [6, 22]. Much of this biological and clinical heterogeneity observed in medulloblastoma is now being explained by the recognition of unique molecular subgroups of the disease, a concept that has been supported for more than a decade now [23].

Hybridization of moderate-to-large series of RNAs isolated from primary medulloblastoma specimens to gene expression microarrays has revolutionized our concept of medulloblastoma as a disease. Based primarily on expression array profiling, numerous studies performed by independent laboratories have reported the existence of discrete molecular subgroups of medulloblastoma [24–28], each characterized by distinct genetics, cytogenetics and transcriptional profiles, as well as patient demographics, tumor phenotype, and clinical behavior (Figs. 9.3 and 9.4) [29].

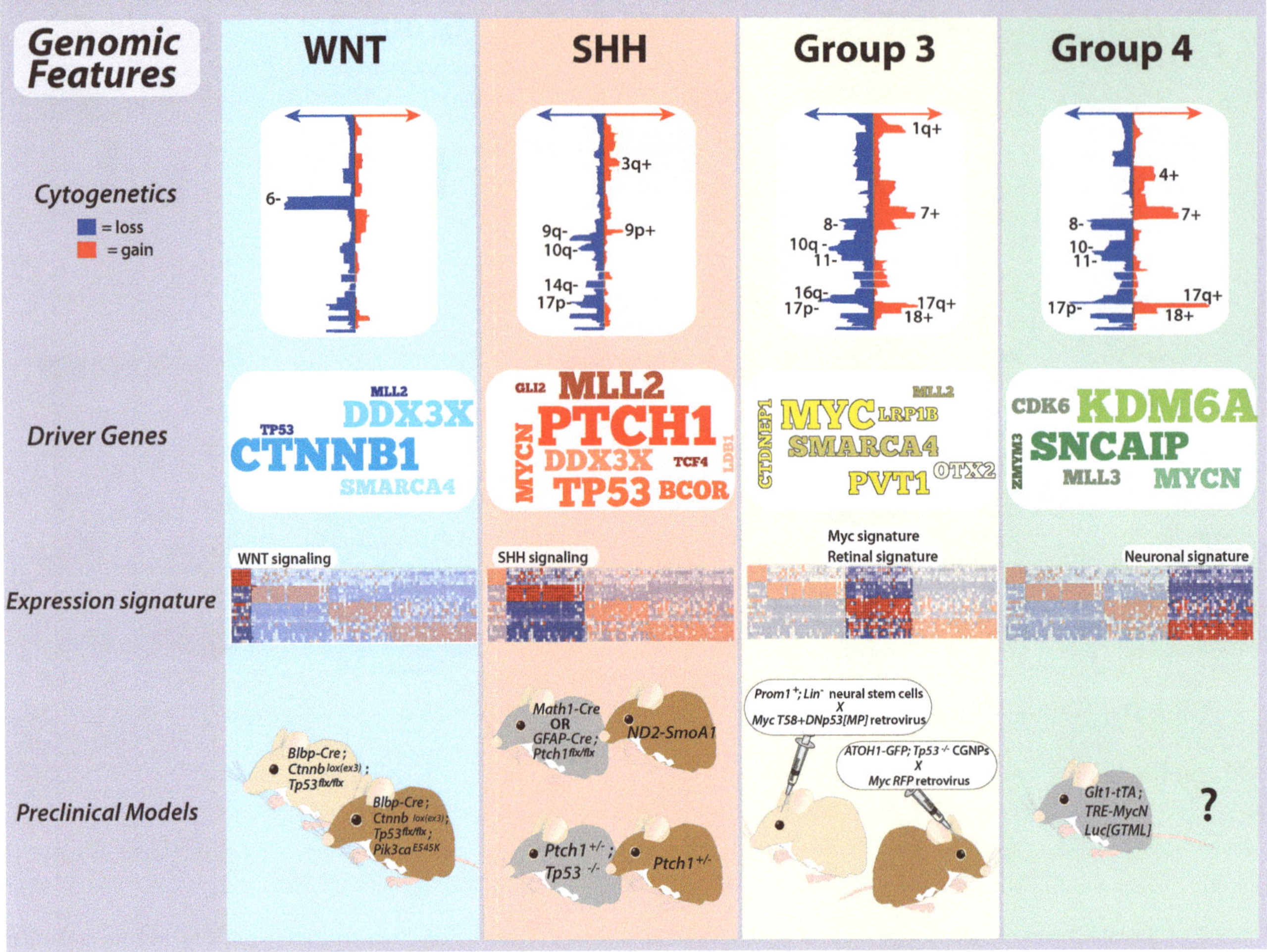

Fig. 9.4. Genomic features of medulloblastoma subgroups. Summary of the genomics of medulloblastoma subgroups, including cytogenetics, prominent driver genes, transcriptional signatures, and available preclinical models.

In late 2010, a consensus meeting attended by leading groups in the medulloblastoma community was held where it was proposed that medulloblastoma should be regarded as consisting of a four-subgroup structure: WNT, SHH, Group 3, and Group 4 [30]. The impact of this consensus report and the studies that precipitated it have changed the way medulloblastoma is both viewed and studied in the basic research setting. Moreover, the implications for the development of clinical trials, revamping patient risk-stratification, and the administration of targeted therapy have been dramatic, all of which are now beginning to take molecular subgroup status into consideration.

WNT Medulloblastoma

The least common of the four consensus medulloblastoma subgroups are those belonging to the WNT subgroup, accounting for just 10–15 % of cases. This subgroup affects a higher than expected proportion of female patients (male:female ratio of ~1:1 compared to an expected ratio of ~1.5:1 for all medulloblastomas) and is predominantly diagnosed in childhood and adolescence, almost never encountered in infants. WNT medulloblastomas are nearly without exception of classic histology and non-metastatic, currently having the best overall prognosis of any patient subgroup with cure rates of almost 100 % [4, 24, 27, 28, 31, 32].

Somatic missense mutations in exon 3 of *CTNNB1* (which encodes β-Catenin) are present in >90 % of WNT medulloblastomas [33]. These mutations constitutively activate β-Catenin and prevent it from being degraded, resulting in its nuclear accumulation and consequent deregulation of WNT target genes. Monosomy 6 is another characteristic genetic feature of WNT subgroup medulloblastomas, highly enriched in this subgroup and found in the vast majority of cases [32, 34]. Immunohistochemistry (IHC) for β-Catenin and fluorescence in situ hybridization (FISH) for chromosome 6 constitute two commonly used "readouts" for WNT subgroup assignment, with either nucleo-positivity for β-Catenin or monosomy 6 acting as capable surrogates for identifying WNT subgroup patients (Fig. 9.5) [35]. More specific assays

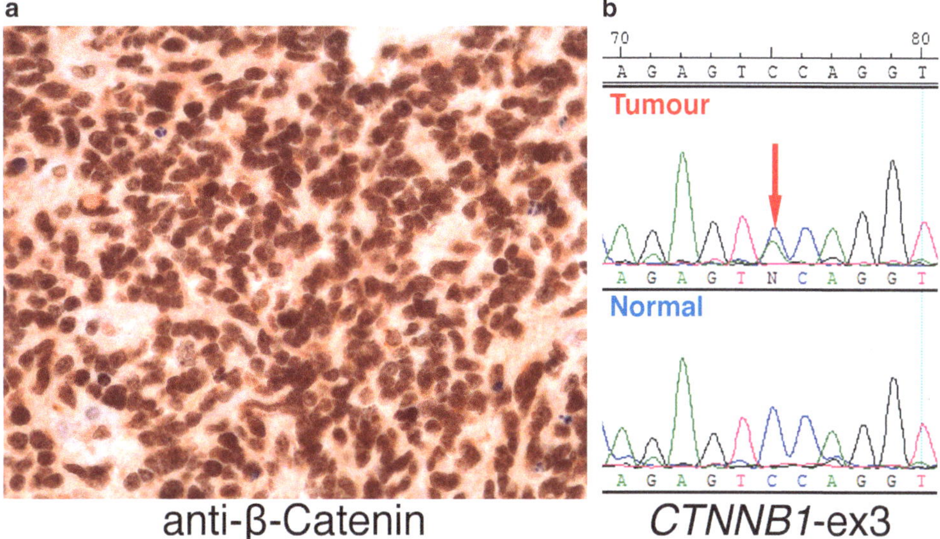

FIG. 9.5. Molecular assays for assignment of WNT medulloblastomas. (**a**) IHC shows strong nucleo-positivity typical of a WNT subgroup medulloblastoma. (**b**) DNA sequencing electropherogram showing a heterozygous *CTNNB1* exon 3 mutation (*red arrow*) present in the tumor DNA of a WNT medulloblastoma (labeled "Tumor") that is absent in matched normal germline control DNA (labeled "Normal") from the same patient.

such as re-sequencing of *CTNNB1* exon 3 performed in combination with additional state-of-the-art molecular profiling methods (discussed below) are now being recommended as more specific and sensitive methods for identifying this important subgroup of medulloblastoma patients.

SHH Medulloblastoma

Medulloblastomas exhibiting aberrant activation of the SHH signaling pathway account for ~25–30 % of cases [32]. In infants (age 3 years or less) and older patients (age 16 years and up), SHH-activated cases predominate, accounting for up to 70 % of patients in these age groups [36]. The gender distribution for SHH subgroup medulloblastomas is comparable to what is seen among all medulloblastoma patients, with an observed male:female ratio of ~1.5:1. True desmoplastic and MBEN histologies appear to be largely restricted to this subgroup [35]; however, large cell/anaplastic (LCA) disease is also encountered, particularly in childhood cases. Metastatic disease (M+) is also observed but relatively uncommon. With respect to patient outcome, SHH cases appear to represent an intermediate prognosis class of patients [32], although specific patient subsets may have highly favorable or disparate clinical outcomes, depending on their underlying genotypes (as will be discussed later) [22, 37].

As was first verified in Gorlin Syndrome patients that develop medulloblastoma, *PTCH1* is the prototypical tumor suppressor in the SHH subgroup, with somatic mutations inactivating PTCH1 confined to this subgroup. *SUFU*, another tumor suppressor functioning as a regulatory component of the SHH signaling pathway, is likewise mutated in this subgroup, both in the germline and somatically [38–40]. Loss of heterozygosity (LOH) on chromosomes 9q and 10q is enriched in SHH medulloblastomas [27, 34], presumably as a mechanism for inactivating the remaining wild-type allele in cases exhibiting *PTCH1* or *SUFU* mutations, respectively. Similar to the use of β-Catenin nucleo-positivity as a biomarker for WNT medulloblastoma, comparable IHC-based methods have been proposed and implemented with modest success for the identification of SHH medulloblastomas, including SFRP1, GLI1, and GAB1, all of which exhibit apparent specificity for this subgroup [27, 28, 35, 41, 42].

Group 3 Medulloblastoma

The generically named Group 3 medulloblastomas account for ~25 % of all cases and appear to be restricted to pediatric patients, with only extremely rare instances reported in adults [42]. There is a male gender bias in Group 3, with an observed male:female ratio of ~2:1. M+ disease is common in Group 3 and has been documented in up to half of these cases. Group 3 subgroup affiliation currently carries with it the most dismal overall survival of the four subgroups, with only ~50 % of these patients or less alive at 5 years from the time of initial diagnosis [32].

Amplification of *MYC* is a characteristic oncogenic event observed in this subgroup, an event that is by and large restricted to Group 3 and found in 15–20 % of cases [34]. Cytogenetic aberrations such as gain of chromosomes 1q and 7, and loss of chromosomes 8p, 11, 16q and i[17]q are commonly observed in Group 3. Although preliminary biomarkers for Group 3 have been suggested (i.e., *MYC* amplification), there are currently no gold-standard single gene/marker assays for assigning medulloblastomas to this subgroup.

Group 4 Medulloblastoma

Group 4 medulloblastomas represent the most common patient subgroup, accounting for 35–40 % of all cases [32]. These tumors occur across all age groups but constitute the most predominant form of the disease in childhood and adolescence. There is a strong gender bias in Group 4, with an observed male:female ratio of ~3:1. Metastatic disease is observed in approximately one-third of Group 4 patients. Similar to the SHH subgroup, Group 4 patients tend to comprise an intermediate outcome subgroup [32], although there is growing evidence for clinical heterogeneity within this large fraction of patients [43].

Cytogenetically, Group 4 medulloblastomas share some commonalities with Group 3, most notably being the highly prevalent i[17]q which is noted in up to 70–80 % of Group 4's. Chromosome X loss in female Group 4 patients is also a frequent occurrence. Compared to other subgroups, Group 4 medulloblastomas remain the least well understood with regards to oncogenic driver genes, although a few interesting novel candidates have emerged from recent genomic studies, as will be discussed in detail below.

Next-Generation Genomics of Medulloblastoma: Assigning Driver Genes to Medulloblastoma Subgroups

Recent technological breakthroughs in the field of genomics have dramatically improved the resolution at which the cancer genome is studied [44, 45]. Application of high-density microarray platforms and next-generation sequencing (NGS) to medulloblastoma has led to the identification of a host of novel candidate genes that are recurrently affected by somatic copy number alterations (SCNAs) or mutation, and sometimes both (Figs. 9.4, 9.6, and 9.7) [33]. Many of these events appear to be enriched or restricted to a particular subgroup and are thus likely playing an integral role in the biology driving the initiation, maintenance, and progression of the subgroup(s) harboring the mutational event. Genes and pathways emerging as important oncogenic drivers in medulloblastoma, including how they are distributed within the subgroups, are described below.

Known Cancer Genes

A number of genes previously implicated in medulloblastoma have now been accurately placed in the context of the molecular subgroups. Several of these candidates were once thought to be rarely affected when studying medulloblastoma as a single entity, but are now considered of higher relevance given their subgroup-specificity and increased frequency within a particular subgroup.

The *TP53* tumor suppressor, classically reported as being somatically mutated in only ~5 % of medulloblastomas, has now been observed to be almost exclusively mutated in WNT and SHH subgroup cases, affecting ~10–15 % of cases from each subgroup [37, 46]. Moreover, germline mutations in *TP53*, the hallmark genetic event causing Li-Fraumeni Syndrome (LFS) [47, 48], a condition predisposing to the development of a variety of different cancers including medulloblastoma, have now been confirmed to be restricted to the SHH subgroup [49], especially in childhood and adolescent patients.

In contrast to the *MYC* proto-oncogene which is amplified exclusively in Group 3, high-level amplifications of *MYCN* are found in both SHH and Group 4 but rarely in Group 3 and never in WNT medulloblastomas [34, 43]. Likewise, copy number gains of *OTX2*, a developmental transcription factor previously implicated in medulloblastoma pathogenesis [50–54], appear to be restricted to Groups 3 and 4 [34, 55], suggesting it plays an important role in the biology of these tumors.

Additional oncogenic copy number alterations showing enrichment in SHH-driven medulloblastoma now include (but are not limited to) amplification of *GLI2*, *MYCL1*, *PPM1D*, *YAP1*, *IGF1R*, *IRS2*, *MDM4*, and *miR-17/92* and focal homozygous deletion of *PTEN* and *PTCH1* [34, 56, 57]. These events collectively suggest that at least three main pathways contribute to the majority of SHH-driven medulloblastomas: SHH signaling, RTK/PI3K signaling, and TP53 signaling [34].

DDX3X

Identified as a common target of recurrent mutation in three parallel NGS studies of medulloblastoma [58–60], *DDX3X* is among the newest candidates to be implicated as an important medulloblastoma driver gene. DDX3X is a DEAD-box RNA helicase that has been shown to play a role in a variety of cellular processes, ranging from chromosome segregation to transcription and translation [61–64]. Mutations in *DDX3X* are confined to either of its two helicase domains and are always non-truncating variants [33], suggesting that these mutations alter the function of DDX3X rather than causing loss-of-function [59, 60]. Approximately half of all WNT cases harbor a *DDX3X* mutation, whereas 10–15 % of SHH cases are likewise mutated. Recent NGS of adult SHH medulloblastomas has revealed a high proportion of *DDX3X* SNVs, suggesting this candidate is particularly important in the biology of adult SHH cases. In contrast, mutations in *DDX3X* are seldomly observed in Groups 3 and 4.

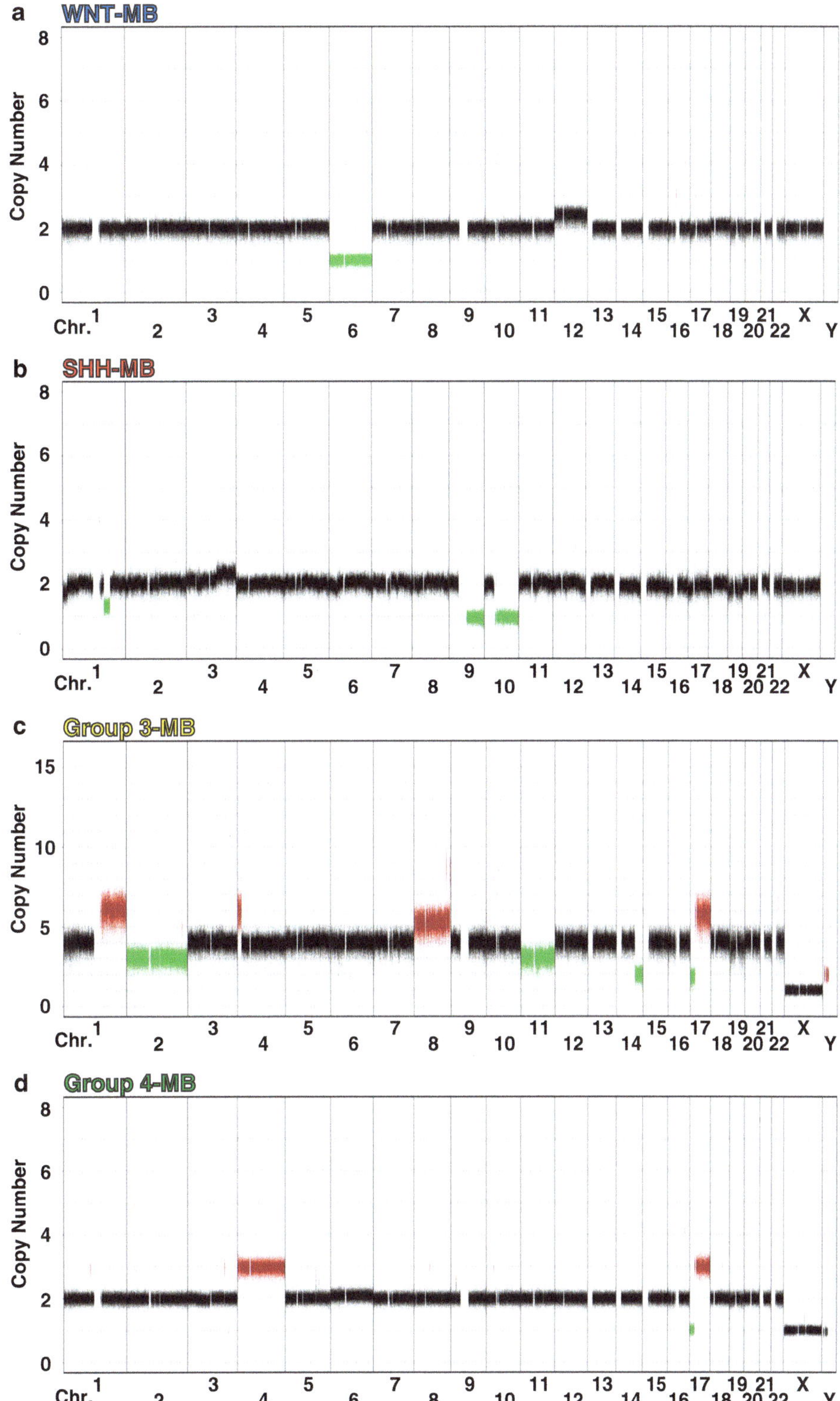

FIG. 9.6. Characteristic cytogenetics of medulloblastoma subgroups. Genome-wide copy number profiles highlighting chromosomal gains and losses typical of each of the four subgroups. (**a**) A WNT subgroup medulloblastoma exhibiting monosomy 6 and an otherwise balanced genome. (**b**) A SHH subgroup medulloblastoma characterized by signature deletions of chromosomes 9q and 10q. (**c**) A Group 3 medulloblastoma with prototypical gains of chromosome 1q and chromosome 8 (including *MYC* amplification), as well as an isochromosome 17q (i[17]q). (**d**) A Group 4 medulloblastoma exhibiting gain of chromosome 4 and i[17]q.

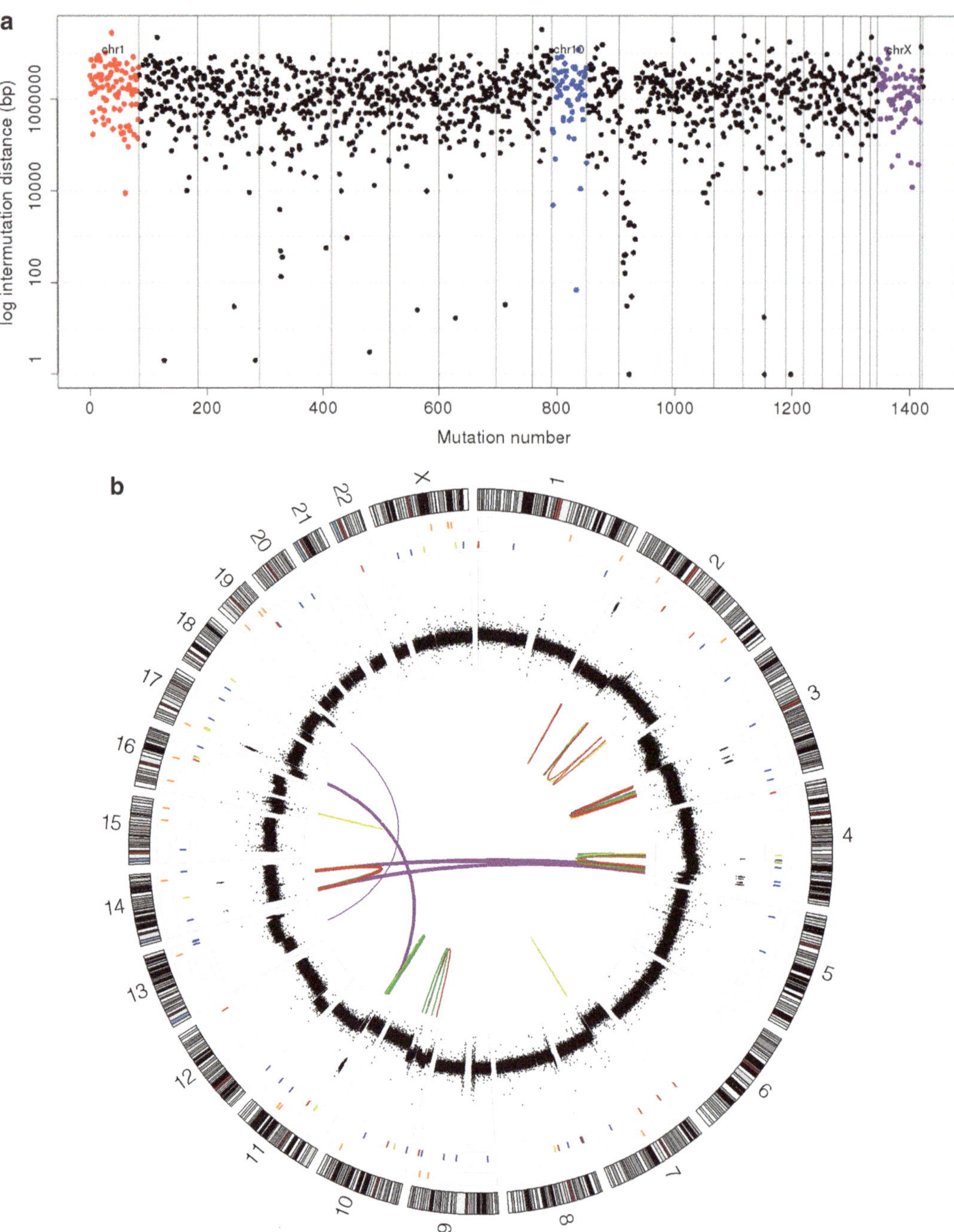

Fig. 9.7. Next-generation sequencing of medulloblastoma. (**a**) Rainfall plot depicting the distribution of somatic mutations (single nucleotide variants; SNVs) across the genome of a SHH subgroup medulloblastoma as determined by NGS. (**b**) Circos plot of NGS data for a SHH subgroup medulloblastoma exhibiting excessive genomic rearrangements and somatic copy number alterations (SCNAs).

Chromatin Modifiers

One of the most unexpected findings disclosed from recent genomic studies of medulloblastoma concerns the high frequency of mutations and copy number alterations affecting chromatin modifiers [33, 65, 66]. In 2009, Northcott and colleagues reported a series of infrequent but recurrent SCNAs targeting histone lysine methyltransferases, histone lysine demethylases, histone acetyltransferases, and chromatin remodelers [67]. A subsequent landmark exon re-sequencing study performed by Parsons et al. identified recurrent and mutually exclusive mutations in histone 3, lysine 4 (H3K4) methyltransferases, *MLL2* and *MLL3*, collectively mutated in ~16 % of surveyed cases [68]. Since these two initial reports implicating deregulation of the chromatin machinery in medulloblastoma, this theme has been further substantiated in all recent medulloblastoma NGS studies, now in the context of molecular subgroups [33, 58–60]. Interestingly, *MLL2* mutations have been confirmed to be more common in WNT and SHH tumors, whereas *MLL3* mutations are more prevalent in Groups 3 and 4. The SWI/SNF family gene *SMARCA4* that encodes BRG1, a component of a multi-protein chromatin-remodeling complex, is recurrently inactivated in WNT and Group 3 medulloblastomas. Similarly, chromatin-modifying genes *LDB1*, *BCOR*, and *LMO4* are targeted either by mutations, copy number alterations, or both exclusively in SHH-driven cases. Finally, *KDM6A*, a histone 3, lysine 27 (H3K27) demethylase, appears to be inactivated by either somatic mutation or focal deletion specifically in Group 4. Moreover, EZH2, which imposes the opposite function of KDM6A, catalyzing the trimethylation of H3K27 (H3K27me^3) is aberrantly over-expressed in Groups 3 and 4, suggesting a propensity for an aberrant H3K27 methylation state in these subgroups [60, 69]. Collectively, this series of recent observations strongly supports the notion that deregulation of the histone code is a key event in medulloblastoma pathogenesis, with somatic alterations occurring in a high proportion of cases across the four subgroups.

Atypical Structural Variation in Medulloblastoma

In addition to the spectrum of genes described above as recurrently mutated or affected by SCNAs, more complex mechanisms of deregulation, including both gene-specific and genome-wide structural rearrangements have been uncovered during the genomics era of medulloblastoma (Fig. 9.8). These recurrent structural variants appear to be common to medulloblastoma and may play an even bigger

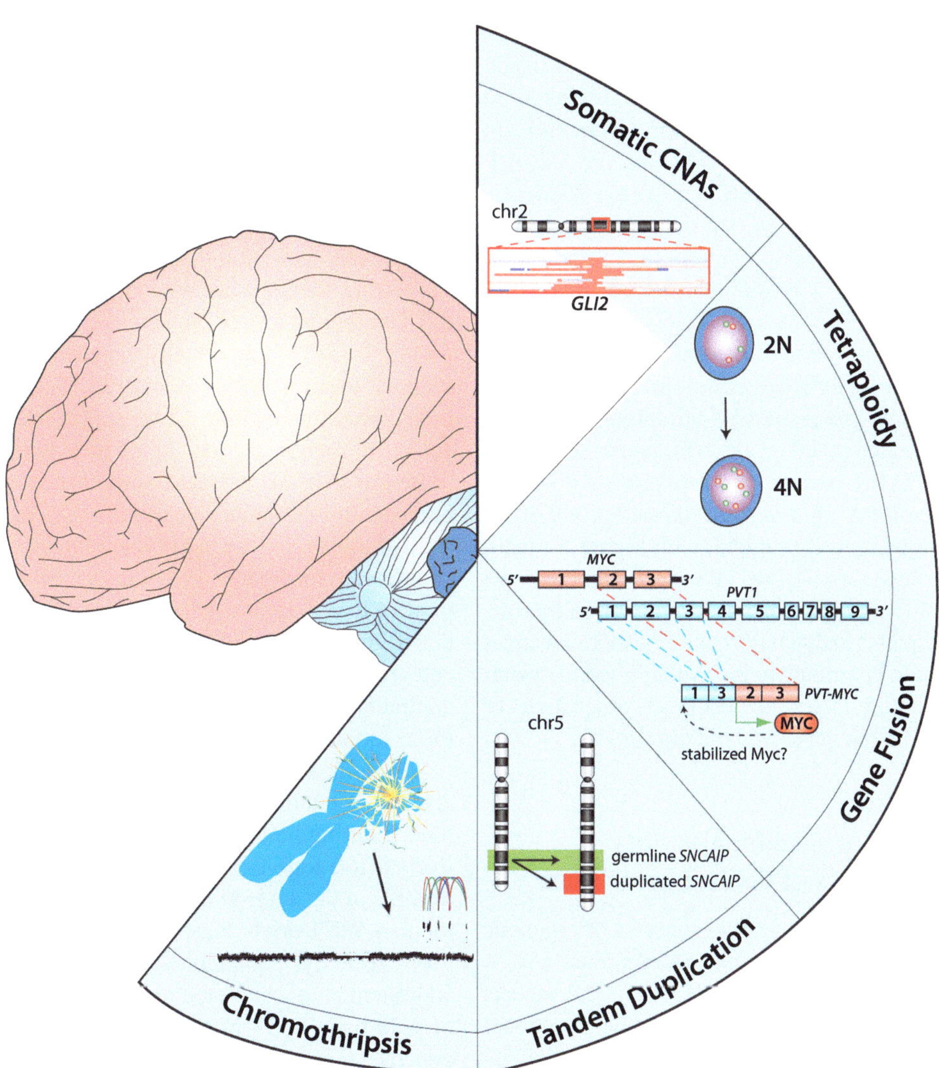

Fig. 9.8. Mechanisms of recurrent structural variation in medulloblastoma. Cartoon showing the different mechanisms responsible for the prominent structural variation reported in medulloblastoma. Depicted types of structural variation include SCNAs, tetraploidy, gene fusions, tandem duplications, and chromothripsis.

role than standard SNVs and SCNAs affecting protein-coding sequences.

NGS of a series of LFS medulloblastomas recently identified massive chromosomal rearrangements known as chromothripsis (Fig. 9.7b) [49]—excessive genomic rearrangements (i.e., inversions, amplifications, deletions) clustered on one or a few chromosomes presumed to have arisen from a single catastrophic DNA breakage/repair event during tumorigenesis [70–72]. This phenomenon was observed in the majority of LFS medulloblastomas analyzed, was specifically enriched in SHH medulloblastoma, and co-occurred with cases harboring either germline or somatic *TP53* mutations [49]. Importantly, chromothripsis observed in these cases often resulted in amplification of known medulloblastoma oncogenes (i.e., *MYCN* and *GLI2*), providing a mechanism for the activation of these critical driver genes.

Using a combination of single nucleotide polymorphism (SNP) arrays and RNA sequencing (RNASeq), Northcott et al. reported *PVT1-MYC* fusion genes as being highly recurrent and specific to *MYC*-amplified Group 3 medulloblastoma [34]. This is the first example of a recurrent fusion gene identified in medulloblastoma and is suspected to potentiate MYC activity by yet an unknown mechanism. In the same study, tandem duplications affecting the *SNCAIP* gene on chromosome 5q were reported in up to ~25 % of a particular Group 4 subtype. *SNCAIP* is a neuronal gene implicated in Parkinson's disease [73, 74]; how these alterations contribute to Group 4 medulloblastoma biology currently remains unclear.

Whole genome duplication (i.e., tetraploidy) has been observed in medulloblastoma karyotypes for more than two decades [75, 76]. Now as a result of NGS, tumor cell ploidy can be readily estimated based on allele frequencies of SNPs and SNVs present in the genome. In a recent report by Jones et al., up to one-third of investigated medulloblastoma genomes were shown to be tetraploid, with higher frequencies noted in Groups 3 and 4 [58]. The significance of the high frequency of tetraploidy observed in medulloblastoma, particularly in Groups 3 and 4, will require further investigation but is thought to contribute to the overall genomic instability (i.e., gains and losses of whole chromosomes or chromosome arms) often noted in these tumors.

Preclinical Models of Medulloblastoma: Validating the Genetics of the Human Disease

Understanding the biological consequences of the genetic and epigenetic events observed in medulloblastoma and its subgroups requires accurate and faithful preclinical models that allow for comprehensive in vitro and in vivo functional studies. A series of established, immortalized medulloblastoma cell lines derived from human patient samples have been in use for the past 20–30 years [77–81]. These models have served as convenient systems for a variety of purposes including, evaluating candidate gene function, investigating genetic, epigenetic, and transcriptional alterations, and testing novel therapies, all in the context of medulloblastoma. Now with the recognition of medulloblastoma subgroups and increasing knowledge of the genetics underlying these subgroups, the validity of these "workhorse" medulloblastoma models has been put into question. Ongoing genomic analysis of these lines suggests they do not faithfully recapitulate the four medulloblastoma subgroups and harbor events not observed in primary medulloblastoma counterparts as a result of their continued evolution during long-term passage in culture [34]. Novel, low-passage lines and medulloblastoma xenograft models that require passaging in the mouse have recently emerged as possible solutions to the caveats associated with immortalized, high-passage cell lines and will likely be more heavily relied upon in the future [82, 83].

An immense amount of knowledge regarding the developmental biology of medulloblastoma has been gained from the use of genetically engineered mouse models [84]. The majority of such murine models generated and studied to date have been driven by activation of the SHH pathway in neuronal progenitor and stem cell populations [85]. Germline inactivation of one copy of the *Ptch1* gene (often referred to as $Ptc^{+/-}$ mice) results in 15–20 % of mice developing cerebellar tumors that are histologically similar to human medulloblastomas and exhibit aberrant SHH pathway activation suggesting they are accurate models of this subgroup [86, 87]. Combining loss of Ptch1 with inactivation of Trp53 (i.e., $Ptc^{+/-}$; $Trp53^{-/-}$) dramatically increases tumor incidence and reduces latency, with up to ~95 % of mice developing medulloblastoma within 12 weeks [88]. Several other SHH-activated mouse models have been generated, including those driven by an activated Smoothened transgene [89–91], homozygous germline deletion of *Ptch1* in specific cell types [92], those driven by administration of SHH ligand with cooperating oncogenes [93–95], and others [96–99]. These models have led to a better understanding of the genetics underlying SHH-driven medulloblastoma, the probable cells-of-origin for this subgroup, and provided the research community with tools for asking an array of questions related to medulloblastoma biology.

Representative models for the remaining subgroups have also been published, providing important clues regarding their differing biologies. Gibson et al. expressed a constitutively active form of β-Catenin (i.e., $Ctnnb1\Delta^{ex3}$) in progenitor cells of the developing hindbrain, successfully generating the first WNT-driven medulloblastoma mouse model [100]. More recently, complementary studies by Pei et al. and Kawauchi et al. combined over-expression of Myc with loss of wild-type Trp53 in orthotopic transplantation models to generate tumors resembling human Group 3 medulloblastoma [101, 102]. Finally, a model relying on transgenic over-expression of Mycn is believed to represent the lone Group 4 medulloblastoma model currently available [103].

As a plethora of new candidate medulloblastoma genes have recently been discovered, it is anticipated that many novel models based on these genes and rational gene combinations will be generated and introduced during the next few years. These models will serve not only to functionally validate events observed in the human disease but also to further progress our understanding of their role in disease biology and evaluate their relevance and utility as potential targets for molecularly informed therapy.

Translational Significance of the Medulloblastoma Genomics Era

Molecular Classification and Risk-Stratification

Medulloblastoma subgroups exhibit highly disparate molecular genetics and clinical characteristics, suggesting they should be treated as different diseases in the clinic. Before such a concept is put into general practice, robust, highly accurate, and efficient methods that are accessible to treating physicians for establishing subgroup assignments are necessary. Novel assays that are gaining an appreciation in this arena include the use of DNA methylation arrays and platforms for measuring the expression of custom gene panels. Both Schwalbe et al. and Hovestadt et al. have recently demonstrated that DNA methylation arrays can be used to assign medulloblastoma subgroups with high confidence, including samples derived from formalin-fixed paraffin embedded (FFPE) material [104, 105]. RNA-based methods such as the nanoString assay have also shown utility at subgrouping of samples preserved in FFPE [106] (Fig. 9.9). Further validation of these methods and potentially others in the setting of medulloblastoma clinical trials is expected in the near future as the interest to subgroup patients in a prospective manner increases.

In light of the excellent prognosis associated with WNT medulloblastoma patients, plans to de-escalate craniospinal radiation or even eliminate it in these patients will be implemented in forthcoming clinical trials. Similarly, prospective stratification of all Group 3 patients into a high-risk treatment category is likewise being considered.

Another subset of patients that appears to be of significant clinical relevance are those with *TP53*-mutated SHH medulloblastomas. Using large retrospective patient cohorts, Zhukova et al. demonstrated that the dismal outcome sometimes attributed to medulloblastomas harboring *TP53* mutation [107] can be explained by considering patient subgroup information [37]. *TP53*-mutated cases within the SHH subgroup exhibit a significantly worse outcome compared to either subgroup-matched non-mutated counterparts or WNT cases likewise harboring *TP53* mutation. Furthermore, the prevalence of chromothripsis and oncogene amplification observed in *TP53*-mutated SHHs suggest these patients should be stratified as a unique risk-group and possibly subjected to treatments tailored for their genotype.

Targeting Medulloblastoma with Rational Therapies

One of the major goals motivating the comprehensive genomic characterization of medulloblastoma is the identification of targets that can be specifically exploited for future treatment of the disease. To date, antagonists of the SHH pathway, acting mainly at the level of SMO, have demonstrated the most promise [108–112]. Compounds such as GDC-0449 from Genentech have shown dramatic although transient tumor regression when administered to patients with metastatic medulloblastoma, with patients eventually becoming resistant to the targeted therapy [111, 113]. Similar acquired resistance has been noted when related SMO antagonists (i.e., LDE-225) have been used to treat mouse models of the disease [110]. Ongoing efforts aim to combine SHH antagonists with additional inhibitory agents targeting cooperating pathways in hopes of achieving an improved and more sustained response to treatment. Furthermore, genomic analysis of human SHH medulloblastomas suggests that not all SHH-driven cases are likely to respond to inhibitors acting at the level of SMO, as subsets of cases such as those exhibiting amplification of downstream pathway components (i.e., *GLI2*) are likely to have primary resistance to these agents [34, 67]. As such, screening patients for both SHH subgroup affiliation and their mutation/copy number status in select SHH pathway genes prior to treatment with the current generation of SHH pathway inhibitors could improve their likelihood of response in the future. In addition, novel approaches targeting pathway components downstream of SMO, including the use of agents inhibiting GLI family transcription factors, are currently being evaluated and may increase the likelihood of response when combined with conventional SHH antagonists [114, 115].

The frequent deregulation of chromatin modifiers in medulloblastoma and the potential consequences of these events on the underlying epigenome make the prospect of epigenetic therapy an attractive possibility for medulloblastoma patients [65, 66]. Histone deacetylase (HDAC) inhibitors such as Vorinostat are currently being evaluated in medulloblastoma clinical trials [116, 117]. Similarly, 3-deazaneplanocin A (DZNep), a potent inhibitor of EZH2, is now being prioritized as an agent to be tested in upcoming clinical trials for medulloblastoma [118]. Similar agents targeting histone-modifying enzymes are presently being evaluated in the research setting and undoubtedly will enter the clinical trials arena for medulloblastoma patients in the near future.

Summary

Considerable advances have recently been made with respect to our understanding of the molecular genetics underlying medulloblastoma (Fig. 9.10). Acknowledgement of unique molecular subgroups and an improved knowledge of the

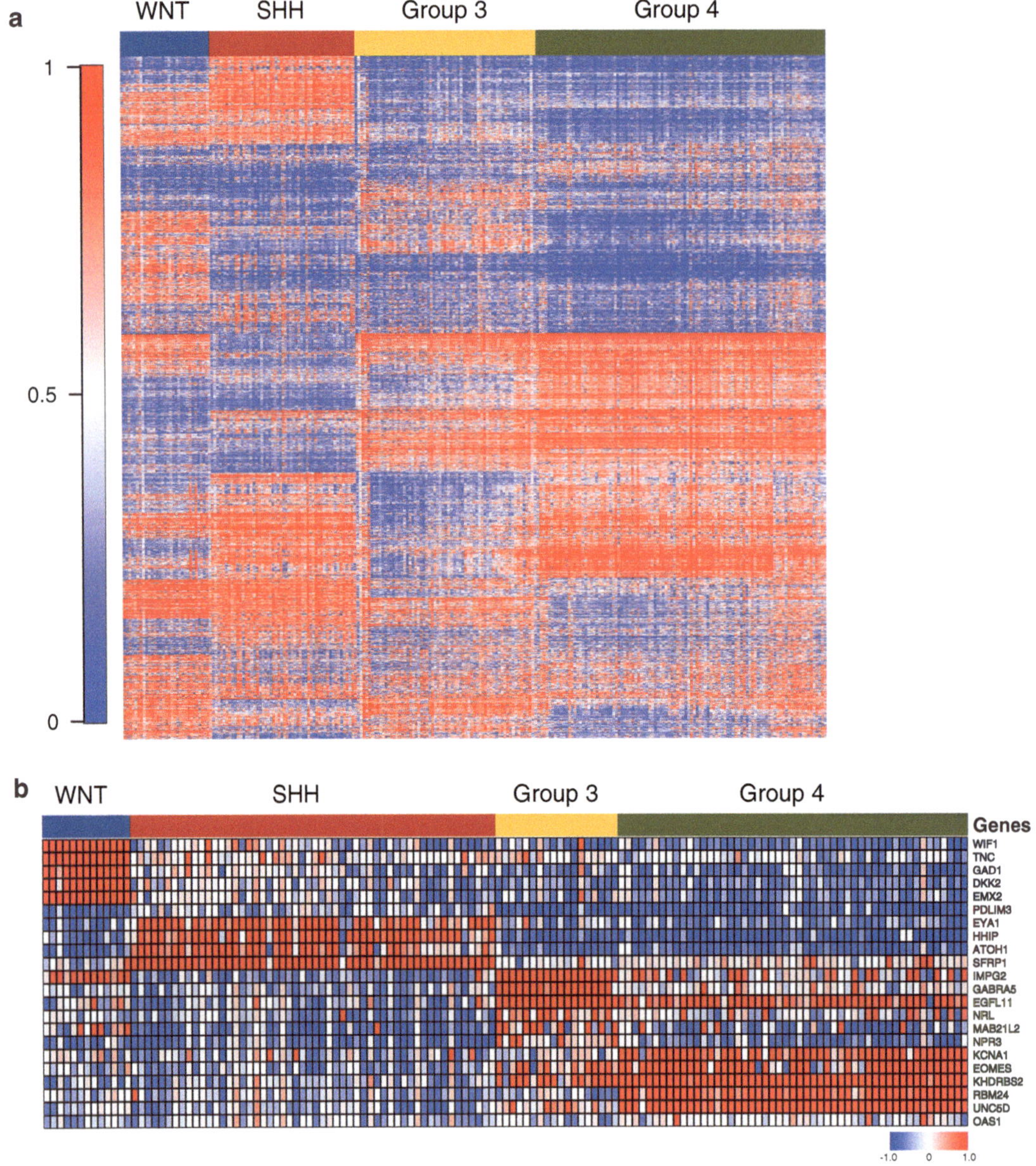

Fig. 9.9. Conventional assays for the molecular classification of medulloblastoma. (**a**) Heatmap of DNA methylation array (Illumina 450K platform) data for >250 primary medulloblastomas classified according to their appropriate molecular subgroup. Data was generated using DNAs extracted from either fresh-frozen tumor tissue or FFPE material. (**b**) Heatmap of gene expression data derived from a custom nanoString assay consisting of 22-signature genes for >100 medulloblastomas classified by molecular subgroup. Data was generated using RNAs extracted from FFPE material.

genes and pathways responsible for their pathogenesis can now at least partially explain the long-recognized biological and clinical heterogeneity encountered in the disease. Application of next-generation genomic platforms to large patient cohorts has identified new driver genes recurrently mutated in specific medulloblastoma subgroups, in addition to recurrent and often complex structural rearrangements, all at base-pair resolution. Additionally, new assays for rapidly confirming subgroup affiliation with pinpoint accuracy have been developed and are now making their way into clinical trials, as the need to progressively subgroup patients in the clinical setting intensifies. As the medulloblastoma research community harnesses the wealth of information gained during the current medulloblastoma "genomics era," new preclinical models faithfully recapitulating the genetics and the biology of the human subgroups are emerging. These new models will serve as valuable tools for the identification, development, and evaluation of rational therapies, bridging the gap between discoveries made in the research laboratory and the future administration of more specific, less-toxic

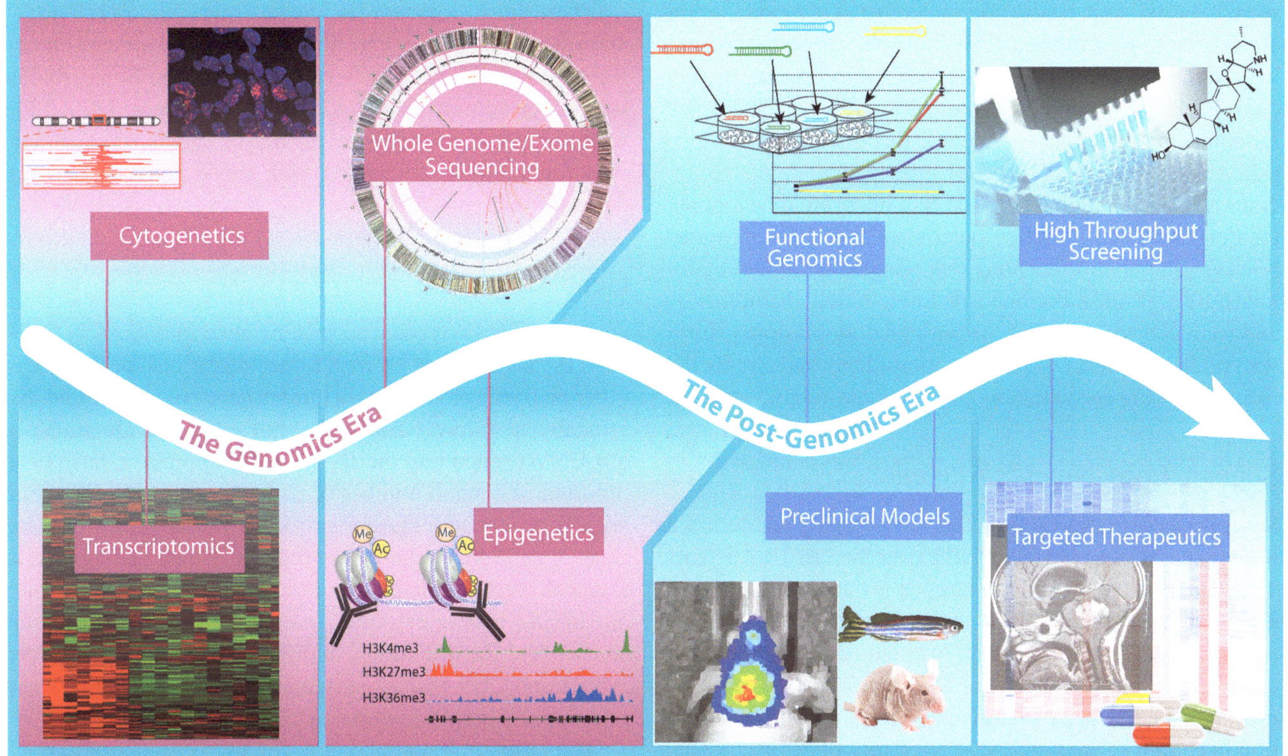

FIG. 9.10. Progression from genomics to the post-genomic era of medulloblastoma. Timeline highlighting the technological approaches being applied in medulloblastoma studies during the current "Genomics Era" and those that will become the focus of the imminent "Post-Genomics Era".

targeted treatment options. It can be anticipated that we are on the verge of an era of personalized medicine for medulloblastoma, whereby patients will be treated with therapies specifically tailored to their underlying genotypes. It is hoped that these novel diagnostic and therapeutic strategies will improve outcomes and quality of life for medulloblastoma patients going forward.

CNS-PNET

Central nervous system primitive neuroectodermal tumor (CNS-PNET, also known as supratentorial PNET to distinguish them from medulloblastoma) is a catch-all term for what is an extremely heterogeneous group of tumors arising in the cerebrum or spinal cord. They are one of the least clearly demarcated entities in terms of their histology, comprising a wide morphological spectrum. The WHO defines them as "An embryonal tumor composed of undifferentiated or poorly differentiated neuroepithelial cells which have the capacity for, or display, divergent differentiation along neuronal, astrocytic, muscular or melanocytic lines" [1]. Four variants of CNS-PNET are described in addition to "not otherwise specified" (NOS), namely: CNS neuroblastoma, CNS ganglioneuroblastoma, medulloepithelioma, and ependymoblastoma (EBL). CNS neuroblastoma is reserved for primitive tumors with solely neuronal differentiation, while ganglioneuroblastoma additionally implies the presence of ganglion cells. A further PNET occurring throughout the brain (including infratentorial locations) and characterized by broad bands of neuropil with true rosettes surrounding lumens, known as embryonal tumor with abundant neuropil and true rosettes (ETANTR), has also been noted but is not yet included in the WHO classification [119]. All of these variants are considered to be of malignancy Grade IV [1].

There is no clear shift in the gender distribution of CNS-PNETs, with a male:female ratio of ~1.2:1. The majority of these tumors occur in children, with a mean age at diagnosis of ~5.5 years [1]. Rarer cases in adults have also been reported, but with an incidence rate approximately one-fifth of that in children [120]. CNS-PNETs diagnosed in older patients are associated with a significantly worse prognosis than those occurring before the age of 40, and also with a worse outcome than for adult medulloblastoma (median survival 16 months for adult CNS-PNET vs. 155 months for medulloblastoma [121]). The latter trend holds true for pediatric cases, with 5-year overall survival typically below 50 % for CNS-PNET compared with 70–80 % for medulloblastoma [122, 123]. Pineal tumors in particular seem to be associated with poor outcomes. Treatment options are also less well defined than those for medulloblastoma, with some evidence that CNS-PNETs are resistant to standard Packer chemotherapy regimens [124], and no clear rationale for molecularly targeted therapies has been proposed. This is especially true for infants, who do not receive craniospinal radiation due to the risk of severe developmental defects. Slightly better outcomes have been reported, however, in patients receiving risk-adapted radiotherapy followed by high-dose cyclophosphamide-based chemotherapy and stem cell rescue [125]. As with medulloblastoma, survivors often experience significant morbidities and a reduction in quality of life due to tumor- and treatment-related sequelae.

Somatic Copy Number Alterations

Several studies have used methods of varying resolution to investigate SCNAs in CNS-PNET over the last 10–15 years. The general picture that has emerged is that these tumors do not typically display any of the common changes seen in medulloblastoma, such as i[17q], but may harbor other changes. Recently, a region of focal amplification on chromosome 19q has been identified as a highly recurrent alteration in certain subsets of CNS-PNET, as will be discussed in more detail in a later section.

One of the earliest studies comparing the cytogenetics of CNS-PNETs to medulloblastoma, for example, noted a higher frequency of chromosome 14q and 19q loss in supratentorial compared with infratentorial tumors, and no 17q gain in the supratentorial cases [126]. Another early report described an amplification of the *TERT* gene in a recurrence of a medulloepithelioma, which was not seen in the primary tumor, suggesting a role in tumor progression [127]. The authors also described increased expression of telomerase as a common finding in CNS-PNET. A lack of 17q gain but recurrent loss of 13q was noted in an array-based study of CNS-PNETs, which also reported amplifications of *PDGFRA/KIT*, *MYB* and 19q, as well as homozygous *CDKN2A/B* deletion [128]. One subsequent report did identify chromosome 17 alterations in 2/10 CNS-PNETs, but again noted that this change was significantly less frequent than in medulloblastoma [129]. The same study reported regions of loss on 1p and gain of 19p as being recurrent in CNS-PNET, and described deletions of *CDKN2A/B* in 7/21 cases examined [129]. Recurrent gain of 19p was confirmed in a more recent study of 29 CNS-PNETs, along with gains on 2p and 1q, which were seen in more than 20 % of cases [130]. Focal loss of *CADPS* on 3p was observed in 28 % of samples, and tumors showing this loss carried a worse prognosis [130]. In addition to *CDKN2A/B* deletions, SCNAs at other key cell-cycle regulatory genes seem to be a relatively common event in CNS-PNET, with 5/20 cases in one study displaying focal amplifications of *CDK4*, *CDK6*, *CCND1*, or *CCND2* [131].

There also appears to be a role for *MYC/MYCN* amplification in CNS-PNET, although there are conflicting reports as to the frequency of these changes. Some studies have reported only single cases with this change [129, 130], while in others it was reported in up to 50 % of cases, and was found to be associated with more aggressive tumor behavior [132].

Gene Mutations

As with SCNAs, reports on specific gene mutations in CNS-PNETs are relatively rare. Some alterations described in other pediatric or adult brain tumors have been identified, but typically at a lower frequency. For example, mutations in *SMARCB1*, encoding the INI1 tumor suppressor, have been reported in a small number of patients originally diagnosed with either medulloblastoma or CNS-PNET [133]. In some cases, a pathology review resulted in a change in diagnosis to atypical teratoid/rhabdoid tumor (AT/RT), for which *SMARCB1* loss is extremely common. The authors of this study noted the difficulties in differential diagnosis between AT/RT and CNS-PNET, particularly in young patients where only limited biopsy material is available.

The issue of potential diagnostic use of mutations which are typically highly specific for one entity, but which are occasionally seen in CNS-PNET, was also raised in a recent report by Gessi et al. [134]. The authors identified mutations at glycine 34 of histone variant H3.3 (encoded by *H3F3A*) in 4/33 CNS-PNETs. This mutation is typically found in hemispheric glioblastomas of older children and young adults, raising the question of whether H3.3 G34-mutant tumors can be defined as a distinct entity.

Mutations in *IDH1*, frequent in adult gliomas, are not common in pediatric patients in general, and also not in pediatric CNS-PNET. It does, however, appear to be a relatively frequent event in adult CNS-PNET (occurring in approximately 15–50 % of cases, although the overall number of tumors investigated remains small) [135–137]. This suggests that adult CNS-PNETs may frequently be related to tumors of a more glial origin, and their relationship to other adult gliomas requires additional investigation. Mutations in *TP53* have also been reported to be relatively frequent in adult CNS-PNET (~40 % in one study, but again with small numbers; [137]), which may further support an astrocytic link. In a similar vein, an entity termed "malignant gliomas with PNET-like component," which shares common molecular features of both malignant glioma and CNS-PNET, has recently been proposed—further highlighting the diagnostic uncertainty in this area [138].

As described in the first part of this chapter, practically all WNT MBs harbor an activating change in *CTNNB1*. Reports of this mutation in CNS-PNET, however, are extremely rare [139, 140]. The frequency of mutations in other genes recently identified as being altered in medulloblastoma (e.g., *DDX3X*, *SMARCA4*, *KDM6A* etc., as outlined above) is not

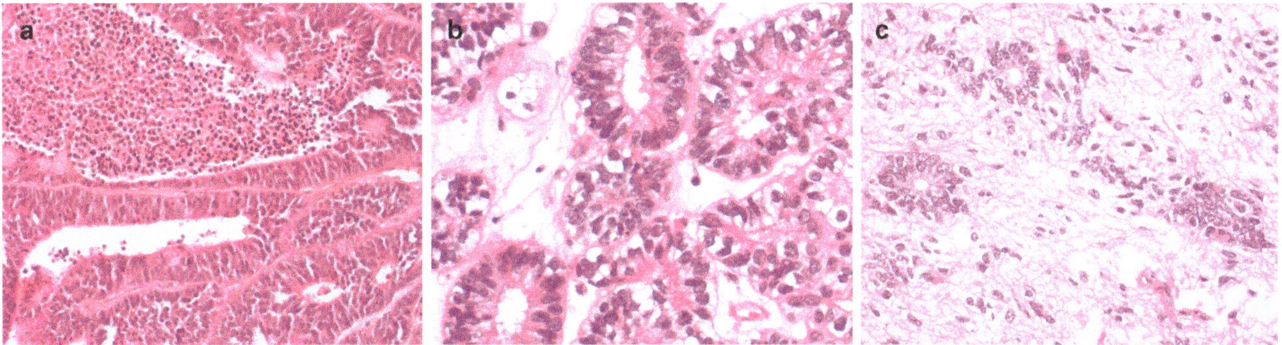

FIG. 9.11. Histological subtypes of CNS-PNET. Representative histology for (**a**) medulloepithelioma, (**b**) ependymoblastoma, and (**c**) ETANTR.

currently known for CNS-PNET. No NGS studies on this entity have been reported at the time of writing, but the results of such studies in the future will be of keen interest.

Signaling Pathways and Molecular Classification

In addition to studies looking at mutations in target genes or focal regions of copy number change, there have also been attempts to investigate deregulated signaling pathways and/or global expression patterns in CNS-PNET. The first seminal study using gene expression arrays looked at a comparison between medulloblastoma, CNS-PNET, AT/RT, and malignant gliomas [23]. This analysis was the first to clearly confirm the hypothesis that medulloblastoma and CNS-PNET do not share a common molecular origin, and display distinct expression signatures.

A possible glial signature in CNS-PNETs, compared with the more neuronal expression pattern in medulloblastoma, was proposed on the basis of a targeted expression analysis looking at various neuroglial developmental genes [141]. The authors identified an up-regulation of SOX2, NOTCH1, ID1, and ASCL1 in CNS-PNET, with higher levels of proneural transcription factors (NEUROD1, NEUROG1) in medulloblastoma.

Some evidence has recently been presented that the WNT/β-catenin pathway may also be playing a role in a proportion of CNS-PNETs [142]. Pathway activation, as assessed by β-catenin IHC, was identified in 11/42 primary CNS-PNETs (26 %). This pathway activation was also associated with a better prognosis among the CNS-PNETs examined (5-years OS 52 % in WNT-activated tumors compared with 13 % otherwise), but not to the extent of the excellent prognosis seen in WNT-activated medulloblastoma (5-years OS >95 %). As noted above, however, the frequency of *CTNNB1* mutation in CNS-PNET is very low, and thus the mechanism of WNT pathway activation is not currently clear.

An important recent study looking at the transcriptional profiles of 51 CNS-PNETs identified subgroups of tumors with differential signaling pathway activation and survival outcomes [143]. Three groups were identified based on their expression signature, showing differences in age and gender distribution, propensity for metastasis, and prognosis. Group 1 tumors showed a "primitive neural" profile, and occurred in young patients with a very poor prognosis. Positive immunohistochemical staining for LIN28A, and frequent presence of focal 19q amplification, suggests that this group may be composed primarily of embryonal tumors with multi-layered rosettes (ETMR), as discussed below. Interestingly, Group 1 was also characterized by a WNT pathway activation signature, and the poor survival of this group is therefore in contrast to the association seen by Rogers et al. [142]. Subgroup 2 tumors were labeled as "oligoneural." They typically showed OLIG2 immunopositivity as well as recurrent *CDKN2A/B* deletion, and a prognosis only slightly better than Group 1 CNS-PNETs, suggesting some similarity with high-grade glial tumors. Group 3 tumors displayed somewhat better outcomes (particularly in children older than 4 years) despite a much higher incidence of metastasis at diagnosis than the other subgroups. They showed a mesenchymal signature, were typically immunonegative for LIN28 and OLIG2 but positive for IGF2, and harbored recurrent loss of chromosome 14 [143]. Further investigation of these subgroups and their implications in terms of diagnostic/prognostic markers and also their cellular origins is clearly warranted.

Medulloepithelioma, Ependymoblastoma, and ETANTR

Medulloepithelioma (characterized by arrangements of neoplastic neuroepithelium mimicking embryonic neural tube, often with multiple lines of differentiation) and EBL (a densely cellular tumor with multi-layered rosettes) are two recognized CNS-PNET variants, which share the presence of rosette structures as a histological feature (Fig. 9.11). Arguably, however, the most fruitful area of research in terms of our molecular genetic understanding of CNS-PNETs in recent years has been in an additional rosette-forming entity

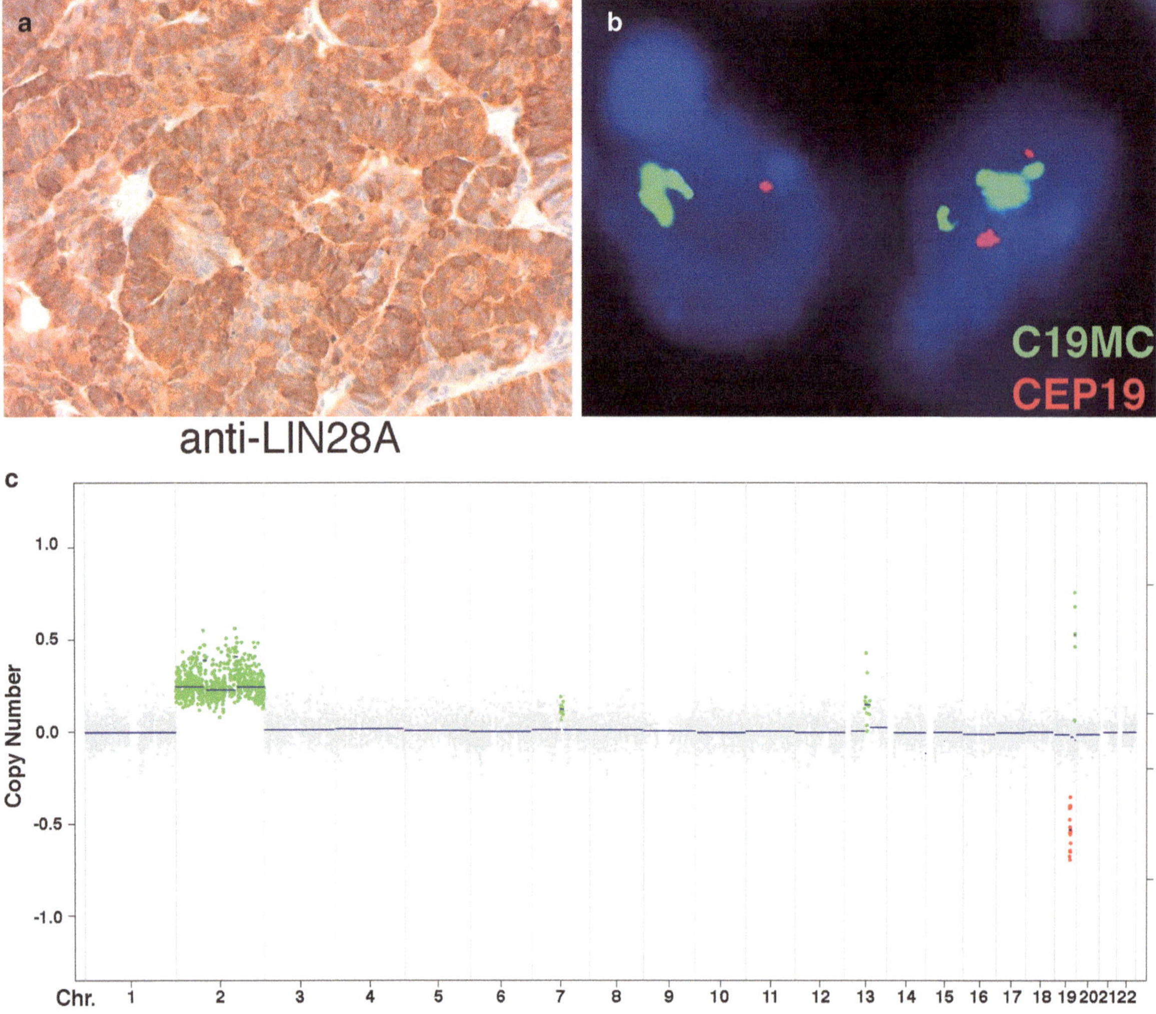

FIG. 9.12. Characteristic molecular features of ETANTR. (**a**) IHC of an ETANTR showing strong immunopositivity for LIN28A. (**b**) An ETANTR possessing signature high-level amplification of the chromosome 19q microRNA cluster (C19MC). (**c**) Genome-wide copy number plot of an ETANTR exhibiting prototypical gain of chromosome 2 and amplification of C19MC.

which is not yet officially recognized by the WHO classification, termed "embryonal tumor with abundant neuropil and true rosettes" (ETANTR) (Fig. 9.11) [119]. This tumor has a distinct histology, typically occurs in infants, can arise throughout the brain (including infratentorially) and is associated with a very poor prognosis [144]. It has recently become apparent that focal amplification of a microRNA cluster on chromosome 19q13 (C19MC), first described in early 2009 [145], is an extremely frequent event in this entity (Fig. 9.12) [143, 146, 147]. Multiple miRNAs within this locus, particularly miR-517c and miR-520g, were found to be strongly up-regulated in 19q13-amplified tumors [146]. Further functional characterization indicated a role for these miRNAs in promoting cell survival and inhibiting differentiation, with oncogenic effects observed both in vitro and in vivo that may partly be mediated by altered WNT pathway signaling [146].

Interestingly, the C19MC amplicon has also been found to be present in a very high proportion of EBLs [146, 147]. This has led to speculation that ETANTR, EBL, and possibly medulloepithelioma may be connected, with similar origins and biology but displaying a spectrum of morphology [148]. Rare reports of recurrent ETANTRs which retained the 19q amplicon but showed altered morphology add a further layer of histological complexity [147, 149]. As such, "embryonal tumor with multi-layered rosettes" (ETMR) has been proposed as an umbrella term to encompass the three entities. Further studies are therefore warranted to determine how closely related these three histological variants are, and whether it may be of diagnostic, prognostic, and potential therapeutic use to consider them as a single entity.

In addition to the C19MC amplification, gain of chromosome 2 is also particularly frequent in these tumors [144–146], but the consequences or targets of this change are not currently known. Other alterations including rare reports of i[17q] have also been described [150].

As noted above, C19MC amplification and chromosome 2 gain were also prominent features of Group 1 tumors according to Picard et al., together with immunopositivity for LIN28A [143]. Immunostaining for this marker has subsequently been shown to be highly specific for embryonal tumors with ependymoblastic rosettes, with diffuse positivity seen in 100 % of cases and not in any other embryonal, glial, or ependymal CNS tumor investigated, making it a valuable diagnostic tool (Fig. 9.12) [151].

Summary

In conclusion, CNS-PNETs are currently much less well characterized or understood in comparison to medulloblastoma and several other pediatric entities. In some respects, they represent a histological "dustbin" to gather all primitive-looking tumors that do not show a clear differentiation down any one defined lineage. What is apparent is that they do not resemble medulloblastoma in terms of their molecular genetic alterations. While 19q amplification seems to define one subset of CNS-PNET, a lack of other common alterations together with the occasional finding of changes thought to be specific for other entities (i.e., *IDH1* and *H3F3A* mutations) suggests a high degree of diagnostic uncertainty for this class of tumors. It will therefore be of great interest to see whether future studies looking at molecular profiles of larger numbers of CNS-PNETs can shed further light on the origins of this heterogeneous group of entities.

References

1. Louis DN, Ohgaki H, Wiestler OD, Cavenee WK. WHO classification of tumors of the central nervous system. LYON: IARC Press; 2007.
2. Jakacki RI, Burger PC, Zhou T, Holmes EJ, Kocak M, Onar A, et al. Outcome of children with metastatic medulloblastoma treated with carboplatin during craniospinal radiotherapy: a Children's Oncology Group Phase I/II study. J Clin Oncol. 2012;30(21):2648–53.
3. Ellison DW, Kocak M, Dalton J, Megahed H, Lusher ME, Ryan SL, et al. Definition of disease-risk stratification groups in childhood medulloblastoma using combined clinical, pathologic, and molecular variables. J Clin Oncol. 2011;29(11):1400–7.
4. Gajjar A, Chintagumpala M, Ashley D, Kellie S, Kun LE, Merchant TE, et al. Risk-adapted craniospinal radiotherapy followed by high-dose chemotherapy and stem-cell rescue in children with newly diagnosed medulloblastoma (St Jude Medulloblastoma-96): long-term results from a prospective, multicentre trial. Lancet Oncol. 2006;7(10):813–20.
5. Giangaspero F, Wellek S, Masuoka J, Gessi M, Kleihues P, Ohgaki H. Stratification of medulloblastoma on the basis of histopathological grading. Acta Neuropathol. 2006;112(1):5–12.
6. Rutkowski S, von Hoff K, Emser A, Zwiener I, Pietsch T, Figarella-Branger D, et al. Survival and prognostic factors of early childhood medulloblastoma: an international meta-analysis. J Clin Oncol. 2010;28(33):4961–8.
7. Brown HG, Kepner JL, Perlman EJ, Friedman HS, Strother DR, Duffner PK, et al. "Large cell/anaplastic" medulloblastomas: a Pediatric Oncology Group Study. J Neuropathol Exp Neurol. 2000;59(10):857–65.
8. Northcott PA, Rutka JT, Taylor MD. Genomics of medulloblastoma: from Giemsa-banding to next-generation sequencing in 20 years. Neurosurg Focus. 2010;28(1):E6.
9. Scheurlen WG, Schwabe GC, Joos S, Mollenhauer J, Sorensen N, Kuhl J. Molecular analysis of childhood primitive neuroectodermal tumors defines markers associated with poor outcome. J Clin Oncol. 1998;16(7):2478–85.
10. Badiali M, Pession A, Basso G, Andreini L, Rigobello L, Galassi E, et al. N-myc and c-myc oncogenes amplification in medulloblastomas. Evidence of particularly aggressive behavior of a tumor with c-myc amplification. Tumori. 1991;77(2):118–21.
11. Giangaspero F, Rigobello L, Badiali M, Loda M, Andreini L, Basso G, et al. Large-cell medulloblastomas. A distinct variant with highly aggressive behavior. Am J Surg Pathol. 1992;16(7):687–93.
12. Aldosari N, Bigner SH, Burger PC, Becker L, Kepner JL, Friedman HS, et al. MYCC and MYCN oncogene amplification in medulloblastoma. A fluorescence in situ hybridization study on paraffin sections from the Children's Oncology Group. Arch Pathol Lab Med. 2002;126(5):540–4.
13. Lamont JM, McManamy CS, Pearson AD, Clifford SC, Ellison DW. Combined histopathological and molecular cytogenetic stratification of medulloblastoma patients. Clin Cancer Res. 2004;10(16):5482–93.
14. Pfister S, Remke M, Benner A, Mendrzyk F, Toedt G, Felsberg J, et al. Outcome prediction in pediatric medulloblastoma based on DNA copy-number aberrations of chromosomes 6q and 17q and the MYC and MYCN loci. J Clin Oncol. 2009;27(10):1627–36.
15. von Hoff K, Hartmann W, von Bueren AO, Gerber NU, Grotzer MA, Pietsch T, et al. Large cell/anaplastic medulloblastoma: outcome according to myc status, histopathological, and clinical risk factors. Pediatr Blood Cancer. 2010;54(3):369–76.
16. Ryan SL, Schwalbe EC, Cole M, Lu Y, Lusher ME, Megahed H, et al. MYC family amplification and clinical risk-factors interact to predict an extremely poor prognosis in childhood medulloblastoma. Acta Neuropathol. 2012;123(4):501–13.
17. Taylor MD, Mainprize TG, Rutka JT. Molecular insight into medulloblastoma and central nervous system primitive neuroectodermal tumor biology from hereditary syndromes: a review. Neurosurgery. 2000;47(4):888–901.
18. Hahn H, Wicking C, Zaphiropoulous PG, Gailani MR, Shanley S, Chidambaram A, et al. Mutations of the human homolog of Drosophila patched in the nevoid basal cell carcinoma syndrome. Cell. 1996;85(6):841–51.
19. Johnson RL, Rothman AL, Xie J, Goodrich LV, Bare JW, Bonifas JM, et al. Human homolog of patched, a candidate gene for the basal cell nevus syndrome. Science. 1996;272(5268):1668–71.
20. Gailani MR, Bale SJ, Leffell DJ, DiGiovanna JJ, Peck GL, Poliak S, et al. Developmental defects in Gorlin syndrome related to a putative tumor suppressor gene on chromosome 9. Cell. 1992;69(1):111–7.

21. Hamilton SR, Liu B, Parsons RE, Papadopoulos N, Jen J, Powell SM, et al. The molecular basis of Turcot's syndrome. N Engl J Med. 1995;332(13):839–47.
22. Garre ML, Cama A, Bagnasco F, Morana G, Giangaspero F, Brisigotti M, et al. Medulloblastoma variants: age-dependent occurrence and relation to Gorlin syndrome—a new clinical perspective. Clin Cancer Res. 2009;15(7):2463–71.
23. Pomeroy SL, Tamayo P, Gaasenbeek M, Sturla LM, Angelo M, McLaughlin ME, et al. Prediction of central nervous system embryonal tumor outcome based on gene expression. Nature. 2002;415(6870):436–42.
24. Cho YJ, Tsherniak A, Tamayo P, Santagata S, Ligon A, Greulich H, et al. Integrative genomic analysis of medulloblastoma identifies a molecular subgroup that drives poor clinical outcome. J Clin Oncol. 2011;29(11):1424–30.
25. Kool M, Koster J, Bunt J, Hasselt NE, Lakeman A, van Sluis P, et al. Integrated genomics identifies five medulloblastoma subtypes with distinct genetic profiles, pathway signatures and clinicopathological features. PLoS One. 2008;3(8):e3088.
26. Thompson MC, Fuller C, Hogg TL, Dalton J, Finkelstein D, Lau CC, et al. Genomics identifies medulloblastoma subgroups that are enriched for specific genetic alterations. J Clin Oncol. 2006;24(12):1924–31.
27. Northcott PA, Korshunov A, Witt H, Hielscher T, Eberhart CG, Mack S, et al. Medulloblastoma comprises four distinct molecular variants. J Clin Oncol. 2011;29(11):1408–14.
28. Remke M, Hielscher T, Korshunov A, Northcott PA, Bender S, Kool M, et al. FSTL5 is a marker of poor prognosis in non-WNT/non-SHH medulloblastoma. J Clin Oncol. 2011;29(29):3852–61.
29. Northcott PA, Korshunov A, Pfister SM, Taylor MD. The clinical implications of medulloblastoma subgroups. Nat Rev Neurol. 2012;8:340–51.
30. Taylor MD, Northcott PA, Korshunov A, Remke M, Cho YJ, Clifford SC, et al. Molecular subgroups of medulloblastoma: the current consensus. Acta Neuropathol. 2012;123(4):465–72.
31. Ellison DW, Onilude OE, Lindsey JC, Lusher ME, Weston CL, Taylor RE, et al. beta-Catenin status predicts a favorable outcome in childhood medulloblastoma: the United Kingdom Children's Cancer Study Group Brain Tumor Committee. J Clin Oncol. 2005;23(31):7951–7.
32. Kool M, Korshunov A, Remke M, Jones DT, Schlanstein M, Northcott PA, et al. Molecular subgroups of medulloblastoma: an international meta-analysis of transcriptome, genetic aberrations, and clinical data of WNT, SHH, Group 3, and Group 4 medulloblastomas. Acta Neuropathol. 2012;123(4):473–84.
33. Northcott PA, Jones DT, Kool M, Robinson GW, Gilbertson RJ, Cho YJ, et al. Medulloblastomics: the end of the beginning. Nat Rev Cancer. 2012;12(12):818–34.
34. Northcott PA, Shih DJ, Peacock J, Garzia L, Morrissy AS, Zichner T, et al. Subgroup-specific structural variation across 1,000 medulloblastoma genomes. Nature. 2012;488(7409):49–56.
35. Ellison DW, Dalton J, Kocak M, Nicholson SL, Fraga C, Neale G, et al. Medulloblastoma: clinicopathological correlates of SHH, WNT, and non-SHH/WNT molecular subgroups. Acta Neuropathol. 2011;121(3):381–96.
36. Northcott PA, Hielscher T, Dubuc A, Mack S, Shih D, Remke M, et al. Pediatric and adult sonic hedgehog medulloblastomas are clinically and molecularly distinct. Acta Neuropathol. 2011;122(2):231–40.
37. Zhukova N, Ramaswamy V, Remke M, Pfaff E, Shih DJ, Martin DC, et al. Subgroup-specific prognostic implications of TP53 mutation in medulloblastoma. J Clin Oncol. 2013;31(23):2927–35.
38. Brugieres L, Remenieras A, Pierron G, Varlet P, Forget S, Byrde V, et al. High frequency of germline SUFU mutations in children with desmoplastic/nodular medulloblastoma younger than 3 years of age. J Clin Oncol. 2012;30(17):2087–93.
39. Brugieres L, Pierron G, Chompret A, Paillerets BB, Di Rocco F, Varlet P, et al. Incomplete penetrance of the predisposition to medulloblastoma associated with germ-line SUFU mutations. J Med Genet. 2010;47(2):142–4.
40. Taylor MD, Liu L, Raffel C, Hui CC, Mainprize TG, Zhang X, et al. Mutations in SUFU predispose to medulloblastoma. Nat Genet. 2002;31(3):306–10.
41. Al-Halabi H, Nantel A, Klekner A, Guiot MC, Albrecht S, Hauser P, et al. Preponderance of sonic hedgehog pathway activation characterizes adult medulloblastoma. Acta Neuropathol. 2011;121(2):229–39.
42. Remke M, Hielscher T, Northcott PA, Witt H, Ryzhova M, Wittmann A, et al. Adult medulloblastoma comprises three major molecular variants. J Clin Oncol. 2011;29(19):2717–23.
43. Korshunov A, Remke M, Kool M, Hielscher T, Northcott PA, Williamson D, et al. Biological and clinical heterogeneity of MYCN-amplified medulloblastoma. Acta Neuropathol. 2012;123(4):515–27.
44. Meyerson M, Gabriel S, Getz G. Advances in understanding cancer genomes through second-generation sequencing. Nat Rev Genet. 2010;11(10):685–96.
45. Stratton MR. Exploring the genomes of cancer cells: progress and promise. Science. 2011;331(6024):1553–8.
46. Pfaff E, Remke M, Sturm D, Benner A, Witt H, Milde T, et al. TP53 mutation is frequently associated with CTNNB1 mutation or MYCN amplification and is compatible with long-term survival in medulloblastoma. J Clin Oncol. 2010;28(35):5188–96.
47. Srivastava S, Zou ZQ, Pirollo K, Blattner W, Chang EH. Germ-line transmission of a mutated p53 gene in a cancer-prone family with Li-Fraumeni syndrome. Nature. 1990;348(6303):747–9.
48. Malkin D, Li FP, Strong LC, Fraumeni Jr JF, Nelson CE, Kim DH, et al. Germ line p53 mutations in a familial syndrome of breast cancer, sarcomas, and other neoplasms. Science. 1990;250(4985):1233–8.
49. Rausch T, Jones DT, Zapatka M, Stutz AM, Zichner T, Weischenfeldt J, et al. Genome sequencing of pediatric medulloblastoma links catastrophic DNA rearrangements with TP53 mutations. Cell. 2012;148(1–2):59–71.
50. Bunt J, Hasselt NE, Zwijnenburg DA, Koster J, Versteeg R, Kool M. Joint binding of OTX2 and MYC in promotor regions is associated with high gene expression in medulloblastoma. PLoS One. 2011;6(10):e26058.
51. Bunt J, Hasselt NE, Zwijnenburg DA, Hamdi M, Koster J, Versteeg R, et al. OTX2 directly activates cell cycle genes and inhibits differentiation in medulloblastoma cells. Int J Cancer. 2012;131:E21–32.

52. Bunt J, de Haas TG, Hasselt NE, Zwijnenburg DA, Koster J, Versteeg R, et al. Regulation of cell cycle genes and induction of senescence by overexpression of OTX2 in medulloblastoma cell lines. Mol Cancer Res. 2010;8(10):1344–57.
53. Boon K, Eberhart CG, Riggins GJ. Genomic amplification of orthodenticle homologue 2 in medulloblastomas. Cancer Res. 2005;65(3):703–7.
54. Di C, Liao S, Adamson DC, Parrett TJ, Broderick DK, Shi Q, et al. Identification of OTX2 as a medulloblastoma oncogene whose product can be targeted by all-trans retinoic acid. Cancer Res. 2005;65(3):919–24.
55. Adamson DC, Shi Q, Wortham M, Northcott PA, Di C, Duncan CG, et al. OTX2 is critical for the maintenance and progression of Shh-independent medulloblastomas. Cancer Res. 2010;70(1):181–91.
56. Fernandez LA, Northcott PA, Dalton J, Fraga C, Ellison D, Angers S, et al. YAP1 is amplified and up-regulated in hedgehog-associated medulloblastomas and mediates Sonic hedgehog-driven neural precursor proliferation. Genes Dev. 2009;23(23):2729–41.
57. Northcott PA, Fernandez LA, Hagan JP, Ellison DW, Grajkowska W, Gillespie Y, et al. The miR-17/92 polycistron is up-regulated in sonic hedgehog-driven medulloblastomas and induced by N-myc in sonic hedgehog-treated cerebellar neural precursors. Cancer Res. 2009;69(8):3249–55.
58. Jones DT, Jager N, Kool M, Zichner T, Hutter B, Sultan M, et al. Dissecting the genomic complexity underlying medulloblastoma. Nature. 2012;488:100–5.
59. Pugh TJ, Weeraratne SD, Archer TC, Pomeranz Krummel DA, Auclair D, Bochicchio J, et al. Medulloblastoma exome sequencing uncovers subtype-specific somatic mutations. Nature. 2012;488:106–10.
60. Robinson G, Parker M, Kranenburg TA, Lu C, Chen X, Ding L, et al. Novel mutations target distinct subgroups of medulloblastoma. Nature. 2012;488:43–8.
61. Pek JW, Kai T. DEAD-box RNA helicase Belle/DDX3 and the RNA interference pathway promote mitotic chromosome segregation. Proc Natl Acad Sci U S A. 2011;108(29):12007–12.
62. Lai MC, Chang WC, Shieh SY, Tarn WY. DDX3 regulates cell growth through translational control of cyclin E1. Mol Cell Biol. 2010;30(22):5444–53.
63. Lai MC, Lee YH, Tarn WY. The DEAD-box RNA helicase DDX3 associates with export messenger ribonucleoproteins as well as tip-associated protein and participates in translational control. Mol Biol Cell. 2008;19(9):3847–58.
64. Rosner A, Rinkevich B. The DDX3 subfamily of the DEAD box helicases: divergent roles as unveiled by studying different organisms and in vitro assays. Curr Med Chem. 2007;14(23):2517–25.
65. Jones DT, Northcott PA, Kool M, Pfister SM. The role of chromatin remodeling in medulloblastoma. Brain Pathol. 2013;23(2):193–9.
66. Batora NV, Sturm D, Jones DT, Kool M, Pfister SM, Northcott PA. Transitioning from genotypes to epigenotypes: why the time has come for medulloblastoma epigenomics. Neuroscience. 2014;264:171–85.
67. Northcott PA, Nakahara Y, Wu X, Feuk L, Ellison DW, Croul S, et al. Multiple recurrent genetic events converge on control of histone lysine methylation in medulloblastoma. Nat Genet. 2009;41(4):465–72.
68. Parsons DW, Li M, Zhang X, Jones S, Leary RJ, Lin JC, et al. The genetic landscape of the childhood cancer medulloblastoma. Science. 2011;331(6016):435–9.
69. Dubuc AM, Remke M, Korshunov A, Northcott PA, Zhan SH, Mendez-Lago M, et al. Aberrant patterns of H3K4 and H3K27 histone lysine methylation occur across subgroups in medulloblastoma. Acta Neuropathol. 2013;125:373–84.
70. Korbel JO, Campbell PJ. Criteria for inference of chromothripsis in cancer genomes. Cell. 2013;152(6):1226–36.
71. Stephens PJ, Greenman CD, Fu B, Yang F, Bignell GR, Mudie LJ, et al. Massive genomic rearrangement acquired in a single catastrophic event during cancer development. Cell. 2011;144(1):27–40.
72. Forment JV, Kaidi A, Jackson SP. Chromothripsis and cancer: causes and consequences of chromosome shattering. Nat Rev Cancer. 2012;12(10):663–70.
73. Kruger R. The role of synphilin-1 in synaptic function and protein degradation. Cell Tissue Res. 2004;318(1):195–9.
74. Eyal A, Engelender S. Synphilin isoforms and the search for a cellular model of lewy body formation in Parkinson's disease. Cell Cycle. 2006;5(18):2082–6.
75. Zerbini C, Gelber RD, Weinberg D, Sallan SE, Barnes P, Kupsky W, et al. Prognostic factors in medulloblastoma, including DNA ploidy. J Clin Oncol. 1993;11(4):616–22.
76. Gajjar AJ, Heideman RL, Douglass EC, Kun LE, Kovnar EH, Sanford RA, et al. Relation of tumor-cell ploidy to survival in children with medulloblastoma. J Clin Oncol. 1993;11(11):2211–7.
77. Jacobsen PF, Jenkyn DJ, Papadimitriou JM. Establishment of a human medulloblastoma cell line and its heterotransplantation into nude mice. J Neuropathol Exp Neurol. 1985;44(5):472–85.
78. Friedman HS, Burger PC, Bigner SH, Trojanowski JQ, Wikstrand CJ, Halperin EC, et al. Establishment and characterization of the human medulloblastoma cell line and transplantable xenograft D283 Med. J Neuropathol Exp Neurol. 1985;44(6):592–605.
79. Friedman HS, Burger PC, Bigner SH, Trojanowski JQ, Brodeur GM, He XM, et al. Phenotypic and genotypic analysis of a human medulloblastoma cell line and transplantable xenograft (D341 Med) demonstrating amplification of c-myc. Am J Pathol. 1988;130(3):472–84.
80. Yamada M, Shimizu K, Tamura K, Okamoto Y, Matsui Y, Moriuchi S, et al. [Establishment and biological characterization of human medulloblastoma cell lines]. No To Shinkei. 1989;41(7):695–702.
81. Pietsch T, Scharmann T, Fonatsch C, Schmidt D, Ockler R, Freihoff D, et al. Characterization of five new cell lines derived from human primitive neuroectodermal tumors of the central nervous system. Cancer Res. 1994;54(12):3278–87.
82. Milde T, Lodrini M, Savelyeva L, Korshunov A, Kool M, Brueckner LM, et al. HD-MB03 is a novel Group 3 medulloblastoma model demonstrating sensitivity to histone deacetylase inhibitor treatment. J Neurooncol. 2012;110:335–48.
83. Zhao X, Liu Z, Yu L, Zhang Y, Baxter P, Voicu H, et al. Global gene expression profiling confirms the molecular fidelity of

primary tumor-based orthotopic xenograft mouse models of medulloblastoma. Neuro Oncol. 2012;14(5):574–83.
84. Gilbertson RJ, Ellison DW. The origins of medulloblastoma subtypes. Annu Rev Pathol. 2008;3:341–65.
85. Wu X, Northcott PA, Croul S, Taylor MD. Mouse models of medulloblastoma. Chin J Cancer. 2011;30(7):442–9.
86. Goodrich LV, Milenkovic L, Higgins KM, Scott MP. Altered neural cell fates and medulloblastoma in mouse patched mutants. Science. 1997;277(5329):1109–13.
87. Wetmore C, Eberhart DE, Curran T. The normal patched allele is expressed in medulloblastomas from mice with heterozygous germ-line mutation of patched. Cancer Res. 2000;60(8):2239–46.
88. Wetmore C, Eberhart DE, Curran T. Loss of p53 but not ARF accelerates medulloblastoma in mice heterozygous for patched. Cancer Res. 2001;61(2):513–6.
89. Hallahan AR, Pritchard JI, Hansen S, Benson M, Stoeck J, Hatton BA, et al. The SmoA1 mouse model reveals that notch signaling is critical for the growth and survival of sonic hedgehog-induced medulloblastomas. Cancer Res. 2004;64(21):7794–800.
90. Hatton BA, Villavicencio EH, Tsuchiya KD, Pritchard JI, Ditzler S, Pullar B, et al. The Smo/Smo model: hedgehog-induced medulloblastoma with 90% incidence and leptomeningeal spread. Cancer Res. 2008;68(6):1768–76.
91. Grammel D, Warmuth-Metz M, von Bueren AO, Kool M, Pietsch T, Kretzschmar HA, et al. Sonic hedgehog-associated medulloblastoma arising from the cochlear nuclei of the brainstem. Acta Neuropathol. 2012;123(4):601–14.
92. Yang ZJ, Ellis T, Markant SL, Read TA, Kessler JD, Bourboulas M, et al. Medulloblastoma can be initiated by deletion of Patched in lineage-restricted progenitors or stem cells. Cancer Cell. 2008;14(2):135–45.
93. Binning MJ, Niazi T, Pedone CA, Lal B, Eberhart CG, Kim KJ, et al. Hepatocyte growth factor and sonic Hedgehog expression in cerebellar neural progenitor cells costimulate medulloblastoma initiation and growth. Cancer Res. 2008;68(19):7838–45.
94. Rao G, Pedone CA, Del Valle L, Reiss K, Holland EC, Fults DW. Sonic hedgehog and insulin-like growth factor signaling synergize to induce medulloblastoma formation from nestin-expressing neural progenitors in mice. Oncogene. 2004;23(36):6156–62.
95. Doucette TA, Yang Y, Pedone C, Kim JY, Dubuc A, Northcott PD, et al. WIP1 enhances tumor formation in a sonic hedgehog-dependent model of medulloblastoma. Neurosurgery. 2012;70(4):1003–10; discussion 1010.
96. Marino S, Vooijs M, van Der Gulden H, Jonkers J, Berns A. Induction of medulloblastomas in p53-null mutant mice by somatic inactivation of Rb in the external granular layer cells of the cerebellum. Genes Dev. 2000;14(8):994–1004.
97. Lee Y, McKinnon PJ. DNA ligase IV suppresses medulloblastoma formation. Cancer Res. 2002;62(22):6395–9.
98. Yan CT, Kaushal D, Murphy M, Zhang Y, Datta A, Chen C, et al. XRCC4 suppresses medulloblastomas with recurrent translocations in p53-deficient mice. Proc Natl Acad Sci U S A. 2006;103(19):7378–83.
99. Frappart PO, Lee Y, Russell HR, Chalhoub N, Wang YD, Orii KE, et al. Recurrent genomic alterations characterize medulloblastoma arising from DNA double-strand break repair deficiency. Proc Natl Acad Sci U S A. 2009;106(6):1880–5.
100. Gibson P, Tong Y, Robinson G, Thompson MC, Currle DS, Eden C, et al. Subtypes of medulloblastoma have distinct developmental origins. Nature. 2010;468(7327):1095–9.
101. Kawauchi D, Robinson G, Uziel T, Gibson P, Rehg J, Gao C, et al. A mouse model of the most aggressive subgroup of human medulloblastoma. Cancer Cell. 2012;21(2):168–80.
102. Pei Y, Moore CE, Wang J, Tewari AK, Eroshkin A, Cho YJ, et al. An animal model of MYC-driven medulloblastoma. Cancer Cell. 2012;21(2):155–67.
103. Swartling FJ, Grimmer MR, Hackett CS, Northcott PA, Fan QW, Goldenberg DD, et al. Pleiotropic role for MYCN in medulloblastoma. Genes Dev. 2010;24(10):1059–72.
104. Schwalbe EC, Williamson D, Lindsey JC, Hamilton D, Ryan SL, Megahed H, et al. DNA methylation profiling of medulloblastoma allows robust subclassification and improved outcome prediction using formalin-fixed biopsies. Acta Neuropathol. 2013;125(3):359–71.
105. Hovestadt V, Remke M, Kool M, Pietsch T, Northcott PA, Fischer R, et al. Robust molecular subgrouping and copy-number profiling of medulloblastoma from small amounts of archival tumor material using high-density DNA methylation arrays. Acta Neuropathol. 2013;125(6):913–6.
106. Northcott PA, Shih DJ, Remke M, Cho YJ, Kool M, Hawkins C, et al. Rapid, reliable, and reproducible molecular subgrouping of clinical medulloblastoma samples. Acta Neuropathol. 2012;123(4):615–26.
107. Tabori U, Baskin B, Shago M, Alon N, Taylor MD, Ray PN, et al. Universal poor survival in children with medulloblastoma harboring somatic TP53 mutations. J Clin Oncol. 2010;28(8):1345–50.
108. Berman DM, Karhadkar SS, Hallahan AR, Pritchard JI, Eberhart CG, Watkins DN, et al. Medulloblastoma growth inhibition by hedgehog pathway blockade. Science. 2002;297(5586):1559–61.
109. Robarge KD, Brunton SA, Castanedo GM, Cui Y, Dina MS, Goldsmith R, et al. GDC-0449-a potent inhibitor of the hedgehog pathway. Bioorg Med Chem Lett. 2009;19(19):5576–81.
110. Buonamici S, Williams J, Morrissey M, Wang A, Guo R, Vattay A, et al. Interfering with resistance to smoothened antagonists by inhibition of the PI3K pathway in medulloblastoma. Sci Transl Med. 2010;2(51):51ra70.
111. Rudin CM, Hann CL, Laterra J, Yauch RL, Callahan CA, Fu L, et al. Treatment of medulloblastoma with hedgehog pathway inhibitor GDC-0449. N Engl J Med. 2009;361(12):1173–8.
112. Peukert S, He F, Dai M, Zhang R, Sun Y, Miller-Moslin K, et al. Discovery of NVP-LEQ506, a second-generation inhibitor of smoothened. ChemMedChem. 2013;8(8):1261–5.
113. Yauch RL, Dijkgraaf GJ, Alicke B, Januario T, Ahn CP, Holcomb T, et al. Smoothened mutation confers resistance to a Hedgehog pathway inhibitor in medulloblastoma. Science. 2009;326(5952):572–4.
114. Kim J, Aftab BT, Tang JY, Kim D, Lee AH, Rezaee M, et al. Itraconazole and arsenic trioxide inhibit Hedgehog pathway activation and tumor growth associated with acquired resistance to smoothened antagonists. Cancer Cell. 2013;23(1):23–34.

115. Kim J, Lee JJ, Gardner D, Beachy PA. Arsenic antagonizes the Hedgehog pathway by preventing ciliary accumulation and reducing stability of the Gli2 transcriptional effector. Proc Natl Acad Sci U S A. 2010;107(30):13432–7.
116. Witt O, Milde T, Deubzer HE, Oehme I, Witt R, Kulozik A, et al. Phase I/II intra-patient dose escalation study of vorinostat in children with relapsed solid tumor, lymphoma or leukemia. Klin Padiatr. 2012;224(6):398–403.
117. Fouladi M, Park JR, Stewart CF, Gilbertson RJ, Schaiquevich P, Sun J, et al. Pediatric phase I trial and pharmacokinetic study of vorinostat: a Children's Oncology Group phase I consortium report. J Clin Oncol. 2010;28(22):3623–9.
118. Gajjar A, Packer RJ, Foreman NK, Cohen K, Haas-Kogan D, Merchant TE. Children's Oncology Group's 2013 blueprint for research: central nervous system tumors. Pediatr Blood Cancer. 2013;60(6):1022–6.
119. Eberhart C, Brat D, Cohen K, Burger P. Pediatric neuroblastic brain tumors containing abundant neuropil and true rosettes. Pediatr Dev Pathol. 2000;3(4):346–52.
120. Smoll NR, Drummond KJ. The incidence of medulloblastomas and primitive neurectodermal tumors in adults and children. J Clin Neurosci. 2012;19(11):1541–4.
121. Gandhi R, Babu R, Cummings TJ, Adamson C. Adult primitive neuroectodermal tumors: the prognostic value of supratentorial location. J Neurooncol. 2013;114(1):141–8.
122. Johnston DL, Keene DL, Lafay-Cousin L, Steinbok P, Sung L, Carret AS, et al. Supratentorial primitive neuroectodermal tumors: a Canadian pediatric brain tumor consortium report. J Neurooncol. 2008;86(1):101–8.
123. Fangusaro J, Finlay J, Sposto R, Ji L, Saly M, Zacharoulis S, et al. Intensive chemotherapy followed by consolidative myeloablative chemotherapy with autologous hematopoietic cell rescue (AuHCR) in young children with newly diagnosed supratentorial primitive neuroectodermal tumor (sPNETs): report of the head start I and II experience. Pediatr Blood Cancer. 2008;50(2):312–8.
124. Biswas S, Burke A, Cherian S, Williams D, Nicholson J, Horan G, et al. Non-pineal supratentorial primitive neuroectodermal tumors (sPNET) in teenagers and young adults: time to reconsider cisplatin based chemotherapy after craniospinal irradiation? Pediatr Blood Cancer. 2009;52(7):796–803.
125. Chintagumpala M, Hassall T, Palmer S, Ashley D, Wallace D, Kasow K, et al. A pilot study of risk-adapted radiotherapy and chemotherapy in patients with supratentorial PNET. Neuro Oncol. 2009;11(1):33–40.
126. Russo C, Pellarin M, Tingby O, Bollen AW, Lamborn KR, Mohapatra G, et al. Comparative genomic hybridization in patients with supratentorial and infratentorial primitive neuroectodermal tumors. Cancer. 1999;86(2):331–9.
127. Fan X, Wang Y, Kratz J, Brat DJ, Robitaille Y, Moghrabi A, et al. hTERT gene amplification and increased mRNA expression in central nervous system embryonal tumors. Am J Pathol. 2003;162(6):1763–9.
128. McCabe M, Ichimura K, Liu L, Plant K, Backlund L, Pearson D, et al. High-resolution array-based comparative genomic hybridization of medulloblastomas and supratentorial primitive neuroectodermal tumors. J Neuropathol Exp Neurol. 2006;65(6):549–61.
129. Pfister S, Remke M, Toedt G, Werft W, Benner A, Mendrzyk F, et al. Supratentorial primitive neuroectodermal tumors of the central nervous system frequently harbor deletions of the CDKN2A locus and other genomic aberrations distinct from medulloblastomas. Genes Chromosomes Cancer. 2007;46(9):839–51.
130. Miller S, Rogers HA, Lyon P, Rand V, Adamowicz-Brice M, Clifford SC, et al. Genome-wide molecular characterization of central nervous system primitive neuroectodermal tumor and pineoblastoma. Neuro Oncol. 2011;13(8):866–79.
131. Li M, Lockwood W, Zielenska M, Northcott P, Ra YS, Bouffet E, et al. Multiple CDK/CYCLIND genes are amplified in medulloblastoma and supratentorial primitive neuroectodermal brain tumor. Cancer Genet. 2012;205(5):220–31.
132. Behdad A, Perry A. Central nervous system primitive neuroectodermal tumors: a clinicopathologic and genetic study of 33 cases. Brain Pathol. 2010;20(2):441–50.
133. Biegel JA, Fogelgren B, Zhou JY, James CD, Janss AJ, Allen JC, et al. Mutations of the INI1 rhabdoid tumor suppressor gene in medulloblastomas and primitive neuroectodermal tumors of the central nervous system. Clin Cancer Res. 2000;6(7):2759–63.
134. Gessi M, Gielen GH, Hammes J, Dorner E, Muhlen AZ, Waha A, et al. H3.3 G34R mutations in pediatric primitive neuroectodermal tumors of central nervous system (CNS-PNET) and pediatric glioblastomas: possible diagnostic and therapeutic implications? J Neurooncol. 2013;112(1):67–72.
135. Balss J, Meyer J, Mueller W, Korshunov A, Hartmann C, von Deimling A. Analysis of the IDH1 codon 132 mutation in brain tumors. Acta Neuropathol. 2008;116(6):597–602.
136. Hayden JT, Fruhwald MC, Hasselblatt M, Ellison DW, Bailey S, Clifford SC. Frequent IDH1 mutations in supratentorial primitive neuroectodermal tumors (sPNET) of adults but not children. Cell Cycle. 2009;8(11):1806–7.
137. Gessi M, Setty P, Bisceglia M, zur Muehlen A, Lauriola L, Waha A, et al. Supratentorial primitive neuroectodermal tumors of the central nervous system in adults: molecular and histopathologic analysis of 12 cases. Am J Surg Pathol. 2011;35(4):573–82.
138. Perry A, Miller CR, Gujrati M, Scheithauer BW, Zambrano SC, Jost SC, et al. Malignant gliomas with primitive neuroectodermal tumor-like components: a clinicopathologic and genetic study of 53 cases. Brain Pathol. 2009;19(1):81–90.
139. Koch A, Waha A, Tonn JC, Sorensen N, Berthold F, Wolter M, et al. Somatic mutations of WNT/wingless signaling pathway components in primitive neuroectodermal tumors. Int J Cancer. 2001;93(3):445–9.
140. Rogers HA, Miller S, Lowe J, Brundler MA, Coyle B, Grundy RG. An investigation of WNT pathway activation and association with survival in central nervous system primitive neuroectodermal tumors (CNS PNET). Br J Cancer. 2009;100(8):1292–302.
141. Phi JH, Kim JH, Eun KM, Wang KC, Park KH, Choi SA, et al. Upregulation of SOX2, NOTCH1, and ID1 in supratentorial primitive neuroectodermal tumors: a distinct differentiation pattern from that of medulloblastomas. J Neurosurg Pediatr. 2010;5(6):608–14.
142. Rogers HA, Ward JH, Miller S, Lowe J, Coyle B, Grundy RG. The role of the WNT/beta-catenin pathway in central nervous system primitive neuroectodermal tumors (CNS PNETs). Br J Cancer. 2013;108(10):2130–41.

143. Picard D, Miller S, Hawkins CE, Bouffet E, Rogers HA, Chan TS, et al. Markers of survival and metastatic potential in childhood CNS primitive neuro-ectodermal brain tumors: an integrative genomic analysis. Lancet Oncol. 2012;13(8):838–48.
144. Gessi M, Giangaspero F, Lauriola L, Gardiman M, Scheithauer BW, Halliday W, et al. Embryonal tumors with abundant neuropil and true rosettes: a distinctive CNS primitive neuroectodermal tumor. Am J Surg Pathol. 2009;33(2):211–7.
145. Pfister S, Remke M, Castoldi M, Bai A, Muckenthaler M, Kulozik A, et al. Novel genomic amplification targeting the microRNA cluster at 19q13.42 in a pediatric embryonal tumor with abundant neuropil and true rosettes. Acta Neuropathol. 2009;117(4):457–64.
146. Li M, Lee KF, Lu Y, Clarke I, Shih D, Eberhart C, et al. Frequent amplification of a chr19q13.41 microRNA polycistron in aggressive primitive neuroectodermal brain tumors. Cancer Cell. 2009;16(6):533–46.
147. Korshunov A, Remke M, Gessi M, Ryzhova M, Hielscher T, Witt H, et al. Focal genomic amplification at 19q13.42 comprises a powerful diagnostic marker for embryonal tumors with ependymoblastic rosettes. Acta Neuropathol. 2010;120(2):253–60.
148. Ceccom J, Bourdeaut F, Loukh N, Rigau V, Milin S, Takin R, et al. Embryonal tumor with multilayered rosettes: diagnostic tools update and review of the literature. Clin Neuropathol. 2014;33:15–22.
149. Woehrer A, Slavc I, Peyrl A, Czech T, Dorfer C, Prayer D, et al. Embryonal tumor with abundant neuropil and true rosettes (ETANTR) with loss of morphological but retained genetic key features during progression. Acta Neuropathol. 2011;122(6):787–90.
150. Fuller C, Fouladi M, Gajjar A, Dalton J, Sanford RA, Helton KJ. Chromosome 17 abnormalities in pediatric neuroblastic tumor with abundant neuropil and true rosettes. Am J Clin Pathol. 2006;126(2):277–83.
151. Korshunov A, Ryzhova M, Jones DT, Northcott PA, van Sluis P, Volckmann R, et al. LIN28A immunoreactivity is a potent diagnostic marker of embryonal tumor with multilayered rosettes (ETMR). Acta Neuropathol. 2012;124(6):875–81.

10 Subependymal Giant Cell Astrocytoma

David H. Harter, Howard L. Weiner, and David Zagzag

Subependymal giant cell astrocytomas (SEGAs) are benign tumors (WHO grade I) that occur almost exclusively in the setting of tuberous sclerosis (TS), a well-defined, multisystem genetic syndrome (Table 10.1). Most commonly originating from the region of the caudate nucleus, these tumors may cause obstruction of cerebrospinal fluid circulation leading to hydrocephalus. Less frequently, they may hemorrhage spontaneously, causing precipitous neurological impairment [1]. Mutations of the *TSC-1* and *TSC-2* genes, both effectors of the mTOR pathway (originally *mammalian* Target of Rapamycin, now formally *mechanistic* Target of Rapamycin), lead to the variably expressed systemic manifestations of TS; cardiac rhabdomyoma, renal angiolipomas, facial adenoma sebaceum, cortical tubers of the brain, and SEGAs. The standard treatment of symptomatic or enlarging SEGAs is surgical excision. Pharmacological effectors of the mTOR pathway, rapamycin (aka sirolimus) and its analogs have recently been shown to induce rapid involution of SEGAs; however, the optimal timing, dosage, safety, and duration of treatment remain areas of active clinical research. SEGAs in the context of TS represent an example of an emerging paradigm: targeted molecular-oncologic therapy.

Incidence and Prevalence

SEGAs (subependymal giant cell tumors) typically occur in the first or second decade of life, predominately, yet not exclusively in patients with TS (tuberous sclerosis). Reports of neo- and prenatal diagnoses illustrate the developmental nature of these tumors [2–5]. Most SEGAs are related to tuberous sclerosis, occurring in approximately 1 per 5,000–10,000 births [6]. Although most SEGAs are associated with TS, the incidence of SEGA is only 5–10 % among patients with TS [7]. A small portion of SEGAs occur without clinical or genetic evidence of TS, or as "forme fruste" of the disorder displaying some characteristics [8]. Tuberous sclerosis occurs across all ethnicities and in both male and female, worldwide estimates are of 1–2 million affected individuals [6].

Genetics and Oncogenesis

Tuberous sclerosis is an autosomal dominant genetic disorder with high penetrance and variable expressivity. The majority of cases are due to de novo mutations, although inherited somatic mutations and gonadal mosaicism may also occur [9]. Somatic mosaicism may result in limited expression of TS. In cases of both spontaneous mutation and gonadal or somatic mosaicism, parental genetic testing may be normal. In cases of gonadal mosaicism, the possibility of transmission to future offspring remains, albeit at an unquantifiable rate. A variety of mutations of within two genes have been identified, TSC1 (chromosome 9) and TSC2 (chromosome 16), both effectors of the mTOR (mechanistic Target of Rapamycin) pathway. Identified aberrations, including mutation and deletion, lead to loss or attenuation of function. Sporadic SEGAs occurring without clinical or genetic evidence of TSC (tuberous sclerosis complex) may be due to dual somatic mutations of TSC1 or TSC2 [10, 11].

The TOR complexes influence many aspects of eukaryote physiology—largely via growth regulation, cell growth, proliferation, and survival (Fig. 10.1) [12]. The mTOR signaling pathway detects and integrates a variety of environmental conditions to regulate growth and homeostasis. Aberrations of the mTOR pathway have been implicated in a wide array of pathological processes including oncogenesis, obesity, type II diabetes, and neurodegenerative conditions. mTOR has been identified as an atypical serinine/threonine protein kinase belonging to the phosphoinositide 3-kinase (PI_3K)-related kinase family. Interacting with other proteins, mTOR forms two complexes: mTOR complex 1 (mTORC1) and mTOR complex 2 (mTORC2). These complexes each have

M.A. Karajannis and D. Zagzag (eds.), *Molecular Pathology of Nervous System Tumors: Biological Stratification and Targeted Therapies*, Molecular Pathology Library 8,
DOI 10.1007/978-1-4939-1830-0_10, © Springer Science+Business Media New York 2015

TABLE 10.1. Diagnostic criteria for tuberous sclerosis complex.

Definite—One primary, two secondary, or one secondary plus two tertiary features
Probable—One secondary, plus one tertiary or three tertiary features
Suspect—One secondary, or two tertiary features
Primary features
Facial angiofibromas[a]
Multiple ungual fibromas[a]
Cortical tuber (histologically confirmed)
Subependymal nodule or giant cell astrocytomas (histologically confirmed)
Multiple calcified subchondral nodules protruding into the ventricle (radiographic evidence)
Multiple retinal astrocytomas[a]
Secondary features
Affected first-degree relative
Cardiac rhabdomyolysis (radiographic or histologic confirmation)
Other retinal hamartoma or achromic patch[a]
Cerebral tubers (radiographic confirmation)
Noncalcified subependymal nodules (radiographically confirmed)
Shagreen patch[a]
Forehead plaque[a]
Pulmonary lymphangiomyomatosis (histologic confirmation)
Renal angiolipoma (radiographic or histologic confirmation)
Renal cysts (histologic confirmation)
Tertiary features
Hypomelanotic macules[a]
"Confetti" skin lesions[a]
Renal cysts (radiographic evidence)
Randomly distributed in a multiparous in the deciduous and/or permanent teeth
Hamartomatous rectal polyps (histologic confirmation)
Bone cysts (radiographic evidence)
Pulmonary lymphangiomyomatosis (radiographic evidence)
Cerebral white matter "migration tracts" or heterotopias (radiographic evidence)
Gingival fibromas[a]
Hamartoma of other organs (histologic confirmation)
Infantile spasms

From Roach ES, Smith M, Huttenlocher P, Bhat M, Alcorn D, Hawley L. Diagnostic criteria: tuberous sclerosis complex. Report of the Diagnostic Criteria Committee of the National Tuberous Sclerosis Association. J Child Neurol 1992;7:221-4, with permission

[a]Histological confirmation not required if the lesion is clinically obvious

independent effectors and effects, as well as differing sensitivities to rapamycin and its analogs [13].

TSC1 (hamartin) and TSC2 (tuberin) form a heterodimer that is a key upstream regulator of mTORC1, functioning as a guanosine triphosphate (GTPase)-activating protein (GAP) for Ras homolog enriched in the brain (Rheb) (Fig. 10.2). The GTP-bound form of Rheb interacts directly with mTORC1, significantly enhancing its kinase activity [13]. TSC1/2 as a Rheb GTPase-activating protein negatively regulates mTORC1 by converting Rheb to its inactive GDP-bound state [14]. TSC1/2 integrates multiple upstream signals that attenuate mTORC1 including growth factors via PI_3k and Ras pathways. The effector kinases of these pathways (Akt/PKB, ERK1/2, RSK1) directly phosphorylate the TSC1/2 dimer to inactivate it, resultantly activating mTORC1 [15]. Cytokines, such as TNFα, may also activate TORC1 by phosphorylation of TSC1/2 via I$\kappa\beta$ kinase β (IKKβ) [16]. The Wnt pathway, a regulator of diverse cellular processes including differentiation, proliferation, and polarity, also modulates mTOR. By inhibiting glycogen synthase kinase 3b, phosphorylation of TSC2 is reduced leading to activation of mTORC1 [17].

Hypoxia, mediated via transcriptional regulation of DNA damage response 1 (REDD1), activates TSC2 function [18]. mTORC1 is activated by DNA damage through a p53-mediated mechanism. The induction of TSC2 and Pten results in downregulation of PI_3K-mTORC1 [19], and also, through induction of Sestrin1/2, activates AMPK [20]. Phosphatidic acid also activates mTORC1 [21].

mTORC1 may also be activated by amino acids (leucine and arginine), which are also required for activation of mTORC1 by some growth factors [22]. The mechanism of mTORC1 activation remains poorly understood, although it has been shown to involve the Rag GTPases and translocation of mTORC1 to the lysosomal surface [23].

Cellular processes regulated by mTORC1 include protein synthesis, lipid synthesis, energy metabolism, cell fate determination, autophagy, and cytoskeletal organization [13]. The role of the mTOR pathway in oncogenesis is evinced by mutations identified in human cancers and cancer syndromes. The loss of p53, a common observation in human cancers, promotes mTORC1 activation. Upstream from mTORC1 and mTORC2, components of the PI_3K pathway are also often mutated in human tumors. Several human cancer syndromes, including TS and neurofibromatosis type I, are defined by mutations in upstream signaling components of mTOR complexes. Dysregulation of translation and protein synthesis downstream of mTORC1 by interaction with initiation factor 4E-binding proteins ($_4$E-BP1/eIF$_4$E) likely plays a significant role in tumorigenesis by promoting cell cycle progression [24]. Another hallmark of proliferating cancer cells, lipid synthesis is regulated by mTOR-PI3K activation of the lipogenic factor SREBP1, which requires mTORC1 signaling [25].

A complex, TSC1-TSC2 (hamartin-tuberin), via GTPase-activating protein acts as a negative regulator of mTORC1, a controller of anabolic processes. Multiple factors and cellular signaling pathways are integrated, leading to phosphorylation events, and resultantly mTORC1 activity [26]. Dysregulated mTOR activity subsequently results in abnormal cellular division and differentiation across tissue types and abnormal cellular enlargement is seen, as is the case in SEGAs.

Clinical Presentation

SEGAs usually present with signs and symptoms of cerebrospinal fluid obstruction due to the encroachment of the foramen of Monro either uni- or bilaterally. The onset of symptoms is usually insidious, with progressive headache,

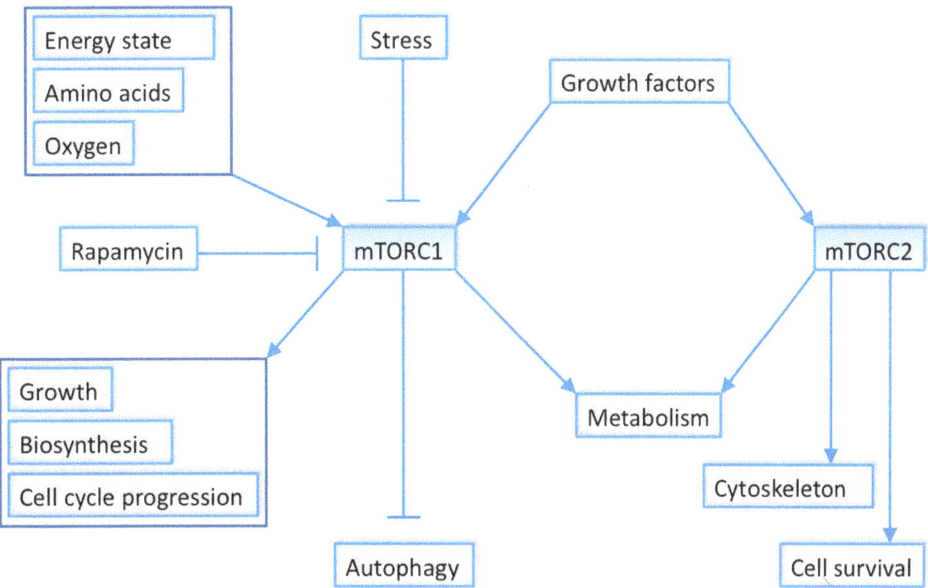

Fig. 10.1. Overview of mTOR1 and mTOR2 interactions and effectors.

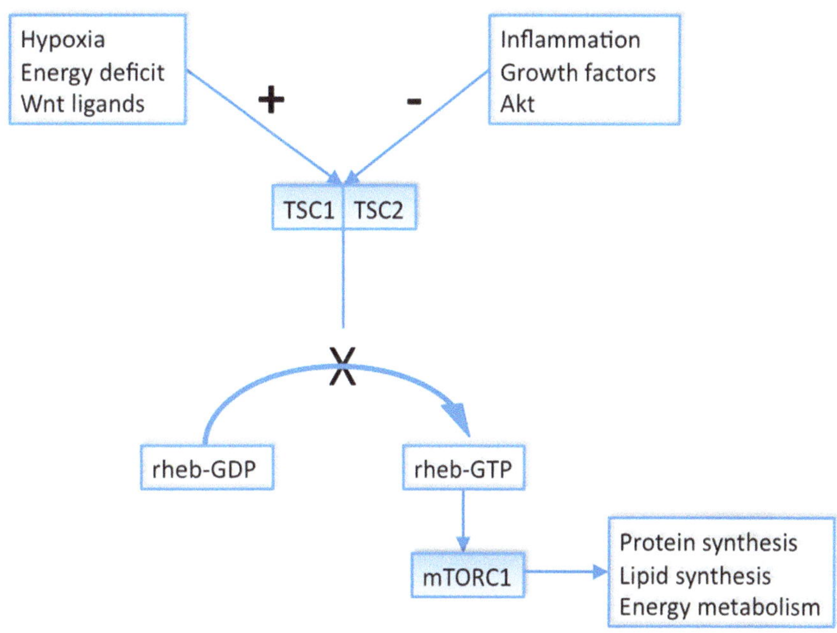

Fig. 10.2. TSC1/2 complex interactions via a Rheb GTPase mediator leading to mTORC1 activation.

cognitive impairment, lethargy and finally, if unrecognized, coma and death. Occasionally, precipitous neurological decline or death due to acute hydrocephalus or intratumoral hemorrhage may occur [27–31]. Clinical history and findings suggestive of tuberous sclerosis may be present; epilepsy and other systemic manifestations may also lead to the diagnosis. SEGAs usually become symptomatic within the first two decades of life.

The diagnosis of TSC is based on clinical examination and confirmed with genetic testing. Cutaneous findings include hypomelanotic macules, facial angiofibromas, and shagreen patches. Oral lesions may include ungula or gingival fibromas. The three hallmark pathologies of TSC in the central nervous system (CNS) are cortical tubers, subependymal nodules, and SEGAs. Functional impairment of effected individuals may be due to seizures, intellectual disability, and/or developmental delay. Renal manifestation may include angiomyolipomas (AML), cysts, and renal cell carcinoma. Cardiac conditions, including rhabdomyoma and arrhythmias may be present. Pulmonary involvement is restricted to lymphangioleiomyomatosis (LAM). Consensus clinical diagnostic criteria (Table 10.1) were developed prior to reliable genetic testing and allow for stratification as *definite, probable, or suspect* TSC [32]. Patients with somatic TSC2 mutations, as a group, are most severely affected. Somatic mutations of TSC1 are less affected [33]. Patients with genetic mosaicism may have localized, minimal, or no clinical evidence of TSC.

Radiographic Characteristics

Location is of primary consideration in the radiologic suspicion of SEGA. Given that the vast majority of these tumors arise within the lateral ventricle in the caudothalamic groove, medial to the posterior caudate nucleus, SEGA should be strongly considered in the differential diagnosis of tumors in this region [34]. Growth on serial neuroimaging differentiates SEGAs from subependymal nodules. The radiologic identification of SEGA may be made on ultrasound (in neonates, and rarely prenates), computed tomography (CT), and magnetic resonance imaging (MRI) [4, 35] (Figs. 10.3 and 10.4).

CT may show uni- or bilateral hyper-dense foci of calcification medial to the genu of the internal capsule (Fig. 10.3). In cases associated with TS, multiple calcifications and subependymal nodules (candle guttering) may be seen along the caudothalamic groove [36]. Ventriculomegaly may be identified unilaterally or bilaterally [37].

MRI characteristics mirror the heterogeneous pathology of SEGAs, with mixed signal intensities on T1- and T2-weighted imaging. SEGAs are usually hypo- and isointense on T1-weighted imaging, and iso- to hyperintense on T2-weighted imaging. Dense contrast enhancement is usually present, although it may occur in a heterogeneous pattern [38]. Calcified portions of the tumor, usually near the base of the tumor, typically appear hypodense on T2-weighted imaging (Fig. 10.4).

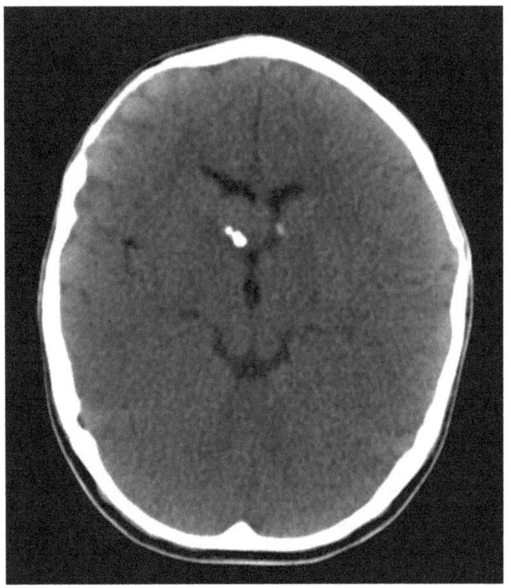

Fig. 10.3. Noncontrast CT scan, 3-year-old with TSC2 mutation. A SEGA is seen on the right, note calcification at the thalamocaudate groove.

Pathology

The origin of almost all SEGAs is the wall of the lateral ventricle, from the region of the posterior caudate/basal ganglia, just medial to the genu of the internal capsule with projection into the frontal horn or body of the lateral ventricle. A focus of dense calcification is often present at the base of the tumor. They are well circumscribed, lobulated, angiomatous, and slow growing. Tumor-related cysts may be present. Malignant transformation is uncommon [39]. SEGAs in other locations have been reported, including the cerebral cortex [40], pineal region [41], and retina [42–44].

Histologically, SEGAs may display a wide range of astrocytic, glial, and neuronal differentiation. Three cell types predominate: small spindle cells, gemistocytic astrocytes, and giant cell with ganglionic features (Fig. 10.5). Mitotic index is usually low and necrosis is an uncommon finding. Nucleoli are usually distinct in all of the cell types and a finely granular chromatin pattern is common. SEGAs may display features associated with malignant potential, pleomorphism, mitotic figures, necrosis, and vascularity; however, true malignant behavior is exceedingly rare [39, 45]. (Table 10.2).

Immunohistochemical staining is variably reactive for S-100 and GFAP—a reflection of the mixed astrocytic/glial composition and heterogeneity of the tumor. Neuronal markers including cytoskeletal components (neurofilaments, MAP2, class III Beta tubulin) and neurosecretory substances (serotonin, Beta endorphin, somatostatin) may also be positive [46]. The presence of both glial and neuronal markers within tumor cells supports the possibility that the originating cells of SEGAs have the potential to differentiate along glioneuronal in addition to neuroendocrine lineage, and to a greater degree than other mixed glioneuronal neoplasms [46]. Reported occurrence of SEGAs in the retina [42–44], with Mueller cell origin capable of dedifferentiation into pluripotent progenitor cell as their putative source, illustrates the potential mechanism of a common progenitor producing multiple cell types.

Treatment Options

The optimal treatment of SEGAs and other TSC-related conditions is an area of intense basic, translational, and clinical research. Recognition of the benign nature of these tumors, along with the potential for long life-expectancy mandates that treatment strategies not only result in long-term disease-free or progression-free survival, but also consider potential long-term complications and cost [47].

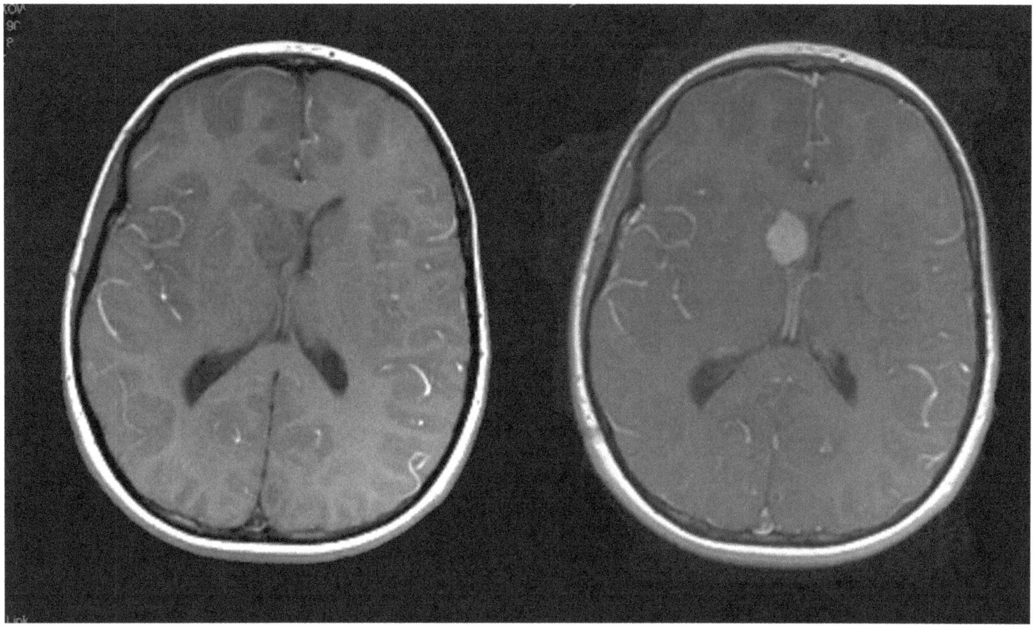

Fig. 10.4. Pre- and postgadolinium T1-weighted axial MRI, 9-year-old with TSC1 mutation. A SEGA is seen on the right, dense contrast enhancement is seen.

Observation

Serial clinic examination and radiologic surveillance are appropriate for incidentally discovered or small, stable, or slowly growing SEGAs. Rapid enlargement is unusual and clinical symptoms that are typically insidious allow for treatment on an elective basis [48–50].

Surgery

Various approaches for resection of SEGAs including craniotomy by transcallosal and transcortical approaches have been the reported. Early operative case series noted significant morbidity and mortality [51–53]. Contemporary series, however, with the aid of microdissection, stereotactic techniques, and modern pediatric neuroanesthetic techniques have significantly improved upon the results of these historical benchmarks [54]. A high rate of gross total resection, with little or no permanent neurological morbidity, can be expected at high-volume surgery centers [55–57]. Tumor recurrence after radiographically confirmed gross or radical subtotal resection is infrequent.

The preferred surgical approach depends upon a number of factors, ventricular size, prior surgery, and surgeon experience. Generally, smaller ventricular size favors a transcallosal approach. Significant ventriculomegally and the presence of an existing frontal resection cavity (i.e., from cortical tuber resection) may favor a transcortical approach. Additionally, success of a purely endoscopic approach via a single frontal burr hole has been reported and may be appropriate for some SEGAs [58].

Medical Therapy

SEGAs are slow-growing tumors with low, if any, potential for malignant transformation [39, 59, 60]. Conventional cytotoxic compounds do not have a role in their treatment. However, targeted medical therapy directed specifically at the implicated signal transduction pathways has emerged as a potentially effective and safe strategy to control SEGAs and other manifestations of TS. Progress in this area was initiated literally with the unearthing of rapamycin.

The discovery of the macrolide compound rapamycin began with a "bioprospecting" expedition to Easter Island ("Rapa Nui" in the native language). A soil sample obtained from the site included the bacterium *Streptomyces hygroscopicus*, from which a secondary metabolite with strong antiproliferative properties was obtained—rapamycin [61]. Eventually, the antifungal properties of rapamycin led to the discovery of its molecular targets—TOR1 and TOR2. Acting to suppress T-function, rapamycin was used in post-transplant patients as an immunosuppressant.

The mechanism of rapamycin and related compounds, known as rapalogs, upon the mTOR pathway is complicated; however, it is known to form a gain-of-function complex with FKBP12, a 12-kDa intracellular protein. This rapamycin-FKBP12 complex inhibits mTOR as component of mTORC1—although the molecular mechanism of this inhibition has not been elucidated. Current theories include impaired structural integrity of mTORC1 [62] and allosteric reduction of the complex's kinase domain activity [63].

The first rapalog approved in the USA was Temsirolimus for advanced renal cell carcinoma. In 2012 Everolimus was

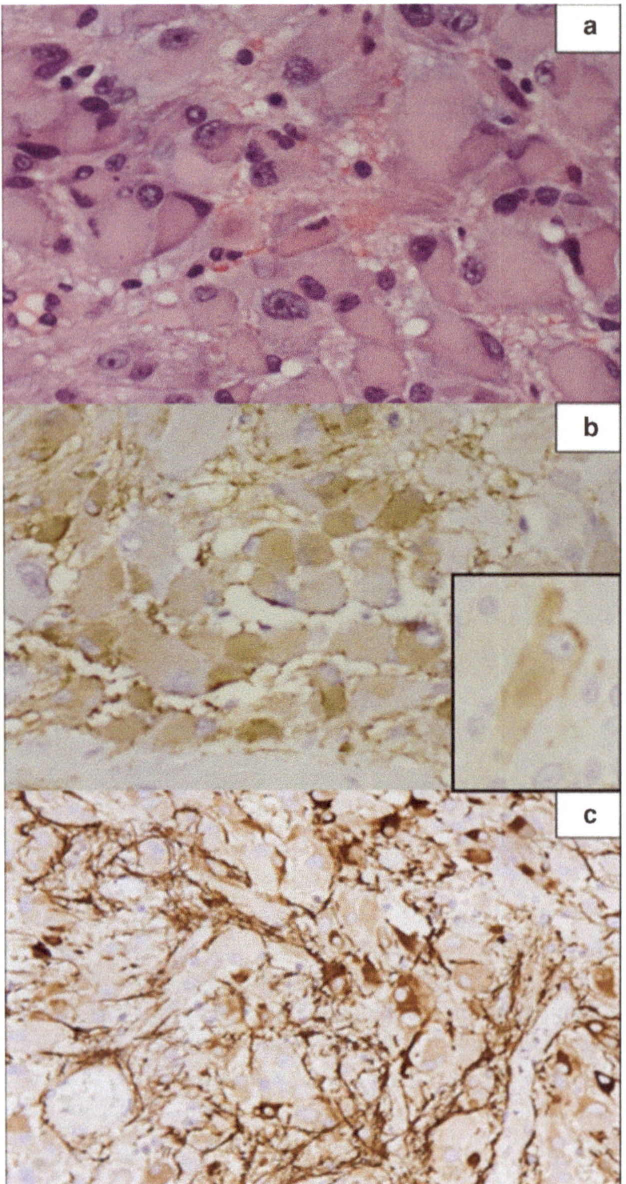

Fig. 10.5. Subependymal giant cell astrocytoma shows large mostly polygonal cells with abundant cytoplasm and often vesicular eccentric nucleus with prominent nucleolus (**a**). The tumor cells share features of glial cells and are immunoreactive for glial fibrillary acidic protein (**b**, **c**) but also have neuronal features and are immunopositive for synaptophysin (*inset*).

Table 10.2. Pathology of subependymal giant cell tumors.

Histology
Low mitotic index
Necrosis uncommon
Calcifications common
Differentiation all multiple lineages—astrocytic, glial, and neuronal
Cell types—gemistocytic astrocytes and giant cell with ganglionic features
Immunohistochemistry
S-100 and GFAP variably reactive
Neuronal markers—neurofilament, MAP2, class III Beta tubulin
Neurosecretory substances (serotonin, Beta endorphin, somatostatin)

approved by the Food and Drug Administration for the treatment of pediatric and adult patients with TSC who have SEGA that requires therapeutic intervention but *cannot be curatively resected* [12]. Case reports, clinical series and clinical trials, including a multicenter, placebo-controlled trial [64–68], have demonstrated ≥50 % volumetric reduction of SEGAs among treated patients. Notably, some trials have also demonstrated a meaningful reduction in seizure frequency during treatment [67, 69]. Common side effects include stomatitis, oral ulceration, and impaired wound healing [66, 70]. Metabolic side effects include hypercholesterolemia, hyperlipidemia, and hyperglycemia [71].

In addition to rapamycin and related compounds, the development of small molecule inhibitors of mTOR kinase activity has been investigated [72, 73]. As adenosine triphosphate (ATP)-competitive inhibitors of mTOR, these molecules block all phosphorylation targets downstream of mTORC1 and mTORC2. As a result, these compounds impair cell growth, proliferation, and tumor formation to a much greater extent than rapamycin, which solely inhibits mTORC1.

Radiosurgery

Stereotactic radiosurgery (SRS) has been used as a primary treatment of SEGAs and for tumor recurrence after initial surgical treatment in a small number of cases. Treatment doses of 13–14 Gee to the 50 % iso dose line have been used [74, 75]. A high rate of local control has been reported; however, instances of tumor progression have been noted, some retreated successfully with SRS, while others required surgical excision [74–76]. The risk of radiation-induced secondary tumors is a concern, especially in young patients, and development of glioblastoma has been reported after radiotherapy for SEGA in TSC [77].

Outcomes

CNS involvement is the leading cause of morbidity and mortality in patients with TSC and is usually related to status epilepticus or SEGAs [78]. Renal disease is the second leading cause of early death [9]. Cardiac or pulmonary involvement is also a potential cause of mortality in TSC [78]. Functionally, poorer cognitive outcomes have been shown for patients with bilateral cortical tubers and early age (<6 months) at the onset of seizures [79]. Tuber count or burden has not been shown to correlate with developmental outcome [80]. Treatment of disorders related to TSC, particularly SEGAs, is likely to undergo a tectonic shift. Rather than palliative and piecemeal strategies, targeted molecular therapies (rapalogs, multi kinase inhibitors, and others) are emerging. These agents may not only control tumor growth, but may also prevent CNS developmental malformations, control or prevent seizures, and ultimately lead to improved quality of life and outcomes.

References

1. Sterman H, Furlan AB, Matushita H, Teixeira MJ. Subependymal giant cell astrocytoma associated with tuberous sclerosis presenting with intratumoral bleeding. Case report and review of literature. Childs Nerv Syst. 2013;29:335–9.
2. Hahn JS, Bejar R, Gladson CL. Neonatal subependymal giant cell astrocytoma associated with tuberous sclerosis: MRI, CT, and ultrasound correlation. Neurology. 1991;41:124–8.
3. Oikawa S, Sakamoto K, Kobayashi N. A neonatal huge subependymal giant cell astrocytoma: case report. Neurosurgery. 1994;35:748–50.
4. Mirkin LD, Ey EH, Chaparro M. Congenital subependymal giant-cell astrocytoma: case report with prenatal ultrasonogram. Pediatr Radiol. 1999;29:776–80.
5. Nabbout R, Santos M, Rolland Y, Delalande O, Dulac O, Chiron C. Early diagnosis of subependymal giant cell astrocytoma in children with tuberous sclerosis. J Neurol Neurosurg Psychiatry. 1999;66:370–5.
6. Osborne JP, Fryer A, Webb D. Epidemiology of tuberous sclerosis. Ann N Y Acad Sci. 1991;615:125–7.
7. Braffman BH, Bilaniuk LT, Naidich TP, et al. MR imaging of tuberous sclerosis: pathogenesis of this phakomatosis, use of gadopentetate dimeglumine, and literature review. Radiology. 1992;183:227–38.
8. Kawahara I, Tsutsumi K, Hirose M, Matsuo Y, Yokoyama H. [Solitary subependymal giant cell astrocytoma: a forme fruste of tuberous sclerosis complex?]. No To Shinkei. 2004;56: 585–91.
9. Northrup H, Koenig MK, Au KS. Tuberous sclerosis complex. In: Pagon RA, Adam MP, Ardinger HH, et al., editors. Gene reviews. Seattle: University of Washington; 1993. http://www.washington.edu/.
10. Ichikawa T, Wakisaka A, Daido S, et al. A case of solitary subependymal giant cell astrocytoma: two somatic hits of TSC2 in the tumor, without evidence of somatic mosaicism. J Mol Diagn. 2005;7:544–9.
11. Kashiwagi N, Yoshihara W, Shimada N, et al. Solitary subependymal giant cell astrocytoma: case report. Eur J Radiol. 2000; 33:55–8.
12. Wander SA, Hennessy BT, Slingerland JM. Next-generation mTOR inhibitors in clinical oncology: how pathway complexity informs therapeutic strategy. J Clin Invest. 2011;121: 1231–41.
13. Laplante M, Sabatini DM. mTOR signaling in growth control and disease. Cell. 2012;149:274–93.
14. Inoki K, Li Y, Xu T, Guan KL. Rheb GTPase is a direct target of TSC2 GAP activity and regulates mTOR signaling. Genes Dev. 2003;17:1829–34.
15. Ma L, Chen Z, Erdjument-Bromage H, Tempst P, Pandolfi PP. Phosphorylation and functional inactivation of TSC2 by Erk implications for tuberous sclerosis and cancer pathogenesis. Cell. 2005;121:179–93.
16. Lee DF, Kuo HP, Chen CT, et al. IKK beta suppression of TSC1 links inflammation and tumor angiogenesis via the mTOR pathway. Cell. 2007;130:440–55.
17. Inoki K, Ouyang H, Zhu T, et al. TSC2 integrates Wnt and energy signals via a coordinated phosphorylation by AMPK and GSK3 to regulate cell growth. Cell. 2006;126:955–68.
18. Brugarolas J, Lei K, Hurley RL, et al. Regulation of mTOR function in response to hypoxia by REDD1 and the TSC1/TSC2 tumor suppressor complex. Genes Dev. 2004;18:2893–904.
19. Stambolic V, MacPherson D, Sas D, et al. Regulation of PTEN transcription by p53. Mol Cell. 2001;8:317–25.
20. Budanov AV, Karin M. p53 target genes sestrin1 and sestrin2 connect genotoxic stress and mTOR signaling. Cell. 2008;134: 451–60.
21. Foster DA. Phosphatidic acid signaling to mTOR: signals for the survival of human cancer cells. Biochim Biophys Acta. 2009;1791:949–55.
22. Hara K, Yonezawa K, Weng QP, Kozlowski MT, Belham C, Avruch J. Amino acid sufficiency and mTOR regulate p70 S6 kinase and eIF-4E BP1 through a common effector mechanism. J Biol Chem. 1998;273:14484–94.
23. Sancak Y, Bar-Peled L, Zoncu R, Markhard AL, Nada S, Sabatini DM. Ragulator-Rag complex targets mTORC1 to the lysosomal surface and is necessary for its activation by amino acids. Cell. 2010;141:290–303.
24. Dowling RJ, Topisirovic I, Alain T, et al. mTORC1-mediated cell proliferation, but not cell growth, controlled by the 4E-BPs. Science. 2010;328:1172–6.
25. Duvel K, Yecies JL, Menon S, et al. Activation of a metabolic gene regulatory network downstream of mTOR complex 1. Mol Cell. 2010;39:171–83.
26. Huang J, Manning BD. The TSC1-TSC2 complex: a molecular switchboard controlling cell growth. Biochem J. 2008;412: 179–90.
27. Kalina P, Drehobl KE, Greenberg RW, Black KS, Hyman RA. Hemorrhagic subependymal giant cell astrocytoma. Pediatr Radiol. 1995;25:66–7.
28. Waga S, Yamamoto Y, Kojima T, Sakakura M. Massive hemorrhage in tumor of tuberous sclerosis. Surg Neurol. 1977;8: 99–101.
29. Stavrinou P, Spiliotopoulos A, Patsalas I, et al. Subependymal giant cell astrocytoma with intratumoral hemorrhage in the absence of tuberous sclerosis. J Clin Neurosci. 2008;15:704–6.
30. Ogiwara H, Morota N. Subependymal giant cell astrocytoma with intratumoral hemorrhage. J Neurosurg Pediatr. 2013; 11:469–72.
31. Mork SJ, Morild I, Giertsen JC. Subependymoma and unexpected death. Forensic Sci Int. 1986;30:275–80.
32. Roach ES, Smith M, Huttenlocher P, Bhat M, Alcorn D, Hawley L. Diagnostic criteria: tuberous sclerosis complex. Report of the Diagnostic Criteria Committee of the National Tuberous Sclerosis Association. J Child Neurol. 1992;7:221–4.
33. Dabora SL, Jozwiak S, Franz DN, et al. Mutational analysis in a cohort of 224 tuberous sclerosis patients indicates increased severity of TSC2, compared with TSC1, disease in multiple organs. Am J Hum Genet. 2001;68:64–80.
34. Barkovich AJ. Pediatric neuroimaging. 3rd ed. Philadelphia: Lippincott, Williams & Wilkins; 2000.
35. Hussain N, Curran A, Pilling D, et al. Congenital subependymal giant cell astrocytoma diagnosed on fetal MRI. Arch Dis Child. 2006;91:520.
36. Katz JS, Milla SS, Wiggins GC, Devinsky O, Weiner HL, Roth J. Intraventricular lesions in tuberous sclerosis complex: a possible association with the caudate nucleus. J Neurosurg Pediatr. 2012;9:406–13.

37. Di Rocco C, Iannelli A, Marchese E. On the treatment of subependymal giant cell astrocytomas and associated hydrocephalus in tuberous sclerosis. Pediatr Neurosurg. 1995;23:115–21.
38. Osborn AG. Diagnostic neuroradiology. 1st ed. St. Louis: Mosby-Year Book; 1994.
39. Grajkowska W, Kotulska K, Jurkiewicz E, et al. Subependymal giant cell astrocytomas with atypical histological features mimicking malignant gliomas. Folia Neuropathol. 2011;49:39–46.
40. Bollo RJ, Berliner JL, Fischer I, et al. Extraventricular subependymal giant cell tumor in a child with tuberous sclerosis complex. J Neurosurg Pediatr. 2009;4:85–90.
41. Dashti SR, Robinson S, Rodgers M, Cohen AR. Pineal region giant cell astrocytoma associated with tuberous sclerosis: case report. J Neurosurg. 2005;102:322–5.
42. Jakobiec FA, Brodie SE, Haik B, Iwamoto T. Giant cell astrocytoma of the retina. A tumor of possible Mueller cell origin. Ophthalmology. 1983;90:1565–76.
43. Margo CE, Barletta JP, Staman JA. Giant cell astrocytoma of the retina in tuberous sclerosis. Retina. 1993;13:155–9.
44. Jung CS, Hubbard II GB, Grossniklaus HE. Giant cell astrocytoma of the retina in a 1-month-old infant. J Pediatr Ophthalmol Strabismus. 2009. doi:10.3928/01913913-20091019-05. Epub 2009 Nov 2.
45. Telfeian AE, Judkins A, Younkin D, Pollock AN, Crino P. Subependymal giant cell astrocytoma with cranial and spinal metastases in a patient with tuberous sclerosis. Case report. J Neurosurg. 2004;100:498–500.
46. Lopes MB, Altermatt HJ, Scheithauer BW, Shepherd CW, VandenBerg SR. Immunohistochemical characterization of subependymal giant cell astrocytomas. Acta Neuropathol. 1996; 91:368–75.
47. Roth J, Roach ES, Bartels U, et al. Subependymal giant cell astrocytoma: diagnosis, screening, and treatment. Recommendations from the International Tuberous Sclerosis Complex Consensus Conference 2012. Pediatr Neurol. 2013; 49:439–44.
48. Ekici MA, Kumandas S, Per H, et al. Surgical timing of the subependymal giant cell astrocytoma (SEGA) with the patients of tuberous sclerosis complex. Turk Neurosurg. 2011;21:315–24.
49. de Ribaupierre S, Dorfmuller G, Bulteau C, et al. Subependymal giant-cell astrocytomas in pediatric tuberous sclerosis disease: when should we operate? Neurosurgery. 2007;60:83–9; discussion 89–90.
50. Clarke MJ, Foy AB, Wetjen N, Raffel C. Imaging characteristics and growth of subependymal giant cell astrocytomas. Neurosurg Focus. 2006;20:E5.
51. Ibrahim I, Young CA, Larner AJ. Fornix damage from solitary subependymal giant cell astrocytoma causing postoperative amnesic syndrome. Br J Hosp Med (Lond). 2009;70:478–9.
52. Jiang T, Jia G, Ma Z, Luo S, Zhang Y. The diagnosis and treatment of subependymal giant cell astrocytoma combined with tuberous sclerosis. Childs Nerv Syst. 2011;27:55–62.
53. Kotulska K, Borkowska J, Roszkowski M, et al. Surgical treatment of subependymal giant cell astrocytoma in tuberous sclerosis complex patients. Pediatr Neurol. 2014;50:307–12.
54. Harter DH, Bassani L, Rodgers SD, et al. A management strategy for intraventricular subependymal giant cell astrocytomas in tuberous sclerosis complex. J Neurosurg Pediatr. 2014;13:21–8.
55. Amin S, Carter M, Edwards RJ, et al. The outcome of surgical management of subependymal giant cell astrocytoma in tuberous sclerosis complex. Eur J Paediatr Neurol. 2013;17:36–44.
56. Lawton MT, Golfinos JG, Spetzler RF. The contralateral transcallosal approach: experience with 32 patients. Neurosurgery. 1996;39:729–34; discussion 734–5.
57. Moavero R, Pinci M, Bombardieri R, Curatolo P. The management of subependymal giant cell tumors in tuberous sclerosis: a clinician's perspective. Childs Nerv Syst. 2011;27:1203–10.
58. Rodgers SD, Bassani L, Weiner HL, Harter DH. Stereotactic endoscopic resection and surgical management of a subependymal giant cell astrocytoma: case report. J Neurosurg Pediatr. 2012;9:417–20.
59. Sharma MC, Ralte AM, Gaekwad S, Santosh V, Shankar SK, Sarkar C. Subependymal giant cell astrocytoma–a clinicopathological study of 23 cases with special emphasis on histogenesis. Pathol Oncol Res. 2004;10:219–24.
60. Nagib MG, Haines SJ, Erickson DL, Mastri AR. Tuberous sclerosis: a review for the neurosurgeon. Neurosurgery. 1984;14:93–8.
61. Loewith R. A brief history of TOR. Biochem Soc Trans. 2011;39:437–42.
62. Kim DH, Sarbassov DD, Ali SM, et al. mTOR interacts with raptor to form a nutrient-sensitive complex that signals to the cell growth machinery. Cell. 2002;110:163–75.
63. Brunn GJ, Fadden P, Haystead TA, Lawrence Jr JC. The mammalian target of rapamycin phosphorylates sites having a (Ser/Thr)-Pro motif and is activated by antibodies to a region near its COOH terminus. J Biol Chem. 1997;272:32547–50.
64. Birca A, Mercier C, Major P. Rapamycin as an alternative to surgical treatment of subependymal giant cell astrocytomas in a patient with tuberous sclerosis complex. J Neurosurg Pediatr. 2010;6:381–4.
65. Franz DN, Leonard J, Tudor C, et al. Rapamycin causes regression of astrocytomas in tuberous sclerosis complex. Ann Neurol. 2006;59:490–8.
66. Franz DN, Belousova E, Sparagana S, et al. Efficacy and safety of everolimus for subependymal giant cell astrocytomas associated with tuberous sclerosis complex (EXIST-1): a multicentre, randomised, placebo-controlled phase 3 trial. Lancet. 2013; 381:125–32.
67. Krueger DA, Care MM, Holland K, et al. Everolimus for subependymal giant-cell astrocytomas in tuberous sclerosis. N Engl J Med. 2010;363:1801–11.
68. Franz DN, Agricola KD, Tudor CA, Krueger DA. Everolimus for tumor recurrence after surgical resection for subependymal giant cell astrocytoma associated with tuberous sclerosis complex. J Child Neurol. 2013;28(5):602–7.
69. Kotulska K, Chmielewski D, Borkowska J, et al. Long-term effect of everolimus on epilepsy and growth in children under 3 years of age treated for subependymal giant cell astrocytoma associated with tuberous sclerosis complex. Eur J Paediatr Neurol. 2013;17(5):479–85.
70. Pengel LH, Liu LQ, Morris PJ. Do wound complications or lymphoceles occur more often in solid organ transplant recipients on mTOR inhibitors? A systematic review of randomized controlled trials. Transpl Int. 2011;24:1216–30.
71. Sivendran S, Agarwal N, Gartrell B, et al. Metabolic complications with the use of mTOR inhibitors for cancer therapy. Cancer Treat Rev. 2014;40(1):190–6.

72. Sini P, James D, Chresta C, Guichard S. Simultaneous inhibition of mTORC1 and mTORC2 by mTOR kinase inhibitor AZD8055 induces autophagy and cell death in cancer cells. Autophagy. 2010;6:553–4.
73. Liu Q, Thoreen C, Wang J, Sabatini D, Gray NS. mTOR mediated anti-cancer drug discovery. Drug Discov Today Ther Strateg. 2009;6:47–55.
74. Park KJ, Kano H, Kondziolka D, Niranjan A, Flickinger JC, Lunsford LD. Gamma Knife surgery for subependymal giant cell astrocytomas. Clinical article. J Neurosurg. 2011;114:808–13.
75. Henderson MA, Fakiris AJ, Timmerman RD, Worth RM, Lo SS, Witt TC. Gamma knife stereotactic radiosurgery for low-grade astrocytomas. Stereotact Funct Neurosurg. 2009;87:161–7.
76. Park YG, Kim EY, Chang JW, Chung SS. Volume changes following gamma knife radiosurgery of intracranial tumors. Surg Neurol. 1997;48:488–93.
77. Matsumura H, Takimoto H, Shimada N, Hirata M, Ohnishi T, Hayakawa T. Glioblastoma following radiotherapy in a patient with tuberous sclerosis. Neurol Med Chir (Tokyo). 1998;38:287–91.
78. Shepherd CW, Gomez MR. Mortality in the Mayo Clinic Tuberous Sclerosis Complex Study. Ann N Y Acad Sci. 1991;615:375–7.
79. Zaroff CM, Barr WB, Carlson C, et al. Mental retardation and relation to seizure and tuber burden in tuberous sclerosis complex. Seizure. 2006;15:558–62.
80. Kaczorowska M, Jurkiewicz E, Domanska-Pakiela D, et al. Cerebral tuber count and its impact on mental outcome of patients with tuberous sclerosis complex. Epilepsia. 2011;52:22–7.

11 Germ Cell Tumors

Girish Dhall, Ashley A. Ibrahim, and Eyas M. Hattab

Abbreviations

AFP	Alpha-fetoprotein
βhCG	β human chorionic gonadotropin
CBTRUS	Central Brain Tumor Registry of the United States
CCKBR	Cholecystokinin B receptor
CGH	Comparative genomic hybridization
CNS	Central nervous system
CSF	Cerebrospinal fluid
FISH	Fluorescent in situ hybridization
GCTs	Germ cell tumors
hPL	Human placental lactogen
JMJD	Jumonji domain-containing
miRNA	microRNA
NGGCTs	Nongerminomatous germ cell tumors
PLAP	Placental alkaline phosphatase
qRT-PCR	Quantitative reverse transcriptase polymerase chain reaction
SNRPN	Small nuclear ribonucleoprotein polypeptide N
WES	Whole exome sequencing
WHO	World Health Organization
YST	Yolk sac tumors

Central nervous system (CNS) germ cell tumors (GCTs) are a rare and heterogeneous group of malignant tumors that occur in children and young adults. According to the Central Brain Tumor Registry of the United States (CBTRUS) 2012 Statistical Report, CNS GCTs accounted for 0.5 % of all CNS tumors in adults, 1.3 % in young adults (ages, 20–34 years), 5.1 % in patients ages 15–19 years, and 3.6 % in patients 0–14 years of age [1]. The incidence of CNS GCTs is much higher in Asian countries where it has been reported to be as high as 9–15 % [2, 3]. CNS GCTs are twice as common in males than in females and 1.5 times more common in whites than in blacks [1]. GCTs typically occur in the gonads but extragonadal sites are more common in children with brain being the most common site in older children. Within the brain, GCTs occur predominantly in the pineal and suprasellar regions with basal ganglia being the third most common location. Approximately 5–10 % of patients have bifocal tumors involving both pineal and suprasellar areas [4].

Pineal tumors tend to be more common in boys while girls have a preponderance of suprasellar tumors. Primary tumors in the suprasellar region and basal ganglia as well as bifocal tumors are more likely to be germinomas whereas nongerminomatous germ cell tumors (NGGCTs) predominate at other sites.

The World Health Organization (WHO) classification of CNS GCTs divides these tumors into germinomas and NGGCTs. NGGCTs include teratoma (mature and immature), teratoma with malignant transformation, yolk sac tumor (YST), embryonal carcinoma, choriocarcinoma, and mixed tumors. While germinomas occur as pure tumors in 60–65 % of cases, nongerminomatous tumors more frequently occur as mixed tumors, which most commonly include germinoma and teratoma along with more malignant elements [5]. Hence, the term NGGCT is a misnomer in this sense and some investigators prefer to use the term mixed malignant germ cell tumors (MMGCT).

Histopathology

Germinoma

The classic germinoma is histologically identical to ovarian dysgerminomas and testicular seminomas comprising large monomorphous tumor cells separated into lobules by thin fibrous septa (Fig. 11.1). The septa contain varying amounts

M.A. Karajannis and D. Zagzag (eds.), *Molecular Pathology of Nervous System Tumors: Biological Stratification and Targeted Therapies*, Molecular Pathology Library 8,
DOI 10.1007/978-1-4939-1830-0_11, © Springer Science+Business Media New York 2015

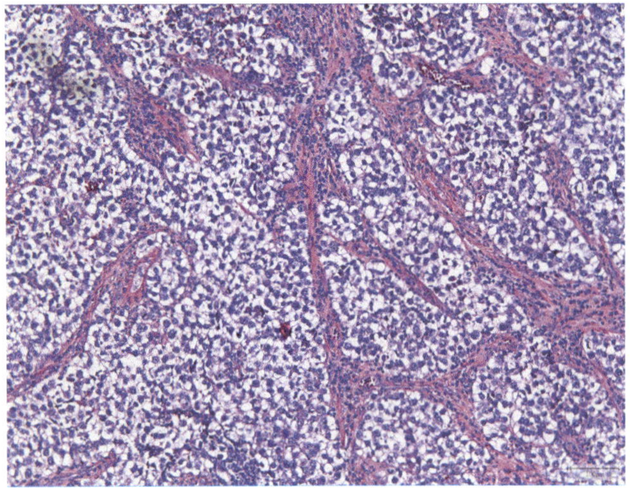

Fig. 11.1. Germinoma. Large monomorphous tumor cells separated into lobules by thin fibrous septa.

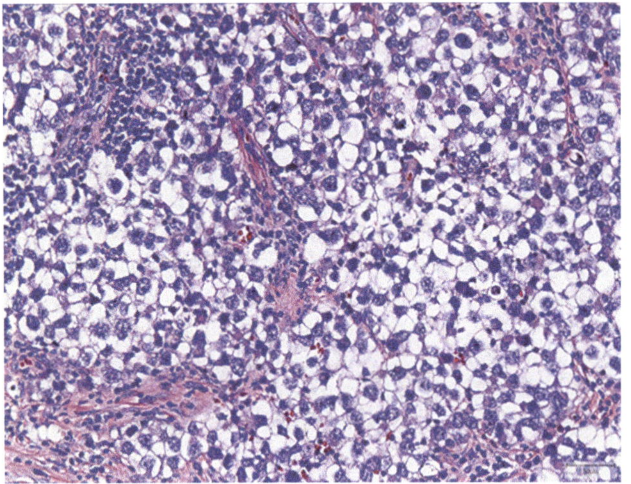

Fig. 11.2. Germinoma. Tumor cells have "squared off" nuclei, abundant clear cytoplasm, and distinct cell borders.

of T lymphocytes and occasionally noncaseating granulomas. In well-preserved, formalin-fixed samples, tumor cells have abundant clear or vacuolated cytoplasm, reflecting their high glycogen content and distinct cell borders. The nuclei are centrally located and have a squared-off appearance (Fig. 11.2). A single conspicuous nucleolus is characteristic. Both individual cell and confluent necrosis can be seen. Calcifications and syncytiotrophoblastic giant cells are additional infrequently encountered phenomena (Fig. 11.3). The latter may be responsible for trace levels of β human chorionic gonadotropin (βhCG) in the cerebrospinal fluid (CSF) but should not be confused with choriocarcinoma where a solid proliferation of syncytiotrophoblasts and cytotrophoblasts is needed for the diagnosis (see below).

Of practical significance is the fact that these tumors are not easily surgically accessible, often yielding very small

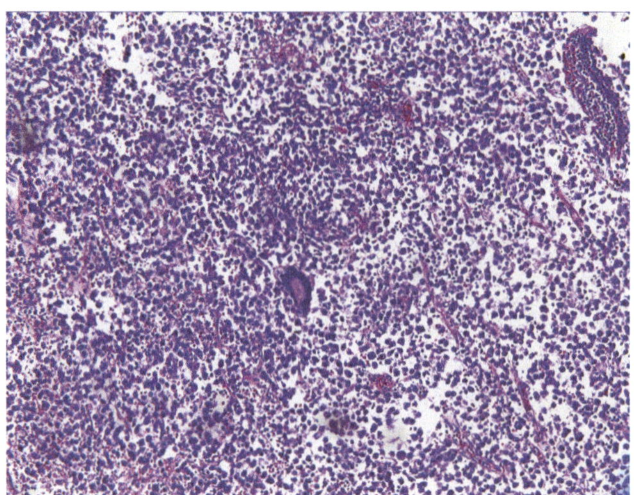

Fig. 11.3. Germinoma. Note the syncytiotrophoblastic giant cell.

samples. As such, in samples where the lymphocytic infiltrate predominates, the diagnostic tumor cells may be obscured and difficult to identify on hematoxylin and eosin-stained sections. Other samples may show an unusual single cell infiltration of the juxtaposed brain parenchyma similar to malignant gliomas or lymphomas. Such scenarios underscore the necessity of routinely employing immunohistochemical studies, including GCT markers, in the work-up of midline CNS lesions.

Yolk Sac Tumor

In contrast to germinomas, yolk sac tumors rarely occur in pure form. More commonly, they are a component of a mixed germ cell tumor. Cytologically, neoplastic cells are large and polygonal in shape with faint eosinophilic or clear cytoplasm and well-defined cytoplasmic borders. Nuclei are moderately atypical, but generally lack marked pleomorphism (Fig. 11.4). Tufts of malignant cuboidal-to-columnar tumor cells surrounding central blood vessels, known as Schiller-Duval bodies, are common though not universal, and not necessary for the diagnosis. The characteristic intercellular and extracellular PAS-positive/diastase-resistant eosinophilic hyaline globules and intercellular longitudinal bands of eosinophilic basement membrane material offer additional diagnostic clues.

Perhaps the most consistent finding in yolk sac tumors is the variety of different morphologic patterns often encountered within the same tumor; a mixture of patterns is the rule (Figs. 11.4 and 11.5). The most common among these is the *reticular* or *microcystic* pattern consisting of cysts lined by a loose network of flattened-to-cuboidal cells. A *macrocystic* pattern is seen when the microcysts coalesce. The *polyvesicular vitelline* pattern displays larger vesicles lined by flat-to-columnar epithelial cells. The *endodermal sinus* pattern shows a predominance of Schiller-Duval bodies and the *papillary* pattern shows papillae rimmed with

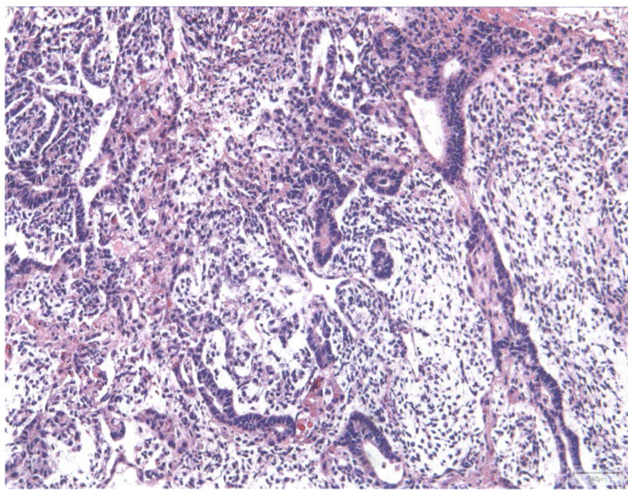

FIG. 11.4. Yolk sac tumor. Microcystic pattern.

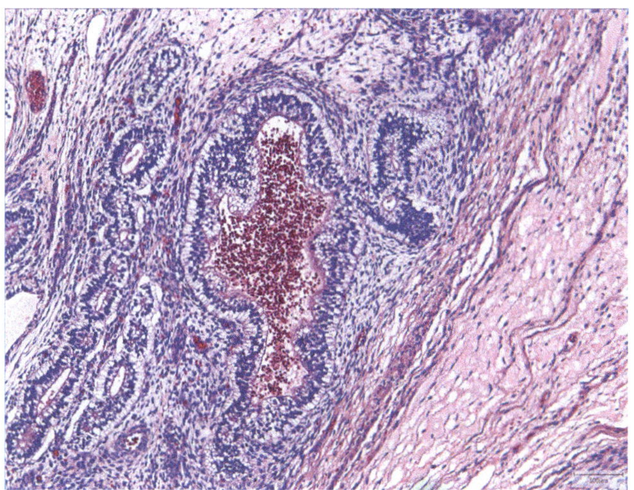

FIG. 11.5. Yolk sac tumor. Glandular pattern.

tumor cells. Clusters of liver-like tumor cells are seen in the *hepatoid* pattern and neoplastic cells embedded in a matrix of basement membrane-rich material are evidence of *parietal* differentiation. *Glandular*, *myxomatous*, *solid*, and *sarcomatoid* patterns are often found in association with the aforementioned patterns.

Embryonal Carcinoma

Tumor cells are highly atypical and are generally larger, more pleomorphic, and more carcinoma-like than those of germinoma (Fig. 11.6). Nuclei are oval-to-round and hyperchromatic with irregular nuclear contours and large single or multiple nucleoli. Their cytoplasm is fairly abundant, somewhat granular, and variably staining. Cytoplasmic borders are not well defined, accounting for the syncytial appearance of the tumor (Fig. 11.7). The malignant cells can be arranged in solid sheets, cords, papillae, or gland-like patterns. The

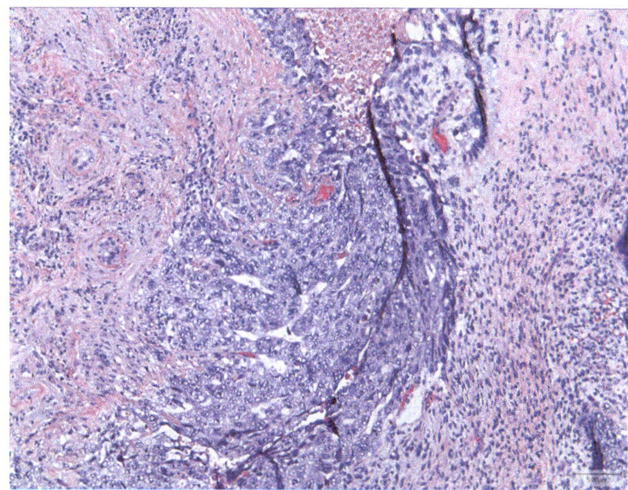

FIG. 11.6. Embryonal carcinoma. Tumor cells are larger than those of germinoma and more carcinoma-like.

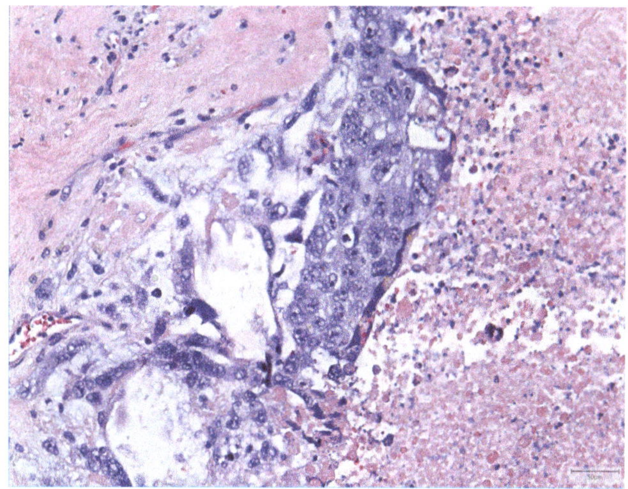

FIG. 11.7. Embryonal carcinoma. Tumor cells show oval-to-round hyperchromatic nuclei with large nucleoli.

so-called *appliqué* pattern, characterized by smudged, degenerate-appearing cells seen towards the periphery of tumor nests, imparts a superficial resemblance to choriocarcinoma. Necrosis is common and the mitotic rate is typically high. As with germinomas, syncytiotrophoblastic giant cells are not an infrequent finding. Small foci of neoplastic poorly differentiated stroma, considered by some investigators to be teratomatous in nature, may accompany embryonal carcinoma and account for chemotherapy failure.

Teratoma

Akin to their gonadal counterparts, teratomas of the CNS can comprise both mature and immature elements. Pure mature teratomas tend to behave in an indolent fashion whereas teratomas occurring as part of a mixed GCT are more aggressive

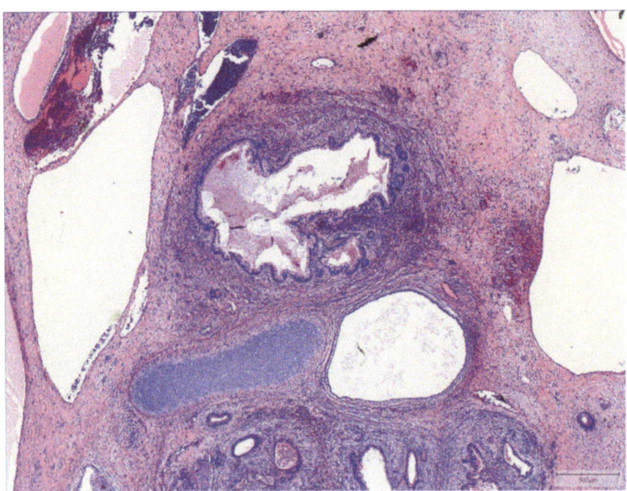

Fig. 11.8 Mature teratoma. Mature teratomas are made up of an admixture of differentiated tissues from more than one germ cell layer.

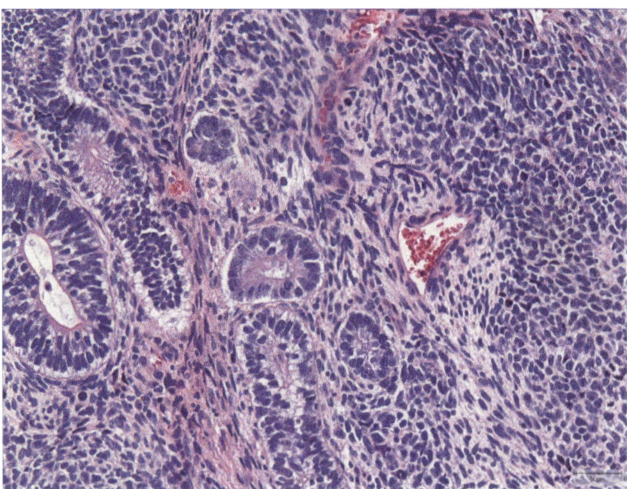

Fig. 11.9. Immature teratoma. Immature teratomas contain tissues that resemble primitive embryonic tissues. Note the immature neuroepithelium.

regardless of their degree of maturity. Their biologic behavior, thus, is likened to that of ovarian teratomas. Congenital teratomas, on the other hand, have a universally poor prognosis regardless of their composition.

Mature Teratoma

Mature teratomas are made up of an admixture of differentiated, adult-type tissues from more than one germ cell layer (Fig. 11.8). Skin and glial tissue are common ectodermal components and enteric, respiratory or transitional type tissues account for endodermal derivation. Focal increased cellularity, mitotic activity, and/or moderate cellular atypia are acceptable and should not prompt a diagnosis of immature teratoma, nor should the presence of "fetal" type tissues (e.g., fetal cartilage). The diagnosis of immaturity, rather, should only be made when tissues closely resemble embryonal (not fetal) type tissues (see below).

Immature Teratoma

Immature teratomas, by definition, contain varying amounts of incompletely differentiated tissues that resemble primitive embryonic tissues (Fig. 11.9). Most commonly, the immature tissue shows neural differentiation with rosette or tubule formation (i.e., primitive or embryonic-type neuroepithelium). Blastomatous-type stroma, consisting of small, round-to-spindled cells with hyperchromatic nuclei, apoptosis, and increased mitoses, is frequently encountered surrounding small, immature glands. Increased mitoses and apoptosis are not features of mature tissue, and can be helpful clues to the identification of immature elements. Any amount of immature component, no matter how small, is sufficient to render the diagnosis of immature teratoma. Following the convention of their ovarian counterparts, some observers choose to quantify the volume of the immature component and assign a grade (grade I–III) based on this volume. While the grading of immature teratomas in the ovary has documented prognostic significance, this has not been proven in the CNS to date. It is worth noting that maturation of a previously treated teratoma is a phenomenon often encountered secondary to effects of chemotherapy and irradiation. Conversely, malignant transformation of mature teratoma after treatment has also been documented [6].

Congenital Teratoma

Congenital teratomas are the most common neonatal brain tumor and, by definition, occur within the first 60 days of life [7, 8]. Although, they are histologically similar to those occurring later in life, key differences exist. First and foremost is their location. In contrast to the infratentorial teratomas of older children, congenital teratomas are predominantly supratentorial. Due to their large size, however, a precise determination of their site of origin is often difficult [9]. Secondly, congenital teratomas are generally pure, either mature or immature. Finally, congenital teratomas carry a dismal prognosis (>90 % mortality rate) while those occurring in older children generally have a much better clinical outcome [8].

Choriocarcinoma

Choriocarcinomas are the most malignant GCTs but are, fortuitously, the least common among the primary tumors. They are extensively hemorrhagic and highly necrotic tumors comprising of two cell types: syncytiotrophoblasts and cytotrophoblasts (Fig. 11.10). Syncytiotrophoblasts are easily recognized as large multinucleated cells with smudged vesicular nuclei and dark eosinophilic-to-amphophilic cytoplasm. Cytotrophoblasts are more uniform and have single

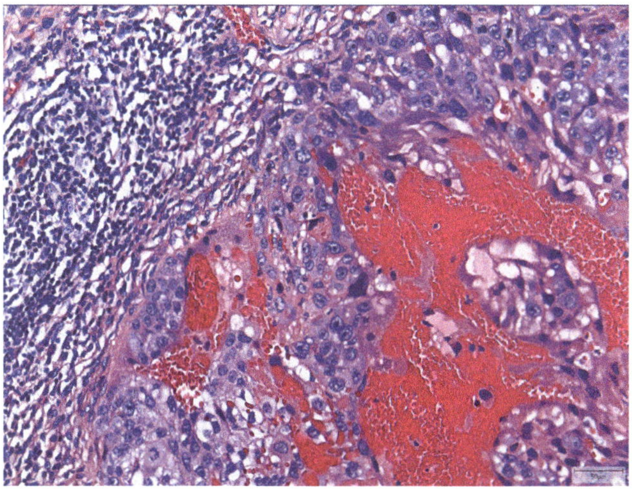

FIG. 11.10 Choriocarcinoma. Tumors show extensive hemorrhage and necrosis with recognizable syncytiotrophoblasts and cytotrophoblasts.

bland nuclei with vesicular chromatin and pale-to-amphophilic cytoplasm. Cytoplasmic borders are distinct. Syncytiotrophoblasts and cytotrophoblasts are arranged in a biphasic plexiform pattern similar to that seen in chorionic villi where sheets of cytotrophoblasts are surrounded (caped) by syncytiotrophoblasts. Mitoses are easily identifiable in the cytotrophoblastic component, but occur only exceptionally in syncytiotrophoblasts. Rarely, the cytotrophoblastic component dominates. This monomorphic pattern, which can be seen following chemotherapy, may be difficult to recognize and often requires immunohistochemical confirmation. As discussed earlier, it is important to recognize that scattered syncytiotrophoblasts are not uncommonly encountered in other GCTs and their presence alone is not diagnostic of choriocarcinoma.

Mixed Germ Cell Tumors

As previously mentioned, mixed germ cell tumors comprise two or more of the previously described histologic variants. The relative percentage of each component should be reported. It is recommended that the tissue be, at minimum, extensively sampled if not entirely embedded to avoid underreporting of a GCT component.

Ancillary Immunohistochemical Studies

Routine use of ancillary immunohistochemical studies is standard of practice in the work-up of primary CNS GCTs. The most historically utilized immunostain in GCTs, placental alkaline phosphatase (PLAP), is now obsolete and has been replaced by superior, more specific and sensitive transcription markers, such as OCT4 [10]. OCT4 preferentially highlights germinomas and embryonal carcinomas and has the added advantage of being a nuclear marker

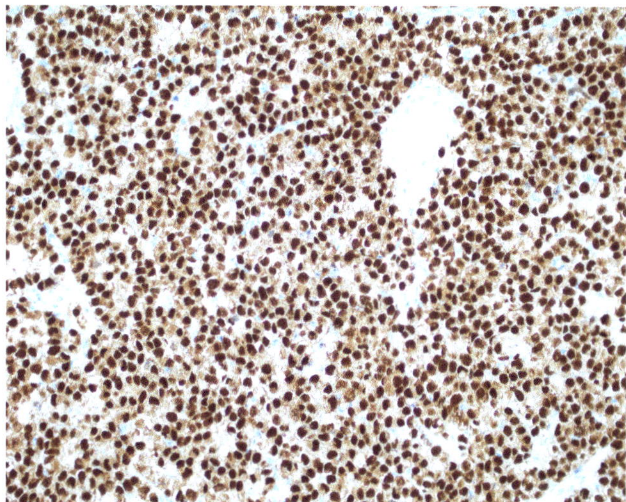

FIG. 11.11. Germinoma. OCT4 immunohistochemistry shows strong nuclear staining.

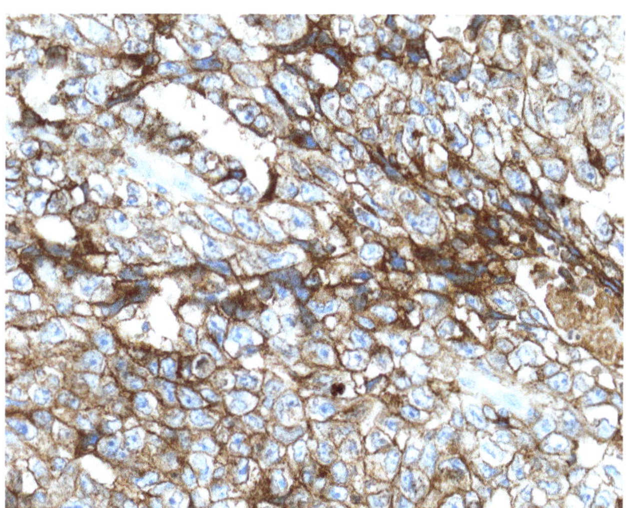

FIG. 11.12. Embryonal carcinoma. CD30 immunostain shows strong membranous staining.

allowing for easier interpretation (Fig. 11.11). CD30 shows strong membranous staining in embryonal carcinomas while other GCTs, including germinomas, are negative (Fig. 11.12). C-kit can also be exploited in the differential diagnosis of embryonal carcinoma versus germinoma as it shows strong and diffuse membranous staining in germinoma but focal or weak cytoplasmic staining in embryonal carcinomas [11–13].

SALL4 appears to be a fairly sensitive and specific pan-germ cell marker and can be used as a screening marker. A recent study by Mei et al. demonstrated 100 % sensitivity for germinomas, embryonal carcinomas, and yolk sac tumors (Fig. 11.13) [14]. Additionally, positive staining was observed in approximately two-thirds of teratomas and

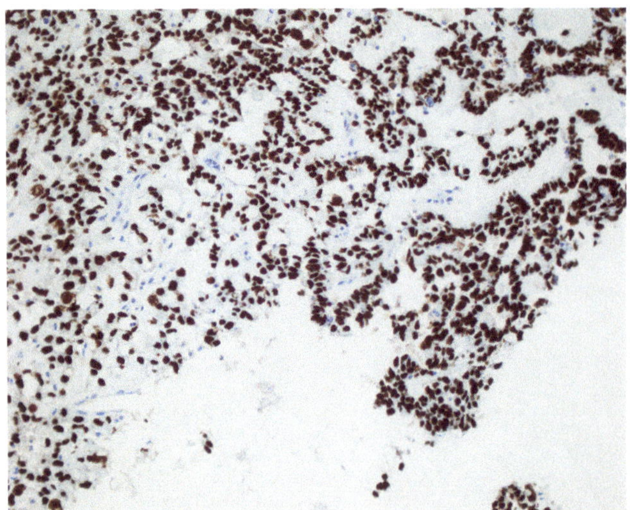

Fig. 11.13. Yolk sac tumor. SALL4, a pan-germ cell marker, shows strong nuclear staining.

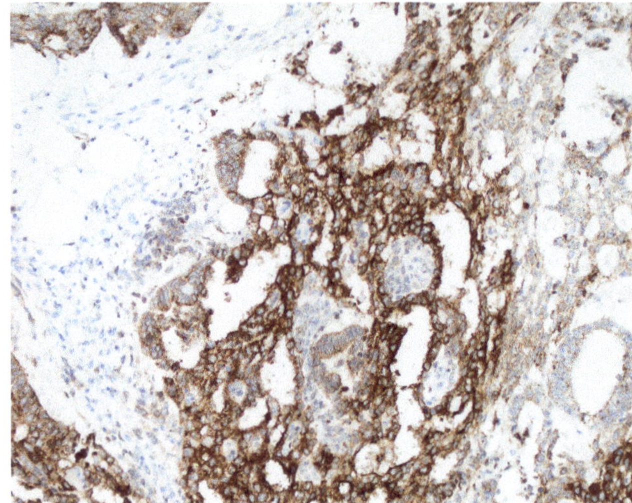

Fig. 11.14. Yolk sac tumor. Glypican 3 immunostain shows cytoplasmic staining.

choriocarcinomas; all non-GCTs were negative for SALL4 staining [14].

Alpha-fetoprotein (AFP) has historically served as the marker of choice for yolk sac tumors. Staining, however, is often focal and patchy and generally varies among the different patterns of tumors. Additionally, abundant background staining is often observed [14]. Glypican-3 is touted as a more superior marker in diagnosing yolk sac tumors of the ovaries and testes. Glypican-3 offers more precise and easy to interpret staining characteristics as well as improved sensitivity (Fig. 11.14) [15]. Studies evaluating glypican-3 staining in CNS yolk sac tumors, however, are limited.

βhCG and human placental lactogen (hPL) strongly stain the syncytiotrophoblastic cells of choriocarcinomas as well as those intermixed with other germ cell tumors [16, 17]. Cytotrophoblastic cells often are weakly positive or negative for these markers. Additionally, cytokeratins can also be used to highlight choriocarcinomas.

Histogenesis

GCTs are thought to arise from progenitor germ cells, mainly due to the facts that the germinoma component resembles progenitor cells very closely, intracranial GCTs resemble their extracranial counterparts morphologically and immunophenotypically, a single tumor can have multiple components (mixed GCTs) suggestive of differentiation of progenitor cells along various lines (embryonic and extraembryonic), and because none of the progenitor cells in the brain share any morphologic features with CNS GCTs. It is hypothesized that aberrant migration of the germ cell progenitors ventrally along the midline is responsible for the predominant midline location of these tumors throughout the body. Both testicular and CNS GCTs have been shown to have overexpression of wild type p53 and MDM2 proteins with a low incidence of TP53 gene mutation and a moderate incidence of MDM2 gene amplification pointing towards a common origin of these tumors [18]. Since $p14^{ARF}$, a protein coded by the *INK4a/ARF* gene locus, functions as a tumor suppressor and regulates the interaction between the MDM2 and p53 proteins by stimulating degradation of MDM2, Iwato et al. further tested for gene mutations in the *INK4a/ARF* gene in 21 CNS GCTs. They found that 71 % of tumors (90 % of germinomas and 55 % of NGGCTs) had either a homozygous deletion (14/15) or a frameshift mutation (1/15) in this gene pointing towards a more central role for this protein in the development of CNS GCTs [19]. More evidence linking germ cell progenitors to CNS GCTs is the lack of methylation seen in gonadal and extragonadal GCTs, since the progenitor cells transiently lose methylation of imprinted genes during migration. Small nuclear ribonucleoprotein polypeptide N (*SNRPN*) is an imprinted gene with complete lack of methylation, which is common to GCTs and progenitor cells. However, Lee et al. showed that lack of methylation of *SNRPN* and other imprinted genes is also seen in neural stem cells in the brain providing an alternate hypothesis about the origin of CNS GCTs [20].

Cytogenetics and Molecular Genetics

Little is known about the molecular biology of CNS GCTs. The overwhelming majority of intracranial GCTs are sporadic; however, a few conditions including Klinefelter syndrome and Down syndrome show higher incidence. Based on the predisposition of GCTs in patients with Klinefelter syndrome, Okada and colleagues studied 25 CNS GCTs with fluorescent in situ hybridization (FISH) for X and Y chromosomes and other chromosomal abnormalities described in systemic GCTs [21]. They found extra copies of the X chromosome in 23 of 25 cases. They showed that extra X chromosomes were hypomethylated in nearly all tumors irrespective of histology, suggesting that these were active X chromosomes with some potential role in the etiology of these tumors [21]. Schneider et al. performed chromosomal comparative genomic hybridization (CGH) analysis on tumor samples from 19 CNS GCT patients (ages, newborn to 25 years; median age, 11.5 years) and then compared these to the CGH profiles of gonadal and extragonadal GCTs. All 15 malignant CNS GCTs had chromosomal imbalance with average number of imbalances being higher in NGGCTs than germinomas and CGH profiles of CNS GCTs being identical to gonadal/extragonadal GCTs. Gain of 12p was the most commonly detected abnormality (11 of 19 tumors and 10 of 15 malignant CNS GCTs). Other chromosomal imbalances detected included 1q gain (1q 21-24) and 8q11-21 gain [22]. In another study, chromosome 12 abnormalities, including 12p gain and isochromosome 12p formation were found at very high frequencies in CNS germinomas (96 % and 57 %, respectively), but only in 20–40 % of cases in others [21–24].

Gene Expression Profiling

Palmer et al. performed gene expression analysis on 27 pediatric malignant GCTs, including 3 CNS GCTs (2 germinomas and 1 YST), and showed that malignant YSTs had a completely different gene expression signature than testicular seminomas [25]. Self-renewing pluripotency genes (*Nanog*, *OCT3/4*, and *UTF*) were overexpressed in seminomas and genes responsible for tumor growth (cholecystokinin B receptor [*CCKBR*]) and differentiation (*KRT19*, *KRT8*, *GATA3*, and *GATA6*), and genes involved in WNT/β-catenin pathway were upregulated in yolk sac tumors. There were no significant differences in gene expression between CNS GCTs of similar histology arising at different sites and different ages within the pediatric age group. In addition, pediatric and adult testicular YSTs exhibited significantly different gene expression signatures suggesting different biologic behavior [25].

MicroRNAs (miRNAs) are responsible for controlling gene expression and also function as oncogenes as well as tumor suppressor genes within tumor cells. Palmer et al. studied miRNA profiles of 32 pediatric GCTs (gonadal and extragonadal), eight control samples, two adult testicular seminomas, and six GCT cell lines [26]. In unsupervised hierarchical clustering analysis, all pediatric GCT samples showed clear separation with seminomas, cell lines, YSTs, and embryonal carcinomas all having clearly different miRNA expression profiles. There was no overlap between malignant and nonmalignant (mature and immature teratoma) GCTs on a heat map based on differentially expressed miRNAs. Nine of the top ten differentially expressed miRNAs belonged to two clusters (miRNA-371 and miRNA-302) and were overexpressed in malignant GCTs compared to nonmalignant GCTs. Similar to gene expression profile, miRNA expression pattern was comparable in various histologic subtypes irrespective of patient age. Both of these miRNA clusters have been shown to be associated with human embryonic stem cells and their overexpression in turn regulates the expression of various transcription factors involved in oncogenesis and malignant progression. They further showed that YSTs and germinomas had a significantly different miRNA expression profile with members of the miRNA-2302 cluster overexpressed in YSTs compared to germinomas resulting in overexpression of transcription factors such as *GATA6*, *GATA3*, *SMARCA1*, and *SOX11*. They further showed that miRNA-451 and miRNA-144 were significantly overexpressed in intracranial compared to extracranial germinomas and miRNA-320, miRNA-487b, and miRNA-491-3p were significantly underexpressed [26].

Murray et al. used TaqMan® quantitative reverse transcriptase polymerase chain reaction (qRT-PCR) to measure miRNA levels in the serum of a 4-year-old boy with a sacrococcygeal mixed GCT with a predominant YST component (AFP 82, 420 kU/L) at diagnosis and followed the levels during treatment. miRNA-71~373 and miRNA-302 were significantly overexpressed in the patient's serum when compared to three healthy controls. miRNA-372 and miRNA-373 levels were 703 and 192 times higher, respectively. The level of miRNA-372 dropped to 5.8-fold higher on day 73 (serum AFP, 5.8), 2.2-fold higher on day 91 (serum AFP, 6), and <1-fold higher on all subsequent follow-up time points (serum AFP, <2) [27]. Terashima and colleagues examined 32 CSF samples from 22 intracranial GCT patients for expression of miRNA-371–373 and miRNA-302–367 clusters. Significantly higher expression levels were found in CSF of GCT patients compared to controls, as well as pretreatment samples compared to those collected during or after treatment. In addition, miRNA-373 expression was significantly higher in germinomas when compared to NGGCTs [28]. These two publications highlighted for the first time the potential for using miRNAs as diagnostic and/or therapeutic biomarkers for CNS GCTs.

Prognostic Stratification and Treatment

The histologic subtype of the tumor remains the best predictor of prognosis in CNS GCTs. Germinomas are sensitive to chemotherapy as well as radiotherapy. Patients with germinoma have been shown to have survival rates in excess of 90 % with craniospinal irradiation (CSI) followed by a boost to the primary site to 50 Gy [29, 30]. However, due to the deleterious long-term side-effects of irradiation on the developing brains of young children, treatment strategies involving upfront chemotherapy along with reduced dose and volume of irradiation have been utilized by multiple cooperative groups all across the world with similar survival statistics.

[31–33] βhCG-producing germinomas (i.e., germinomas with syncytiotrophoblasts) have been shown by some to have a higher recurrence rate than for pure germinomas, justifying a more aggressive treatment approach [34, 35]. However, other studies have shown no difference [36]. The current Children's Oncology Group (COG) study, ACNS1123, is utilizing a treatment approach using carboplatin and etoposide for four cycles followed by low-dose ventricular field irradiation (1,800 cGy whole ventricular irradiation with a boost to a total dose of 3,000 cGy to the primary site) for patients with non-disseminated disease in the pineal or the suprasellar region.

Unlike germinomas, CNS NGGCTs are more resistant to therapy and using irradiation-only strategies resulted in survival figures of only 20–40 % at 5 years [4, 37, 38]. Chemotherapy combined with irradiation is currently considered the standard of care for NGGCTs, with the exception of mature teratomas. Recently closed COG study, ACNS0122, treated CNS NGGCT patients with six cycles of chemotherapy (cycles of carboplatin and etoposide alternating with cycles of ifosfamide and etoposide) followed by full-dose CSI to 3,600 cGy and a boost of 5,400 cGy to the primary tumor site, which resulted in 2-year event-free survival (EFS) and overall survival (OS) of 84 % and 93 %, respectively. Patients with localized disease who achieved a complete response (CR) or partial response (PR; >65 % reduction in the size of the primary tumor radiologically and negative tumor markers) had a 2-year EFS and OS of 91.6 % and 98 %, respectively [39]. Based on these results, the currently open COG study, ACNS1123, is attempting to reduce the dose and field of irradiation (from 3,600 cGy CSI to 3,000 cGy ventricular field irradiation) in patients who achieve either a CR or PR to induction chemotherapy (similar to ACNS0122). Mature teratomas are treated by total surgical resection with 5-year survival rates as high as 93 % [35]. Patients with immature teratomas often require additional therapy following gross total resection. Some recommend the use of local or partial brain field radiation while others advocate aggressive surgical resection alone for "low-grade" immature teratomas and adjuvant chemotherapy and radiotherapy for those with "high-grade" histology [40, 41]. Massive intracranial congenital teratomas are almost universally fatal.

Molecular Signaling Pathways and Targeted Therapies

Japanese intracranial GCT consortium performed whole exome sequencing (WES) on 33 CNS GCTs. *KIT* mutations were the most commonly found abnormality, predominantly in germinomas. Mutations in *MTOR*, *NF1*, and *EGFR* genes were found in tumors negative for *KIT* mutations [42]. Wang et al. performed WES on 28 CNS GCTs (12 germinomas, 12 NGGCTs, and 4 mixed GCTs) [43]. *KIT* mutations were present in 38 % of cases with mutations in *KIT* and *RAS* being mutually exclusive. Mutations in tumor suppressor genes such as *TP53*, *PTEN*, and *PTCH1* were found in 21 % of cases. The authors reported for the first time a significant enrichment in Jumonji domain-containing (*JMJD*) genes in 39 % of the cases [43]. *JMJD* family proteins are a group of histone demethylases that are involved in fundamental processes such as transcription regulation and DNA repair [44]. Fukushima et al. screened 52 CNS GCTs (30 germinomas, 9 teratomas, 12 mixed GCTs, and 1 YST) for mutations in genes involved in MAPK pathway and detected mutations only in *KIT* and *RAS* genes [45]. These mutations were more frequent in germinomas (60 %) versus NGGCTs and were again mutually exclusive. Interestingly, c-kit expression by immunohistochemistry was present in all germinomas regardless of the mutation status [45]. These studies demonstrating alterations in several signal transduction pathways that might play a role in the pathogenesis of CNS GCTs might provide molecular targets for development of novel therapeutic agents in the future.

Osorio and colleagues reported on six patients with CNS GCTs (five pure germinomas and one mixed CNS GCT with predominant germinoma components), who were treated with dasatinib (KIT inhibitor) in an effort to avoid irradiation and/or to delay recurrence [46]. The study could not directly assess the efficacy of dasatinib in this population, since most patients received dasatinib while they were in a minimal residual disease state, i.e., no evaluable target lesions on imaging. However, only 33 % of patients received irradiation in conventional dosing, suggesting a possible role for targeted therapy with KIT inhibitors in combination with chemotherapy with or without irradiation [46].

References

1. Dolecek TA, Propp JM, Stroup NE, Kruchko C. CBTRUS statistical report: primary brain and central nervous system tumors diagnosed in the United States in 2005–2009. Neuro Oncol. 2012;14 Suppl 5:v1–49.
2. Kamoshima Y, Sawamura Y. Update on current standard treatments in central nervous system germ cell tumors. Curr Opin Neurol. 2010;23(6):571–5.
3. Matsutani M, Sano K, Takakura K, Fujimaki T, Nakamura O, Funata N, et al. Primary intracranial germ cell tumors: a clinical analysis of 153 histologically verified cases. J Neurosurg. 1997;86(3):446–55.
4. Jennings MT, Gelman R, Hochberg F. Intracranial germ-cell tumors: natural history and pathogenesis. J Neurosurg. 1985;63(2):155–67.
5. Rosenblum MK, Nakazato Y, Matsutani M. CNS germ cell tumors. In: Louis DN, Oghaki H, Wiestler OD, Cavenee WK, editors. WHO classification of tumours of the central nervous system. 4th ed. Lyon: IARC Press; 2007. p. 197–204.
6. Motzer RJ, Amsterdam A, Prieto V, Sheinfeld J, Murty VV, Mazumdar M, et al. Teratoma with malignant transformation: diverse malignant histologies arising in men with germ cell tumors. J Urol. 1998;159(1):133–8.

7. Raisanen JM, Davis RL. Congenital brain tumors. Pathology (Phila). 1993;2(1):103–16.
8. Isaacs Jr H. I. Perinatal brain tumors: a review of 250 cases. Pediatr Neurol. 2002;27(4):249–61.
9. Buetow PC, Smirniotopoulos JG, Done S. Congenital brain tumors: a review of 45 cases. AJR Am J Roentgenol. 1990;155(3):587–93.
10. Hattab EM, Tu PH, Wilson JD, Cheng L. OCT4 immunohistochemistry is superior to placental alkaline phosphatase (PLAP) in the diagnosis of central nervous system germinoma. Am J Surg Pathol. 2005;29(3):368–71.
11. Hattab EM, Tu P, Wilson JD, Cheng L. C-kit and HER2/neu expression in primary intracranial germinoma (abstract). J Neuropathol Exp Neurol. 2004;63(5):547.
12. Iczkowski KA, Butler SL, Shanks JH, Hossain D, Schall A, Meiers I, et al. Trials of new germ cell immunohistochemical stains in 93 extragonadal and metastatic germ cell tumors. Hum Pathol. 2008;39(2):275–81.
13. Takeshima H, Kaji M, Uchida H, Hirano H, Kuratsu J. Expression and distribution of c-kit receptor and its ligand in human CNS germ cell tumors: a useful histological marker for the diagnosis of germinoma. Brain Tumor Pathol. 2004;21(1):13–6.
14. Mei K, Liu A, Allan RW, Wang P, Lane Z, Abel TW, et al. Diagnostic utility of SALL4 in primary germ cell tumors of the central nervous system: a study of 77 cases. Mod Pathol. 2009;22(12):1628–36.
15. Zynger DL, McCallum JC, Luan C, Chou PM, Yang XJ. Glypican 3 has a higher sensitivity than alpha-fetoprotein for testicular and ovarian yolk sac tumour: immunohistochemical investigation with analysis of histological growth patterns. Histopathology. 2010;56(6):750–7.
16. Ho DM, Liu HC. Primary intracranial germ cell tumor. Pathologic study of 51 patients. Cancer. 1992;70(6):1577–84.
17. Inoue HK, Naganuma H, Ono N. Pathobiology of intracranial germ-cell tumors: immunochemical, immunohistochemical, and electron microscopic investigations. J Neurooncol. 1987;5(2):105–15.
18. Iwato M, Tachibana O, Tohma Y, et al. Molecular analysis for p53 and mdm2 in intracranial germ cell tumors. Acta Neuropathol. 2000;99:21–5.
19. Iwato M, Tachibana O, Tohma Y, et al. Alterations of the INK4a/ARF locus in human intracranial germ cell tumors. Cancer Res. 2000;60:2113–5.
20. Lee SH, Appleby V, Jeyapalan JN, Palmer RD, Nicholson JC, Sottile V, et al. Variable methylation of the imprinted gene, SNRPN, supports a relationship between intracranial germ cell tumours and neural stem cells. J Neurooncol. 2011;101(3):419–28.
21. Okada Y, Nishikawa R, Matsutani M, Louis DN. Hypomethylated X chromosome gain and rare isochromosome 12p in diverse intracranial germ cell tumors. J Neuropathol Exp Neurol. 2002;61(6):531–8.
22. Schneider DT, Zahn S, Sievers S, Alemazkour K, Reifenberger G, Wiestler OD, et al. Molecular genetic analysis of central nervous system germ cell tumors with comparative genomic hybridization. Mod Pathol. 2006;19(6):864–73.
23. Rickert CH, Simon R, Bergmann M, Dockhorn-Dworniczak B, Paulus W. Comparative genomic hybridization in pineal germ cell tumors. J Neuropathol Exp Neurol. 2000;59(9):815–21.
24. Hattab EM, Zhang SB, Wilson JD, Tu PH, Cheng L. Chromosome 12p abnormalities in germinoma of the central nervous system: A FISH analysis of 23 cases (abstract). Brain Pathol. 2006;16 Suppl 1:S155.
25. Palmer RD, Barbosa-Morais NL, Gooding EL, Muralidhar B, Thornton CM, Pett MR, et al. Pediatric malignant germ cell tumors show characteristic transcriptome profiles. Cancer Res. 2008;68(11):4239–47.
26. Palmer RD, Murray MJ, Saini HK, van Dongen S, Abreu-Goodger C, Muralidhar B, et al. Malignant germ cell tumors display common microRNA profiles resulting in global changes in expression of messenger RNA targets. Cancer Res. 2010;70(7):2911–23.
27. Murray MJ, Halsall DJ, Hook CE, Williams DM, Nicholson JC, Coleman N. Identification of microRNAs From the miR-371~373 and miR-302 clusters as potential serum biomarkers of malignant germ cell tumors. Am J Clin Pathol. 2011;135(1):119–25.
28. Terashima KS J, Luan J, Yu A, Suzuki T, Nishikawa R, Matsutani M, et al., eds. microRNA 371-373 and 302A in cerebrospinal fluid are potential tumor-derived biomarkers for intracranial germ cell tumors. 3rd International CNS Germ Cell Tumor Symposium; Cambridge; 2013.
29. Shibamoto Y, Abe M, Yamashita J, Takahashi M, Hiraoka M, Ono K, et al. Treatment results of intracranial germinoma as a function of the irradiated volume. Int J Radiat Oncol Biol Phys. 1988;15(2):285–90.
30. Aoyama H, Shirato H, Kakuto Y, Inakoshi H, Nishio M, Yoshida H, et al. Pathologically-proven intracranial germinoma treated with radiation therapy. Radiother Oncol. 1998;47(2):201–5.
31. Khatua S, Dhall G, O'Neil S, Jubran R, Villablanca JG, Marachelian A, et al. Treatment of primary CNS germinomatous germ cell tumors with chemotherapy prior to reduced dose whole ventricular and local boost irradiation. Pediatr Blood Cancer. 2010;55(1):42–6.
32. Matsutani M. Long-term followup of germinomas treated by ventricular irradiation with 24 Gy and concurrently administered carboplatin and etoposide chemotherapy [abstract GCT 02]. Neuro Oncol. 2010;12(6):ii28.
33. Calaminus G, Kortmann R, Worch J, Nicholson JC, Alapetite C, Garre ML, et al. SIOP CNS GCT 96: final report of outcome of a prospective, multinational nonrandomized trial for children and adults with intracranial germinoma, comparing craniospinal irradiation alone with chemotherapy followed by focal primary site irradiation for patients with localized disease. Neuro Oncol. 2013;15(6):788–96.
34. Sawamura Y, Ikeda J, Shirato H, Tada M, Abe H. Germ cell tumours of the central nervous system: treatment consideration based on 111 cases and their long-term clinical outcomes. Eur J Cancer. 1998;34(1):104–10.
35. Sano K. So-called intracranial germ cell tumours: are they really of germ cell origin? Br J Neurosurg. 1995;9(3):391–401.
36. Ogawa K, Shikama N, Toita T, Nakamura K, Uno T, Onishi H, et al. Long-term results of radiotherapy for intracranial germinoma: a multi-institutional retrospective review of 126 patients. Int J Radiat Oncol Biol Phys. 2004;58(3):705–13.
37. Dearnaley DP, A'Hern RP, Whittaker S, Bloom HJ. Pineal and CNS germ cell tumors: Royal Marsden Hospital experience 1962–1987. Int J Radiat Oncol Biol Phys. 1990;18(4):773–81.
38. Hoffman HJ, Otsubo H, Hendrick EB, Humphreys RP, Drake JM, Becker LE, et al. Intracranial germ-cell tumors in children. J Neurosurg. 1991;74(4):545–51.

39. Goldman S, Bouffet E, Fisher G, Wharam MD, Shaw D, Chuba PJ, et al. A phase II trial of neoadjuvant chemotherapy +/- second-look surgery prior to radiotherapy for non-germinomatous germ cell tumors (NGGCT): Children's Oncology Group Study ACNS0122 [abstract GCT 06]. Neuro Oncol. 2010;12(6):ii29.
40. Aoyama H, Shirato H, Yoshida H, Hareyama M, Nishio M, Yanagisawa T, et al. Retrospective multi-institutional study of radiotherapy for intracranial non-germinomatous germ cell tumors. Radiother Oncol. 1998;49(1):55–9.
41. Phi JH, Kim SK, Park SH, Hong SH, Wang KC, Cho BK. Immature teratomas of the central nervous system: is adjuvant therapy mandatory? J Neurosurg. 2005;103(6 Suppl):524–30.
42. Ichimura K, Fukushima S, Totoki Y, et al., eds. Exome sequencing of intracranial germ cell tumours. 3rd International CNS Germ Cell Tumor Symposium; Cambridge; 2013.
43. Wang L, Terashima K, Yamaguchi S, et al., eds. Exome sequencing of CNS germ cell tumors reveals frequent mutations in KIT and KRAS pathways and JMJD genes. 3rd International CNS Germ Cell Tumor Symposium; Cambridge; 2013.
44. Tian X, Fang J. Current perspectives on histone demethylases. Acta Biochim Biophys Sin (Shanghai). 2007;39(2):81–8.
45. Fukushima S, Otsuka A, Suzuki T, et al., eds. Mutually exclusive mutations of c-kit and RAS are associated with chromosomal instability in primary intracranial germinomas. 3rd International CNS Germ Cell Tumor Symposium; Cambridge; 2013.
46. Osorio DS, Finlay JL, Dhall G, Goldman S, Eisenstat D, Brown RJ. Feasibility of dasatinib in children and adolescents with new or recurrent central nervous system germinoma. Pediatr Blood Cancer. 2013;60(9):E100–2.

12 Choroid Plexus Tumors

Sriram Venneti, Martin Hasselblatt, Johannes E. Wolff, and Alexander R. Judkins

Definition

Choroid plexus tumors (CPTs) are neoplasms derived from the choroid plexus epithelium of the brain. Three types have been described. (1) Choroid plexus papilloma (CPP), with delicate fibrovascular connective tissue covered by a single layer of epithelial cells with round or oval monomorphic nuclei defined as WHO grade I tumors [1] (Fig. 12.1b). (2) Atypical choroid plexus papillomas (APPs) are characterized by increased mitotic activity and are WHO grade II tumors. [1] (Fig. 12.1c). A mitotic index of two or more mitoses per 10 randomly selected high power fields (HPFs) (one HPF corresponding to 0.23 mm^2) can be used to establish the diagnosis of APP [2]. (3) Choroid plexus carcinomas (CPCs) are characterized by frank histological signs of malignancy, including at least four of the following five features: (a) frequent mitoses (usually greater than 5 per 10 HPFs), (b) increased cellular density, (c) nuclear pleomorphism, (d) blurring of the papillary pattern, and (e) necrosis (Figs. 12.1d and 12.2). These tumors correspond to WHO grade III [1].

Clinical Features

Epidemiology

CPTs are rare, representing between 4 and 9 % of brain tumors in population-based studies [3, 4]. The typical age of presentation is the first year of life. However, CPTs can occur as rare congenital brain tumors [5, 6] and in adults, including the elderly [7–9]. These tumors also occur in other species including canines [10–14]. While most tumors are sporadic, CPTs are reported in: Li–Fraumeni syndrome (discussed below), pediatric patients with large melanocytic skin lesions [15], Pierpont syndrome [16], hypermelanosis Ito [17], and Aicardi syndrome [18]. CPPs can also be seen in von Hippel–Lindau disease [19], but it is not known if loss of the VHL allele contributes to the pathogenesis of these tumors. It is possible that these abnormalities indicate rare pathways of tumorigenesis that are yet to be elucidated.

Clinical Presenting Features

Raised intracranial pressure by hydrocephalus is the main presenting feature of CPTs [20, 21]. Other presenting symptoms may include blindness, non-focal symptoms such as convulsions [20] or focal signs such as hemiparesis [22, 23]. Large amounts of cerebral spinal fluid (CSF) production may also be encountered even when a drain or shunt is placed [24]. Sometimes highly vascularized tumors present as acute intracranial hemorrhage without previous symptoms [25]. Tumor locations in the cerebello-pontine angle may result in more specific signs such as unilateral rhinorrhea and otorrhea [26], or trigeminal neuralgia [27].

Imaging and Tumor Localization

The typical imaging characteristics of CPTs include intraventricular location and contrast enhancement indicating a high degree of vascularization. Invasion of brain tissue is a characteristic finding for CPCs as opposed to CPPs. CPTs are more common in the lateral ventricles [28] than in the third or fourth ventricles [29]. The cerebello-pontine angle is a typical location when the tumor originates in the choroid plexus of the fourth ventricle [30]. Ectopic locations unrelated to the ventricles/choroid plexus have also been described [23, 31–34]. Lateral ventricle tumors are more frequent in infants, while cerebello-pontine angle tumors occur more frequently in adults [30]. An unusual feature of CPTs is that even WHO grade I and II tumors have the potential to metastasize [35–39]. The typical metastatic route is through the CSF [39, 40], often to the spine but also with surprising frequency to the internal ear canals, pituitary stalk, and interpeduncular fossa [41]. Metastases can occur sometimes many years after primary tumor resection. Imaging of the entire craniospinal axis is recommended [40, 42, 43]. Rarely, hematogeneous metastases can occur to other

M.A. Karajannis and D. Zagzag (eds.), *Molecular Pathology of Nervous System Tumors: Biological Stratification and Targeted Therapies*, Molecular Pathology Library 8,
DOI 10.1007/978-1-4939-1830-0_12,

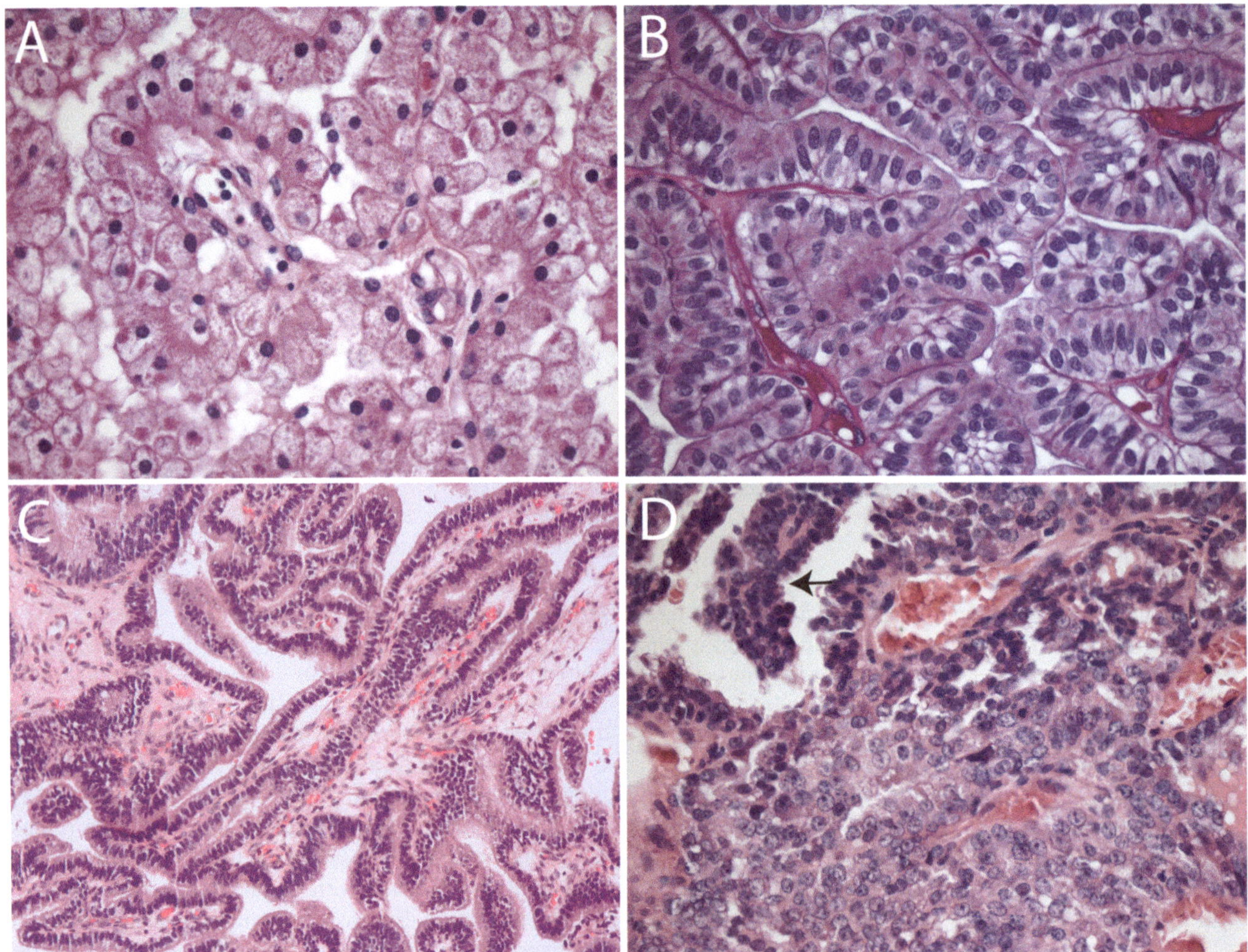

Fig. 12.1. *Histologic features of normal choroid plexus and choroid plexus tumors*. (**a**) Normal choroid plexus demonstrating typical "cobblestone" appearance (40×). (**b**) Choroid plexus papilloma, in contrast to normal choroid plexus in 2A, displays more elongated/columnar cells crowded in a pseudostratified manner and a smooth rather than cobblestone appearance (40×). (**c**) Atypical choroid plexus papilloma, with increased cellularity and focal blurring of the papillary architecture (20×). (**d**) Choroid plexus carcinoma showing focal papillary architecture (*arrow*) adjacent to an area where the papillary architecture is more blurred (40×).

parts of the brain [44], abdomen [45], bone [46, 47], and lung [48]. Abdominal seeding has been described in patients with ventricular-peritoneal shunts [49].

Imaging techniques for CPTs differ in several aspects from that for other brain tumors. As CPTs are the most frequent brain tumors detected on prenatal ultrasound [50–53], ultrasound remains an important diagnostic tool until the fontanels close [6, 51, 54]. On magnetic resonance imaging (MRI), CPTs show inhomogeneity on T2-weighted images, and moderate to marked contrast enhancement. Diagnostic specificity increases when age and intraventricular location are considered. Contrast enhancement, a common finding in these tumors, might be related to the rich vascular stroma. However, extraventricular tumors might not demonstrate contrast enhancement [34]. Differentiating the degree of malignancy on MRI can be difficult. Nevertheless, some general patterns may be observed. CPPs are usually irregular, lobulated, and solid-cystic masses, whereas CPC may present as a poorly defined, mixed-intensity mass [55]. Extensive peritumoral edema and necrosis is more frequent in CPC than in CPP [56, 57]. A thin capsule may be seen in CPP [55].

More recently, nuclear medicine methods and molecular imaging may improve diagnostic ability and also address challenging clinical issues including how to distinguish between tumor and postsurgical scars/postradiation pseudoprogression. For example, sestamibi, an agent that accumulates in mitochondria, has been used to distinguish CPTs from other brain tumors or postsurgical scars [58–62].

Pathology and Diagnostics

Macroscopy

CPTs appear macroscopically as space-occupying lesions located in the ventricles and, less commonly, in extraventricular locations. Grossly, CPPs are well demarcated with a cauliflower-like appearance. They may be attached to the

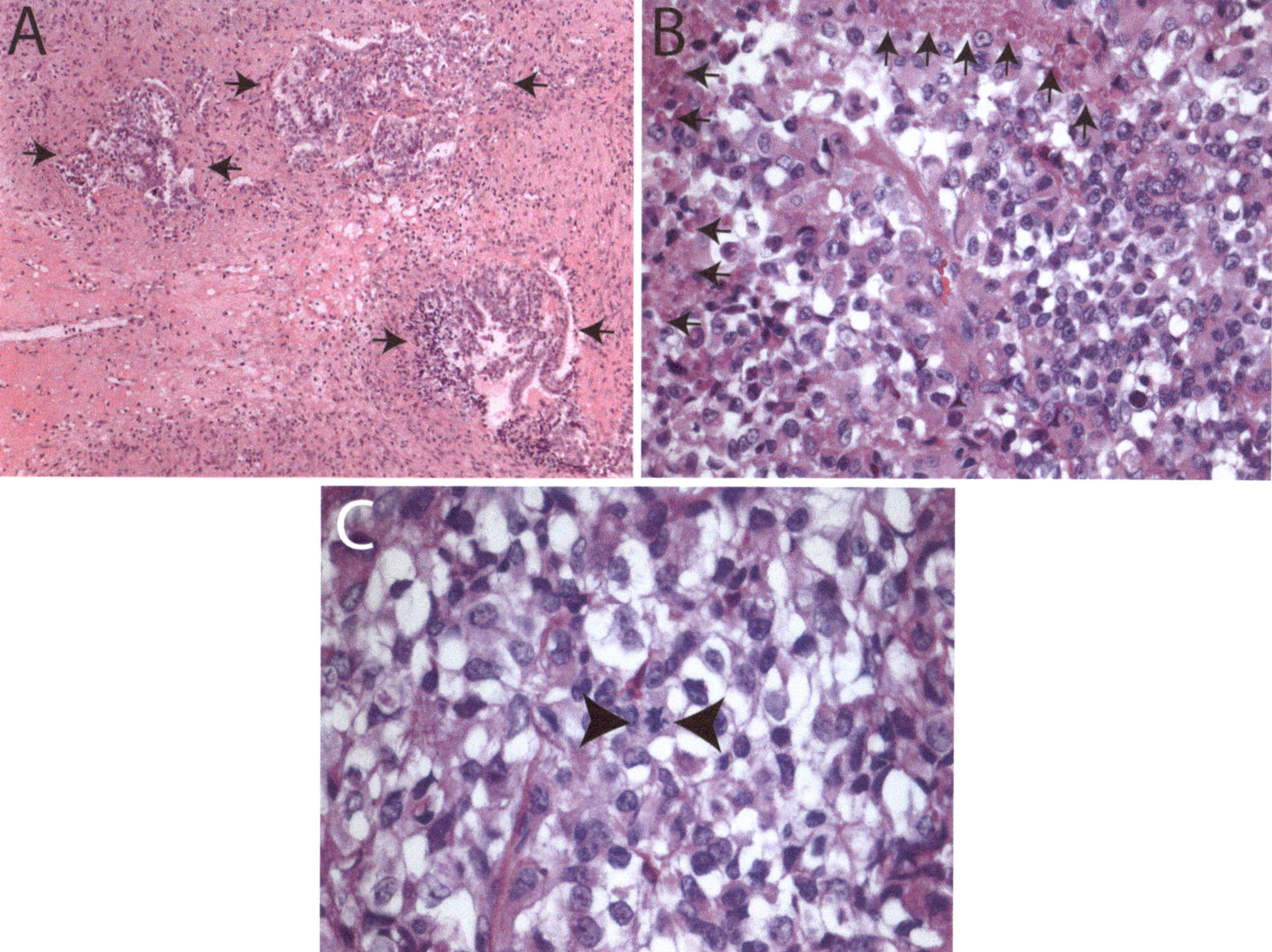

FIG. 12.2. *Histologic features of choroid plexus carcinomas.* (**a**) Choroid plexus carcinoma invading surrounding brain tissue (*arrows*, 10×). (**b**) Choroid plexus carcinoma exhibiting increased cellularity, nuclear pleomorphism, blurring of papillary architecture, and focal areas of necrosis (*arrows*, 40×). (**c**) Choroid plexus carcinoma showing loss of papillary architecture, increased cellularity, nuclear pleomorphism, and a mitotic figure between *arrowheads* (63×).

ventricular wall. CPCs usually show varying degrees of invasion into the surrounding brain. High vascularity and hemorrhages are frequent.

Histopathology

CPTs are typically comprised of epithelial cells with a round or oval nucleus and small amount of surrounding cytoplasm. CPTs are fragile, and drop metastases due to CSF spread are not uncommon [63]. Key cytologic features of CPTs in the CSF include variably sized clusters to frank papillary fragments, and cells that retain epithelial features such as sharply defined cell borders [43, 64].

Specific features of the different CPTs are described below, but from a practical point of view, these tumors can be histologically classified by where they fall along the spectrum of three key histologic features: (1) growth pattern—papillary to solid, (2) mitotic activity/cellular atypia—few or none/absent to moderate/moderate to severe, (3) necrosis—little to none or prominent.

CPPs, the least malignant of CPTs, are composed of delicate fibrovascular connective tissue fronds covered by a single layer of epithelial cells with round or oval monomorphic nuclei (Fig. 12.1b). CPPs can be distinguished from normal choroid plexus (Fig. 12.1a) by an overall increased amount of choroid plexus epithelium with flatter papillae (compared to the typical cobbled stone appearance of normal choroid plexus) comprising cells with increased nuclear to cytoplasmic ratios (Fig. 12.1a, b). These cells rest upon a basement membrane that can be elucidated with special stains for collagen. Mitotic activity is extremely low. Brain invasion, high cellularity, necrosis, nuclear pleomorphism, and focal blurring of thc papillary pattern are unusual, but may occur and should prompt the consideration of APP. Rarely, CPPs acquire unusual histological features, including oncocytic change, mucinous degeneration, melanization as well as formation of bone, cartilage, adipose tissue, or neuropil islands. CSF-mediated metastases can occur despite the histologic classification of WHO grade I [38].

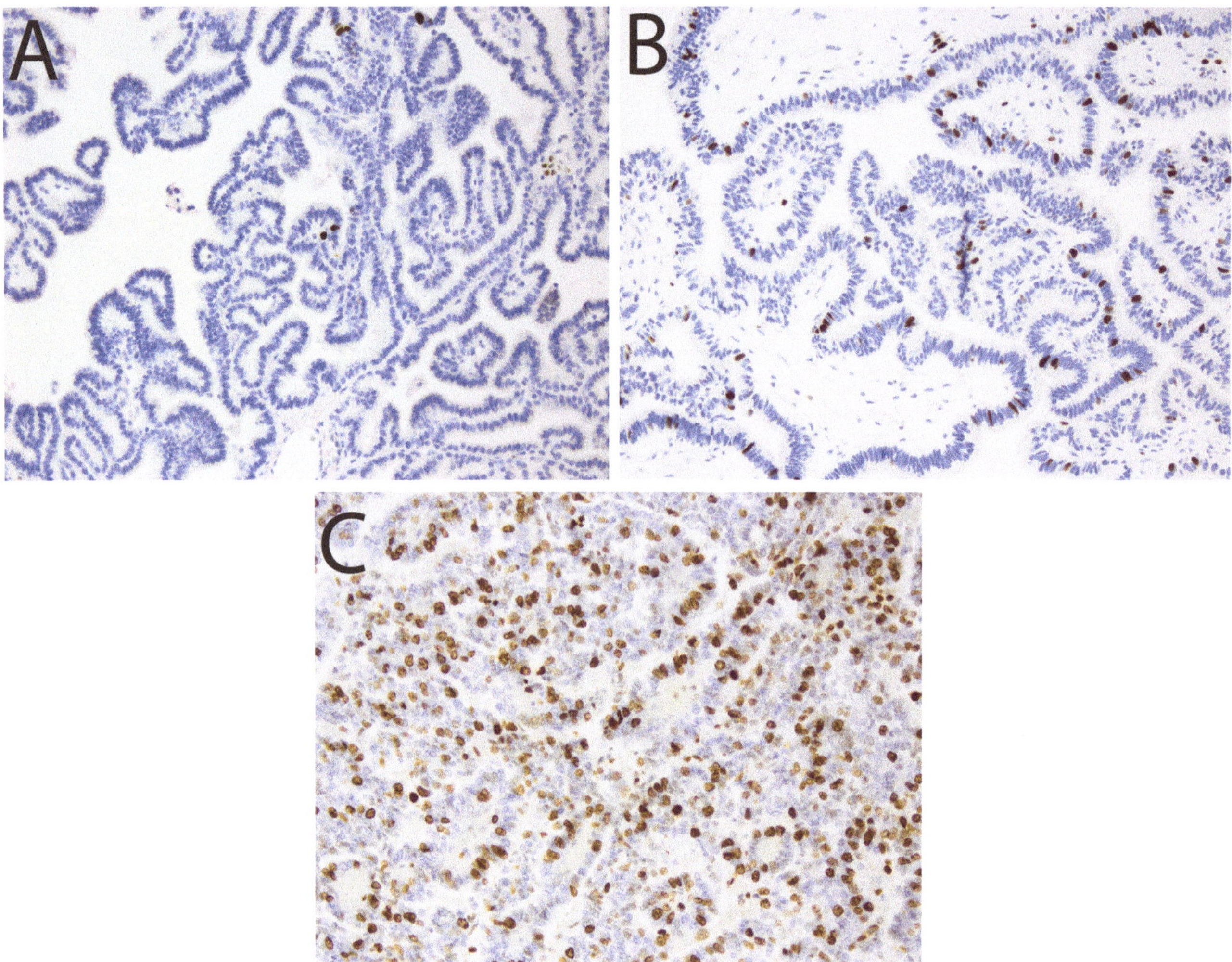

Fig. 12.3. *Proliferative activity in choroid plexus tumors.* Immunostains for Ki67/MIB1 illustrating: (**a**) Choroid plexus papilloma with low mitotic index (20×). (**b**) Atypical choroid plexus papilloma, with intermediate proliferative activity (20×). (**c**) Choroid plexus carcinoma, showing high Ki67/MIB1 labeling (20×).

An intermediate grade CPT, the atypical choroid plexus papilloma (APP) is recognized by the WHO (Grade II) (Figs. 12.1c and 12.3b). These tumors are defined by the presence of two or more mitoses per ten HPFs in what otherwise appears to be a CPP [1, 2]. Additional histologic features that have been reported in APP by some authors include increased cellularity, nuclear pleomorphism, solid growth, and necrosis. However, none of these features are required for the diagnosis of APP and the isolated occurrence of atypical histological features does not automatically imply malignancy.

CPC is a high-grade (WHO III) tumor of the choroid plexus that demonstrates frank signs of malignancy. In contrast to lower grade CPTs, CPCs demonstrate at least four of the following five features (1) frequent mitoses (Fig. 12.2C, typically more than 5 per 10 HPF), (2) increased cellular density (Figs. 12.1d and 12.2 b, c), (3) nuclear pleomorphism (Figs. 12.1d and 12.2b, c), (4) blurring of the papillary pattern (Figs. 12.1d and 12.2b, c), and (5) necrosis (Fig. 12.2b). Invasion of adjacent brain tissue by CPC is common (Fig. 12.2a). In CPCs that are truly anaplastic, identification of epithelial features may become quite challenging.

Immunohistochemistry

CPTs demonstrate expression of a wide range of immunohistochemical markers, a reminder that despite their epithelial appearance, these cells have a neuroepithelial developmental origin. The typical, though variably expressed, pattern includes S-100 protein, synaptophysin, vimentin, cytokeratins (Fig. 12.4d), glial fibrillary acidic protein (GFAP) (Fig. 12.4c), and transthyretin (TTR) (Fig. 12.4a) [65–67]. While TTR is expressed in normal choroid plexus and in many CPTs, it is unfortunately nonspecific and therefore unreliable as a precise marker of choroid plexus origins in any given tumor. However, immunohistochemical detection for membranous expression of the inward rectifier potassium channel Kir7.1 is considered specific for CPT [68] (Fig. 12.5). The Ki67/MIB index can be helpful in refining tumor grade [69] (Fig. 12.3).

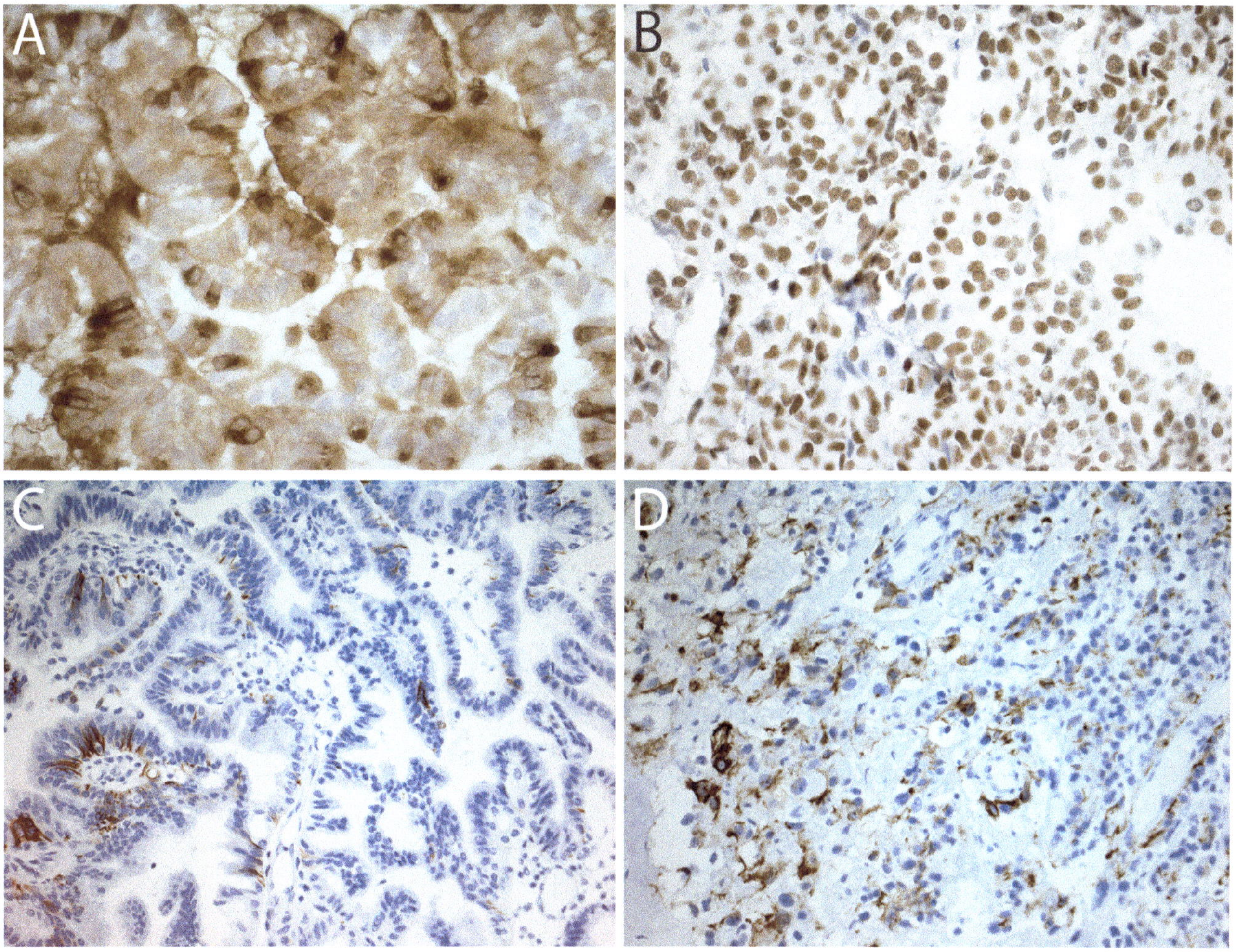

Fig. 12.4. *Immunohistochemical analyses in choroid plexus tumors*. (**a**) Immunostain for transthyretin in a choroid plexus papilloma showing diffuse positivity (40×). (**b**) SMARCB1 immunostain in a choroid plexus carcinoma showing strong nuclear positivity (40×). Retained SMARCB1 staining helps differentiate these tumors from AT/RT, which show loss of SMARCB1 expression. (**c**) Focal GFAP expression in a choroid plexus carcinoma (20×). (**d**) Cytokeratin stain (AE1-3) in a choroid plexus carcinoma showing focal immunoreactivity (20×).

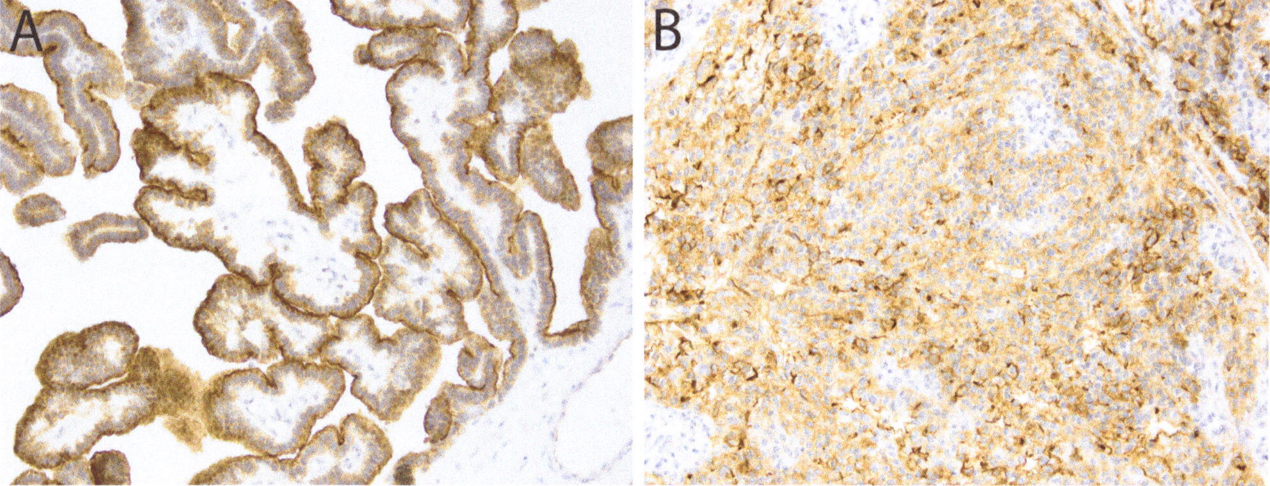

Fig. 12.5. *Immunohistochemistry for Kir7.1 in choroid plexus tumors*. Membranous staining for Kir7.1 in a choroid plexus papilloma (**a**, 20×) and a choroid plexus carcinoma (**b**, 20×).

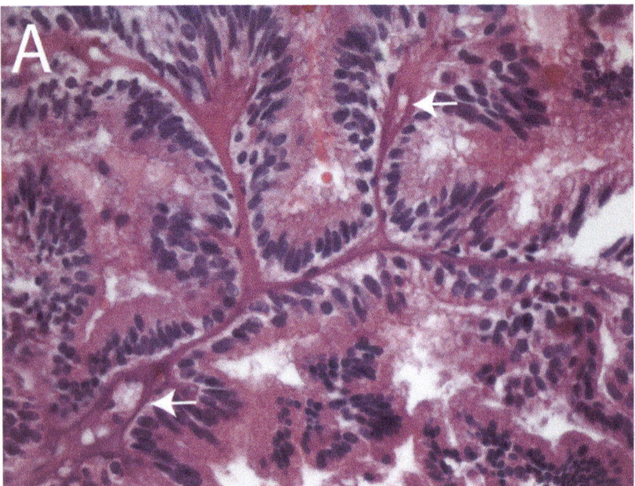

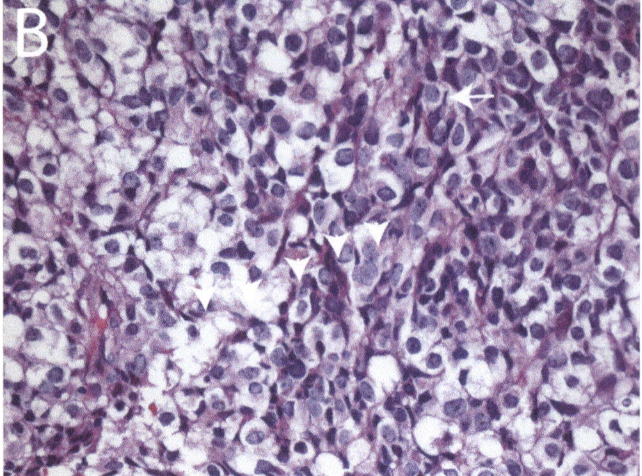

FIG. 12.6. *Histologic mimics encountered in choroid plexus tumors*. (**a**) Choroid plexus papilloma showing elongated tumor cells arranged focally around blood vessels reminiscent of an ependymoma (40×). (**b**) Choroid plexus carcinoma with perinuclear halos surrounding tumor cells mimicking an oligodendroglial neoplasm (40×).

Histological Differential Diagnosis

Depending on the age group, the differential diagnosis of CPTs includes atypical teratoid/rhabdoid tumor (AT/RT), central nervous system (CNS), primitive neuroectodermal tumors (PNET), papillary ependymoma, oligodendroglioma, neurocytoma, papillary tumor of the pineal region (PTPR), and metastases [70–75]. However, the first differential diagnosis to consider is normal choroid plexus. Typically, normal choroid plexus can be distinguished readily enough when the lesion is entirely papillary, with papillae that are not overly cellular and which exhibit a cobblestone surface, and the absence of mitoses (Figs. 12.1a, b). Further, normal choroid plexus epithelial cells express SERCA3, but SERCA3 expression is decreased in CPTs [76].

AT/RT frequently arises in the differential diagnosis, especially in young children [77]. While AT/RT may occasionally demonstrate poorly differentiated epithelial structures, this histologic pattern is generally quite rare. When such cases do arise, the diagnosis may be resolved by immunohistochemical staining for expression of SMARCB1, which is retained in all CPTs (Fig. 12.4b) [73], as well as choroid plexus marker Kir7.1, which stains the majority of CPC but not AT/RT (Fig. 12.5) [78].

Occasionally in pediatric cases, a supratentorial PNET, particularly the medulloepithelioma, may enter into the differential diagnosis. These tumors can usually be distinguished on histologic grounds; they have tubular structures rather than papillary architecture and comprise cells with embryonal rather than epithelial features. Furthermore, medulloepithelioma is characterized by 19q13.42 amplification and LIN28 expression, linking these rare tumors to embryonal tumor with abundant neuropil and true rosettes (ETANTR) [79, 80]. Cribriform neuroepithelial tumor (CRINET) is a rare tumor characterized by cribriform strands and well-defined surfaces, which may be misinterpreted as CPC. Unlike the majority of CPC, however, CRINET is characterized by SMARCB1 loss as well as EMA staining of surfaces [79]. In contrast to AT/RT, prognosis of CRINET seems to be relatively favorable [81].

Papillary ependymomas share the intraventricular location and confusion may arise in CPPs with elongated tumor cells that may give the appearance of overlapping histopathological features (Fig. 12.6a). One important clue to the differential diagnosis is the presence of a delicate basement membrane in CPTs, a feature consistently lacking in ependymomas. While GFAP may be present in both, it is generally stronger and more diffuse in ependymomas. Rarely, synchronous appearance of CPT and ependymoma has been described [82, 83]. PTPR has to be considered in children and young adults with tumors of third ventricular location. The majority of PTPRs can be distinguished from CPTs by absent staining for epithelial membrane antigen and Kir7.1, as well as the presence of distinct MAP-2 immunoreactivity [68].

The endolymphatic sac tumor (ELST) is a low-grade carcinoma originating in the ear. These extremely rare tumors are capable of invading the cerebello-pontine angle and might be mistaken for CPTs in this region. Kir7.1 and EAAT-1 (glutamate transporter) are typically positive in CPTs but absent in ELSTs [84]. The choroid plexus is a common site for metastases and this should be considered in any adult with CPTs. Renal cell carcinoma [85], thyroid carcinoma [86, 87], and cholangiocellular carcinoma [88] primaries have all been reported.

Pathogenesis and Molecular Genetics

Pathogenesis

CPTs were the first models for virally induced brain tumors. Simian Virus 40 (SV40), which naturally infects Asian macaques, has been shown to induce CPTs. The virus is capable of transforming human choroid cells in vitro [89–91] and creates CPTs in hamsters and mice in vivo [92–97]. Transgenic mice harboring the SV40 large T-antigen gene develop CPPs by 80–90 days [98, 99]. SV40 is frequently found in human CPTs [100–103]. The T-antigen of the SV40 virus binds to tumor suppressor genes such as p53 [104] and pRB [99]. This suggests virus-induced tumorigenesis. However, an unintended natural experiment that occurred when the vaccine for poliomyelitis was contaminated with the SV40 virus in India did not produce clear evidence of increased incidence of CPTs. It still remains to be conclusively established if SV40 induces CPTs in humans.

Only limited data are available regarding molecular genetic alterations in CPT. Using comparative genomic hybridization, gains of chromosomes 5, 7, and 9 as well as losses of chromosomes 10 and 22q could be demonstrated in CPP. In contrast, CPC mainly showed gains of chromosomes 1, 4, 12, and 20 as well as losses of 5, 18, and 22q [105]. These findings could be extended using high-resolution methods, showing recurrent copy number gains of chromosomes 1, 2, 4, 12, and 20 as well as losses of chromosomes 5, 6, 16, 18, 19, and 22 in CPC. Clustering analysis separated choroid plexus carcinomas into two groups: one characterized by marked losses and the other characterized by gains across the chromosomes. Chromosomal losses of 9, 19p, and 22q were significantly more frequent in younger children (<36 months), whereas gains on chromosomes 7 and 19, and chromosome arms 8q, 14q, and 21q prevailed in older patients [106].

The involvement of the *TP53* tumor suppressor gene in CPT patients was first suggested by the occurrence of CPC in families with Li–Fraumeni syndrome [107–109], and by the observation of p53 inactivation in tumor tissues [69]. A Canadian group reported a large CPT population with p53 alterations [110]. A Brazilian study confirmed these finding on a larger scale [111–113] for a specific mutation *TP53* mutation: R337H. This *TP53* mutation is also linked to adreno-cortical carcinoma. Interestingly, high-resolution single nucleotide polymorphism (SNP) array analysis did reveal extremely high total structural variation in *TP53-mutated* CPC tumor genomes compared with *TP53* wild-type tumors and CPPs [110]. However, in the absence of *TP53* germline mutations CPTs may still arise through the same pathway driven by somatic mutations [114]. Even though a close association between *TP53* mutation status and nuclear accumulation of p53 protein is often claimed [110], the majority of CPTs show only weak and focal nuclear staining, suggesting that p53 immunohistochemistry might not be a reliable indicator of *TP53* mutations in these tumors.

Other molecular events in the pathogenesis of CPT are not yet as well characterized. *TP53* mutations are unlikely to be the only event in the pathogenesis of CPTs. Patients with multiple resections show progression of CPTs with a tendency to increasing degrees of malignancy [40], and CPTs may arise from teratomas [115], indicating an accumulation of events leading to the final phenotype. Several other pathways have been suggested to be operative in the biology of CPTs. In mice, over-expression of notch3 initiated the formation of CPTs [116]. Some evidence suggests alterations of notch signaling also occur in human CPT [116, 117].

By comparing gene expression profiles obtained from human CPP cells with that of nonneoplastic choroid plexus epithelial cells, the transcription factor TWIST1 was identified to be highly expressed in CPP and also promoted proliferation and invasion in vitro [118]. Amplification and activating mutations of tyrosine receptor signaling pathways play an important role in the biology of human cancer. In CPC, amplification and over-expression of PDGF receptors has been described [119]. Furthermore, in immortalized choroid plexus epithelial cells, PDGF-BB exhibited a time- and dose-dependent proliferative response, which was significantly attenuated by the tyrosine-kinase inhibitor imatinib [120], providing a rationale for the development of treatments targeting PDGF receptor signaling in CPT.

The role of epigenetic alterations in CPT is also poorly understood. In pediatric brain tumors, human telomerase reverse transcriptase (hTERT) promoter methylation has been shown to be associated with tumor progression and poor prognosis. Methylation of the hTERT promoter has also been reported in the majority of CPCs [121]. The clinical utility of these findings for CPCs remain to be elucidated. Similarly, the prognostic and predictive role of MGMT promoter methylation, which occurs frequently in CPTs [122], remains to be determined.

Clinical Aspects and Treatments

Prognosis and Current Treatment

Due to the low incidence of CPTs, few randomized trials have been conducted [123, 124]. Most data come from individual case reports [50, 125], case series [23, 58, 126–129], or systematic literature reviews [130–133]. These data suggest that histological classification appears to be the most reliable prognostic parameter [134, 135]. Patients with CPPs have long-term survival rates exceeding 95 % when completely resected. In contrast, CPCs in patients treated with surgical resection and radiation therapy have 5-year survival rates of approximately 60 %. Primary and metastatic CPC in infants from Li–Fraumeni families fare even worse, with 5-year survival rates of less than 5 % [130].

Tumor resection is of very high therapeutic value in CPTs [28, 135–141]. In particular, gross total resection was found to be of significant prognostic value in meta-analyses, [130, 134, 141] thereby confirming the institutional experiences of many groups [23, 124, 142]. Meta analyses also confirmed the value of a second resection [143]. However, attempts at radical resection should be made with caution, since the high vascularity of these tumors also translates into a high rate of intratumoral bleeding [136], and other surgical complications such as tension pneumoventricle [144] and hyperacute disseminated intravascular coagulation [145]. Newer surgical techniques might reduce morbidity and mortality. These include endoscopic [137] and combined endoscopic and microsurgical approaches [146]. For tumors of the foramen of Luschka, a telovelar approach has been proposed [147]. Preoperative embolization may reduce the operative risk [6, 50, 148, 149]. In one case the tumor regressed after embolization without the need for resection [150]. Similarly, preoperative intensive chemotherapy may reduce the risk for intraoperative hemorrhage even when the size of the tumor does not shrink significantly [151].

Radiation therapy can increase survival of CPTs in patients old enough to receive therapeutic doses [129, 130, 134, 152, 153]. For example, CPPs may be sensitive to radiation therapy [39] and CPCs may show a survival benefit with craniospinal irradiation [152]. However, long-term sequelae of radiation are particular devastating for the developing brains of young children and limit the use of this modality.

Chemotherapy improved survival rates at least in the subgroup of incompletely resected CPC [42, 132]. The five most frequently used drugs are cisplatin, vincristine, cyclophosphamide, carboplatin, and etoposide. Of those, etoposide (VP16) was most frequently used in protocols and had the most convincing survival benefit in various multivariate analyses [133]. More recently reports suggest temozolomide is less promising [125]. In a prospective clinical trial, CPT-SIOP-2000, cyclophosphamide was found equally effective to carboplatin. As a result of these experiences, the benefit of chemotherapy (including high-dose chemotherapy recently reported for an adult patient [154] is becoming more widely accepted, at least for young children [135, 153, 155, 156]. However, intensive chemotherapy is associated with its own risks, and fatal complications have been described [136]. These studies highlight the need for better targeted and less toxic agents.

The influence of germline *TP53* mutations on prognosis and efficacy of treatment remains controversial. A large series of patients treated mainly with intensive chemotherapy including ifosfamide etoposide carboplatin (ICE) show a significantly worse prognosis in patients with Li–Fraumeni syndrome [110]. A second report of patients treated with various chemotherapeutic protocols, among them head start III, described long-term survivors among the Li–Fraumeni population [157]. However, data from the Brazilian family with *TP53*-R337H mutations failed to show statistically significant differences in survival on treatment [111]. Finally, in the international CPT study, there was no significant difference between Li–Fraumeni and non-Li–Fraumeni families. These differences in results prompt further prospective evaluations.

Unique biological features of CPTs may provide leads to novel therapeutic approaches. The blood–brain barrier is located typically in the vascular wall and is characterized by tight junctions between endothelial cells. In contrast, choroid plexus capillaries are leaky. As this feature of leaky blood vessels is maintained in CPTs, systemic medication may reach tumor cells even among the most differentiated CPTs without hindrance from the blood–brain barrier. The normal choroid plexus also functions as an immunological gate to the CNS, including interferon-γ signal mediated entry of circulating leucocytes for immune surveillance [158], and IL-6 production [159]. It is possible that these immune pathways could be leveraged to develop novel therapeutic approaches against CPTs in the future.

Summary

CPTs are tumors arising from the choroid plexus and based on histologic criteria are classified as CPP, APP, and CPC, which correspond to WHO grades I, II, and III, respectively. CPTs occur in all ages but are more common in childhood, peaking in incidence during the first decade of life. Histological grading remains a key prognostic factor and several ancillary immunohistochemical tests can aid in establishing their diagnoses. CPPs are usually treated with surgical resection, whereas a combination of surgical resection and/or chemo/radiation therapy may be used for higher-grade tumors. The biology of CPTs is poorly understood. Factors implicated in the pathogenesis of CPTs include alterations in p53- and SV40-induced viral transformation. However, the molecular genetics of CPT initiation and progression have not been otherwise elucidated and should provide fruitful avenues for future research.

References

1. Louis DN, Ohgaki H, Wiestler OD, Cavenee WK, Burger PC, Jouvet A, Scheithauer BW, Kleihues P. The 2007 WHO classification of tumours of the central nervous system. Acta Neuropathol. 2007;114:97–109.
2. Jeibmann A, Hasselblatt M, Gerss J, Wrede B, Egensperger R, Beschorner R, Hans VH, Rickert CH, Wolff JE, Paulus W. Prognostic implications of atypical histologic features in choroid plexus papilloma. J Neuropathol Exp Neurol. 2006;65:1069–73.
3. Zulch, ed. Brain tumors: their biology and pathology. New York: Springer; 1957.
4. Stagno V, Mugamba J, Ssenyonga P, Kaaya BN, Warf BC. Presentation, pathology, and treatment outcome of brain

tumors in 172 consecutive children at CURE Children's hospital of Uganda. The predominance of the visible diagnosis and the uncertainties of epidemiology in sub-Saharan Africa. Childs Nerv Syst. 2014;30:137–46.
5. Wilhelm M, Hirsch W, Merkenschlager A, Stepan H, Geyer C, Kiess W. A rare case of congenital choroid plexus carcinoma. Pediatr Hematol Oncol. 2012;29:643–6.
6. Ditz C, Nowak G, Koch C, Merz H, Tronnier V. Atypical choroid plexus papilloma in a newborn: prenatal diagnosis, preoperative tumor embolization, and resection. J Neurol Surg A Cent Eur Neurosurg. 2013;74:59–63.
7. Jusue-Torres I, Ortega-Zufiria JM, Tamarit-Degenhardt M, Poveda-Nunez PD. Atypical choroid plexus papilloma in adults: case report and literature review. Neurocirugia. 2012;23:116–21.
8. Kishore S, Negi G, Meena H, Anuradha K, Pathak PV, Bansal K. Choroid plexus carcinoma in an adult. J Neurosci Rural Pract. 2012;3:71–3.
9. Umredkar AA, Chhabra R, Bal A, Das A. Choroid plexus papilloma of the fourth ventricle in a septuagenarian. J Neurosci Rural Pract. 2012;3:402–4.
10. Kurtz HJ, Hanlon GF. Choroid plexus papilloma in a dog. Vet Pathol. 1971;8:91–5.
11. Ribas JL, Mena H, Braund KG, Sesterhenn IA, Toivio-Kinnucan M. A histologic and immunocytochemical study of choroid plexus tumors of the dog. Vet Pathol. 1989;26:55–64.
12. Steiss JE, Cox NR, Knecht CD. Electroencephalographic and histopathologic correlations in eight dogs with intracranial mass lesions. Am J Vet Res. 1990;51:1286–91.
13. Ohashi F, Kotani T, Onishi T, Katamoto H, Nakata E, Fritz-Zieroth B. Magnetic resonance imaging in a dog with choroid plexus carcinoma. J Vet Med Sci. 1993;55:875–6.
14. Pastorello A, Constantino-Casas F, Archer J. Choroid plexus carcinoma cells in the cerebrospinal fluid of a Staffordshire Bull Terrier. Vet Clin Pathol. 2010;39:505–10.
15. Kinsler VA, Aylett SE, Coley SC, Chong WK, Atherton DJ. Central nervous system imaging and congenital melanocytic naevi. Arch Dis Child. 2001;84:152–5.
16. Vadivelu S, Edelman M, Schneider SJ, Mittler MA. Choroid plexus papilloma and Pierpont syndrome. J Neurosurg Pediatr. 2013;11:115–8.
17. Morigaki R, Pooh KH, Shouno K, Taniguchi H, Endo S, Nakagawa Y. Choroid plexus papilloma in a girl with hypomelanosis of Ito. J Neurosurg Pediatr. 2012;10:182–5.
18. Frye RE, Polling JS, Ma LC. Choroid plexus papilloma expansion over 7 years in Aicardi syndrome. J Child Neurol. 2007;22:484–7.
19. Blamires TL, Maher ER. Choroid plexus papilloma. A new presentation of von Hippel-Lindau (VHL) disease. Eye (Lond). 1992;6(Pt 1):90–2.
20. Bleggi-Torres LF, Urban LA, Antoniuk A, Carboni P, Ramina R, Gugelmin ES. Choroid plexus carcinoma: report of 15 cases. Arq Neuropsiquiatr. 2000;58:505–11.
21. Jaiswal S, Vij M, Mehrotra A, Kumar B, Nair A, Jaiswal AK, Behari S, Jain VK. Choroid plexus tumors: a clinico-pathological and neuro-radiological study of 23 cases. Asian J Neurosurg. 2013;8:29–35.
22. Mishra A, Srivastava C, Singh SK, Chandra A, Ojha BK. Choroid plexus carcinoma: case report and review of literature. J Pediatr Neurosci. 2012;7:71–3.
23. Pendleton C, Olivi A, Jallo GI, Quinones-Hinojosa A. Unique challenges faced by pediatric neurosurgeon Harvey Cushing in 1909 at Johns Hopkins: a choroid plexus tumor of the lateral ventricle mimicking a cerebellar lesion. Childs Nerv Syst. 2011;27:1145–8.
24. Phi JH, Shin CH, Wang KC, Park SH, Kim SK. Catastrophic electrolyte imbalance caused by excessive production and overdrainage of cerebrospinal fluid in an infant with choroid plexus papilloma. Childs Nerv Syst. 2011;27:1153–6.
25. Maimone G, Ganau M, Nicassio N, Paterniti S. Paratrigonal choroid plexus papilloma presenting with satellite multiple supra- and infratentorial hemorrhages. Neuroanatomical basis and pathological hypothesis. Int J Surg Case Rep. 2013;4:239–42.
26. Kinoshita Y, Wasita B, Akatsuka K, Kambe A, Kurosaki M, Watanabe T. Choroid plexus papilloma presenting with cerebrospinal fluid rhinorrhea and otorrhea: case report. Neurol Med Chir (Tokyo). 2010;50:930–3.
27. Jia DZ, Zhou MD, Jiang YQ, Li G. Trigeminal neuralgia caused by a choroid plexus papilloma of the cerebellopontine angle: case report and review of the literature. J Int Med Res. 2010;38:289–92.
28. Ogiwara H, Dipatri Jr AJ, Alden TD, Bowman RM, Tomita T. Choroid plexus tumors in pediatric patients. Br J Neurosurg. 2012;26:32–7.
29. Mahta A, Kim RY, Kesari S. Fourth ventricular choroid plexus papilloma. Med Oncol. 2012;29:1285–6.
30. Khoddami M, Gholampour Shahaboddini R. Choroid plexus papilloma of the cerebellopontine angle. Arch Iran Med. 2010;13:552–5.
31. Ma YH, Ye K, Zhan RY, Wang LJ. Primary choroid plexus papilloma of the sellar region. J Neurooncol. 2008;88:51–5.
32. Bian LG, Sun QF, Wu HC, Jiang H, Sun YH, Shen JK. Primary choroid plexus papilloma in the pituitary fossa: case report and literature review. Acta Neurochir (Wien). 2011;153:851–7.
33. Imai M, Tominaga J, Matsumae M. Choroid plexus papilloma originating from the cerebrum parenchyma. Surg Neurol Int. 2011;2:151.
34. Xiao A, Xu J, He X, You C. Extraventricular choroid plexus papilloma in the brainstem. J Neurosurg Pediatr. 2013;12:247–50.
35. Leys D, Pasquier F, Lejeune JP, Lesoin F, Petit H, Delandsheer JM. Benign choroid plexus papilloma. 2 local recurrences and intraventricular seeding. Neurochirurgie. 1986;32:258–61.
36. Domingues RC, Taveras JM, Reimer P, Rosen BR. Foramen magnum choroid plexus papilloma with drop metastases to the lumbar spine. AJNR Am J Neuroradiol. 1991;12:564–5.
37. Enomoto H, Mizuno M, Katsumata T, Doi T. Intracranial metastasis of a choroid plexus papilloma originating in the cerebellopontine angle region: a case report. Surg Neurol. 1991;36:54–8.
38. McEvoy AW, Galloway M, Revesz T, Kitchen ND. Metastatic choroid plexus papilloma: a case report. J Neurooncol. 2002;56:241–6.
39. Zachary G, George J, Jaishri B, Peter B, Stephanie T. Management of disseminated choroid plexus papilloma: a case study. Pediatr Blood Cancer. 2014;61:562–3.
40. Stuivenvolt M, Mandl E, Verheul J, Fleischeuer R, Tijssen CC. Atypical transformation in sacral drop metastasis from posterior fossa choroid plexus papilloma. BMJ Case Rep. 2012;2012.

41. Al-Abdullah AA, Abu-Amero KK, Hellani A, Alkhalidi H, Bosley TM. Choroid plexus papilloma metastases to both cerebellopontine angles mimicking neurofibromatosis type 2. J Neurol. 2011;258:504–6.
42. Menon G, Nair SN, Baldawa SS, Rao RB, Krishnakumar KP, Gopalakrishnan CV. Choroid plexus tumors: an institutional series of 25 patients. Neurol India. 2010;58:429–35.
43. Savage NM, Crosby JH, Reid-Nicholson MD. The cytologic findings in choroid plexus carcinoma: report of a case with differential diagnosis. Diagn Cytopathol. 2012;40(1):1–6.
44. Allen J, Wisoff J, Helson L, Pearce J, Arenson E. Choroid plexus carcinoma—responses to chemotherapy alone in newly diagnosed young children. J Neurooncol. 1992;12:69–74.
45. Geerts Y, Gabreels F, Lippens R, Merx H, Wesseling P. Choroid plexus carcinoma: a report of two cases and review of the literature. Neuropediatrics. 1996;27:143–8.
46. Hayakawa I, Fujiwara K, Tsuchida T, Aoki M. Choroid plexus carcinoma with metastasis to bone (author's transl). No Shinkei Geka. 1979;7:815–8.
47. Valladares JB, Perry RH, Kalbag RM. Malignant choroid plexus papilloma with extraneural metastasis. Case report. J Neurosurg. 1980;52:251–5.
48. Sheridan M, Besser M. Fatal pulmonary embolism by tumor during resection of a choroid plexus papilloma: case report. Neurosurgery. 1994;34:910–2. discussion 912.
49. McCallum S, Cooper K, Franks DN. Choroid plexus carcinoma. Cytologic identification of malignant cells in ascitic fluid. Acta Cytol. 1988;32:263–6.
50. Hartge DR, Axt-Fliedner R, Weichert J. Prenatal diagnosis and successful postnatal therapy of an atypical choroid plexus papilloma-Case report and review of literature. J Clin Ultrasound. 2010;38:377–83.
51. Anselem O, Mezzetta L, Grange G, Zerah M, Benard C, Marcou V, Fallet-Bianco C, Adamsbaum C, Tsatsaris V. Fetal tumors of the choroid plexus: is differential diagnosis between papilloma and carcinoma possible? Ultrasound Obstet Gynecol. 2011;38:229–32.
52. Vassallo M, Maruotti GM, Quarantelli M, Pastore G, Paladini D. Choroid plexus carcinoma: prenatal characterization by 3-dimensional sonography and magnetic resonance imaging, perinatal management, and natural history. J Ultrasound Med. 2012;31:337–9.
53. Renna MD, Pisani P, Conversano F, Perrone E, Casciaro E, Renzo GC, Paola MD, Perrone A, Casciaro S. Sonographic markers for early diagnosis of fetal malformations. World J Radiol. 2013;5:356–71.
54. Lysyy O, Puzhevsky A, Strauss S. Choroid plexus papilloma in an infant: ultrasound diagnosis. Eur J Pediatr. 2012;171:1717–8.
55. Zhang TJ, Yue Q, Lui S, Wu QZ, Gong QY. MRI findings of choroid plexus tumors in the cerebellum. Clin Imaging. 2011;35:64–7.
56. Yan C, Xu Y, Feng J, Sun C, Zhang G, Shi J, Hao P, Wu Y, Lin B. Choroid plexus tumours: classification, MR imaging findings and pathological correlation. J Med Imaging Radiat Oncol. 2013;57:176–83.
57. Vandesteen L, Drier A, Galanaud D, Clarencon F, Leclercq D, Karachi C, Dormont D. Imaging findings of intraventricular and ependymal lesions. J Neuroradiol. 2013;40:229–44.
58. Wolff JE, Myles T, Pinto A, Rigel JE, Angyalfi S, Kloiber R. Detection of choroid plexus carcinoma with Tc-99m sestamibi: case report and review of the literature. Med Pediatr Oncol. 2001;36:323–5.
59. Kirton A, Kloiber R, Rigel J, Wolff J. Evaluation of pediatric CNS malignancies with (99m)Tc-methoxyisobutylisonitrile SPECT. J Nucl Med. 2002;43:1438–43.
60. Subbiah V, Ketonen L, Bruner JM, Nunez R, Weinberg J, Wolff JE. 99mTc-sestamibi scan differentiates tumor from other contrast enhancing tissue in choroid plexus tumors. J Pediatr Hematol Oncol. 2010;32:160–2.
61. Finnema SJ, Stepanov V, Ettrup A, Nakao R, Amini N, Svedberg M, Lehmann C, Hansen M, Knudsen GM, Halldin C. Characterization of [C]Cimbi-36 as an agonist PET radioligand for the 5-HT and 5-HT receptors in the nonhuman primate brain. Neuroimage. 2013;84C:342–53.
62. Korchi AM, Garibotto V, Ansari M, Merlini L. Pseudoprogression after proton beam irradiation for a choroid plexus carcinoma in pediatric patient: MRI and PET imaging patterns. Childs Nerv Syst. 2013;29:509–12.
63. Wieczorek V, Kluge H, Linke E, Zimmermann K, Kuehn H-J, Witte O, Isenmann S Pathological CSF cell findings in primary and metastatic CNS tumor, malignant lymphoma and leukemia. In: Atlas of CSF Cytology; 2007, p 79.
64. Berger P. Smears and frozen sections in surgical neuropathology: a manual. Baltimore: PB Medical Publishing; 2009.
65. Muthuphei MN. Divergent differentiation in choroid plexus papilloma. An immunohistochemical study of five cases. Cent Afr J Med. 1995;41:103–4.
66. Megerian CA, Pilch BZ, Bhan AK, McKenna MJ. Differential expression of transthyretin in papillary tumors of the endolymphatic sac and choroid plexus. Laryngoscope. 1997;107:216–21.
67. Hayashi H, Aoki M, Tsugu H, Hirakawa K, Yoshino S, Fukushima T, Inoue T, Nabeshima K. A case of choroid plexus papilloma with stromal sclerosis and indistinct papillary structures. Brain Tumor Pathol. 2012;29:37–42.
68. Hasselblatt M, Bohm C, Tatenhorst L, Dinh V, Newrzella D, Keyvani K, Jeibmann A, Buerger H, Rickert CH, Paulus W. Identification of novel diagnostic markers for choroid plexus tumors: a microarray-based approach. Am J Surg Pathol. 2006;30:66–74.
69. Vajtai I, Varga Z, Bodosi M, Voros E. Melanotic papilloma of the choroid plexus: report of a case with implications for pathogenesis. Noshuyo Byori. 1995;12:151–4.
70. Rorke LB, Packer R, Biegel J. Central nervous system atypical teratoid/rhabdoid tumors of infancy and childhood. J Neurooncol. 1995;24:21–8.
71. Burger PC, Yu IT, Tihan T, Friedman HS, Strother DR, Kepner JL, Duffner PK, Kun LE, Perlman EJ. Atypical teratoid/rhabdoid tumor of the central nervous system: a highly malignant tumor of infancy and childhood frequently mistaken for medulloblastoma: a Pediatric Oncology Group study. Am J Surg Pathol. 1998;22:1083–92.
72. Judkins AR, Mauger J, Ht A, Rorke LB, Biegel JA. Immunohistochemical analysis of hSNF5/INI1 in pediatric CNS neoplasms. Am J Surg Pathol. 2004;28:644–50.
73. Judkins AR, Burger PC, Hamilton RL, Kleinschmidt-DeMasters B, Perry A, Pomeroy SL, Rosenblum MK, Yachnis

AT, Zhou H, Rorke LB, Biegel JA. INI1 protein expression distinguishes atypical teratoid/rhabdoid tumor from choroid plexus carcinoma. J Neuropathol Exp Neurol. 2005;64:391–7.
74. Judkins AR, Eberhart CG, Wesseling P Atypical teratoid/rhabdoid tumor. WHO classification of tumors of the central nervous system. 2007; 4:147–149.
75. Tripathy K, Misra A, Misra D, Pujari S, Nayak M, Rath J. Melanotic choroid plexus carcinoma of the posterior fossa. J Clin Neurol. 2011;7:105–6.
76. Ghezali LA, Arbabian A, Jeibmann A, Hasselblatt M, Hallaert GG, Van den Broecke C, Gray F, Brouland JP, Varin-Blank N, Papp B (2013) Loss of endoplasmic reticulum calcium pump expression in choroid plexus tumours. Neuropathol Appl Neurobiol. 2013; [Epub ahead of print].
77. Schittenhelm J, Nagel C, Meyermann R, Beschorner R. Atypical teratoid/rhabdoid tumors may show morphological and immunohistochemical features seen in choroid plexus tumors. Neuropathology. 2011;31:461–7.
78. Hasselblatt M, Blumcke I, Jeibmann A, Rickert CH, Jouvet A, van de Nes JA, Kuchelmeister K, Brunn A, Fevre-Montange M, Paulus W. Immunohistochemical profile and chromosomal imbalances in papillary tumours of the pineal region. Neuropathol Appl Neurobiol. 2006;32:278–83.
79. Ibrahim GM, Huang A, Halliday W, Dirks PB, Malkin D, Baskin B, Shago M, Hawkins C. Cribriform neuroepithelial tumour: novel clinicopathological, ultrastructural and cytogenetic findings. Acta Neuropathol. 2011;122:511–4.
80. Korshunov A Sturm D, Ryzhova M, et al. Embryonal tumor with abundant neuropil and true rosettes (ETANTR), ependymoblastoma, and medulloepithelioma share molecular similarity and comprise a single clinicopathological entity. Acta Neuropathol. 2013; [Epub ahead of print].
81. Hasselblatt M, Oyen F, Gesk S, Kordes U, Wrede B, Bergmann M, Schmid H, Fruhwald MC, Schneppenheim R, Siebert R, Paulus W. Cribriform neuroepithelial tumor (CRINET): a nonrhabdoid ventricular tumor with INI1 loss and relatively favorable prognosis. J Neuropathol Exp Neurol. 2009;68:1249–55.
82. Bollo RJ, Zagzag D, Samadani U. Synchronous choroid plexus papilloma of the fourth ventricle and ependymoma of the filum terminale: case report. Neurosurgery. 2010;67:E1454–9; discussion E1459.
83. Hayashi Y, Mohri M, Nakada M, Hamada J. Ependymoma and choroid plexus papilloma as synchronous multiple neuroepithelial tumors in the same patient: a case report and review of literature. Neurosurgery. 2011;68:E1144–7; discussion E1147.
84. Schittenhelm J, Roser F, Tatagiba M, Beschorner R. Diagnostic value of EAAT-1 and Kir7.1 for distinguishing endolymphatic sac tumors from choroid plexus tumors. Am J Clin Pathol. 2012;138:85–9.
85. Siomin V, Lin JL, Marko NF, Barnett GH, Toms SA, Chao ST, Angelov L, Vogelbaum MA, Navaratne K, Suh JH, Weil RJ. Stereotactic radiosurgical treatment of brain metastases to the choroid plexus. Int J Radiat Oncol Biol Phys. 2011;80:1134–42.
86. Kitagawa Y, Higuchi F, Abe Y, Matsuda H, Kim P, Ueki K. Metastasis to the choroid plexus from thyroid cancer: case report. Neurol Med Chir (Tokyo). 2013;53(11):832–6.
87. Manzil FF, Bender LW, Scott JW. Evaluation of rare choroid plexus metastasis from papillary thyroid carcinoma with multimodality imaging. Clin Nucl Med. 2014;39(6):551–3.
88. Kurisu K, Kamoshima Y, Terasaka S, Kobayashi H, Kubota K, Houkin K. A case of metastatic choroid plexus tumor from cholangiocellular carcinoma. No Shinkei Geka. 2011;39:991–7.
89. Shein HM, Enders JF, Levinthal JD. Transformation induced by simian virus 40 in human renal cell cultures. II. Cell-virus relationships. Proc Natl Acad Sci U S A. 1962;48:1350–7.
90. Carruba G, Dallapiccola B, Brinchi V, de Giuli MC. Ultrastructural and biological characterization of human choroid cell cultures transformed by Simian Virus 40. In Vitro. 1983;19:443–52.
91. Carruba G, Dallapiccola B, Mantegazza P, Garaci E, Micara G, Radaelli A, De Giuli MC. Transformation of human choroid cells in vitro by SV40. Ultrastructural and cytogenetic analysis of cloned cell lines. J Submicrosc Cytol. 1984;16:459–70.
92. Kirschstein RL, Gerber P. Ependymomas produced after intracerebral inoculation of SV40 into new-born hamsters. Nature. 1962;195:299–300.
93. Davis LE, Nager GT, Johnson RT. Experimental viral infections of the inner ear. II. Simian virus 40 induced tumors of the temporal bone. Ann Otol Rhinol Laryngol. 1979;88:198–204.
94. Brinster RL, Chen HY, Messing A, van Dyke T, Levine AJ, Palmiter RD. Transgenic mice harboring SV40 T-antigen genes develop characteristic brain tumors. Cell. 1984;37:367–79.
95. Small JA, Blair DG, Showalter SD, Scangos GA. Analysis of a transgenic mouse containing simian virus 40 and v-myc sequences. Mol Cell Biol. 1985;5:642–8.
96. Reynolds RK, Hoekzema GS, Vogel J, Hinrichs SH, Jay G. Multiple endocrine neoplasia induced by the promiscuous expression of a viral oncogene. Proc Natl Acad Sci U S A. 1988;85:3135–9.
97. Enjoji M, Iwaki T, Hara H, Sakai H, Nawata H, Watanabe T. Establishment and characterization of choroid plexus carcinoma cell lines: connection between choroid plexus and immune systems. Jpn J Cancer Res. 1996;87:893–9.
98. Cho HJ, Seiberg M, Georgoff I, Teresky AK, Marks JR, Levine AJ. Impact of the genetic background of transgenic mice upon the formation and timing of choroid plexus papillomas. J Neurosci Res. 1989;24:115–22.
99. Chen J, Tobin GJ, Pipas JM, Van Dyke T. T-antigen mutant activities in vivo: roles of p53 and pRB binding in tumorigenesis of the choroid plexus. Oncogene. 1992;7:1167–75.
100. Tabuchi K, Kirsch WM, Low M, Gaskin D, Van Buskirk J, Maa S. Screening of human brain tumors for SV40-related T antigen. Int J Cancer. 1978;21:12–7.
101. Bergsagel DJ, Finegold MJ, Butel JS, Kupsky WJ, Garcea RL. DNA sequences similar to those of simian virus 40 in ependymomas and choroid plexus tumors of childhood. N Engl J Med. 1992;326:988–93.
102. Lednicky JA, Garcea RL, Bergsagel DJ, Butel JS. Natural simian virus 40 strains are present in human choroid plexus and ependymoma tumors. Virology. 1995;212:710–7.
103. Martini F, Iaccheri L, Lazzarin L, Carinci P, Corallini A, Gerosa M, Iuzzolino P, Barbanti-Brodano G, Tognon M. SV40

early region and large T antigen in human brain tumors, peripheral blood cells, and sperm fluids from healthy individuals. Cancer Res. 1996;56:4820–5.

104. Palmiter RD, Chen HY, Messing A, Brinster RL. SV40 enhancer and large-T antigen are instrumental in development of choroid plexus tumours in transgenic mice. Nature. 1985;316:457–60.

105. Rickert CH, Wiestler OD, Paulus W. Chromosomal imbalances in choroid plexus tumors. Am J Pathol. 2002;160:1105–13.

106. Ruland V, Hartung S, Kordes U, Wolff JE, Paulus W, Hasselblatt M. Choroid plexus carcinomas are characterized by complex chromosomal alterations related to patient age and prognosis. Genes Chromosomes Cancer. 2014;53(5):373–80.

107. Garber JE, Burke EM, Lavally BL, Billett AL, Sallan SE, Scott RM, Kupsky W, Li FP. Choroid plexus tumors in the breast cancer-sarcoma syndrome. Cancer. 1990;66:2658–60.

108. Yuasa H, Tokito S, Tokunaga M. Primary carcinoma of the choroid plexus in Li-Fraumeni syndrome: case report. Neurosurgery. 1993;32:131–3; discussion 133–134.

109. Kleihues P, Schauble B, zur Hausen A, Esteve J, Ohgaki H. Tumors associated with p53 germline mutations: a synopsis of 91 families. Am J Pathol. 1997;150:1–13.

110. Tabori U, Shlien A, Baskin B, Levitt S, Ray P, Alon N, Hawkins C, Bouffet E, Pienkowska M, Lafay-Cousin L, Gozali A, Zhukova N, Shane L, Gonzalez I, Finlay J, Malkin D. TP53 alterations determine clinical subgroups and survival of patients with choroid plexus tumors. J Clin Oncol. 2010;28:1995–2001.

111. Custodio G, Taques GR, Figueiredo BC, Gugelmin ES, Oliveira Figueiredo MM, Watanabe F, Pontarolo R, Lalli E, Torres LF. Increased incidence of choroid plexus carcinoma due to the germline TP53 R337H mutation in southern Brazil. PLoS One. 2011;6:e18015.

112. Seidinger AL, Mastellaro MJ, Paschoal Fortes F, Godoy Assumpcao J, Aparecida Cardinalli I, Aparecida Ganazza M, Correa Ribeiro R, Brandalise SR, Dos Santos AS, Yunes JA. Association of the highly prevalent TP53 R337H mutation with pediatric choroid plexus carcinoma and osteosarcoma in southeast Brazil. Cancer. 2011;117:2228–35.

113. Giacomazzi J, Selistre SG, Rossi C, Alemar B, Santos-Silva P, Pereira FS, Netto CB, Cossio SL, Roth DE, Brunetto AL, Zagonel-Oliveira M, Martel-Planche G, Goldim JR, Hainaut P, Camey SA, Ashton-Prolla P. Li-Fraumeni and Li-Fraumeni-like syndrome among children diagnosed with pediatric cancer in Southern Brazil. Cancer. 2013;119(24):4341–9.

114. Lv SQ, Song YC, Xu JP, Shu HF, Zhou Z, An N, Huang QL, Yang H. A novel TP53 somatic mutation involved in the pathogenesis of pediatric choroid plexus carcinoma. Med Sci Monit. 2012;18:CS37–41.

115. Dessauvagie BF, Ruba S, Robbins PD. Choroid plexus papilloma arising in a mature cystic teratoma of a 32-year-old female. Pathology. 2013;45:88–9.

116. Dang L, Fan X, Chaudhry A, Wang M, Gaiano N, Eberhart CG. Notch3 signaling initiates choroid plexus tumor formation. Oncogene. 2006;25:487–91.

117. Beschorner R, Waidelich J, Trautmann K, Psaras T, Schittenhelm J. Notch receptors in human choroid plexus tumors. Histol Histopathol. 2013;28:1055–63.

118. Hasselblatt M, Mertsch S, Koos B, Riesmeier B, Stegemann H, Jeibmann A, Tomm M, Schmitz N, Wrede B, Wolff JE, Zheng W, Paulus W. TWIST-1 is overexpressed in neoplastic choroid plexus epithelial cells and promotes proliferation and invasion. Cancer Res. 2009;69:2219–23.

119. Nupponen NN, Paulsson J, Jeibmann A, Wrede B, Tanner M, Wolff JE, Paulus W, Ostman A, Hasselblatt M. Platelet-derived growth factor receptor expression and amplification in choroid plexus carcinomas. Mod Pathol. 2008;21:265–70.

120. Koos B, Paulsson J, Jarvius M, Sanchez BC, Wrede B, Mertsch S, Jeibmann A, Kruse A, Peters O, Wolff JE, Galla HJ, Soderberg O, Paulus W, Ostman A, Hasselblatt M. Platelet-derived growth factor receptor expression and activation in choroid plexus tumors. Am J Pathol. 2009;175:1631–7.

121. Castelo-Branco P, et al. Methylation of the TERT promoter and risk stratification of childhood brain tumours: an integrative genomic and molecular study. Lancet Oncol. 2013;14:534–42.

122. Hasselblatt M, Muhlisch J, Wrede B, Kallinger B, Jeibmann A, Peters O, Kutluk T, Wolff JE, Paulus W, Fruhwald MC. Aberrant MGMT (O6-methylguanine-DNA methyltransferase) promoter methylation in choroid plexus tumors. J Neurooncol. 2009;91:151–5.

123. Wolff J (2008) Chroid plexus tumoren. In: Korinthenberg + Ritter: Pädiatrische Hämatologie und Onkologie ISBN: 3-540-03702-0 2:2.

124. Wolff JE, Finlay JL. Choroid plexus tumors. In: Carroll WL, Finlay JL, editors. Cancer in children. Sudbury: Jones & Bartlett; 2009.

125. Misaki K, Nakada M, Mohri M, Hayashi Y, Hamada J. MGMT promoter methylation and temozolomide response in choroid plexus carcinoma. Brain Tumor Pathol. 2011;28:259–63.

126. Asai A, Hoffman HJ, Hendrick EB, Humphreys RP, Becker LE. Primary intracranial neoplasms in the first year of life. Childs Nerv Syst. 1989;5:230–3.

127. Packer RJ, Perilongo G, Johnson D, Sutton LN, Vezina G, Zimmerman RA, Ryan J, Reaman G, Schut L. Choroid plexus carcinoma of childhood. Cancer. 1992;69:580–5.

128. Berger C, Thiesse P, Lellouch-Tubiana A, Kalifa C, Pierre-Kahn A, Bouffet E. Choroid plexus carcinomas in childhood: clinical features and prognostic factors. Neurosurgery. 1998;42:470–5.

129. Sun MZ, Oh MC, Ivan ME, Kaur G, Safaee M, Kim JM, Phillips JJ, Auguste KI, Parsa AT. Current management of choroid plexus carcinomas. Neurosurg Rev. 2014;37(2):179–92. discussion 192.

130. Wolff JE, Sajedi M, Coppes MJ, Anderson RA, Egeler RM. Radiation therapy and survival in choroid plexus carcinoma. Lancet. 1999;353:2126.

131. Wolff JE, Gnekow AK, Kortmann RD, Pietsch T, Urban C, Graf N, Kuhl J. Preradiation chemotherapy for pediatric patients with high-grade glioma. Cancer. 2002;94:264–71.

132. Wrede B, Liu P, Wolff JE. Chemotherapy improves the survival of patients with choroid plexus carcinoma: a meta-analysis of individual cases with choroid plexus tumors. J Neurooncol. 2007;85:345–51.

133. Berrak SG, Liu DD, Wrede B, Wolff JE. Which therapy works better in choroid plexus carcinomas? J Neurooncol. 2011;103:155–62.

134. Wolff J. International choroid plexus tumor initiative. Med Ped Oncol. 2002;39:76.
135. Koh EJ, Wang KC, Phi JH, Lee JY, Choi JW, Park SH, Park KD, Kim IH, Cho BK, Kim SK. Clinical outcome of pediatric choroid plexus tumors: retrospective analysis from a single institute. Childs Nerv Syst. 2014;30(2):217–25.
136. Lafay-Cousin L, Keene D, Carret AS, Fryer C, Brossard J, Crooks B, Eisenstat D, Johnston D, Larouche V, Silva M, Wilson B, Zelcer S, Bartels U, Bouffet E. Choroid plexus tumors in children less than 36 months: the Canadian Pediatric Brain Tumor Consortium (CPBTC) experience. Childs Nerv Syst. 2011;27:259–64.
137. Meng H, Feng H, Zhang L, Wang J. Endoscopic removal of a cystic choroid plexus papilloma of the third ventricle: a case report and review of the literature. Clin Neurol Neurosurg. 2011;113:582–5.
138. Mizowaki T, Nagashima T, Yamamoto K, Kawamura A, Yoshida M, Kohmura E. Optimized surgical approach to third ventricular choroid plexus papillomas of young children based on anatomical variations. World Neurosurg. 2013; pii: S1878-8750(13)00458-0.
139. Safaee M, Oh MC, Sughrue ME, Delance AR, Bloch O, Sun M, Kaur G, Molinaro AM, Parsa AT. The relative patient benefit of gross total resection in adult choroid plexus papillomas. J Clin Neurosci. 2013;20:808–12.
140. Safaee M, Clark AJ, Bloch O, Oh MC, Singh A, Auguste KI, Gupta N, McDermott MW, Aghi MK, Berger MS, Parsa AT. Surgical outcomes in choroid plexus papillomas: an institutional experience. J Neurooncol. 2013;113:117–25.
141. Sun MZ, Ivan ME, Clark AJ, Oh MC, Delance AR, Oh T, Safaee M, Kaur G, Bloch O, Molinaro A, Gupta N, Parsa AT. Gross total resection improves overall survival in children with choroid plexus carcinoma. J Neurooncol. 2014;116(1):179–85.
142. Wrede B, Peters Ove Peter Thall, Hasselblatt Martin, Pietsch Torsten, Kortmann Rolf-D., Warmuth-Metz Monika, Mahajan Anita, Lucia Leskova, Xuemei Wang, Wolff Johannes EA (2009) CPT-SIOP-2000 study: Interim results January 2009. Turkish Journal of Cancer 2009: http://wwwturkjcancerorg/archivephp3
143. Wrede B, Liu P, Ater J, Wolff JE. Second surgery and the prognosis of choroid plexus carcinoma—results of a meta-analysis of individual cases. Anticancer Res. 2005;25:4429–33.
144. Goncalves MB, Nunes CF, Melo Jr JO, Guimaraes RD, Klescoski Jr J, Landeiro JA. Tension pneumoventricle after resection of a fourth ventricle choroid plexus papilloma: an unusual postoperative complication. Surg Neurol Int. 2012;3:116.
145. Moiyadi AV, Jalali R, Menon S. Hyperacute disseminated intravascular coagulation following surgery for a choroid plexus carcinoma in a child. Neurol India. 2010;58:485–6.
146. Reddy D, Gunnarsson T, Scheinemann K, Provias JP, Singh SK. Combined staged endoscopic and microsurgical approach of a third ventricular choroid plexus papilloma in an infant. Minim Invasive Neurosurg. 2011;54:264–7.
147. Lee CC, Lin CF, Yang TF, Hsu SP, Chen HH, Chen SC, Shih YH. Telovelar approach for choroid plexus papilloma in the foramen of Luschka: a safe way using a neuromonitor. Clin Neurol Neurosurg. 2012;114:249–53.
148. Trivelato FP, Manzato LB, Rezende MT, Barroso PM, Faleiro RM, Ulhoa AC. Preoperative embolization of choroid plexus papilloma with Onyx via the anterior choroidal artery: technical note. Childs Nerv Syst. 2012;28:1955–8.
149. Haliasos N, Brew S, Robertson F, Hayward R, Thompson D, Chakraborty A. Preoperative embolisation of choroid plexus tumours in children: part I-does the reduction of perioperative blood loss affect the safety of subsequent surgery? Childs Nerv Syst. 2013;29:65–70.
150. Wind JJ, Bell RS, Bank WO, Myseros JS. Treatment of third ventricular choroid plexus papilloma in an infant with embolization alone. J Neurosurg Pediatr. 2010;6:579–82.
151. Lafay-Cousin L, Mabbott DJ, Halliday W, Taylor MD, Tabori U, Kamaly-Asl ID, Kulkarni AV, Bartels U, Greenberg M, Bouffet E. Use of ifosfamide, carboplatin, and etoposide chemotherapy in choroid plexus carcinoma. J Neurosurg Pediatr. 2010;5:615–21.
152. Mazloom A, Wolff JE, Paulino AC. The impact of radiotherapy fields in the treatment of patients with choroid plexus carcinoma. Int J Radiat Oncol Biol Phys. 2010;78:79–84.
153. Bettegowda C, Adogwa O, Mehta V, Chaichana KL, Weingart J, Carson BS, Jallo GI, Ahn ES. Treatment of choroid plexus tumors: a 20-year single institutional experience. J Neurosurg Pediatr. 2012;10:398–405.
154. Samuel TA, Parikh J, Sharma S, Giller CA, Sterling K, Kapoor S, Pirkle C, Jillella A. Recurrent adult choroid plexus carcinoma treated with high-dose chemotherapy and syngeneic stem cell (bone marrow) transplant. J Neurol Surg A Cent Eur Neurosurg. 2013;74 Suppl 1:e149–54.
155. Addo NK, Kamaly-Asl ID, Josan VA, Kelsey AM, Estlin EJ. Preoperative vincristine for an inoperable choroid plexus papilloma: a case discussion and review of the literature. J Neurosurg Pediatr. 2011;8:149–53.
156. Mosleh O, Tabori U, Bartels U, Huang A, Schechter T, Bouffet E. Successful treatment of a recurrent choroid plexus carcinoma with surgery followed by high-dose chemotherapy and stem cell rescue. Pediatr Hematol Oncol. 2013;30:386–91.
157. Gozali AE, Britt B, Shane L, Gonzalez I, Gilles F, McComb JG, Krieger MD, Lavey RS, Shlien A, Villablanca JG, Erdreich-Epstein A, Dhall G, Jubran R, Tabori U, Malkin D, Finlay JL. Choroid plexus tumors; management, outcome, and association with the Li-Fraumeni syndrome: the Children's Hospital Los Angeles (CHLA) experience, 1991–2010. Pediatr Blood Cancer. 2012;58:905–9.
158. Kunis G, Baruch K, Rosenzweig N, Kertser A, Miller O, Berkutzki T, Schwartz M. IFN-gamma-dependent activation of the brain's choroid plexus for CNS immune surveillance and repair. Brain. 2013;136:3427–40.
159. Zhang X, Wu C, Song J, Gotte M, Sorokin L. Syndecan-1, a cell surface proteoglycan, negatively regulates initial leukocyte recruitment to the brain across the choroid plexus in murine experimental autoimmune encephalomyelitis. J Immunol. 2013;191:4551–61.

13 Atypical Teratoid Rhabdoid Tumors

Sriram Venneti, Ganjam V. Kalpana, Alexander R. Judkins, and Sharon L. Gardner

Definition

Atypical teratoid/rhabdoid tumors (AT/RTs) correspond to World Health Organization grade IV tumors occurring predominantly in infants and young children. These tumors are classically associated with the presence of primitive neuroectodermal cells, variably prominent rhabdoid cells, and have evidence of differentiation along several different lines including neuronal, glial, epithelial, and mesenchymal lineages. They are characterized by biallelic genetic alteration of the *SMARCB1* gene (also referred to as *SNF5/BAF47/INI1*), resulting in loss of SMARCB1 protein expression.

Clinical Features

AT/RTs are highly malignant tumors encountered predominantly, though not exclusively, in young children. These tumors were first described in the mid-1980s [1–3]. It has been challenging to determine the exact incidence of these tumors, since until recently they were often misclassified as other central nervous system (CNS) embryonal tumors. However, since the discovery of presence of *SMARCB1* alterations in these tumors, routine immunohistochemistry analysis has replaced fluorescence in situ hybridization (FISH) to demonstrate the absence of the SMARCB1 protein in these tumors, enabling more accurate diagnostics and a clear-cut molecular genetic distinction from other CNS tumors. The incidence of AT/RT is approximately 1–2 % of CNS tumors in children <21 years of age but rises to 10–20 % in those <3 years of age [4, 5]. Recent retrospective studies from national tumor registries have estimated the median age of children initially diagnosed with AT/RT to be between 1 and 2 years of age [6, 7].

AT/RTs have been described to occur throughout the central nervous system. However, these tumors are most commonly located in the infratentorial region in infants and more often supratentorially in older children [5, 8]. In addition, the incidence of metastatic disease at diagnosis is higher in patients <3 years of age. Seeding along cerebrospinal fluid pathways has been reported in up to 20 % of patients at presentation [9]. Because of the predominant tumor location within the posterior fossa, affected children typically present with symptoms including vomiting, lethargy, and failure to thrive, while headache and hemiplegia are more commonly seen in older patients with cerebral hemispheric tumors.

Rhabdoid Tumor Predisposition syndrome (RTPS) is a complex familial disorder seen predominantly in infants. RTPS results in increased susceptibility to development of AT/RT, malignant rhabdoid tumors (MRT) outside the CNS, schwannomas, choroid plexus carcinoma, central primitive neuroectodermal tumor, and medulloblastoma (MB) [10, 11]. Approximately 30–35 % of infants and children diagnosed with MRT may show RTPS [10, 12–14]. The genetics of RTPS are discussed below.

Histopathology

Macroscopy

Many AT/RTs share macroscopic characteristics with other CNS embryonal tumors such as MB and primitive neuroectodermal tumor (PNET). They are bulky tumors, often well demarcated from the surrounding brain. While typically soft in consistency and pink to tan in color (Fig. 13.1), the presence of firm whitish areas may indicate the presence of mesenchymal differentiation. AT/RT may be heterogeneous with cystic, necrotic, and hemorrhagic regions (Fig. 13.1). Neuroimaging studies are similar to those seen in patients with PNET and MB. These tumors are typically iso- to slightly hyperintense by fluid-attenuated inversion recovery (FLAIR) with restricted diffusion. Most tumors are contrast enhancing and up to a quarter of them demonstrate radiographic evidence of leptomeningeal dissemination.

M.A. Karajannis and D. Zagzag (eds.), *Molecular Pathology of Nervous System Tumors: Biological Stratification and Targeted Therapies*, Molecular Pathology Library 8,
DOI 10.1007/978-1-4939-1830-0_13, © Springer Science+Business Media New York 2015

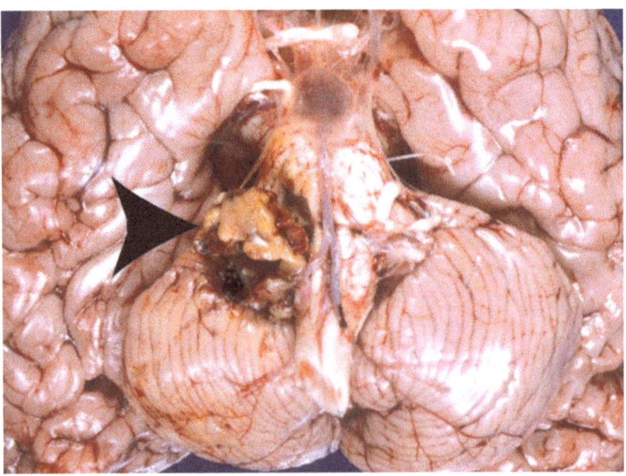

Fig. 13.1 Gross image of AT/RT. Tumor (pink to tan mass) with areas of hemorrhage and necrosis located at the cerebellopontine angle

Histopathology

AT/RTs can be quite heterogeneous and are sometimes difficult to recognize solely on the basis of histopathology. The most striking feature in many cases is the presence of neoplastic cells with rhabdoid features: large cytologically atypical cells with irregular and well-defined cell borders eccentrically placed large nuclei with vesicular chromatin and prominent eosinophilic nucleoli, and abundant pink cytoplasm sometimes containing an eosinophilic cytoplasmic inclusion (Fig. 13.2). In practice, the appearance of these cells often falls along a spectrum, ranging from cells with classic rhabdoid features, to cells with epithelioid features (less striking nuclear atypia and large amounts of pale eosinophilic cytoplasm). Frequently, these cells can exhibit prominent cytoplasmic vacuolar degeneration (Fig. 13.2b). In whatever form they appear, these large cells are rarely the sole or even predominant histopathological feature in AT/RT. Typically, these cells are encountered in small collections or are interspersed among the more numerous primitive neuroectodermal tumor cells (Fig. 13.3). However, it is important to recognize that a relatively diverse range of histopathological patterns may be encountered in AT/RT. Mesenchymal differentiation in these tumors most commonly appears as areas with prominent spindle cell features (Fig. 13.4a) and accumulation of extracellular mucopolysaccharide (Fig. 13.4b). Variable degrees of epithelial differentiation may also be encountered in AT/RT (Fig. 13.5). This is the least common histopathological pattern seen in AT/RT and can manifest as poorly differentiated glandular structures, papillary structures, or poorly differentiated ribbons and cords of cells with epithelial features. Occasionally in the latter case, abundant mucopolysaccharide-rich material separates the nests and cords of tumors in a pattern reminiscent of chordoma. Irrespective of the histopathological pattern, mitotic figures are generally abundant in AT/RT. Both karyorrhexis and areas of geographic necrosis are commonly encountered [8, 9, 15, 16].

Differential Diagnosis

The differential diagnosis of AT/RT includes MB, CNS PNET, pineoblastoma, anaplastic ependymoma, choroid plexus carcinoma, and germ cell tumors [9, 15, 17–19]. Particular care must be taken to avoid confusing anaplastic/large cell MB for AT/RT and vice versa. Misdiagnosis can generally be avoided with attention to a few critical details.

First, at the cytologic level, anaplastic/large cell MB show a range of nuclear features that while overlapping with AT/RT in some regards, generally fail to recapitulate the vesicular chromatin-staining pattern typical of these tumors. While they are variably prominent, at least some proportion of rhabdoid tumor cells demonstrates prominent eosinophilic nucleoli. These are not encountered in anaplastic/large cell MB except in the rare case with predominant or exclusively large cell features; these tumors lack the vesicular chromatin staining and variability seen in AT/RT.

Second, evaluation of the cytoplasmic features is extremely helpful. The presence of tumor cells with rhabdoid cytoplasmic inclusions is reassuring. However, the prominence of such cells within any given case can be extremely variable. This may be a function of biology, sampling, or both. In cases where no classic rhabdoid cells are encountered, it is critical to recognize the presence of poorly preserved rhabdoid tumor cells. The presence of scattered cells with large poorly preserved nuclei, vacuolar cytoplasmic degeneration, and prominent well-defined cell borders may be the only histologic evidence of an AT/RT. In other cases, it is the presence of cells with epithelioid or vaguely epithelioid features that alerts the pathologist to the presence of an AT/RT.

Finally, it is important to evaluate the overall histologic pattern for clues to the presence of an AT/RT. In many cases the overall growth pattern may appear essentially indistinguishable from a classic MB or CNS PNET. However, in some cases it is possible to recognize features suggestive of epithelial differentiation in what is otherwise an unremarkable MB or CNS PNET. These features include evidence of epithelial (the presence of poorly differentiated glandular and epithelial structures or the growth of tumor cells in small nests and cords) and/or mesenchymal structures [most often a spindle cell growth pattern (Fig. 13.4a), but occasionally tumors show evidence of more advanced mesenchymal differentiation including the presence of bone and cartilage]. Finally, the accumulation of extracellular myxohyaline material (Fig. 13.4b) in a CNS embryonal tumor is a histologic feature that should raise the differential diagnosis of AT/RT.

Among the non-CNS embryonal neoplasms, there are several features that deserve consideration in the differential

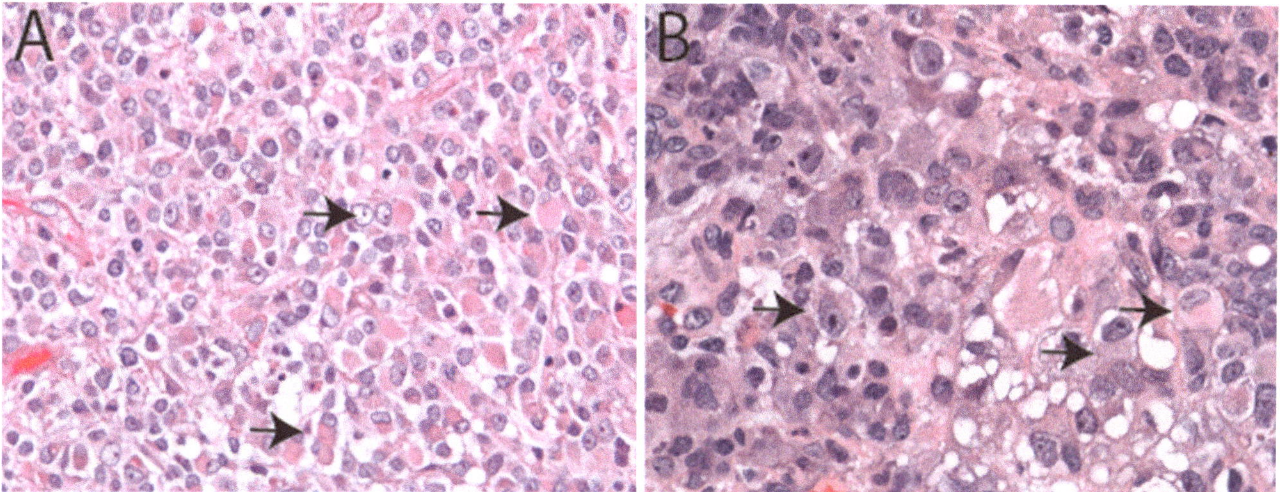

Fig. 13.2 Classic rhabdoid morphology in AT/RT. H&E sections (20×, **a**, and 40×, **b**) illustrating classic rhabdoid tumor cells in AT/RT characterized by large cells with eccentrically placed nuclei with vesicular chromatin and abundant pink cytoplasm sometimes containing an eosinophilic cytoplasmic inclusion (*arrows*). Vacuolar cytoplasmic degeneration typical of ATR/RT in (**b**)

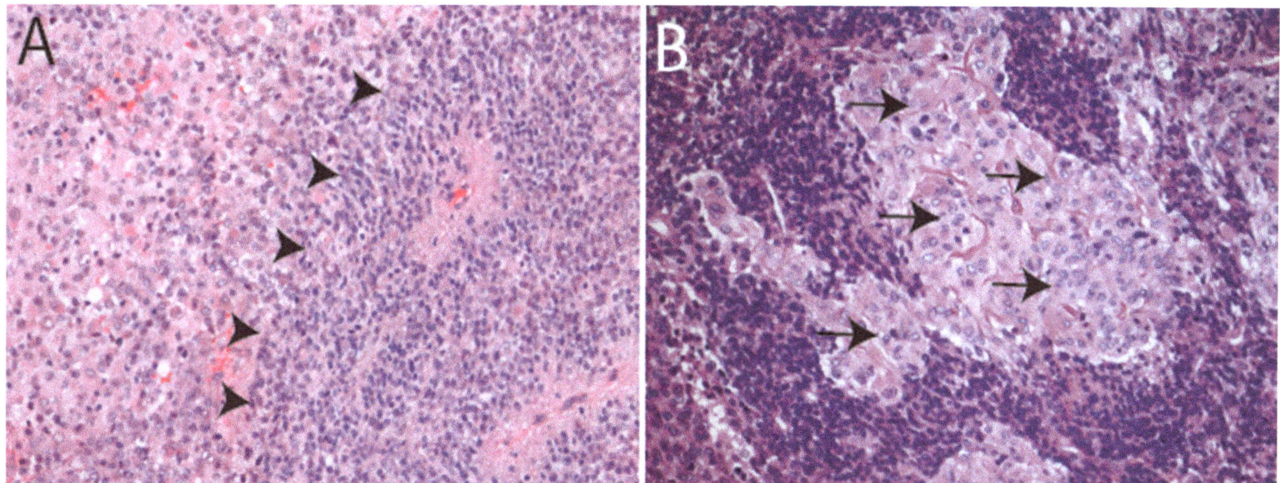

Fig. 13.3 Primitive neuroectodermal features in AT/RT. H&E sections showing primitive neuroectodermal component (*arrowheads* in **a**, 20×) with adjacent rhabdoid areas (*arrows* in **b**, 40×)

diagnosis of AT/RT. Anaplastic ependymomas in the posterior fossa can resemble AT/RT due to their high cellularity and necrosis. It is not uncommon to encounter areas where AT/RTs undermine and appear to grow into the choroid plexus. Combined with occasional papillary features or cells arranged in cord-like structures resembling poorly differentiated epithelial structures, choroid plexus carcinomas should be considered in the differential diagnosis. Prominent spindle cell pattern may resemble a sarcoma and glandular or epithelial differentiations may suggest a teratoma or metastatic carcinoma. In the pineal and other midline locations, germ cell tumors should also enter into the differential diagnosis. Immunohistochemical studies and molecular testing can play a pivotal role in helping the pathologist refine the diagnosis in such cases.

Immunohistochemistry

Immunohistochemical staining for the SMARCB1 protein has been shown to be a highly sensitive and specific tool for detecting the presence of alterations in the *SMARCB1* gene on chromosome 22q11.2 (Judkins et al., 2004). In addition to SMARCB1, immunohistochemical expression of several other markers may play an important role in the diagnosis of

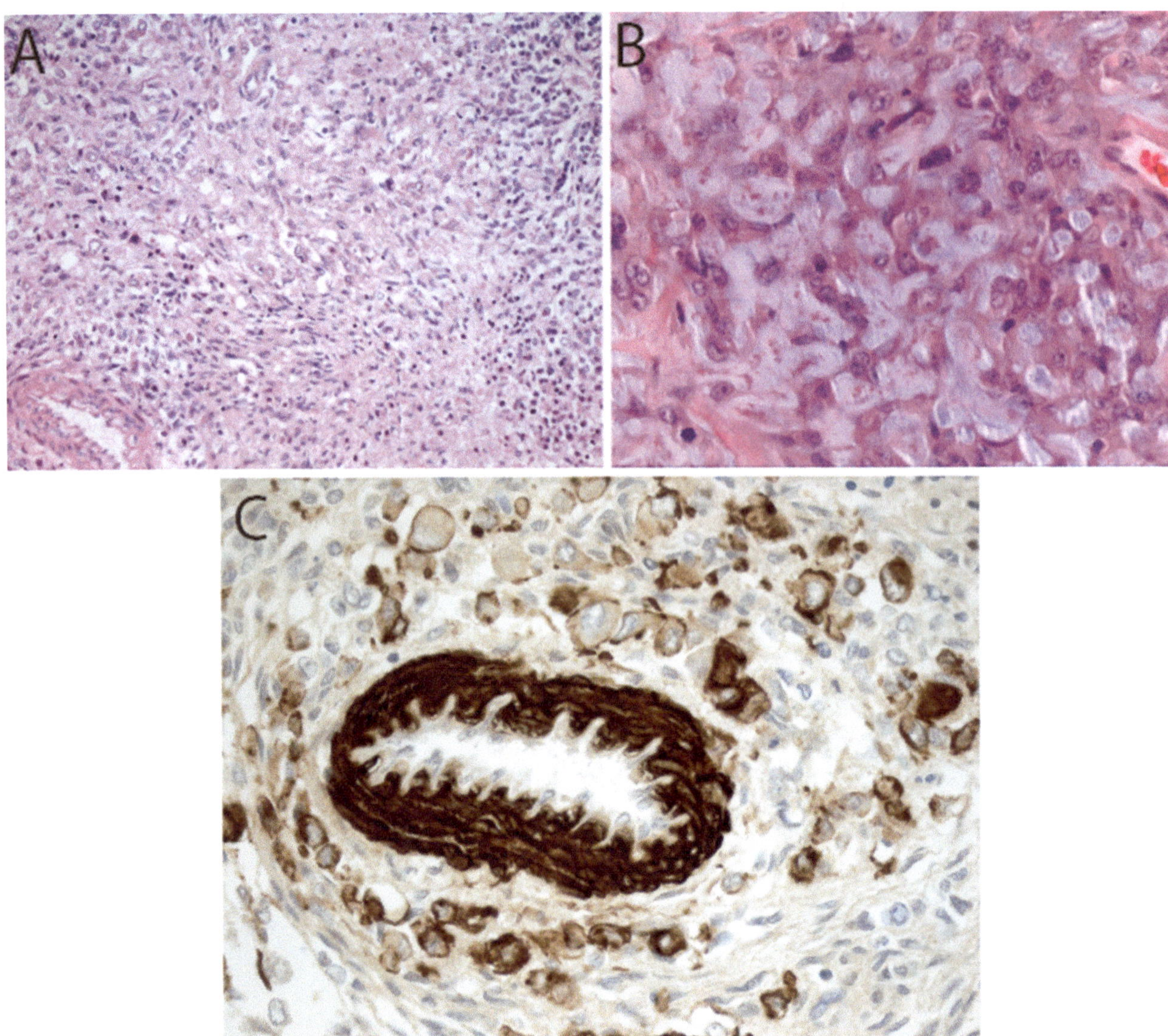

Fig. 13.4 Mesenchymal differentiation in AT/RT. H&E sections showing spindle cell component (20×, **a**) and extracellular mucopolysaccharide accumulation (40×, **b**) in AT/RT. Immunostain for smooth muscle antigen (SMA, 40×) showing staining in vessel wall and tumor cells

AT/RT. The heterogeneity in appearance of AT/RT and suggestion of differentiation along multiple cell lineages is reflected in the polyphenotypic immunostaining profile characteristic of these tumors. AT/RTs demonstrate almost universal expression of smooth muscle antigen (SMA, Fig. 13.4c), epithelial membrane antigen (EMA, Fig. 13.5b) and vimentin (Figs. 13.5a). While the latter stain is of limited specificity, it can occasionally prove a useful tool for demonstrating the presence of hard to detect rhabdoid cells. The combined expression of mesenchymal (SMA, Fig. 13.4c) and epithelial markers (EMA, Fig. 13.5b) is unique for AT/RT among other CNS tumors. Expression of glial fibrillary acid protein (GFAP, Fig. 13.6a) and neuronal markers including neurofilament protein (NFP), synaptophysin (SYN, Fig. 13.6b, and NeuN is typically seen in up to about 75 % of AT/RT. Cytokeratin markers such as AE1.3 are also positive in some AT/RT, though typically they are not as frequently expressed as the other markers discussed above [8, 9]. Classical germ cell markers such as placental alkaline phosphatase (PLAP), β–human chorionic gonadotropin (β–HCG) and octomer-binding transcription factor (OCT-4) may be negative. However, other germ cell markers such as Sal-like protein-4 (SALL4), sex determining region Y-box 2 (SOX2) and Nanog may be positive suggesting the potential for pluripotency in these tumors [20]. The expression of these various markers is highly variable from case to case and may reflect the complex biology of these tumors and their ability to differentiate along multiple lineages.

Loss of SMARCB1 expression in tumor cells enables differentiation of AT/RT from other CNS tumors, which dem-

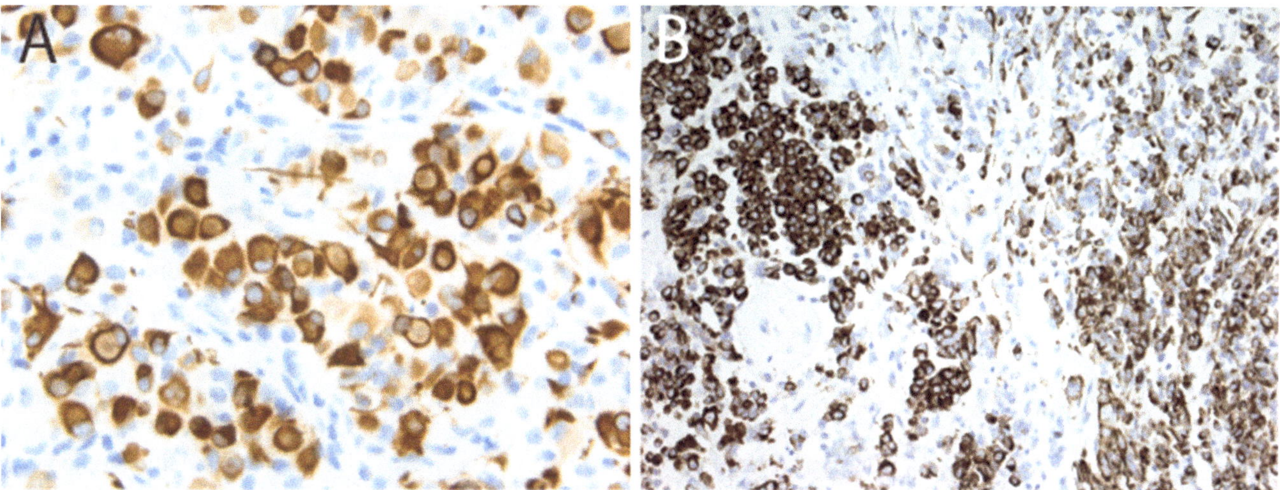

FIG. 13.5 Vimentin and epithelial membrane antigen expression in AT/RT. Immunostains for vimentin (**a**, 20×) and epithelial membrane antigen (EMA, 40×, showing membranous staining, (**b**) in AT/RT

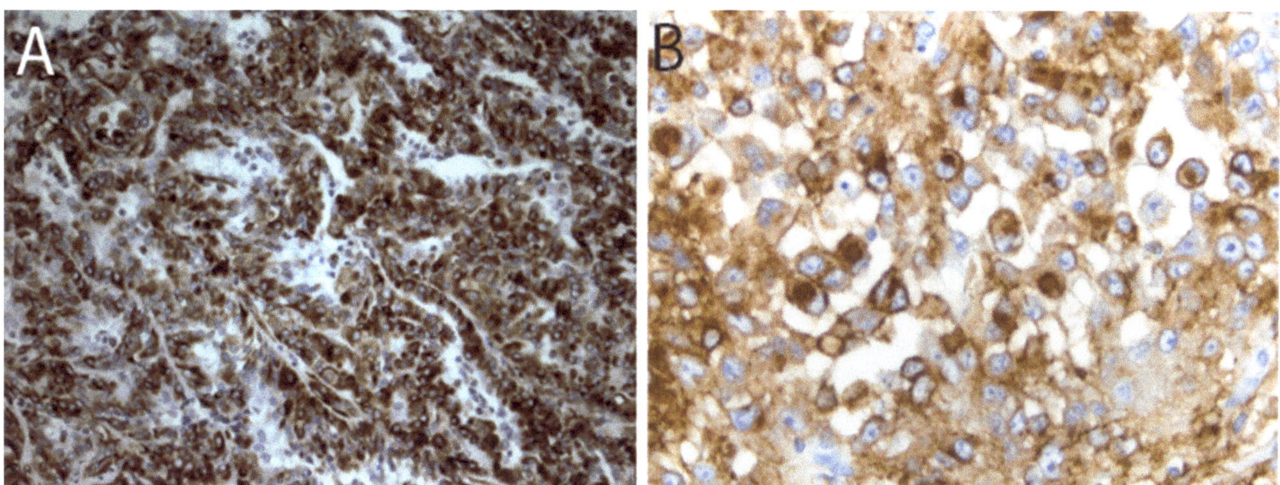

FIG. 13.6 Neuroglial markers in AT/RT. Immunostains for glia fibrillary acidic protein (GFAP, 40×, **a**) and synaptophysin (SYN, 20×, **b**) in AT/RT

onstrate retained expression of SMARCB1 (Fig. 13.7). Correct interpretation of SMARCB1 immunohistochemical staining is aided by the fact that SMARCB1 is a ubiquitously expressed nuclear protein and therefore it demonstrates positive immunostaining in endothelial cells and infiltrating tumor lymphocytes (Fig. 13.7). The loss of expression of SMARCB1 in these cells, as well as the failure of the stain to be expressed in any adjacent normal tissues, should signal to the pathologist the need to repeat the SMARCB1 immunohistochemical staining.

As a result of the utility of SMARCB1, combined with the histopathological diversity of AT/RT, it has become the standard of care to stain all CNS embryonal neoplasms with SMARCB1. By so doing, cases of previously unrecognized AT/RT have been reported in some institutions [21]. Routine application of SMARCB1 immunostaining has led to the recognition of loss of expression in other tumor types including CNS low-grade tumors undergoing malignant transformation (ganglioglioma, pleomorphic xanthoastrocytoma) [22, 23] as well as extra-CNS tumors including epithelioid sarcoma, extraskeletal myxoid chondrosarcoma, renal medullary carcinoma, and epithelioid malignant peripheral nerve sheath tumor [24–26]. The pathogenic role, if any, of loss of SMARCB1 in these non-rhabdoid tumors remains to be determined. It is particularly critical that the neuropathologist who makes the diagnosis of AT/RT recognizes that at least a third of all newly diagnosis AT/RTs are attributable to a germline mutation [12] (see below). It is therefore essential that a referral for genetic counseling and testing be made for the patient and their family.

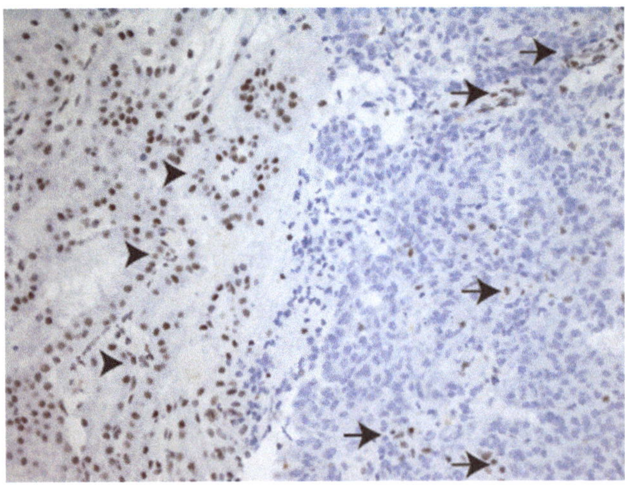

Fig. 13.7 Loss of SMARCB1 staining in AT/RT. Immunostain for SMARCB1 (20×), showing loss of SMARCB1 expression in tumor cells. As an internal control, there is preserved SMARCB1 staining in adjacent choroid plexus (*arrow heads*) and intra-tumoral endothelial cells and infiltrating lymphocytes (*arrows*)

Cytogenetics and Molecular Genetics

Molecular Genetics

SMARCB1 is a tumor suppressor gene biallelically mutated in >95 % of all AT/RTs [27–30]. SMARCB1 is also referred to as: (1) INI1 (Integrase Interactor 1) as the mammalian homologue was first discovered as an HIV-1 integrase-binding protein, (2) BAF47 (BRG1-associated factor 47), and (3) hSNF5 (human sucrose non-fermenting) [31]. SMARCB1 is a component of the mammalian chromatin remodeling SWI/SNF (Switch/Sucrose Non-Fermentable) complex, which reorganizes and/or repositions nucleosomes in an ATP-dependent manner [32]. This complex is believed to be a critical epigenetic regulator for normal development and maintenance of tissue-specific gene expression [33].

The subunits of the SWI/SNF complex are grouped into two major subfamilies: (1) BAF (BRG1 or hBRM-associated factor) complex and (2) PBAF (Polybromo-associated BAF) [34–41]. Among the subunits, there are four core components that are present in all versions of the SWI/SNF complex including: (1) the ATPase enzymatic subunits SMARCA2 (hBRM, hBrahma) or SMARCA4 (BRG1, or Brahma-related gene 1), (2) SMARCB1 (INI1/SNF5/BAF47), (3) SMARCC1 (BAF155), and (4) SMARCC2 (BAF170).

Mutations in almost all subunits of the SWI/SNF complex have been identified in many human cancers [42–44]. SMARCB1 is biallelically inactivated in >95 % of MRT but is variably mutated in other cancer types (discussed below), suggesting that the function of SMARCB1 through SWI/SNF is essential for protecting a specific cell type from becoming cancerous and preventing the genesis of rhabdoid tumors including AT/RT [45].

Mutational Spectrum of SMARCB1 Found in AT/RT

Notwithstanding their histological and immunohistochemical diversity, nearly all AT/RTs involve mutation, deletion, or loss of expression of the *SMARCB1* gene. Approximately 70 % MRT arise due to biallelic loss of the *SMARCB1* tumor suppressor, and an additional 20–25 % exhibit loss of SMARCB1 function due to reduced RNA or protein expression [12].

Several studies have defined the spectrum of *SMARCB1* mutations within AT/RT. These studies have shown that approximately 40 % of *SMARCB1* mutations are homozygous deletions, frequently associated with chromosomal rearrangements of 22q11 [3, 46, 47]. In addition to homozygous deletion of *SMARCB1*, 96 coding-sequence mutations were identified in nine exons of the *SMARCB1* gene among 119 ATRT tumor samples analyzed [12].

These mutations occurred with the highest frequency in exons 5 and 9 in AT/RT, while mutations within exon 8 have yet to be detected, and mutations in exons 1 and 3 are largely underrepresented [12, 48]. The majority of coding-sequence mutations (48/96) were single base-pair point mutations, 47 of which were nonsense mutations predicting premature truncation of the protein, and one of which was a missense mutation in exon 9 [12]. The second-most frequent (31/96) type of mutation was deletion and appeared to be localized to a few spots within *SMARCB1*; 20 were found within exon 9 and 14 involved deletion of one of four cytosines in bases 1,145–1,148, and six involved deletion of one of two guanines at position 1,143 or 1,144 [12]. The remaining mutations identified were duplications of 4–19 bases (7/96), insertions (6/96), and intragenic deletions of one or two exons (4/96) [12]. In addition to coding-sequence mutations, a mutation affecting splicing of the *SMARCB1* transcript has also been identified: an A to G mutation in intron 5, which disrupts the splice acceptor site [49].

Most mutations discussed were likely somatic mutations, however; a study on 49 tumor and matched blood DNA samples showed that 33 % (16/49) mutations were germline [12]. These germline mutations were coding-sequence mutations resulting in introduction of a premature stop codon found within exons 2, 4, 5, 6, and 7 [12].

Some of the mutations identified occur repeatedly in different MRT samples indicating possible hot-spots for mutation [12, 48]. Examples include the cytosine deletion at the 3′ end of the *SMARCB1* coding sequence (detected in ten different AT/RTs) and C601T (p. Arg201x, found in 12 RTs), and C472T (p. Arg158x, found in seven different tumors). Interestingly, the C601T and C472T mutations have also been identified as germline mutations in families with rhabdoid tumor predisposition syndrome (RTPS) [47]. Other germline mutations identified in RTPS included deletions and insertions causing frame shifts, nonsense mutations, missense mutations, and mutations affecting splicing of the *SMARCB1* transcript [11, 47, 50–54]. Notably, many of the

SMARCB1 mutations associated with RTPS are *de novo* germline mutations [11, 47]. LOH is common in RTPS, causing loss of the second allele of *SMARCB1* [11, 47, 50].

Exome analysis has revealed that the genomes of these cancers are remarkably simple, showing extremely low rate of mutations with loss of SMARCB1 being the primary recurrent event [55]. This observation is consistent with the data that mouse models with heterozygous deletions of *SMARCB1* gene develop a high frequency of tumors with early onset resembling AT/RT with loss of heterozygosity (LOH) at the *SMARCB1* locus [56].

Rarely, other components of SWI/SNF may be implicated in the development of AT/RT. There are a few exceptions to the above observations. There are reports indicating that tumors that exhibit typical AT/RT features showed the presence of intact *SMARCB1* gene and protein, but show nonsense mutation and inactivation of *SMARCA4* [57]. Conversely, recently, there has been an explosion of data describing pathological SMARCB1 mutations/loss of expression in several other tumor types including schwannoma, epithelioid MPNST, epithelioid sarcoma, extraskeletal myxoid chondrosarcoma, synovial sarcoma, pediatric undifferentiated sarcoma, renal medullary carcinoma, small cell undifferentiated variant of hepatoblastoma and myoepithelial carcinoma, and schwannomatosis [26, 58–68]. The role of SMARCB1 mutation/loss in these tumors remains to be clearly established.

Molecular Diagnosis

The ubiquitous expression of SMARCB1 and its loss in nearly all AT/RTs makes it a powerful target as a diagnostic tool. Immunohistochemical analysis for loss of SMARCB1 expression was shown to effectively establish the diagnosis of AT/RT and distinguish MRTs from other pediatric soft tissue tumors [18, 19, 69]. Earlier studies demonstrated that AT/RTs could be distinguished from other histologically similar CNS tumors by cytogenetic studies using FISH of chromosome region 22q11.2 to visualize loss of *SMARCB1* locus [70]. Additionally, quantitative real-time PCR (q-RT-PCR) can be performed when DNA of the tumor tissues are available to determine the presence of missense and non-synonymous mutations in the exons of *SMARCB1* gene.

Prognostic Stratification and Treatments

Prognosis and Treatment

The treatment of children with AT/RT presents several challenges. These tumors are very aggressive and often resistant to even the most intensive therapies. In addition, because these tumors are more commonly found in very young children, treatment modalities such as craniospinal irradiation are not always an option.

Chemotherapy

One of the earliest regimens resulting in long-term survival even in young children with AT/RT incorporated the approach used by the rhabdomyosarcoma group for patients with parameningeal tumors known as Intergroup Rhabdomyosarcoma Study-III (IRS-III). Weinblatt and Kochen treated a patient with a CNS rhabdoid tumor who underwent gross total resection of the tumor followed by 4,140 cGy focal irradiation and intensive chemotherapy using the IRS-III regimen [71]. The patient was alive and without evidence of disease 4.5 years at the time of the report. Olson et al. published their results on three additional patients with AT/RT using a similar approach [72].

Chi et al. published one of the largest prospective studies to date incorporating the IRS III chemotherapy into an intensive multimodality treatment approach [73]. They reported the results of 20 children newly diagnosed with AT/RT treated between 2004 and 2006. The 2-year progression-free survival rate was 53 ± 13 % with an overall survival rate of 70 ± 10 %.

High Dose Chemotherapy

Finlay et al. have used a strategy known as Head Start therapy for very young children newly diagnosed with malignant brain tumors including AT/RT. This approach uses high dose chemotherapy with autologous stem cell reinfusion in order to avoid or at least postpone the use of irradiation in very young children. The initial report included patients treated on Head Start I and Head Start II [74]. Patients enrolled on Head Start I received 5 cycles of induction chemotherapy with cisplatin, vincristine (during the first 3 cycles), cyclophosphamide, and etoposide. This was followed by a single course of high dose chemotherapy including carboplatin, thiotepa, and etoposide with autologous stem cell reinfusion. Head Start II had identical therapy except for the addition of high dose methotrexate with each induction course. One patient received craniospinal irradiation following autologous stem cell reinfusion, but prior to relapse. At the time of the report, there were three patients treated on Head Start II who were event-free survivors 42+, 54+, and 67+ months following diagnosis without radiation therapy.

Lafay-Cousin et al. have recently reported the experience of the Canadian Brain Tumor Consortium. This was a retrospective review of children treated between 1995 and 2007 [75]. The majority of the patients were <36 months of age and over 1/3 had metastatic disease. . Of the 40 patients who were treated, 22 received standard dose chemotherapy and 18 received high dose chemotherapy with autologous stem cell reinfusion. Adjuvant radiation therapy was administered to 15 patients and nine received intrathecal chemotherapy. Children who received high dose chemotherapy had a 2-year overall survival of 60 ± 12.6 % compared to 21.7 ± 8.5 % for those treated with standard dose chemotherapy. Half of the survivors did not receive any irradiation.

Radiation Therapy

The group from St. Jude Children's Research Hospital has investigated the role of radiation therapy in a retrospective review of patients with AT/RT treated at their institution between 1987 and 2007 [76]. The timing and field of irradiation were age- and risk dependent with the youngest patients receiving irradiation at least a month or more following resection and usually limited to the involved-field. Cox regression modeling revealed that overall survival in their cohort was adversely affected by disease progression prior to irradiation, time from diagnosis to start of irradiation and age at diagnosis. They concluded that early postoperative irradiation is important for local control particularly in patients without evidence of metastatic disease at diagnosis.

The Children's Oncology Group has recently closed accrual to a study for children newly diagnosed with AT/RT. This is a single arm study which incorporated high dose methotrexate during induction and consolidation with triple high dose chemotherapy using carboplatin and thiotepa following the previous infant brain tumor study, CCG99703. Radiation therapy was administered between induction and consolidation to children >6 months of age with localized posterior fossa tumors and to those >12 months of age with supratentorial disease. The remaining patients received irradiation following consolidation. Although the study was closed for a year as a result of a toxic pulmonary death, accrual was recently completed and results should be available shortly.

Molecular Signaling Pathways

AT/RTs are relatively free of the genomic instability and widespread accumulation of mutations that are common in many cancers [55]. However, since SMARCB1 is a component of the SWI/SNF complex, its loss may result in modifications of the epigenome that result in large expression changes which may lead to the development of tumors. It has been demonstrated that SWI/SNF regulates transcription of approximately 2–10 % of cellular genes [77].

The SWI/SNF complex mediates both activation and repression of transcription by chromatin remodeling. The exact function of SMARCB1 within SWI/SNF complex is not understood. However, SMARCB1 is one of the subunits that may bridge the interaction of SWI/SNF with specific transcription factors. For example, SMARCB1 interacts with cMYC and the SWI/SNF complex is required for the transactivation functions of cMYC [78]. Another transcription factor that has been shown to bind to SMARCB1 is Hedgehog-Gli1 transcription factor. Inactivation of SMARCB1 may lead to disruption of specific nucleosome patterning and occupancy with accompanying gene expression changes [79].

Loss of SMARCB1 results in a widespread but specific deregulation of genes and pathways important for the cell cycle, differentiation, senescence, or apoptosis, all with tumorigenic potential. Gene expression profile studies carried out to define the changes in transcriptome that occur when SMARCB1 is reintroduced into SMARCB1-null MRT cells identified downstream effectors and several pathways and genes important for normal cell division and homeostasis [80–82]. Genes upregulated by SMARCB1 tend to be antiproliferative or involved in inducing senescence and differentiation, while genes repressed by SMARCB1 tend to be involved in cell cycle progression [82–84]. Several important cell cycle regulatory genes are over-expressed in AT/RT due to loss of SMARCB1 including *Cyclin D1* and *Aurora A* [84–86]. Experimental studies in murine models and human RT cell lines have demonstrated that *Cyclin D1* is a key regulator of AT/RT tumor cell growth and that abrogation of *Cyclin D1* leads to complete loss of tumor formation in genetically engineered *smarcb1*± heterozygous mouse models [84, 85, 87]. Furthermore, reintroduction of SMARCB1 leads to induction of senescence [85, 88–90].

In mammalian cells SMARCB1 loss results in transcriptional activation of EZH2 gene, a polycomb gene (PcG) protein and a component of the mammalian polycomb complex, PRC2 as well as in repression and increased H3K27-trimethylation of polycomb targets [91]. It thus appears that SMARCB1 represses and EZH2 activates stem cell-associated programs [91]. This is consistent with the observation that there is frequent activation/upregulation of PcG proteins and frequent inactivation of SWI/SNF components in human cancers [91, 92]. Thus it appears that SWI/SNF modulates the expression and activities of PcG complex to maintain the epigenome and proper expression of cellular genes required for preventing tumor formation [91, 92].

Molecular Targeted Therapies

Although a few children with AT/RT are long-term survivors following therapy with surgery, intensive chemotherapy, and irradiation, new treatment modalities are desperately needed. Current treatments are very toxic and largely ineffective. Several groups are trying to develop more targeted therapy by focusing on unique aspects of these tumors.

As previously noted, the majority of AT/RTs have biallelic inactivation of the SMARCB1 gene. Many investigators are trying to develop therapy directed towards the effects of the loss of this gene. Kalpana et al. were one of the first teams to study downstream targets of the loss of the SMARCB1 gene [82]. They used cDNA microarray analyses to identify downstream targets and then defined the functional significance of these targets. They found that SMARCB1 activated interferon-stimulated genes and repressed polo-like kinase 1 suggesting that interferon and down modulation of polo-like kinase 1 may be potential therapeutic options.

This same group has suggested that cyclin D1 could be a valuable target since loss of SMARCB1 results in derepression of cyclin D1 and rhabdoid tumors are very dependent on

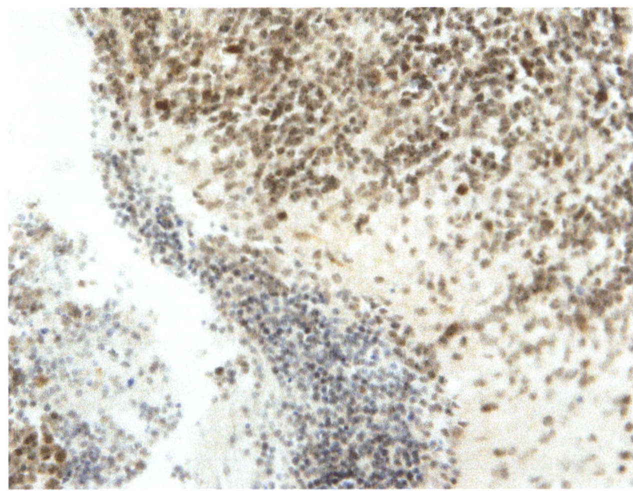

Fig. 13.8 Expression of downstream effector, Aurora Kinase A (*AURKA*) in AT/RT: Aurora Kinase A (*AURKA*) is upregulated in primary human AT/RTs. A primary human AT/RT subjected to immunohistochemical analysis using α-Aurora A antibodies. The tumor cells are strongly positive for AURKA expression (*stained brown*). However, the tumor adjacent normal brain granular cells (blue due to the nuclear stain) are negative for AURKA staining (From Lee S, Cimica V, Ramachandra N, Zagzag D, Kalpana GV (2011) Aurora A Is a Repressed Effector Target of the Chromatin Remodeling Protein INI1/hSNF5 Required for Rhabdoid Tumor Cell Survival. Cancer Res 71:3225–3235, with permission)

cyclin D1 for survival [87]. Furthermore, the same group identified *Aurora Kinase A* (*AURKA*) as a repressed downstream target of SMARCB1 and demonstrated that AT/RT tumors that are deficient in SMARCB1 over-express Aurora A (Fig. 13.8) [86]. Furthermore, this group demonstrated that siRNA-mediated knockdown of *AURKA* leads to mitotic catastrophe and cell death in RT tumor cell lines [86]. Histone deacetylase inhibitors have been shown to decrease cyclin D1 expression [93]. Several different histone deacetylase inhibitors have been shown to alter gene expression and inhibit AT/RT cell growth in vitro and in xenografts [94–96].

Hertwig et al. found that loss of SMARCB1 resulted in an increased sensitivity to phosphorylation of a cytoplasmic unfolded protein response component, eIF2α [97]. They showed that bortezomib, a proteasome inhibitor FDA approved for multiple myeloma, resulted in increased apoptosis of SMARCB1 knockdown cells.

Ogino et al. were one of the first groups to suggest a role of insulin growth factor (IGF) II and insulin growth factor receptor (IGFR) in the pathogenesis of AT/RT [98]. They used immunohistochemistry to demonstrate cytoplasmic positivity for IGFII and cytoplasmic and membranous expression of IGFRI.

D'cunja et al. also used immunohistochemistry to confirm the expression of IGF-1R on 8/8 AT/RT primary tumors [99]. IGF-1R antisense oligonucleotides were used in two AT/RT cell lines resulting in significant downregulation of IGF-1R mRNA and protein expression, apoptosis and increased sensitivity to the chemotherapy drugs doxorubicin and cisplatin.

Arcaro et al. found increased expression of IGF-1R and insulin receptor on AT/RT cell lines compared with normal brain tissue [100]. They found that the AT/RT cells secreted insulin, which potently activated Akt. Inhibitors of the insulin receptor as well as the PI3K/Akt pathway impaired AT/RT growth and proliferation.

Darr et al. also noted persistent Akt activation in Smarcb-1-deficient tumor cells as a result of PI3K-mediated signaling [101]. They, too, were able to prevent proliferation of the Smarcb-1-deficient cells in vitro through inhibition of Akt and inhibited the development of xenografted tumors in their mouse model.

The Pediatric Oncology Experimental Therapeutics Investigators Consortium has used a panel of large drug libraries to identify potential drug therapies for a number of different pediatric tumors [102]. They have recently published their evaluation of three AT/RT cell lines. Their screening studies revealed that agents which altered a number of pathways including Erb2, mTOR, proteasomes, Hsp90, Polo-like kinases, and Aurora kinases were cytotoxic to all three cell lines. Additional studies with the FDA-approved tyrosine kinase inhibitor, lapatinib, revealed cytotoxicity in vitro, in xenografts and in combination with IGF-1R inhibitors.

Although several targeted therapies have been tested in vitro and in animal models, very few have been tested in humans. The Children's Oncology Group recently conducted a phase I/II study using the Aurora kinase A inhibitor MLN8237 in children with a variety of solid tumors. Other investigators have recently begun to use this agent in children with recurrent or progressive AT/RT [103]. Although dosing and safety data are available, efficacy results are pending.

Summary

AT/RTs are characterized by alterations in the SMARCB1 gene and are primarily seen in the pediatric age group. These tumors may demonstrate a wide spectrum of histopathologic features that raises important differential diagnostic considerations. Assessment of molecular alterations in SMARCB1 is vital to the diagnosis of AT/RT and can be performed by immunohistochemistry for the SMARCB1 protein or by molecular tests such as FISH or PCR. We discuss the various molecular alterations seen in SMARCB1 in AT/RT, which include somatic and germline mutations. The pathogenesis of AT/RT is not completely understood but loss of SMARCB1 can contribute to tumor formation by affecting various cellular processes including cell cycle proteins such as Cyclin D1 and the epigenome by altering the transcriptional activity of EZH2 in the regulation of stem cell-associated programs.

While the prognosis for patients with AT/RT remains poor, there are several current regimens available to treat patients that target a variety of different pathways and biological processes.

References

1. Bonnin JM, Rubinstein LJ, Palmer NF, Beckwith JB. The association of embryonal tumors originating in the kidney and in the brain. A report of seven cases. Cancer. 1984;54: 2137–46.
2. Biggs PJ, Garen PD, Powers JM, Garvin AJ. Malignant rhabdoid tumor of the central nervous system. Hum Pathol. 1987; 18:332–7.
3. Biegel JA, Kalpana G, Knudsen ES, Packer RJ, Roberts CW, Thiele CJ, Weissman B, Smith M. The role of INI1 and the SWI/SNF complex in the development of rhabdoid tumors: meeting summary from the workshop on childhood atypical teratoid/rhabdoid tumors. Cancer Res. 2002;62:323–8.
4. Hilden JM, Meerbaum S, Burger P, Finlay J, Janss A, Scheithauer BW, Walter AW, Rorke LB, Biegel JA. Central nervous system atypical teratoid/rhabdoid tumor: results of therapy in children enrolled in a registry. J Clin Oncol. 2004;22:2877–84.
5. Tekautz TM, Fuller CE, Blaney S, Fouladi M, Broniscer A, Merchant TE, Krasin M, Dalton J, Hale G, Kun LE, Wallace D, Gilbertson RJ, Gajjar A. Atypical teratoid/rhabdoid tumors (ATRT): improved survival in children 3 years of age and older with radiation therapy and high-dose alkylator-based chemotherapy. J Clin Oncol. 2005;23(7):1491–9.
6. Woehrer A, Slavc I, Waldhoer T, Heinzl H, Zielonke N, Czech T, Benesch M, Hainfellner JA, Haberler C, Austrian Brain Tumor R. Incidence of atypical teratoid/rhabdoid tumors in children: a population-based study by the Austrian Brain Tumor Registry, 1996–2006. Cancer. 2010;116:5725–32.
7. von Hoff K, Hinkes B, Dannenmann-Stern E, von Bueren AO, Warmuth-Metz M, Soerensen N, Emser A, Zwiener I, Schlegel PG, Kuehl J, Fruhwald MC, Kortmann RD, Pietsch T, Rutkowski S. Frequency, risk-factors and survival of children with atypical teratoid rhabdoid tumors (AT/RT) of the CNS diagnosed between 1988 and 2004, and registered to the German HIT database. Pediatr Blood Cancer. 2011;57:978–85.
8. Rorke LB, Packer RJ, Biegel JA. Central nervous system atypical teratoid/rhabdoid tumors of infancy and childhood: definition of an entity. J Neurosurg. 1996;85:56–65.
9. Judkins AR, Eberhart CG, Wesseling P. Atypical teratoid/rhabdoid tumor. WHO classification of tumors of the central nervous system.2007; 4:147–149.
10. Sevenet N, Sheridan E, Amram D, Schneider P, Handgretinger R, Delattre O. Constitutional mutations of the hSNF5/INI1 gene predispose to a variety of cancers. Am J Hum Genet. 1999;65:1342–8.
11. Lee HY, Yoon CS, Sevenet N, Rajalingam V, Delattre O, Walford NQ. Rhabdoid tumor of the kidney is a component of the rhabdoid predisposition syndrome. Pediatr Dev Pathol. 2002;5:395–9.
12. Biegel JA. Molecular genetics of atypical teratoid/rhabdoid tumor. Neurosurg Focus. 2006;20:E11.
13. Bourdeaut F, et al. Frequent hSNF5/INI1 germline mutations in patients with rhabdoid tumor. Clin Cancer Res. 2011;17: 31–8.
14. Eaton KW, Tooke LS, Wainwright LM, Judkins AR, Biegel JA. Spectrum of SMARCB1/INI1 mutations in familial and sporadic rhabdoid tumors. Pediatr Blood Cancer. 2011;56:7–15.
15. Rorke LB, Packer R, Biegel J. Central nervous system atypical teratoid/rhabdoid tumors of infancy and childhood. J Neurooncol. 1995;24:21–8.
16. Bhattacharjee M, Hicks J, Langford L, Dauser R, Strother D, Chintagumpala M, Horowitz M, Cooley L, Vogel H. Central nervous system atypical teratoid/rhabdoid tumors of infancy and childhood. Ultrastruct Pathol. 1997;21:369–78.
17. Burger PC, Yu IT, Tihan T, Friedman HS, Strother DR, Kepner JL, Duffner PK, Kun LE, Perlman EJ. Atypical teratoid/rhabdoid tumor of the central nervous system: a highly malignant tumor of infancy and childhood frequently mistaken for medulloblastoma: a Pediatric Oncology Group study. Am J Surg Pathol. 1998;22:1083–92.
18. Judkins AR, Mauger J, Ht A, Rorke LB, Biegel JA. Immunohistochemical analysis of hSNF5/INI1 in pediatric CNS neoplasms. Am J Surg Pathol. 2004;28:644–50.
19. Judkins AR, Burger PC, Hamilton RL, Kleinschmidt-DeMasters B, Perry A, Pomeroy SL, Rosenblum MK, Yachnis AT, Zhou H, Rorke LB, Biegel JA. INI1 protein expression distinguishes atypical teratoid/rhabdoid tumor from choroid plexus carcinoma. J Neuropathol Exp Neurol. 2005;64: 391–7.
20. Venneti S, Le P, Martinez D, Xie SX, Sullivan LM, Rorke-Adams LB, Pawel B, Judkins AR. Malignant rhabdoid tumors express stem cell factors, which relate to the expression of EZH2 and Id proteins. Am J Surg Pathol. 2011;35:1463–72.
21. Haberler C, Laggner U, Slavc I, Czech T, Ambros IM, Ambros PF, Budka H, Hainfellner JA. Immunohistochemical analysis of INI1 protein in malignant pediatric CNS tumors: Lack of INI1 in atypical teratoid/rhabdoid tumors and in a fraction of primitive neuroectodermal tumors without rhabdoid phenotype. Am J Surg Pathol. 2006;30:1462–8.
22. Allen JC, Judkins AR, Rosenblum MK, Biegel JA. Atypical teratoid/rhabdoid tumor evolving from an optic pathway ganglioglioma: case study. Neuro Oncol. 2006;8:79–82.
23. Chacko G, Chacko AG, Dunham CP, Judkins AR, Biegel JA, Perry A. Atypical teratoid/rhabdoid tumor arising in the setting of a pleomorphic xanthoastrocytoma. J Neurooncol. 2007;84: 217–22.
24. Cheng JX, Tretiakova M, Gong C, Mandal S, Krausz T, Taxy JB. Renal medullary carcinoma: rhabdoid features and the absence of INI1 expression as markers of aggressive behavior. Mod Pathol. 2008;21:647–52.
25. Kohashi K, Oda Y, Yamamoto H, Tamiya S, Oshiro Y, Izumi T, Taguchi T, Tsuneyoshi M. SMARCB1/INI1 protein expression in round cell soft tissue sarcomas associated with chromosomal translocations involving EWS: a special reference to SMARCB1/INI1 negative variant extraskeletal myxoid chondrosarcoma. Am J Surg Pathol. 2008;32:1168–74.
26. Hornick JL, Dal Cin P, Fletcher CD. Loss of INI1 expression is characteristic of both conventional and proximal-type epithelioid sarcoma. Am J Surg Pathol. 2009;33:542–50.
27. Rosty C, Peter M, Zucman J, Validire P, Delattre O, Aurias A. Cytogenetic and molecular analysis of a t(1;22)(p36;q11.2)

in a rhabdoid tumor with a putative homozygous deletion of chromosome 22. Genes Chromosomes Cancer. 1998;21: 82–9.
28. Sawyer JR, Goosen LS, Swanson CM, Tomita T, de Leon GA. A new reciprocal translocation (12;22)(q24.3;q11.2-12) in a malignant rhabdoid tumor of the brain. Cancer Genet Cytogenet. 1998;101:62–7.
29. Versteege I, Sevenet N, Lange J, Rousseau-Merck MF, Ambros P, Handgretinger R, Aurias A, Delattre O. Truncating mutations of hSNF5/INI1 in aggressive paediatric cancer. Nature. 1998;394:203–6.
30. Biegel JA, Zhou JY, Rorke LB, Stenstrom C, Wainwright LM, Fogelgren B. Germ-line and acquired mutations of INI1 in atypical teratoid and rhabdoid tumors. Cancer Res. 1999;59: 74–9.
31. Kalpana GV, Marmon S, Wang W, Crabtree GR, Goff SP. Binding and stimulation of HIV-1 integrase by a human homolog of yeast transcription factor SNF5. Science. 1994;266:2002–6.
32. Clapier CR, Cairns BR. The biology of chromatin remodeling complexes. Annu Rev Biochem. 2009;78:273–304.
33. Ho L, Crabtree GR. Chromatin remodelling during development. Nature. 2010;463:474–84.
34. Cote J, Quinn J, Workman JL, Peterson CL. Stimulation of Gal4 derivative binding to nucleosomal DNA by the yeast Swi/Snf complex. Science. 1994;265:53–60.
35. Kwon H, Imbalzano AN, Khavari PA, Kingston RE, Green MR. Nucleosome disruption and enhancement of activator binding by a human Sw1/Snf complex. Nature. 1994;370:477–81.
36. Cairns BR, Henry NL, Kornberg RD. TFG3/TAF30/ANC1, a component of the yeast SWI/SNF complex that is similar to the leukemogenic proteins ENL and AF-9. Mol Cell Biol. 1996;16:3308–16.
37. Cairns BR, Levinson RS, Yamamoto KR, Kornberg RD. Essential role of Swp73p in the function of yeast Swi/Snf complex. Genes Dev. 1996;10:2131–44.
38. Papoulas O, Beek SJ, Moseley SL, McCallum CM, Sarte M, Shearn A, Tamkun JW. The Drosophila trithorax group proteins BRM, ASH1 and ASH2 are subunits of distinct protein complexes. Development. 1998;125:3955–66.
39. Nie ZQ, Xue WT, Yang DF, Zhou S, Deroo BJ, Archer TK, Wang WD. A specificity and targeting subunit of a human SWI/SNF family-related chromatin-remodeling complex. Mol Cell Biol. 2000;20:8879–88.
40. Mohrmann L, Langenberg K, Krijgsveld J, Kal AJ, Heck AJR, Verrijzer CP. Differential targeting of two distinct SWI/SNF-related Drosophila chromatin-remodeling complexes. Mol Cell Biol. 2004;24:3077–88.
41. Wang Z, Zhai WG, Richardson JA, Olson EN, Meneses JJ, Firpo MT, Kang CH, Skarnes WC, Tjian R. Polybromo protein BAF180 functions in mammalian cardiac chamber maturation. Genes Dev. 2004;18:3106–16.
42. Hargreaves DC, Crabtree GR. ATP-dependent chromatin remodeling: genetics, genomics and mechanisms. Cell Res. 2011;21:396–420.
43. Wilson BG, Roberts CW. SWI/SNF nucleosome remodellers and cancer. Nat Rev Cancer. 2011;11:481–92.
44. Wang X, Haswell JR, Roberts CW. Molecular pathways: SWI/SNF (BAF) complexes Are frequently mutated in cancer—mechanisms and potential therapeutic insights. Clin Cancer Res. 2013;20(1):21–7.
45. Shain AH, Pollack JR. The spectrum of SWI/SNF mutations, ubiquitous in human cancers. PLoS One. 2013;8:e55119.
46. Rousseau-Merck MF, Versteege I, Legrand I, Couturier J, Mairal A, Delattre O, Aurias A. hSNF5/INI1 inactivation is mainly associated with homozygous deletions and mitotic recombinations in rhabdoid tumors. Cancer Res. 1999;59:3152–6.
47. Sevenet N, Lellouch-Tubiana A, Schofield D, Hoang-Xuan K, Gessler M, Birnbaum D, Jeanpierre C, Jouvet A, Delattre O. Spectrum of hSNF5/INI1 somatic mutations in human cancer and genotype-phenotype correlations. Hum Mol Genet. 1999;8:2359–68.
48. Biegel JA, Tan L, Zhang F, Wainwright L, Russo P, Rorke LB. Alterations of the hSNF5/INI1 gene in central nervous system atypical teratoid/rhabdoid tumors and renal and extra-renal rhabdoid tumors. Clin Cancer Res. 2002;8:3461–7.
49. Uno K, Takita J, Yokomori K, Tanaka Y, Ohta S, Shimada H, Gilles FH, Sugita K, Abe S, Sako M, Hashizume K, Hayashi Y. Aberrations of the hSNF5/INI1 gene are restricted to malignant rhabdoid tumors or atypical teratoid/rhabdoid tumors in pediatric solid tumors. Genes Chromosomes Cancer. 2002;34: 33–41.
50. Taylor MD, Gokgoz N, Andrulis IL, Mainprize TG, Drake JM, Rutka JT. Familial posterior fossa brain tumors of infancy secondary to germline mutation of the hSNF5 gene. Am J Hum Genet. 2000;66:1403–6.
51. Fernandez C, Bouvier C, Sevenet N, Liprandi A, Coze C, Lena G, Figarella-Branger D. Congenital disseminated malignant rhabdoid tumor and cerebellar tumor mimicking medulloblastoma in monozygotic twins—Pathologic and molecular diagnosis. Am J Surg Pathol. 2002;26:266–70.
52. Fujisawa H, Takabatake Y, Fukusato T, Tachibana O, Tsuchiya Y, Yamashita J. Molecular analysis of the rhabdoid predisposition syndrome in a child: a novel germline hSNF5/INI1 mutation and absence of c-myc amplification. J Neurooncol. 2003;63:257–62.
53. Janson K, Nedzi LA, David O, Schorin M, Walsh JW, Bhattacharjee M, Pridjian G, Tan L, Judkins AR, Biegel JA. Predisposition to atypical teratoid/rhabdoid tumor due to an inherited INI1 mutation. Pediatr Blood Cancer. 2006;47:279–84.
54. Ammerlaan ACJ, Houben MPWA, Tijssen CC, Wesseling P, Hulsebos TJM. Secondary meningioma in a long-term survivor of atypical teratoid/rhabdoid tumour with a germline INI1 mutation. Childs Nerv Syst. 2008;24:855–7.
55. Lee RS, Stewart C, Carter SL, Ambrogio L, Cibulskis K, Sougnez C, Lawrence MS, Auclair D, Mora J, Golub TR, Biegel JA, Getz G, Roberts CW. A remarkably simple genome underlies highly malignant pediatric rhabdoid cancers. J Clin Invest. 2012;122:2983–8.
56. Roberts CW, Biegel JA. The role of SMARCB1/INI1 in development of rhabdoid tumor. Cancer Biol Ther. 2009;8:412–6.
57. Hasselblatt M, Gesk S, Oyen F, Rossi S, Viscardi E, Giangaspero F, Giannini C, Judkins AR, Fruhwald MC, Obser

T, Schneppenheim R, Siebert R, Paulus W. Nonsense mutation and inactivation of SMARCA4 (BRG1) in an atypical teratoid/rhabdoid tumor showing retained SMARCB1 (INI1) expression. Am J Surg Pathol. 2011;35:933–5.
58. Modena P, Lualdi E, Facchinetti F, Galli L, Teixeira MR, Pilotti S, Sozzi G. SMARCB1/INI1 tumor suppressor gene is frequently inactivated in epithelioid sarcomas. Cancer Res. 2005;65:4012–9.
59. Kohashi K, Izumi T, Oda Y, Yamamoto H, Tamiya S, Taguchi T, Iwamoto Y, Hasegawa T, Tsuneyoshi M. Infrequent SMARCB1/INI1 gene alteration in epithelioid sarcoma: a useful tool in distinguishing epithelioid sarcoma from malignant rhabdoid tumor. Hum Pathol. 2009;40:349–55.
60. Sullivan LM, Folpe AL, Pawel BR, Judkins AR, Biegel JA. Epithelioid sarcoma is associated with a high percentage of SMARCB1 deletions. Mod Pathol. 2013;26:385–92.
61. Hulsebos TJ, Plomp AS, Wolterman RA, Robanus-Maandag EC, Baas F, Wesseling P. Germline mutation of INI1/SMARCB1 in familial schwannomatosis. Am J Hum Genet. 2007;80:805–10.
62. Boyd C, Smith MJ, Kluwe L, Balogh A, Maccollin M, Plotkin SR. Alterations in the SMARCB1 (INI1) tumor suppressor gene in familial schwannomatosis. Clin Genet. 2008;74: 358–66.
63. Sestini R, Bacci C, Provenzano A, Genuardi M, Papi L. Evidence of a four-hit mechanism involving SMARCB1 and NF2 in schwannomatosis-associated schwannomas. Hum Mutat. 2008;29:227–31.
64. Swensen JJ, Keyser J, Coffin CM, Biegel JA, Viskochil DH, Williams MS. Familial occurrence of schwannomas and malignant rhabdoid tumour associated with a duplication in SMARCB1. J Med Genet. 2009;46:68–72.
65. Hollmann TJ, Hornick JL. INI1-deficient tumors: diagnostic features and molecular genetics. Am J Surg Pathol. 2011;35: E47–63.
66. Kalamarides M, et al. Neurofibromatosis 2011: a report of the Children's Tumor Foundation annual meeting. Acta Neuropathol. 2012;123:369–80.
67. Smith MJ, Walker JA, Shen Y, Stemmer-Rachamimov A, Gusella JF, Plotkin SR. Expression of SMARCB1 (INI1) mutations in familial schwannomatosis. Hum Mol Genet. 2012;21:5239–45.
68. Smith MJ, Wallace AJ, Bowers NL, Rustad CF, Woods CG, Leschziner GD, Ferner RE, Evans DG. Frequency of SMARCB1 mutations in familial and sporadic schwannomatosis. Neurogenetics. 2012;13:141–5.
69. Hoot AC, Russo P, Judkins AR, Perlman EJ, Biegel JA. Immunohistochemical analysis of hSNF5/INI1 distinguishes renal and extra-renal malignant rhabdoid tumors from other pediatric soft tissue tumors. Am J Surg Pathol. 2004;28: 1485–91.
70. Bruch LA, Hill DA, Cai DX, Levy BK, Dehner LP, Perry A. A role for fluorescence in situ hybridization detection of chromosome 22q dosage in distinguishing atypical teratoid/rhabdoid tumors from medulloblastoma/central primitive neuroectodermal tumors. Hum Pathol. 2001;32:156–62.
71. Weinblatt M, Kochen J. Rhabdoid tumor of the central nervous system. Med Pediatr Oncol. 1992;20:258.
72. Olson TA, Bayar E, Kosnik E, Hamoudi AB, Klopfenstein KJ, Pieters RS, Ruymann FB. Successful treatment of disseminated central nervous system malignant rhabdoid tumor. J Pediatr Hematol Oncol. 1995;17:71–5.
73. Chi SN, Zimmerman MA, Yao X, Cohen KJ, Burger P, Biegel JA, Rorke-Adams LB, Fisher MJ, Janss A, Mazewski C, Goldman S, Manley PE, Bowers DC, Bendel A, Rubin J, Turner CD, Marcus KJ, Goumnerova L, Ullrich NJ, Kieran MW. Intensive multimodality treatment for children with newly diagnosed CNS atypical teratoid rhabdoid tumor. J Clin Oncol. 2009;27:385–9.
74. Gardner SL, Asgharzadeh S, Green A, Horn B, McCowage G, Finlay J. Intensive induction chemotherapy followed by high dose chemotherapy with autologous hematopoietic progenitor cell rescue in young children newly diagnosed with central nervous system atypical teratoid rhabdoid tumors. Pediatr Blood Cancer. 2008;51:235–40.
75. Lafay-Cousin L, Hawkins C, Carret AS, Johnston D, Zelcer S, Wilson B, Jabado N, Scheinemann K, Eisenstat D, Fryer C, Fleming A, Mpofu C, Larouche V, Strother D, Bouffet E, Huang A. Central nervous system atypical teratoid rhabdoid tumours: the Canadian Paediatric Brain Tumour Consortium experience. Eur J Cancer. 2012;48:353–9.
76. Panandiker ASP, Merchant TE, Beltran C, Wu SJ, Sharma S, Boop FA, Jenkins JJ, Helton KJ, Wright KD, Broniscer A, Kun LE, Gajjar A. Sequencing of local therapy affects the pattern of treatment failure and survival in children with atypical teratoid rhabdoid tumors of the central nervous system. Int J Radiat Oncol Biol Phys. 2012;82:1756–63.
77. Martens JA, Winston F. Recent advances in understanding chromatin remodeling by Swi/Snf complexes. Curr Opin Genet Dev. 2003;13:136–42.
78. Cheng SW, Davies KP, Yung E, Beltran RJ, Yu J, Kalpana GV. c-MYC interacts with INI1/hSNF5 and requires the SWI/SNF complex for transactivation function. Nat Genet. 1999;22: 102–5.
79. Tolstorukov MY, Sansam CG, Lu P, Koellhoffer EC, Helming KC, Alver BH, Tillman EJ, Evans JA, Wilson BG, Park PJ, Roberts CWM. Swi/Snf chromatin remodeling/tumor suppressor complex establishes nucleosome occupancy at target promoters. Proc Natl Acad Sci U S A. 2013;110:10165–70.
80. Medjkane S, Novikov E, Versteege I, Delattre O. The tumor suppressor hSNF5/INI1 modulates cell growth and actin cytoskeleton organization. Cancer Res. 2004;64:3406–13.
81. Vries RG, Bezrookove V, Zuijderduijn LM, Kia SK, Houweling A, Oruetxebarria I, Raap AK, Verrijzer CP. Cancer-associated mutations in chromatin remodeler hSNF5 promote chromosomal instability by compromising the mitotic checkpoint. Genes Dev. 2005;19:665–70.
82. Morozov A, Lee SJ, Zhang ZK, Cimica V, Zagzag D, Kalpana GV. INI1 induces interferon signaling and spindle checkpoint in rhabdoid tumors. Clin Cancer Res. 2007;13:4721–30.
83. Betz BL, Strobeck MW, Reisman DN, Knudsen ES, Weissman BE. Re-expression of hSNF5/INI1/BAF47 in pediatric tumor cells leads to G1 arrest associated with induction of p16ink4a and activation of RB. Oncogene. 2002;21:5193–203.
84. Tsikitis M, Zhang Z, Edelman W, Zagzag D, Kalpana GV. Genetic ablation of Cyclin D1 abrogates genesis of rhabdoid tumors resulting from Ini1 loss. Proc Natl Acad Sci U S A. 2005;102:12129–34.
85. Zhang ZK, Davies KP, Allen J, Zhu L, Pestell RG, Zagzag D, Kalpana GV. Cell cycle arrest and repression of cyclin D1

transcription by INI1/hSNF5. Mol Cell Biol. 2002;22: 5975–88.
86. Lee S, Cimica V, Ramachandra N, Zagzag D, Kalpana GV. Aurora A is a repressed effector target of the chromatin remodeling protein INI1/hSNF5 required for rhabdoid tumor cell survival. Cancer Res. 2011;71:3225–35.
87. Smith ME, Das BC, Kalpana GV. In vitro activities of novel 4-HPR derivatives on a panel of rhabdoid and other tumor cell lines. Cancer Cell Int. 2011;11:34.
88. Reincke BS, Rosson GB, Oswald BW, Wright CF. INI1 expression induces cell cycle arrest and markers of senescence in malignant rhabdoid tumor cells. J Cell Physiol. 2003;194: 303–13.
89. Oruetxebarria I, Venturini F, Kekarainen T, Houweling A, Zuijderduijn LM, Mohd-Sarip A, Vries RG, Hoeben RC, Verrijzer CP. P16INK4a is required for hSNF5 chromatin remodeler-induced cellular senescence in malignant rhabdoid tumor cells. J Biol Chem. 2004;279:3807–16.
90. Chai J, Charboneau AL, Betz BL, Weissman BE. Loss of the hSNF5 gene concomitantly inactivates p21CIP/WAF1 and p16INK4a activity associated with replicative senescence in A204 rhabdoid tumor cells. Cancer Res. 2005;65: 10192–8.
91. Wilson BG, Wang X, Shen X, McKenna ES, Lemieux ME, Cho YJ, Koellhoffer EC, Pomeroy SL, Orkin SH, Roberts CW. Epigenetic antagonism between polycomb and SWI/SNF complexes during oncogenic transformation. Cancer Cell. 2010;18:316–28.
92. Alimova I, Birks DK, Harris PS, Knipstein JA, Venkataraman S, Marquez VE, Foreman NK, Vibhakar R. Inhibition of EZH2 suppresses self-renewal and induces radiation sensitivity in atypical rhabdoid teratoid tumor cells. Neuro Oncol. 2013;15: 149–60.
93. Alao JP, Stavropoulou AV, Lam EWF, Coombes RC, Vigushin DM. Histone deacetylase inhibitor, Trichostatin A induces ubiquitin-dependent cyclin D1 degradation in MCF-7 breast cancer cells. Mol Cancer. 2006;5.
94. Graham C, Tucker C, Creech J, Favours E, Billups CA, Liu TB, Fouladi M, Freeman BB, Stewart CF, Houghton PJ. Evaluation of the antitumor efficacy, pharmacokinetics, and pharmacodynamics of the histone deacetylase inhibitor depsipeptide in childhood cancer models in vivo. Clin Cancer Res. 2006;12:223–34.
95. Furchert S, Jung M, Loidl A, Jurgens H, Fruhald MC. Inhibitors of histone deacteylases as potential therapeutics for high-risk medulloblastoma and atypical teratoid/rhabdoid tumors. Neuro Oncol. 2007;9:197.
96. Knipstein JA, Birks DK, Donson AM, Alimova I, Foreman NK, Vibhakar R. Histone deacetylase inhibition decreases proliferation and potentiates the effect of ionizing radiation in atypical teratoid/rhabdoid tumor cells. Neuro Oncol. 2012;14: 175–83.
97. Hertwig F, Meyer K, Braun S, Ek S, Spang R, Pfenninger CV, Artner I, Prost G, Chen X, Biegel JA, Judkins AR, Englund E, Nuber UA. Definition of genetic events directing the development of distinct types of brain tumors from postnatal neural stem/progenitor cells. Cancer Res. 2012;72:3381–92.
98. Ogino S, Kubo S, Abdul-Karim FW, Cohen ML. Comparative immunohistochemical study of insulin-like growth factor II and insulin-like growth factor receptor type 1 in pediatric brain tumors. Pediatr Dev Pathol. 2001;4:23–31.
99. D'Cunja J, Shalaby T, Rivera P, von Buren A, Patti R, Heppner FL, Arcaro A, Rorke-Adams LB, Phillips PC, Grotzer MA. Antisense treatment of IGF-IR induces apoptosis and enhances chemosensitivity in central nervous system atypical teratoid/rhabdoid tumours cells. Eur J Cancer. 2007;43:1581–9.
100. Arcaro A, Doepfner KT, Boller D, Guerreiro AS, Shalaby T, Jackson SP, Schoenwaelder SM, Delattre O, Grotzer MA, Fischer B. Novel role for insulin as an autocrine growth factor for malignant brain tumour cells. Biochem J. 2007;406:57–66.
101. Darr J, Klochendler A, Isaac S, Eden A. Loss of IGFBP7 expression and persistent AKT activation contribute to SMARCB1/Snf5-mediated tumorigenesis. Oncogene. 2013; 33(23):3024–32.
102. Singh A, Lun X, Jayanthan A, Obaid H, Ruan Y, Strother D, Chi SN, Smith A, Forsyth P, Narendran A. Profiling pathway-specific novel therapeutics in preclinical assessment for central nervous system atypical teratoid rhabdoid tumors (CNS ATRT): favorable activity of targeting EGFR- ErbB2 signaling with lapatinib. Mol Oncol. 2013;7:497–512.
103. Ginn KF, Gajjar A. Atypical teratoid rhabdoid tumor: current therapy and future directions. Front Oncol. 2012;2:114.

14 Hemangioblastoma

Jasmeet Chadha Singh and David Zagzag

Hemangioblastomas are slow-growing, but highly vascular tumors that arise in specific regions of the central nervous system (CNS) and retina. They constitute about 0.9 % of total brain tumors [1]. Hemangioblastomas may occur sporadically, or as tumors associated with von Hippel–Lindau syndrome (vHL) in about 35–40 % of patients [1–3]. In some series, as much as 80 % of hemangioblastomas are associated with vHL.

Genetics

vHL syndrome is associated with a germline mutation in the *VHL* gene on chromosome 3p25. However, according to the genetic "two-hit hypothesis" proposed by Knudson, tumorigenesis requires a second somatic inactivation of the other *VHL* allele.

Other than mutations in *VHL*, there is a paucity of data regarding other genetic hits in hemangioblastomas that might contribute to tumorigenesis. Sprenger et al. performed comparative genomic hybridization (CGH) of ten sporadic hemangioblastomas and found that the most common genetic aberrations in sporadic tumors are loss of chromosome 3 (70 %), loss of chromosome 6 (50 %), loss of chromosome 9 (30 %), loss of 18q (30 %), and gain of chromosome 19 (30 %). Based on the frequencies and co-occurrence of these genetic changes, they hypothesized that the loss of chromosome 3 is an early event in oncogenesis in sporadic hemangioblastomas, followed by loss of chromosome 6 and subsequently chromosomes 9 and 18q, and lastly by the gain of chromosome 19 [4]. In another study, CGH results of 7 vHL-associated and 16 sporadic hemangioblastomas were compared. Mutations in the *VHL* gene on 3p25-56 were found in 100 % of hereditary hemangioblastomas, but only in 30 % of sporadic tumors. Conversely, complete loss of chromosome 3 occurred more commonly in sporadic hemangioblastomas (69 %) than in vHL-associated hemangioblastomas (14 %). Thus, it can be concluded that sporadic mutation in the *VHL* gene is not the primary oncogenic event in sporadic hemangioblastomas [5].

Epigenetic and other means of somatic inactivation of *VHL* are also being investigated. It has been proposed that inactivation of promoter CpG islands, due to hypermethylation, leads to transcriptional silencing of *VHL* [6].

Prowse et al. examined 53 vHL-related tumors, including 30 renal cell carcinomas (RCCs), 15 hemangioblastomas, 5 pheochromocytomas and 3 pancreatic tumors, for genetic changes such as LOH (loss of heterozygosity), intragenic somatic mutations as well as DNA hypermethylation. In this series, hypermethylation of the vHL gene was detected in 33 % of tumors (6 out of 18 tumors; 2 RCCs and 4 hemangioblastomas). Two tumors, both hemangioblastomas, showed intragenic somatic mutations in a wild-type gene [6].

In a subsequent study, Rickert et al. performed CGH of 20 hemangioblastomas (one vHL and the remainder sporadic), which revealed that the most common cytogenetic changes associated with hemangioblastomas include the loss of chromosomes 19, 6, and 22q, which are seen in 35 %, 30 %, and 15 % of patients, respectively, and the loss of chromosome 6 being significantly associated with the cellular variant. Loss of chromosome 3 was uncommon in this series of sporadic hemangioblastomas, in contrast to the earlier studies by Sprenger et al. [7].

Lemeta et al. suggested that LOH at 6q is common and concurrent with 3p loss in sporadic hemangioblastomas [8]. This finding was subsequently confirmed by other studies [4, 7, 9]. The same authors subsequently demonstrated high prevalence of LOH at the ZAC-1 tumor suppressor gene region located on 6q24-25. Moreover, they also demonstrated that promoter methylation of ZAC-1 leads to epigenetic silencing of the gene in 90 % of tumors [10].

CGH has demonstrated that the reticular and cellular variants of hemangioblastoma have different cytogenetic profiles, with the loss of chromosome 6 significantly associated with the cellular variants [7].

M.A. Karajannis and D. Zagzag (eds.), *Molecular Pathology of Nervous System Tumors: Biological Stratification and Targeted Therapies*, Molecular Pathology Library 8,
DOI 10.1007/978-1-4939-1830-0_14,

Pathogenesis

vHL tumorigenesis can be mediated by both hypoxia-induced factor (HIF) and non-HIF-mediated mechanisms. HIF-1 is a heterodimeric transcriptional factor that regulates genes which respond to changes in oxygen levels in tissues [11, 12]. It is composed of HIF-1α and HIF-1β subunits [13]. Levels of HIF-1α are upregulated under hypoxic conditions and, by translocation into the nucleus and dimerization with HIF-1β, activate genes that promote angiogenesis (VEGF), erythropoiesis (EPO), nitric oxide synthesis (NOS), and glucose transport (GLUT-1). However, under normoxic conditions, HIF-1α undergoes ubiquitin-mediated degradation in the proteosomes, which are mediated by vHL protein [14–19]. The vHL protein binds to HIF-1α only after it undergoes oxygen-dependent hydroxylation of the proline residues 402 or 564 or both by members of the Elongin family (EGlN) [15, 18–21]. EGlN1 is the primary HIF-1 hydroxylase while EGlN2 and EGlN3 play compensatory roles under certain conditions [22]. However, when vHL is mutated, HIF-1α will not undergo degradation and remains constitutionally active [23]. This promotes tumorigenesis by increased transcriptional activation of genes that promote angiogenesis and other growth factors.

It has also been demonstrated that vHL is critical for cellular [24] differentiation during development and its inactivation causes developmental arrest [25] and protracted cellular differentiation [26]. The cell of origin in hemangioblastoma is an embryologically arrested hemangioblast derived from the mesoderm, which retains its multipotent properties and ability to differentiate into both red blood cells and blood vessel endothelium [27, 28]. Accordingly, foci of extramedullary hematopoeisis have been detected in hemangioblastomas. Vortmeyer et al. have detected the presence of fetal hemoglobin in these areas of extramedullary hematopoeisis, suggesting that the vHL deletion leads to primitive hematopoeisis [25, 26]. Moreover, co-expression of Epo and Epo receptor on these hemangioblasts represents a key event in vHL deficiency and further promotes tumor growth via autocrine and paracrine stimulation [25]. Developmentally arrested structural elements composed of hemangioblast progenitor cells have been demonstrated in the cerebella of *VHL*-mutated patients [29]. Hemangioblastic activity in the nervous system occurs in the embryonic stage [30] and hence its presence in adult brain depicts persistence of developmentally arrested hemangioblastic cells. vHL disease produces developmental aberrations giving rise to angiomesenchymal tumorlets resembling hemangioblastomas in the human CNS [31]. More recently, the pleuripotent vHL deficient cells in hemangioblastomas have been demonstrated to give rise to mast cells via the c-Kit signaling pathway. Accordingly, mast cells from tumor samples of patients exhibited LOH in the VHL alleles when compared with the peripheral blood lymphocytes [32].

Pathology

Macroscopically, hemangioblastoma is a well-circumscribed tumor, with both solid and cystic components. The tumor appears yellow in color due to its high lipid content.

Microscopically, the tumor has two components: a network of capillaries lined by hyperplastic endothelial cells with intervening vacuolated stromal cells, which have pale cytoplasms, pleomorphic nuclei and high lipid content. Mitoses are conspicuously absent [33]. A recent study of 156 tumors reports that tumor architecture relates to the size of the tumor; with smaller tumors (<8 mm^3) composed of mesenchymal architecture comprising of a network of capillaries, while the larger tumors composed of enlarged stromal cells clustered in groups (Fig. 14.1) [26]. The stromal cell, which is the tumor cell in hemangioblastoma, is an embryologically arrested hemangioblast derived from the mesoderm that retains its multipotent properties as well as the ability to differentiate into both red blood cells and blood vessel endothelium. The stromal cells are immunoreactive for cytokeratin, S-100, NSE (neuron specific enolase), actin, GFAP (glial fibrillary acid protein), vimentin, and EMA (epithelial membrane antigen). The stromal and capillary endothelial cells express different surface adhesion molecules suggesting different cells of origin. The capillary endothelial cells express endothelium associated adhesion molecules such as ICAM-1, ICAM-2, PECAM, ELAM, and VCAM-1. The stromal cells express neuronal cell adhesion molecule (NCAM), which further supports its mesenchymal origin. Since NCAM is also expressed by metastatic renal cell cancer to the CNS, its expression by hemangioblastoma can present as a diagnostic challenge [34, 35]. The stromal cells also stain negatively for von Willebrand factor, a marker of endothelial origin [36]. Brachyury, a protein transcription product of the T box gene, which regulates the formation of mesoderm, is expressed in the cytoplasm of stromal cells and is highly specific for hemangioblastoma, distinguishing it from morphologically similar lesions such as metastatic clear cell renal cell cancer and angiomatous meningioma [37, 38].

Histologically, hemangioblastomas are classified into two variants: the more common reticular variant (composed of proliferating vascular elements) and the rare cellular variant (composed of epitheloid clusters of stromal cells), which are associated with greater GFAP positivity, higher proliferation index, and probability of recurrence [39].

Receptors for cellular growth factors including proangiogenic factors, such as epidermal growth factor receptor (EGFR), platelet derived growth factor receptor (PDGFR), placental growth factor receptor (PFG-1), and vascular endothelial growth factor receptor (VEGF), are expressed on tumor cells in hemangioblastomas [40]. However, unlike malignant gliomas, the VEGF expression does not correlate with the vascular density as indicated by the expression of

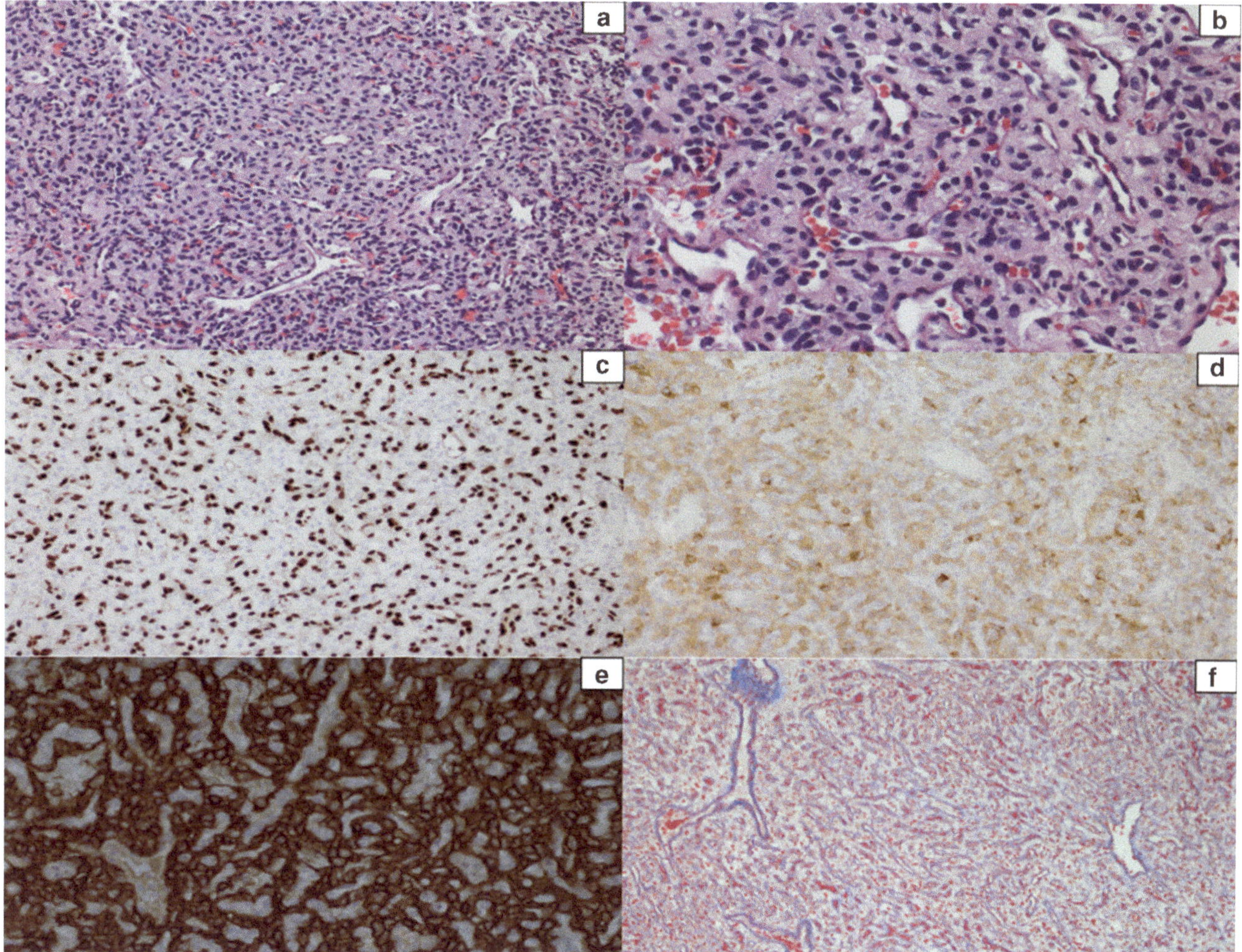

FIG. 14.1. (**a**, **b**) H&E, (**c**) ERG, (**d**) Inhibin, (**e**) Carbomic anhydrase and (**f**) Azocarmine. (**a**) H&E stain shows a highly vascular neoplasm. The tumor is composed of vascular cells and cells with round nuclei designated as "stromal" cells. (**b**) Higher power reveals numerous vascular channels (v) and interspersed stromal cells are seen. Note the nuclear pseudoinclusion in a stromal cell (*arrowhead*). (**c**): ERG immunohistochemistry. Note the intense nuclear staining in vascular cells; (**d**, **e**) Inhibin and carbonic anhydrase immunohistochemistry. Note the intense staining in stromal cells (**f**) Azocarmine stain highlights vascular channels (**a**, **f**, ×50; **b–d**, and **e**, ×100).

CD34-positive endothelial cells. This suggests that pro-angiogenic factors other than VEGF probably contribute to the intense tumor vascularity [41].

Clinical Features

Hemangioblastomas most commonly arise in the CNS especially, but not exclusively, in the posterior fossa. The frequent sites of occurrence in the order of commonality are cerebellum, dorsal part of the spinal cord, brainstem, and retina (Figs. 14.2 and 14.3) [42–44]. The most common site of occurrence of hemangioblastomas in the spinal cord is the thoracic region, followed by cervical and lumbar (48 %, 36 % and 16 %, respectively) [45]. Spinal cord and brainstem hemangioblastomas are frequently associated with tumors at other sites and especially cerebellar hemangioblastomas; in turn, however, cerebellar hemangioblastomas are less frequently associated with tumors at the other sites, suggesting that the spinal cord/brainstem hemangioblastomas are the accompanying manifestation of the latter [46, 47]. Supratentorial (cerebral, sellar/suprasellar, intraventricular) hemangioblastomas are rare [48–50]. It is sometimes difficult to differentiate supratentorial hemangioblastoma from meningioma [38, 51]. Occasionally, hemangioblastomas may arise in extraneural sites such as bone, soft tissue, skin, liver, pancreas, and kidney [52–55].

One-third of hemangioblastomas are associated with the vHL syndrome. The spectrum of tumors [56] associated with vHL is broad and includes hemangioblastomas, renal cell

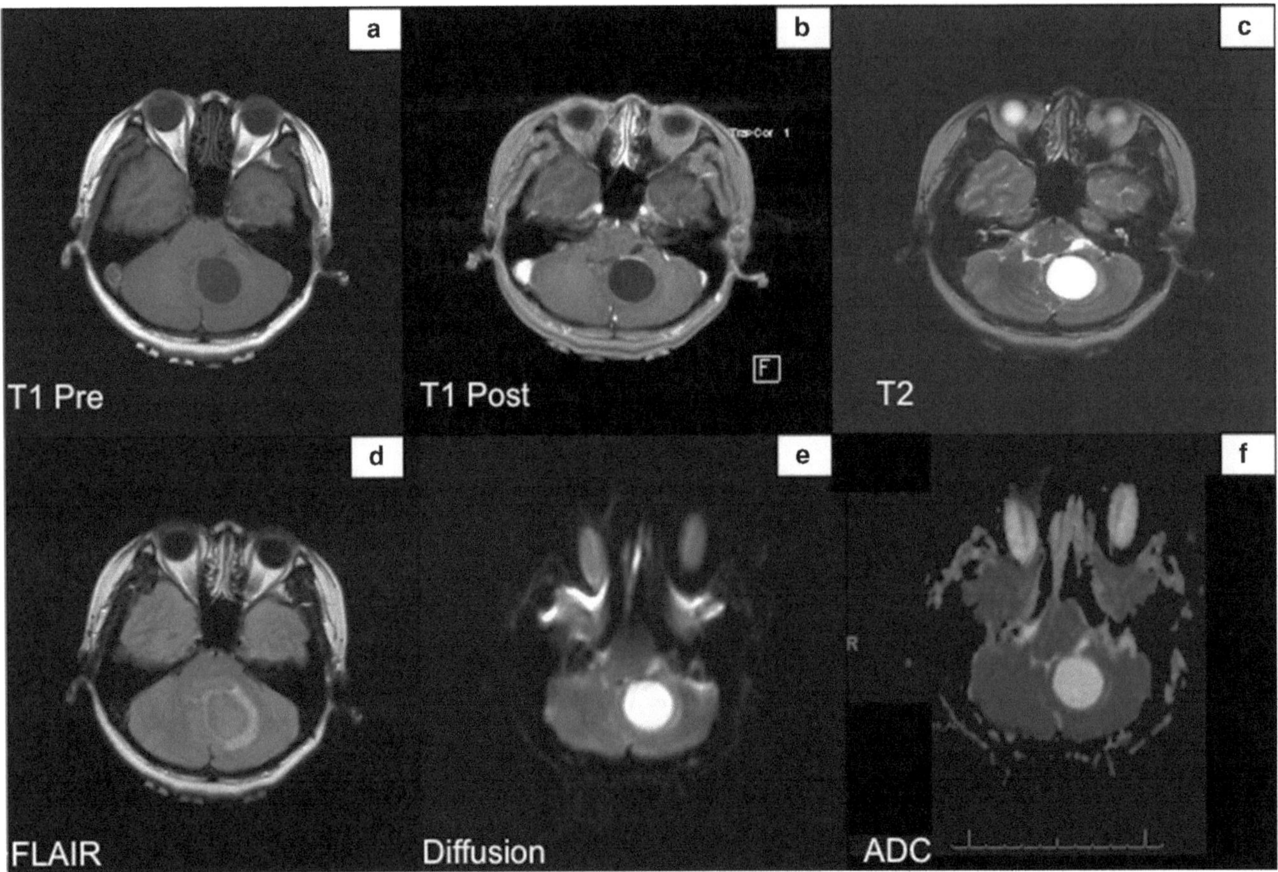

Fig. 14.2 MRI shows the tumor within the inferior medial left cerebellum. Lesion in isointense with the adjacent brain parenchyma on the T1 weighted sequences (Panel **a**), hyperintense on T2 weighted sequence (Panel **c**), and avidly enhances gadolinium (Panel **b**). Diffusion weighted sequence does not demonstrate hyperintense signal within the mass (Panels **e** and **f**)

carcinomas [57, 58], pheochromocytomas [59], extra-adrenal paragangliomas [60, 61], retinal angiomas [62–64], neuroendocrine pancreatic tumors [65–69], papillary cystadenomas of the epididymis [70] and broad uterine ligament [71], as well as endolymphatic sac tumors (ELSTs) of the middle ear [72–74]. vHL-mutated patients with hemangioblastomas are generally younger and present with multiple tumors, while the non-vHL-associated tumors are seen in older patients and are usually solitary.

Based on clinical manifestations, vHL is classified into type 1 and type 2. Type 1 vHL is not associated with pheochromocytoma while type 2 is. Type 2 is further divided into type 2A, 2B, and 2C. vHL-type 2b is associated with high incidence of hemangioblastoma and pheochromocytoma [44, 75–77].

Since patients with vHL syndrome are predisposed to developing multiple hemangioblastomas and require specialized surveillance and treatment, it is imperative to correctly diagnose vHL as early as possible. Genetic testing for vHL in addition to a comprehensive family history should be considered standard practice for all patients with CNS hemangioblastomas, especially those diagnosed under 30 years of age. Clinical screening of vHL-associated tumors consists of complete neuraxis imaging with magnetic resonance imaging (MRI) of the brain and entire spine, MRI of the abdomen, retinoscopy, and measurement of urine catecholamines. Some authors have suggested ophthalmologic screening for family members of vHL disease for early detection of retinal hemangioblastomas [78].

Hemangioblastomas are considered benign tumors, but can cause significant neurological deficits depending on their size and location. Headache, vomiting, cerebellar symptoms, and cranial nerve involvement may be the presenting features. Posterior fossa tumors can also cause cerebrospinal fluid (CSF) flow obstruction leading to hydrocephalus [79, 80]. Patients with spinal cord tumors may present with progressive scoliosis and radicular symptoms until the tumor is large enough to cause weakness. Onset of retinal hemangioblastomas can start prior to 10 years of age until 30 years, after which the risk gradually decreases. It usually presents with unilateral involvement [77]. Hemangioblastomas exhibit a stuttering growth pattern, i.e., there are periods of growth followed by periods of quiescence, which may be as long as 2 years. Indications for treatment relate to the

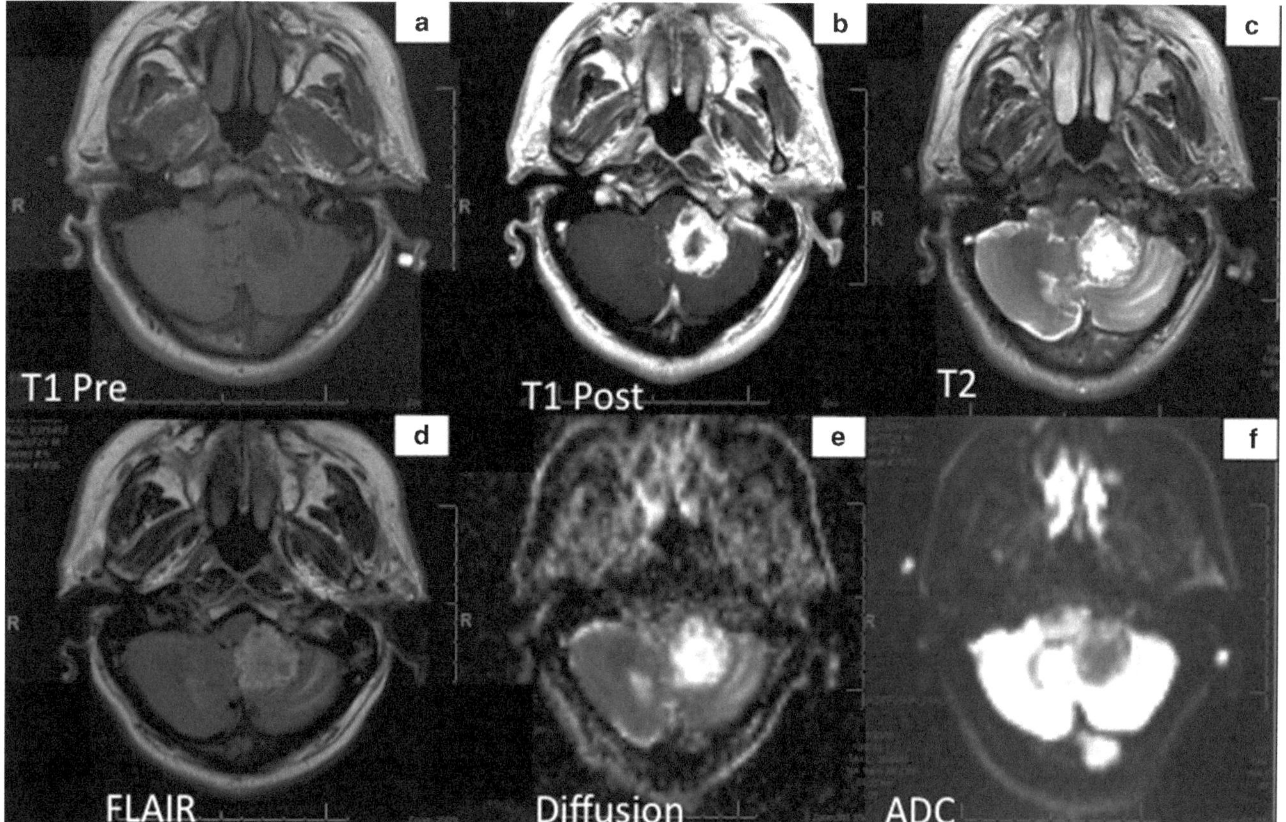

FIG. 14.3. MRI shows the tumor that appears as an irregular thick-walled mass in the region of the left cerebellar tonsil, which enhances intensely with gadolinium (Panel **b**). Mass in predominantly T1 hypointense (panel **a**) but contains several areas of T2 hyperintensity indicating hemorrhagic component (Panel **c**). Diffusion studies show hyperintensity relative to the contralateral white matter (Panels **e** and **f**).

patient's symptoms and tumor size, location, and rate of progression [81]. It is quite common for spinal cord hemangioblastomas to present with syrinx formation [82]. Occurrence of erythrocytosis with male predominance is common in hemangioblastomas due to production of erythropoietin [83, 84]. Due to their arteriovenous malformation-like vascularization, solid hemangioblastomas present a unique neurosurgical challenge [85].

There have been numerous clinical reports of worsening of vHL-associated hemangioblastomas in pregnancy, leading to progressive neurological deficits and obstructive hydrocephalus [86–90]. However, in the first prospective study comparing the rate of tumor growth in pregnant versus the nonpregnant cohorts with vHL-associated hemangioblastomas, Ye et al. observed that there were no differences in tumor growth rate, peritumoral cyst growth and the need for surgery. However, this was a small study with only 27 patients in the pregnancy cohort and it is possible that patients who chose to become pregnant were already in a better state of health leading to selection bias [91].

Imaging

Hemangioblastomas show post-contrast enhancement on computed tomogram (CT) scans and T1-weighed MRI. Imaging studies show the typical appearance of a cyst with mural nodule in approximately 60 % of cases. The nodular portion shows flow voids in the T1 and T2-weighted sequences. Generally, the cysts are slightly hyperintense compared to CSF in T1-weighted images. Both the nodule and the cyst appear bright on T2 and fluid attenuated inversion recovery (FLAIR) sequences [92].

Treatment

While most neurosurgeons agree that surgical intervention of symptomatic hemangioblastomas is required, controversy arises in dealing with asymptomatic hemangioblastomas, which commonly occur in patients with vHL syndrome. Unlike other benign intracranial tumors that exhibit a slow, progressive growth pattern, hemangioblastomas often have prolonged periods of growth arrest, thus making their natural course difficult to predict [81]. For asymptomatic, radiographically stable tumors, no treatment may be recommended. When asymptomatic tumors show progression on imaging only, the best time for intervention may be difficult to determine [93–96]. Similar to patients with other tumor predisposition syndromes, the optimal clinical management of vHL requires a specialist who oversees and coordinates a multidisciplinary plan of care, including appropriate screening tests.

From a therapeutic perspective, surgical removal remains the treatment of choice for hemangioblastomas and has been successfully employed for cerebellar [97], spinal [98, 99], and brainstem [94, 100] hemangioblastomas. Preoperative cerebral angiography helps surgeons determine the nature of the tumor vascular supply. Following diagnostic imaging, pretreatment with dexamethasone for several days is generally recommended. Intraoperative bleeding increases with tumor size, making en bloc resection of larger tumors difficult. However, modern microsurgical techniques are used to identify feeding vessels and thus help minimize intraoperative bleeding. Dissection should be carried out along the external surface of the tumor in the gliotic brain-tumor interface, to avoid entering the tumor, thus preventing brisk hemorrhage from the hemangioblastoma. The tumor-associated cysts are non-neoplastic and consist of compressed glial tissue, which collapses on its own once the associated tumor is removed. Postoperative complications include temporary worsening of neurological deficits, new neurological deficits, which may or may not resolve during follow-up, cranial postoperative infection, hydrocephalus and aseptic meningitis [101]. A postoperative contrast-enhanced MRI is routinely obtained to verify extent of resection. If no residual is noted, tumor recurrence is rare.

More recently, stereotactic radiosurgery is also being employed with encouraging results especially in spinal hemangioblastomas [102–105]. One advantage of radiosurgery is the ability to treat multiple lesions in a single treatment setting. In a series of 9 patients with 20 spinal hemangioblastomas, 4-year tumor overall and solid tumor control rates with stereotactic radiosurgery were as high as 90 % and 95 %, respectively [106]. In other studies, however, patients with multiple hemangioblastomas associated with vHL syndrome were found to less likely exhibit tumor control after treatment with radiation therapy compared to single sporadic hemangioblastomas [107, 108]. In general, smaller tumor volumes and higher doses of radiation (median 16 Gy) confer a better tumor control [109].

In contrast to surgery and radiation therapy, there is a paucity of data on systemic treatment of hemangioblastomas. Since hemangioblastomas are highly vascular, systemic anti-angiogenic therapies are being investigated as an alternative to surgery, particularly in vHL patients with multiple tumors. Several vHL patients have been treated with semaxanib, a multi-tyrosine kinase inhibitor predominantly active against VEGFR-2. Although disease stabilization outside the CNS was observed in some patients, most of the treatment responses were limited to retinal hemangioblastomas [110]. In a clinical trial for vHL patients with sunitinib, which predominantly targets VEGFR and PDGFR, antitumor activity was seen against renal cell carcinoma, but not hemangioblastomas [111]. EGFR, which is overexpressed and activated in hemangioblastomas, represents an additional attractive target for therapeutic intervention and study in future clinical trials [112]. There have been case reports on the use of anti-angiogenic agents such as bevacizumab [113], pazopanib [114], sunitinib [115], thalidomide [116], and interferon [117] with limited success. However, no prospective clinical trials using these agents have been conducted to date.

Prognosis

Gross total tumor resection was a predictor of prolonged progression-free survival (PFS) in one series [118]. Poor prognostic factors include poor performance status [101], multiple hemangioblastomas, retinal hemangioblastomas, and presence of solid rather than cystic tumors. The risk of recurrence in the future is higher if the age of diagnosis is younger than 40 years with primary sites being the brainstem and spinal cord [119].

Acknowledgment The authors thank Dr Ajax George, Department of Radiology, NYU Langone Medical Center, for providing MRI images.

References

1. Surawicz TS, Mccarthy BJ, Kupelian V, Jukich PJ, Bruner JM, Davis FG. Descriptive epidemiology of primary brain and CNS tumors: results from the Central Brain Tumor Registry of the United States, 1990–1994. Neuro Oncol. 1999;1:14–25.
2. Richard S, Beigelman C, Gerber S, van Effenterre R, Gaudric A, Sahel M, Binaghi M, DE Kersaint-Gilly A, Houtteville JP, Brunon JP, et al. Does hemangioblastoma exist outside von Hippel-Lindau disease? Neurochirurgie. 1994;40:145–54.
3. Sora S, Ueki K, Saito N, Kawahara N, Shitara N, Kirino T. Incidence of von Hippel-Lindau disease in hemangioblastoma patients: the University of Tokyo Hospital experience from 1954–1998. Acta Neurochir (Wien). 2001;143:893–6.
4. Sprenger SH, Gijtenbeek JM, Wesseling P, Sciot R, van Calenbergh F, Lammens M, Jeuken JW. Characteristic chromosomal aberrations in sporadic cerebellar hemangioblastomas revealed by comparative genomic hybridization. J Neurooncol. 2001;52:241–7.
5. Gijtenbeek JM, Jacobs B, Sprenger SH, Eleveld MJ, van Kessel AG, Kros JM, Sciot R, van Calenbergh F, Wesseling P, Jeuken JW. Analysis of von hippel-lindau mutations with comparative genomic hybridization in sporadic and hereditary hemangioblastomas: possible genetic heterogeneity. J Neurosurg. 2002;97:977–82.
6. Prowse AH, Webster AR, Richards FM, Richard S, Olschwang S, Resche F, Affara NA, Maher ER. Somatic inactivation of the VHL

gene in Von Hippel-Lindau disease tumors. Am J Hum Genet. 1997;60:765–71.
7. Rickert CH, Hasselblatt M, Jeibmann A, Paulus W. Cellular and reticular variants of hemangioblastoma differ in their cytogenetic profiles. Hum Pathol. 2006;37:1452–7.
8. Lemeta S, Pylkkanen L, Sainio M, Niemela M, Saarikoski S, Husgafvel-Pursiainen K, Bohling T. Loss of heterozygosity at 6q is frequent and concurrent with 3p loss in sporadic and familial capillary hemangioblastomas. J Neuropathol Exp Neurol. 2004; 63:1072–9.
9. Lemeta S, Salmenkivi K, Pylkkanen L, Sainio M, Saarikoski ST, Arola J, Heikkila P, Haglund C, Husgafvel-Pursiainen K, Bohling T. Frequent loss of heterozygosity at 6q in pheochromocytoma. Hum Pathol. 2006;37:749–54.
10. Lemeta S, Jarmalaite S, Pylkkanen L, Bohling T, Husgafvel-Pursiainen K. Preferential loss of the nonimprinted allele for the ZAC1 tumor suppressor gene in human capillary hemangioblastoma. J Neuropathol Exp Neurol. 2007;66:860–7.
11. Lonergan KM, Iliopoulos O, Ohh M, Kamura T, Conaway RC, Conaway JW, Kaelin Jr WG. Regulation of hypoxia-inducible mRNAs by the von Hippel-Lindau tumor suppressor protein requires binding to complexes containing elongins B/C and Cul2. Mol Cell Biol. 1998;18:732–41.
12. Simon MC, Keith B. The role of oxygen availability in embryonic development and stem cell function. Nat Rev Mol Cell Biol. 2008;9:285–96.
13. Wang GL, Semenza GL. Purification and characterization of hypoxia-inducible factor 1. J Biol Chem. 1995;270:1230–7.
14. Kaelin Jr WG. The von Hippel-Lindau protein, HIF hydroxylation, and oxygen sensing. Biochem Biophys Res Commun. 2005; 338:627–38.
15. Kamura T, Sato S, Iwai K, Czyzyk-Krzeska M, Conaway RC, Conaway JW. Activation of HIF1alpha ubiquitination by a reconstituted von Hippel-Lindau (VHL) tumor suppressor complex. Proc Natl Acad Sci U S A. 2000;97:10430–5.
16. Semenza GL. Regulation of cancer cell metabolism by hypoxia-inducible factor 1. Semin Cancer Biol. 2009;19:12–6.
17. Cockman ME, Masson N, Mole DR, Jaakkola P, Chang GW, Clifford SC, Maher ER, Pugh CW, Ratcliffe PJ, Maxwell PH. Hypoxia inducible factor-alpha binding and ubiquitylation by the von Hippel-Lindau tumor suppressor protein. J Biol Chem. 2000;275:25733–41.
18. Tanimoto K, Makino Y, Pereira T, Poellinger L. Mechanism of regulation of the hypoxia-inducible factor-1 alpha by the von Hippel-Lindau tumor suppressor protein. EMBO J. 2000;19: 4298–309.
19. Ohh M, Park CW, Ivan M, Hoffman MA, Kim TY, Huang LE, Pavletich N, Chau V, Kaelin WG. Ubiquitination of hypoxia-inducible factor requires direct binding to the beta-domain of the von Hippel-Lindau protein. Nat Cell Biol. 2000;2:423–7.
20. Ivan M, Kondo K, Yang H, Kim W, Valiando J, Ohh M, Salic A, Asara JM, Lane WS, Kaelin Jr WG. HIFalpha targeted for VHL-mediated destruction by proline hydroxylation: implications for O2 sensing. Science. 2001;292:464–8.
21. Kaelin WG. Proline hydroxylation and gene expression. Annu Rev Biochem. 2005;74:115–28.
22. Kaelin Jr WG. Cancer and altered metabolism: potential importance of hypoxia-inducible factor and 2-oxoglutarate-dependent dioxygenases. Cold Spring Harb Symp Quant Biol. 2011;76: 335–45.
23. Maxwell PH, Wiesener MS, Chang GW, Clifford SC, Vaux EC, Cockman ME, Wykoff CC, Pugh CW, Maher ER, Ratcliffe PJ. The tumour suppressor protein VHL targets hypoxia-inducible factors for oxygen-dependent proteolysis. Nature. 1999;399: 271–5.
24. Haase VH. The VHL tumor suppressor in development and disease: functional studies in mice by conditional gene targeting. Semin Cell Dev Biol. 2005;16:564–74.
25. Vortmeyer AO, Frank S, Jeong SY, Yuan K, Ikejiri B, Lee YS, Bhowmick D, Lonser RR, Smith R, Rodgers G, Oldfield EH, Zhuang Z. Developmental arrest of angioblastic lineage initiates tumorigenesis in von Hippel-Lindau disease. Cancer Res. 2003;63:7051–5.
26. Shively SB, Beltaifa S, Gehrs B, Duong H, Smith J, Edwards NA, Lonser R, Raffeld M, Vortmeyer AO. Protracted haemangioblastic proliferation and differentiation in von Hippel-Lindau disease. J Pathol. 2008;216:514–20.
27. Park DM, Zhuang Z, Chen L, Szerlip N, Maric I, Li J, Sohn T, Kim SH, Lubensky IA, Vortmeyer AO, Rodgers GP, Oldfield EH, Lonser RR. von Hippel-Lindau disease-associated hemangioblastomas are derived from embryologic multipotent cells. PLoS Med. 2007;4:e60.
28. Glasker S, Smith J, Raffeld M, Li J, Oldfield EH, Vortmeyer AO. VHL-deficient vasculogenesis in hemangioblastoma. Exp Mol Pathol. 2014;96(2):162–7.
29. Shively SB, Falke EA, Li J, Tran MG, Thompson ER, Maxwell PH, Roessler E, Oldfield EH, Lonser RR, Vortmeyer AO. Developmentally arrested structures preceding cerebellar tumors in von Hippel-Lindau disease. Mod Pathol. 2011;24:1023–30.
30. Gering M, Rodaway AR, Gottgens B, Patient RK, Green AR. The SCL gene specifies haemangioblast development from early mesoderm. EMBO J. 1998;17:4029–45.
31. Vortmeyer AO, Yuan Q, Lee YS, Zhuang Z, Oldfield EH. Developmental effects of von Hippel-Lindau gene deficiency. Ann Neurol. 2004;55:721–8.
32. Merrill MJ, Edwards NA, Lonser RR. Hemangioblastoma-associated mast cells in von Hippel-Lindau disease are tumor derived. Blood. 2013;121:859–60.
33. Frosch MP, A. D., Girolami UD 2010. The central nervous system. In: Perkins, J. (ed.) Robbins and Cotran Pathologic Basis of Disease, Eighth Edition.
34. Bohling T, Maenpaa A, Timonen T, Vantunen L, Paetau A, Haltia M. Different expression of adhesion molecules on stromal cells and endothelial cells of capillary hemangioblastoma. Acta Neuropathol. 1996;92:461–6.
35. Omulecka A, Lach B, Alwasiak J, Gregor A. Immunohistochemical and ultrastructural studies of stromal cells in hemangioblastoma. Folia Neuropathol. 1995;33:41–50.
36. Mccomb RD, Jones TR, Pizzo SV, Bigner DD. Localization of factor VIII/von Willebrand factor and glial fibrillary acidic protein in the hemangioblastoma: implications for stromal cell histogenesis. Acta Neuropathol. 1982;56:207–13.
37. Barresi V, Vitarelli E, Branca G, Antonelli M, Giangaspero F, Barresi G. Expression of brachyury in hemangioblastoma: potential use in differential diagnosis. Am J Surg Pathol. 2012;36:1052–7.
38. Takeuchi H, Hashimoto N, Kitai R, Kubota T. A report of supratentorial leptomeningeal hemangioblastoma and a literature review. Neuropathology. 2008;28:98–102.
39. Hasselblatt M, Jeibmann A, Gerss J, Behrens C, Rama B, Wassmann H, Paulus W. Cellular and reticular variants of haemangioblastoma revisited: a clinicopathologic study of 88 cases. Neuropathol Appl Neurobiol. 2005;31:618–22.
40. Bohling T, Hatva E, Kujala M, Claesson-Welsh L, Alitalo K, Haltia M. Expression of growth factors and growth factor receptors in capillary hemangioblastoma. J Neuropathol Exp Neurol. 1996;55:522–7.
41. Vaquero J, Zurita M, Coca S, Salas C, Oya S. Expression of vascular endothelial growth factor in cerebellar hemangioblastomas does not correlate with tumor angiogenesis. Cancer Lett. 1998; 132:213–7.

42. Constans JP, Meder F, Maiuri F, Donzelli R, Spaziante R, DE Divitiis E. Posterior fossa hemangioblastomas. Surg Neurol. 1986;25:269–75.
43. Stein AA, Schilp AO, Whitfield RD. The histogenesis of hemangioblastoma of the brain. A review of twenty-one cases. J Neurosurg. 1960;17:751–61.
44. Lonser RR, Glenn GM, Walther M, Chew EY, Libutti SK, Linehan WM, Oldfield EH. von Hippel-Lindau disease. Lancet. 2003;361: 2059–67.
45. Wanebo JE, Lonser RR, Glenn GM, Oldfield EH. The natural history of hemangioblastomas of the central nervous system in patients with von Hippel-Lindau disease. J Neurosurg. 2003;98: 82–94.
46. Oken MM, Creech RH, Tormey DC, Horton J, Davis TE, Mcfadden ET, Carbone PP. Toxicity and response criteria of the Eastern Cooperative Oncology Group. Am J Clin Oncol. 1982;5: 649–55.
47. Mills SA, Oh MC, Rutkowski MJ, Sughrue ME, Barani IJ, Parsa AT. Supratentorial hemangioblastoma: clinical features, prognosis, and predictive value of location for von Hippel-Lindau disease. Neuro Oncol. 2012;14:1097–104.
48. Lonser RR, Butman JA, Kiringoda R, Song D, Oldfield EH. Pituitary stalk hemangioblastomas in von Hippel-Lindau disease. J Neurosurg. 2009;110:350–3.
49. Neumann HP, Eggert HR, Scheremet R, Schumacher M, Mohadjer M, Wakhloo AK, Volk B, Hettmannsperger U, Riegler P, Schollmeyer P, et al. Central nervous system lesions in von Hippel-Lindau syndrome. J Neurol Neurosurg Psychiatry. 1992; 55:898–901.
50. Peyre M, David P, van Effenterre R, Francois P, Thys M, Emery E, Redondo A, Decq P, Aghakhani N, Parker F, Tadie M, Lacroix C, Bhangoo R, Giraud S, Richard S. Natural history of supratentorial hemangioblastomas in von Hippel-Lindau disease. Neurosurgery. 2010;67:577–87; discussion 587.
51. Sharma RR, Cast IP, O'brien C. Supratentorial haemangioblastoma not associated with Von Hippel Lindau complex or polycythaemia: case report and literature review. Br J Neurosurg. 1995; 9:81–4.
52. Jiang JG, Rao Q, Xia QY, Tu P, Lu ZF, Shen Q, Zhang RS, Yu B, Zhou XJ, Shi SS, Shi QL. Sporadic hemangioblastoma of the kidney with PAX2 and focal CD10 expression: report of a case. Int J Clin Exp Pathol. 2013;6:1953–6.
53. Nonaka D, Rodriguez J, Rosai J. Extraneural hemangioblastoma: a report of 5 cases. Am J Surg Pathol. 2007;31:1545–51.
54. Deb P, Pal S, Dutta V, Srivastava A, Bhargava A, Yadav KK. Adrenal haemangioblastoma presenting as phaeochromocytoma: a rare manifestation of extraneural hemangioblastoma. Endocr Pathol. 2012;23:187–90.
55. Rao Q, Chen JY, Wang JD, Ma HH, Zhou HB, Lu ZF, Zhou XJ. Renal cell carcinoma in children and young adults: clinicopathological, immunohistochemical, and VHL gene analysis of 46 cases with follow-up. Int J Surg Pathol. 2011;19:170–9.
56. Frantzen C, Links, TP, Giles, RH. 1993 Von Hippel-Lindau Disease. GeneReviews® [Internet]. 1993–2014. 2000.
57. Seizinger BR, Rouleau GA, Ozelius LJ, Lane AH, Farmer GE, Lamiell JM, Haines J, Yuen JW, Collins D, Majoor-Krakauer D, et al. Von Hippel-Lindau disease maps to the region of chromosome 3 associated with renal cell carcinoma. Nature. 1988; 332:268–9.
58. Fleming S. Genetics of kidney tumours. Forum (Genova). 1998;8:176–84.
59. Kolackov K, Tupikowski K, Bednarek-Tupikowska G. Genetic aspects of pheochromocytoma. Adv Clin Exp Med. 2012;21: 821–9.
60. Raygada M, Pasini B, Stratakis CA. Hereditary paragangliomas. Adv Otorhinolaryngol. 2011;70:99–106.
61. Burnichon N, Abermil N, Buffet A, Favier J, Gimenez-Roqueplo AP. The genetics of paragangliomas. Eur Ann Otorhinolaryngol Head Neck Dis. 2012;129:315–8.
62. Salazar R, Gonzalez-Castano C, Rozas P, Castro J. Retinal capillary hemangioma and von Hippel-Lindau disease: diagnostic and therapeutic implications. Arch Soc Esp Oftalmol. 2011;86: 218–21.
63. Mettu P, Agron E, Samtani S, Chew EY, Wong WT. Genotype-phenotype correlation in ocular von Hippel-Lindau (VHL) disease: the effect of missense mutation position on ocular VHL phenotype. Invest Ophthalmol Vis Sci. 2010;51:4464–70.
64. Wong WT, Agron E, Coleman HR, Tran T, Reed GF, Csaky K, Chew EY. Clinical characterization of retinal capillary hemangioblastomas in a large population of patients with von Hippel-Lindau disease. Ophthalmology. 2008;115:181–8.
65. Speisky D, Duces A, Bieche I, Rebours V, Hammel P, Sauvanet A, Richard S, Bedossa P, Vidaud M, Murat A, Niccoli P, Scoazec JY, Ruszniewski P, Couvelard A. Molecular profiling of pancreatic neuroendocrine tumors in sporadic and Von Hippel-Lindau patients. Clin Cancer Res. 2012;18:2838–49.
66. Lecumberri Pascual E. [Associated gastroenteropancreatic neuroendocrine tumours to familiar syndromes]. Endocrinol Nutr. 2009;56 Suppl 2:10–5.
67. Erlic Z, Ploeckinger U, Cascon A, Hoffmann MM, von Duecker L, Winter A, Kammel G, Bacher J, Sullivan M, Isermann B, Fischer L, Raffel A, Knoefel WT, Schott M, Baumann T, Schaefer O, Keck T, Baum RP, Milos I, Muresan M, Peczkowska M, Januszewicz A, Cupisti K, Tonjes A, Fasshauer M, Langrehr J, von Wussow P, Agaimy A, Schlimok G, Lamberts R, Wiech T, Schmid KW, Weber A, Nunez M, Robledo M, Eng C, Neumann HP. Systematic comparison of sporadic and syndromic pancreatic islet cell tumors. Endocr Relat Cancer. 2010;17:875–83.
68. Shen HC, Adem A, Ylaya K, Wilson A, He M, Lorang D, Hewitt SM, Pechhold K, Harlan DM, Lubensky IA, Schmidt LS, Linehan WM, Libutti SK. Deciphering von Hippel-Lindau (VHL/Vhl)-associated pancreatic manifestations by inactivating Vhl in specific pancreatic cell populations. PLoS One. 2009;4:e4897.
69. Starker LF, Carling T. Molecular genetics of gastroenteropancreatic neuroendocrine tumors. Curr Opin Oncol. 2009;21:29–33.
70. Glasker S, Tran MG, Shively SB, Ikejiri B, Lonser RR, Maxwell PH, Zhuang Z, Oldfield EH, Vortmeyer AO. Epididymal cystadenomas and epithelial tumourlets: effects of VHL deficiency on the human epididymis. J Pathol. 2006;210:32–41.
71. Shen T, Zhuang Z, Gersell DJ, Tavassoli FA. Allelic deletion of VHL gene detected in papillary tumors of the broad ligament, epididymis, and retroperitoneum in von Hippel-Lindau disease patients. Int J Surg Pathol. 2000;8:207–12.
72. Megerian CA, Mckenna MJ, Nuss RC, Maniglia AJ, Ojemann RG, Pilch BZ, Nadol Jr JB. Endolymphatic sac tumors: histopathologic confirmation, clinical characterization, and implication in von Hippel-Lindau disease. Laryngoscope. 1995;105:801–8.
73. Manski TJ, Heffner DK, Glenn GM, Patronas NJ, Pikus AT, Katz D, Lebovics R, Sledjeski K, Choyke PL, Zbar B, Linehan WM, Oldfield EH. Endolymphatic sac tumors. A source of morbid hearing loss in von Hippel-Lindau disease. JAMA. 1997;277:1461–6.
74. Hamazaki S, Yoshida M, Yao M, Nagashima Y, Taguchi K, Nakashima H, Okada S. Mutation of von Hippel-Lindau tumor suppressor gene in a sporadic endolymphatic sac tumor. Hum Pathol. 2001;32:1272–6.
75. Tootee A, Hasani-Ranjbar S. Von hippel-lindau disease: a new approach to an old problem. Int J Endocrinol Metab. 2012; 10:619–24.
76. Kaelin Jr WG. The von Hippel-Lindau gene, kidney cancer, and oxygen sensing. J Am Soc Nephrol. 2003;14:2703–11.
77. Shuin T, Yamasaki I, Tamura K, Okuda H, Furihata M, Ashida S. von Hippel-Lindau disease: molecular pathological basis, clinical

criteria, genetic testing, clinical features of tumors and treatment. Jpn J Clin Oncol. 2006;36:337–43.

78. Hasani-Ranjbar S, Amoli MM, Ebrahim-Habibi A, Haghpanah V, Hejazi M, Soltani A, Larijani B. Mutation screening of VHL gene in a family with malignant bilateral pheochromocytoma: from isolated familial pheochromocytoma to von Hippel-Lindau disease. Fam Cancer. 2009;8:465–71.
79. Kuwahara T, Muraki M, Kitamura S, Tuchiya N, Ninchoji T, Uemura K. A case of hydrocephalus with hypacusis due to hemangioblastoma. No Shinkei Geka. 1991;19:385–9.
80. Jeffreys R. Clinical and surgical aspects of posterior fossa haemangioblastomata. J Neurol Neurosurg Psychiatry. 1975;38: 105–11.
81. Ammerman JM, Lonser RR, Dambrosia J, Butman JA, Oldfield EH. Long-term natural history of hemangioblastomas in patients with von Hippel-Lindau disease: implications for treatment. J Neurosurg. 2006;105:248–55.
82. Kanno H, Yamamoto I, Nishikawa R, Matsutani M, Wakabayashi T, Yoshida J, Shitara N, Yamasaki I, Shuin T. Spinal cord hemangioblastomas in von Hippel-Lindau disease. Spinal Cord. 2009;47:447–52.
83. Trimble M, Caro J, Talalla A, Brain M. Secondary erythrocytosis due to a cerebellar hemangioblastoma: demonstration of erythropoietin mRNA in the tumor. Blood. 1991;78:599–601.
84. Jeffreys RV, Napier JA, Reynolds SH. Erythropoietin levels in posterior fossa haemangioblastoma. J Neurol Neurosurg Psychiatry. 1982;45:264–6.
85. Rachinger J, Buslei R, Prell J, Strauss C. Solid haemangioblastomas of the CNS: a review of 17 consecutive cases. Neurosurg Rev. 2009;32:37–47; discussion 47–8.
86. Drapkin AJ, Rose WS. Cerebellar hemangioblastoma during pregnancy. Neurosurgery. 1989;24:298–9.
87. Delisle MF, Valimohamed F, Money D, Douglas MJ. Central nervous system complications of von Hippel-Lindau disease and pregnancy; perinatal considerations: case report and literature review. J Matern Fetal Med. 2000;9:242–7.
88. Erdogan B, Sen O, Aydin MV, Bagis T, Bavbek M. Cerebellar hemangioblastoma in pregnancy. A case report. J Reprod Med. 2002;47:864–6.
89. Hayden MG, Gephart R, Kalanithi P, Chou D. Von Hippel-Lindau disease in pregnancy: a brief review. J Clin Neurosci. 2009; 16:611–3.
90. Kasarskis EJ, Tibbs PA, Lee C. Cerebellar hemangioblastoma symptomatic during pregnancy. Neurosurgery. 1988;22:770–2.
91. Ye DY, Bakhtian KD, Asthagiri AR, Lonser RR. Effect of pregnancy on hemangioblastoma development and progression in von Hippel-Lindau disease. J Neurosurg. 2012;117:818–24.
92. Raz E, Zagzag D, Saba L, Mannelli L, di Paolo PL, D'ambrosio F, Knopp E. Cyst with a mural nodule tumor of the brain. Cancer Imaging. 2012;12:237–44.
93. van Velthoven V, Reinacher PC, Klisch J, Neumann HP, Glasker S. Treatment of intramedullary hemangioblastomas, with special attention to von Hippel-Lindau disease. Neurosurgery. 2003; 53:1306–13; discussion 1313–4.
94. Weil RJ, Lonser RR, Devroom HL, Wanebo JE, Oldfield EH. Surgical management of brainstem hemangioblastomas in patients with von Hippel-Lindau disease. J Neurosurg. 2003;98: 95–105.
95. Lonser RR, Weil RJ, Wanebo JE, Devroom HL, Oldfield EH. Surgical management of spinal cord hemangioblastomas in patients with von Hippel-Lindau disease. J Neurosurg. 2003;98: 106–16.
96. Vaganovs P, Bokums K, Miklasevics E, Plonis J, Zarina L, Geldners I, Gardovskis J, Vjaters E. Von hippel-lindau syndrome: diagnosis and management of hemangioblastoma and pheochromocytoma. Case Rep Urol. 2013;2013:624096.
97. Jagannathan J, Lonser RR, Smith R, Devroom HL, Oldfield EH. Surgical management of cerebellar hemangioblastomas in patients with von Hippel-Lindau disease. J Neurosurg. 2008; 108:210–22.
98. Lonser RR, Oldfield EH. Microsurgical resection of spinal cord hemangioblastomas. Neurosurgery. 2005;57:372–6; discussion 372–6.
99. Mehta GU, Asthagiri AR, Bakhtian KD, Auh S, Oldfield EH, Lonser RR. Functional outcome after resection of spinal cord hemangioblastomas associated with von Hippel-Lindau disease. J Neurosurg Spine. 2010;12:233–42.
100. Wind JJ, Bakhtian KD, Sweet JA, Mehta GU, Thawani JP, Asthagiri AR, Oldfield EH, Lonser RR. Long-term outcome after resection of brainstem hemangioblastomas in von Hippel-Lindau disease. J Neurosurg. 2011;114:1312–8.
101. Pavesi G, Feletti A, Berlucchi S, Opocher G, Martella M, Murgia A, Scienza R. Neurosurgical treatment of von Hippel-Lindau-associated hemangioblastomas: benefits, risks and outcome. J Neurosurg Sci. 2008;52:29–36.
102. Chang SD, Meisel JA, Hancock SL, Martin DP, Mcmanus M, Adler Jr JR. Treatment of hemangioblastomas in von Hippel-Lindau disease with linear accelerator-based radiosurgery. Neurosurgery. 1998;43:28–34; discussion 34–5.
103. Daly ME, Choi CY, Gibbs IC, Adler Jr JR, Chang SD, Lieberson RE, Soltys SG. Tolerance of the spinal cord to stereotactic radiosurgery: insights from hemangioblastomas. Int J Radiat Oncol Biol Phys. 2011;80:213–20.
104. Chang UK, Lee DH. Stereotactic radiosurgery for spinal neoplasms: current status and future perspective. J Neurosurg Sci. 2013;57:87–101.
105. Moss JM, Choi CY, Adler Jr JR, Soltys SG, Gibbs IC, Chang SD. Stereotactic radiosurgical treatment of cranial and spinal hemangioblastomas. Neurosurgery. 2009;65:79–85; discussion 85.
106. Selch MT, Tenn S, Agazaryan N, Lee SP, Gorgulho A, de Salles AA. Image-guided linear accelerator-based spinal radiosurgery for hemangioblastoma. Surg Neurol Int. 2012;3:73.
107. Sayer FT, Nguyen J, Starke RM, Yen CP, Sheehan JP. Gamma knife radiosurgery for intracranial hemangioblastomas—outcome at 3 years. World Neurosurg. 2011;75:99–105; discussion 45–8.
108. Asthagiri AR, Mehta GU, Zach L, Li X, Butman JA, Camphausen KA, Lonser RR, Lonser RR. Prospective evaluation of radiosurgery for hemangioblastomas in von Hippel-Lindau disease. Neuro Oncol. 2010;12:80–6.
109. Patrice SJ, Sneed PK, Flickinger JC, Shrieve DC, Pollock BE, Alexander 3rd E, Larson DA, Kondziolka DS, Gutin PH, Wara WM, Mcdermott MW, Lunsford LD, Loeffler JS, Loeffler JS. Radiosurgery for hemangioblastoma: results of a multiinstitutional experience. Int J Radiat Oncol Biol Phys. 1996; 35:493–9.
110. Madhusudan S, Deplanque G, Braybrooke JP, Cattell E, Taylor M, Price P, Tsaloumas MD, Moore N, Huson SM, Adams C, Frith P, Scigalla P, Harris AL. Antiangiogenic therapy for von Hippel-Lindau disease. JAMA. 2004;291:943–4.
111. Matin SF, McCutcheon IE, Gombos DS, et al. Treatment of VHL patients with sunitinib: clinical outcomes and translational studies. J Clin Oncol. 2010;28:15s; suppl; abstr 3040.
112. Chen GJ, Karajannis MA, Newcomb EW, Zagzag D. Overexpression and activation of epidermal growth factor receptor in hemangioblastomas. J Neurooncol. 2010;99:195–200.
113. Riklin C, Seystahl K, Hofer S, Happold C, Winterhalder R, Weller M. Antiangiogenic treatment for multiple CNS hemangioblastomas. Onkologie. 2012;35:443–5.

114. Kim BY, Jonasch E, Mccutcheon IE. Pazopanib therapy for cerebellar hemangioblastomas in von Hippel-Lindau disease: case report. Target Oncol. 2012;7:145–9.
115. Reyes-Botero G, Gallego Perez-Larraya J, Sanson M. Sporadic CNS hemangioblastomatosis, response to sunitinib and secondary polycythemia. J Neurooncol. 2012;107:439–40.
116. Sardi I, Sanzo M, Giordano F, Buccoliero AM, Mussa F, Arico M, Genitori L. Monotherapy with thalidomide for treatment of spinal cord hemangioblastomas in a patient with von Hippel-Lindau disease. Pediatr Blood Cancer. 2009;53:464–7.
117. Niemela M, Maenpaa H, Salven P, Summanen P, Poussa K, Laatikainen L, Jaaskelainen J, Joensuu H. Interferon alpha-2a therapy in 18 hemangioblastomas. Clin Cancer Res. 2001;7: 510–6.
118. Garces-AMBROSSI GL, Mcgirt MJ, Mehta VA, Sciubba DM, Witham TF, Bydon A, Wolinksy JP, Jallo GI, Gokaslan ZL. Factors associated with progression-free survival and long-term neurological outcome after resection of intramedullary spinal cord tumors: analysis of 101 consecutive cases. J Neurosurg Spine. 2009;11:591–9.
119. Kanno H, Kuratsu J, Nishikawa R, Mishima K, Natsume A, Wakabayashi T, Houkin K, Terasaka S, Shuin T. Clinical features of patients bearing central nervous system hemangioblastoma in von Hippel-Lindau disease. Acta Neurochir (Wien). 2013;155:1–7.

15
Schwannomas

Matthias A. Karajannis and Anat Stemmer-Rachamimov

Schwannomas are benign tumors arising from Schwann cells, named after the German physiologist Theodor Schwann. Schwann cells, or neurolemmocytes, are glial cells that play a number of important roles in peripheral nerve biology, including nerve development, myelination, metabolism, conduction, and repair. The majority of schwannomas arise sporadically, i.e., in patients without a positive family history and no identifiable tumor predisposition syndrome. Schwannomas arise from cranial, spinal, or peripheral nerves and small myelinated nerves in the skin or viscera. The most commonly affected cranial nerve is the eighth cranial nerve, near the vestibular ganglion (vestibular schwannoma, VS), followed by the fifth (trigeminal schwannoma) [1]. VS represents one of the most common intracranial tumor, and the incidence of sporadic VS in the United States is approximately 3,000 per year [1].

Schwannomas arising from spinal nerve roots have a predilection for the sensory (dorsal) roots with the lumbosacral and cauda equina regions most commonly affected. The peripheral nerves most affected are in the flexor surfaces of the upper and lower limbs: the ulnar and peroneal nerves. Rarely, schwannomas occur within the parenchyma of the brain or spinal cord [2] where the tumors are presumed to arise from small myelinated peripheral nerve fibers that accompany vessels into the parenchyma or from aberrant peripheral nerve fibers [3, 4].

Known hereditary tumor predisposition syndromes associated with schwannomas include *neurofibromatosis type 2* (*NF2*), *schwannomatosis*, and *Carney's complex*.

NF2 is caused by inactivation of the *NF2* gene located on chromosome 22q [5, 6]. The *NF2* gene product, Merlin, is a unique tumor suppressor in that it functions both at the cell cortex and in the nucleus [7].

NF2 patients typically develop progressive hearing loss in adolescence or young adulthood due to bilateral vestibular schwannomas (VS), but also develop schwannomas at other locations throughout the nervous system. Patients with *schwannomatosis* suffer from multiple, often painful schwannomas, but with rare exceptions, do not develop VS and meningiomas, which are common in NF2 [8–10]. The disease is familial in approximately 15 % of the patients only, and follows an autosomal dominant mode of inheritance. Germline mutations in *SMARCB1* [11–13], a gene that is also involved in rhabdoid tumor predisposition syndrome (RPDS), can be identified in approximately 50 % of familial and <10 % of sporadic patients [14]. A recent study identified mutations in the *LZTR1* gene, another tumor suppressor, in the majority of patients with schwannomatosis that did not have germline alterations in *SMARCB1* [15].

Carney's complex is an autosomal dominant multiple neoplasia syndrome. The diagnosis is made if two or more major manifestations of the syndrome are present. Major manifestations include skin lesions (lentiginis, blue nevi, and cutaneous myxomas), cardiac myxoma, endocrine manifestations (hyperplasias and adenomas of adrenal and pituitary), and psammomatous melanocytic schwannomas [16–18]. Schwannomas in Carney's complex patients most frequently arise in the paraspinal sympathetic chain or the gastrointestinal tract, although they may occur anywhere in the peripheral nervous system. Inactivating mutations in the regulatory subunit type 1 alpha gene (*PRKAR1A*) located at 17q22-24 can be identified in approximately 30 % of Carney's complex patients [19, 20].

Historically, the mainstay of treatment for schwannomas has included surgery and radiation therapy, both of which have major drawbacks. Although surgical resection is effective at tumor control, serious complications depending on tumor size and location are common, such as disfigurement and further loss of neurologic function. Stereotactic radiosurgery (SRS) or fractionated radiation therapy (RT) have been proposed as alternatives. SRS has the largest clinical experience in VS management with published outcomes, including for NF2 [21, 22]. However, its safety and efficacy in the NF2 population has not been established in patients with large VS and significant hearing impairment and there is concern about long-term efficacy. The risk for a radiation-induced secondary malignancy has also been raised, although

M.A. Karajannis and D. Zagzag (eds.), *Molecular Pathology of Nervous System Tumors: Biological Stratification and Targeted Therapies*, Molecular Pathology Library 8,
DOI 10.1007/978-1-4939-1830-0_15,

rare [23, 24]. For a subset of NF2 patients with unilateral hearing only and progressive hearing loss due to a growing ipsilateral VS, surgical resection will most likely result in total deafness. SRS as currently performed at doses of 12–13 Gy, can maintain hearing in some patients, but clinical studies show that hearing commonly declines after 5 years [22]. Over the recent years, our increasing understanding of the biology of NF2 mutant tumors, including schwannomas, has opened avenues for preclinical and clinical development of molecular targeted medical therapies for schwannomas. As a result, some of these therapies have begun to show promise in the clinic, and novel agents are being actively developed in a growing number of preclinical studies and clinical trials.

Pathology and Histopathology

Schwannomas are benign (WHO Grade I) peripheral nerve sheath tumors that are composed of neoplastic Schwann cells. Other terms that may be used as synonyms for schwannomas include neurinoma and neurilemmoma. The term neuroma should not be used as synonym for schwannomas, as it implies a non-neoplastic process, such as a traumatic neuroma, Morton's neuroma [1].

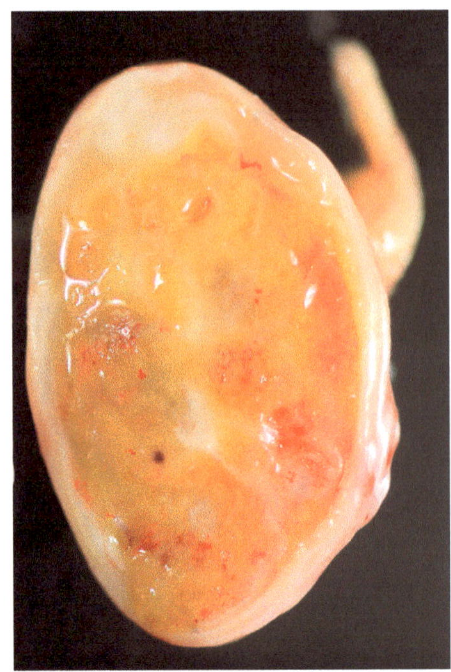

Fig. 15.1. Macroscopic features of a schwannoma: encapsulated mass, associated with a nerve, with homogenous yellow/tan cut surface

Macroscopic Findings

Most schwannomas are globoid, encapsulated, discrete masses. The capsule consists of the epineurium of the nerve in which the tumor arises. The nerve of origin may sometimes be observed entering and/or exiting the tumor mass (Fig. 15.1). The tumor size and shape are dictated by the site of origin: tumors arising in spinal nerve roots often have a "dumbbell" shape with a narrow center, where the tumor is confined within the nerve foramen, and two enlarged extremities where it is unconfined in the extra and intra spinal compartments. Schwannomas that arise in the mediastinum or retroperitoneum where space is not confined, may reach large dimensions and develop degenerative cystic changes.

The cut surface of schwannomas appears tan and homogenous (Fig. 15.1). There may be white areas (fibrosis) or yellow areas which represent fat infiltration or sheets of lipid laden macrophages. In some cases (especially in large tumors) there may be areas of hemorrhage or cystic degeneration.

In some cases, especially in the skin and viscera, schwannomas may grow in a plexiform pattern, expanding and replacing the nerve of origin, in a similar pattern to plexiform neurofibromas.

Histological Features

Most schwannomas have the conventional (classic) histological features. However, other patterns of growth and histological patterns may be seen, especially in association with tumor syndromes (see below) and may be misdiagnosed as other tumor types.

Conventional Schwannomas

The histological appearance of conventional schwannomas is of a benign spindle cell tumor with sharply demarcated margins (encapsulated). Nerve axons and perineurial cells are often present at the periphery of the tumor, and can be highlighted with immunostaining for Neurofilament and Claudin 1, respectively. In contrast with neurofibromas, very few axons (if any) are present within the tumor.

A biphasic pattern with compact (Antoni A) and loose (Antoni B) areas is a characteristic feature (Fig. 15.2). The proportions of these areas vary, and in some tumors only one type will be present. Diagnosis based on the loose (Antoni B) areas can be difficult as the histological features are nonspecific. The hallmark of schwannomas is the formation of nuclear palisades around nuclear free areas (Verocay bodies) which may at times form elongated ribbons (Fig. 15.3) or clusters where tumor cells form groups of "streaming" elongated, narrow nuclei. Longstanding tumors may display degenerative changes such as cysts and sheets of lipid laden macrophages. Some schwannomas may have large clusters of "back to back" large hyalinized vessels mimicking vascular malformations, often associated with thrombosis and hemosiderin-laden macrophages. Another type of degenerative change in schwannomas is the presence of scattered

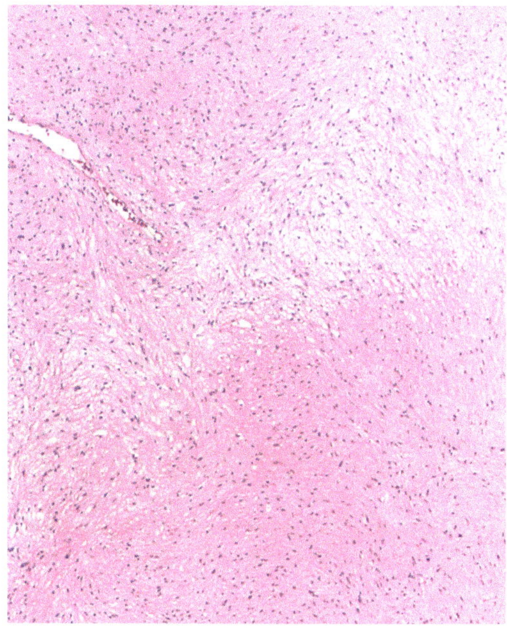

Fig. 15.2. Conventional schwannoma (H&E): Antoni A (compact) and Antoni B (loose, pale) areas are classic features in schwannomas

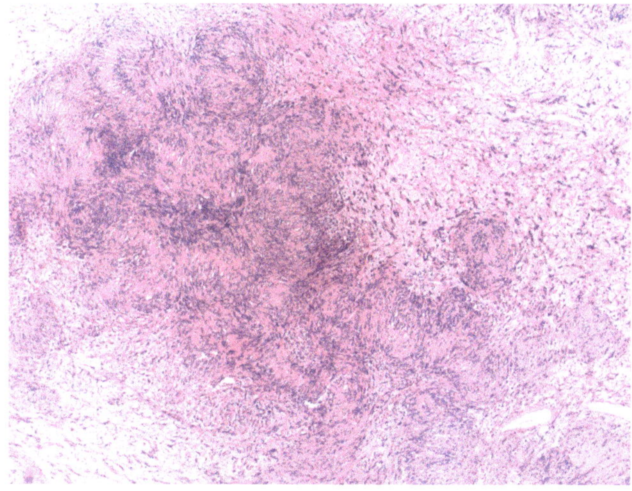

Fig. 15.3. Conventional schwannoma (H&E): Verocay bodies are characteristic of schwannomas and are nuclear palisades around nuclear free areas

large, atypical, hyperchromatic nuclei ("ancient change") which are not indicative of malignant transformation.

Cellular Schwannomas

Cellular schwannomas are characterized by dense cellularity with intersecting fascicles or patternless growth, and lack of the histological hallmarks of conventional schwannomas. The characteristic biphasic (Antoni A/Antoni B) pattern and Verocay bodies are not present and the tumor is often composed of compact (Antoni A) areas only. In addition to hypercellularity, the tumors may display mitotic activity, nuclear atypia, and necrosis (Fig. 15.4). However, despite the presence of these worrisome histological features, cellular schwannomas are benign, and although recurrence rate is variable, they are slow growing and never metastasize [25–27].

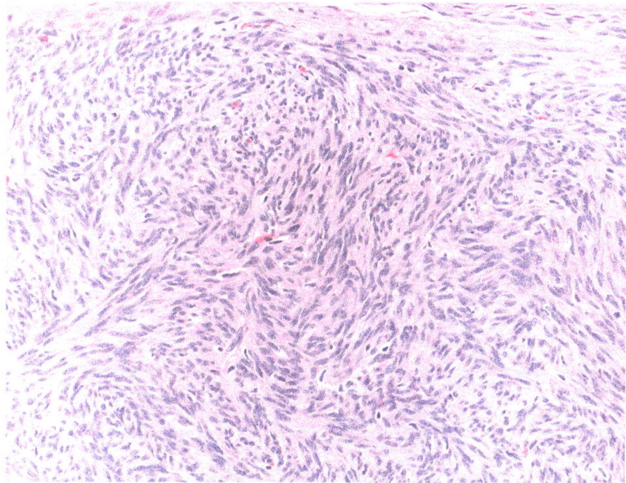

Fig. 15.4. Cellular schwannoma (H&E): Dense cellularity, fascicular growth pattern and scattered mitotic figs. in a cellular schwannoma

The lack of the classical histological features and the presence of dense cellularity and mitoses may prompt a diagnosis of malignancy. The differential diagnosis includes sarcomas such as leiomyosarcoma, or malignant peripheral nerve sheath tumor (MPNST). Helpful distinguishing features that support the diagnosis of cellular schwannoma include the presence of a peripheral capsule, diffuse S100 positivity and collagen IV expression.

Plexiform Schwannomas

Plexiform schwannomas grow within the nerve, expanding and replacing it along its course, so it appears grossly like a rope; a similar pattern as the better known plexiform neurofibromas, with which they may be confused (Fig. 15.5).

Plexiform schwannomas are most common in the skin but may also occur in soft tissue or major peripheral nerves [28–30]. In contrast to other schwannoma subtypes, plexiform schwannomas are often non-encapsulated and may infiltrate adjacent soft tissue, encasing nerves and skin adnexa. Furthermore, entrapped axons are often present within the tumor mass, features that mimic plexiform neurofibromas [31].

Plexiform schwannomas may be associated with NF2 or schwannomatosis; there is no association with NF1 [32, 33]. In contrast to plexiform neurofibromas, there is no risk of malignant transformation. Helpful for the histological diagnosis of plexiform schwannomas are the presence of conventional schwannoma features (Verocay bodies, Antoni A/ Antoni B areas) and diffuse S100 positivity.

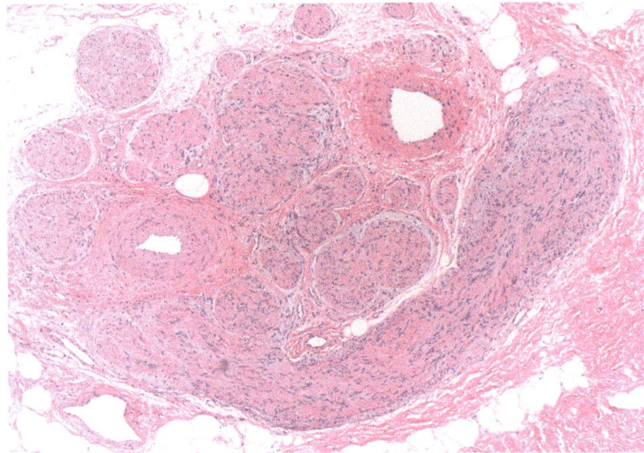

Fig. 15.5. Plexiform schwannomas (H&E): plexiform schwannomas grow along the nerve, expanding and replacing it

Melanotic Schwannomas

Melanotic schwannomas are rare and distinct tumors that are composed of neoplastic Schwann cells that contain melanin. The tumors appear as pigmented, circumscribed masses. Melanotic schwannomas are of two types: non-psammomatous and psammomatous, defined by the presence of psammoma bodies (concentrically laminated bodies that are PAS positive). Non-psammomatous melanotic schwannnomas are benign. In contrast, half of the psammomatous melanotic schwannomas are associated with Carney's complex and may undergo malignant transformation [16, 17, 34]. Therefore, in the case of psammomatous melanotic schwannomas, the possibility of an underlying Carney's syndrome should be investigated.

Melanotic schwannomas lack the classical features of conventional schwannomas (Antoni A/Antoni B areas, Verocay bodies, vascular clusters) and are often composed of large, epitheloid cells, with large round/oval nuclei and prominent nucleoli (Fig. 15.6). The differential diagnosis of melanocytic schwannomas is with melanocytic lesions; melanocytoma and melanoma (primary and metastatic). Electron microscopy may be helpful. Positive collagen IV immunostaining and a rich reticulin network can support the diagnosis of schwannoma.

Sporadic and Syndromic Schwannomas

The great majority (90 %) of schwannomas are single, sporadic tumors [35]. However, schwannomas may also occur as part of the clinical manifestations in patients with an underlying genetic predisposition (syndromic).

In a study in which the histological features of solitary sporadic schwannomas were compared to schwannomas associated with NF2; some histological features were found to be more common in sporadic/solitary schwannomas. In particular, solitary schwannomas were found to have prominent vascular clusters that mimic vascular malformations ("back to back" vessels with thick hyalinized walls or dilated sinusoidal vessels), thrombosis, and inflammation (Fig. 15.7) [36]. In addition, a more recent study found that in contrast to the mosaic pattern seen in NF-associated schwannomas (NF2 and schwannomatosis), most solitary/sporadic schwannomas retain INI1 expression and appear diffusely positive [37] (see below).

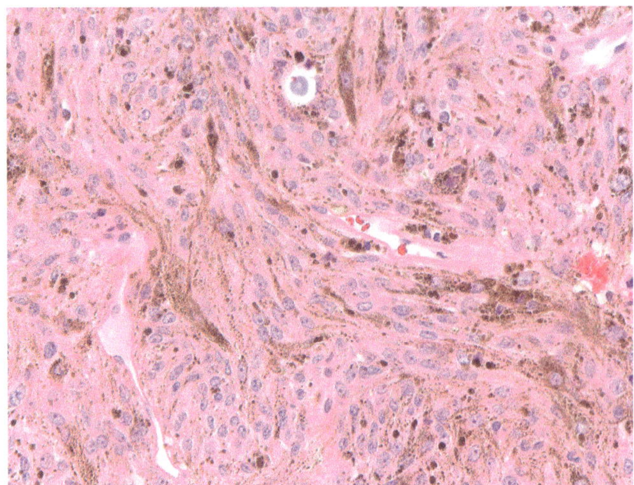

Fig. 15.6. Melanotic Scwhannoma: Melanotic schwannomas are composed of pigmented Schwann cells, and may contain psammoma bodies

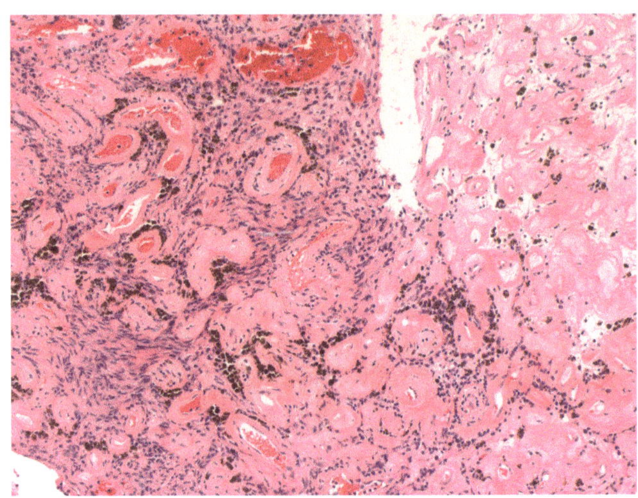

Fig. 15.7. Sporadic/solitary Schwannoma: Clustered thick hyalinized blood vessels mimicking vascular malformations are a common finding in solitary/sporadic schwannomas

Syndromic Schwannomas

The syndromes associated with multiple schwannomas include NF2, schwannomatosis and Carney's Syndrome.

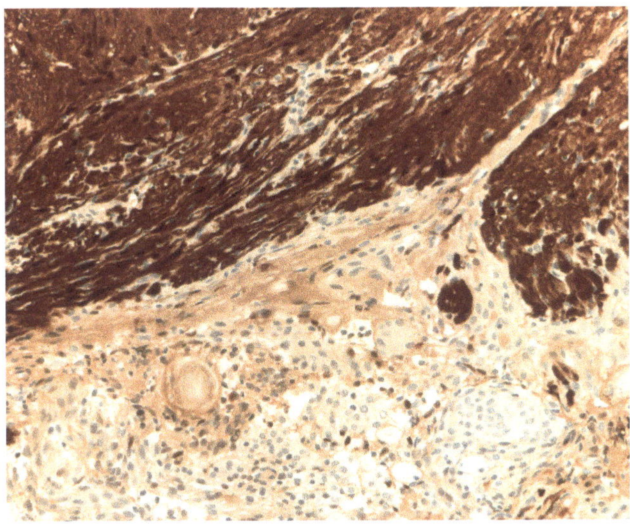

Fig. 15.8. Schwannoma/meningioma collision tumor (S100 immunostain): a collision tumor composed of schwannoma (on the *right*, immunopositive for S100) and meningioma (on the *left*, S100 negative) is pathognomonic of NF2

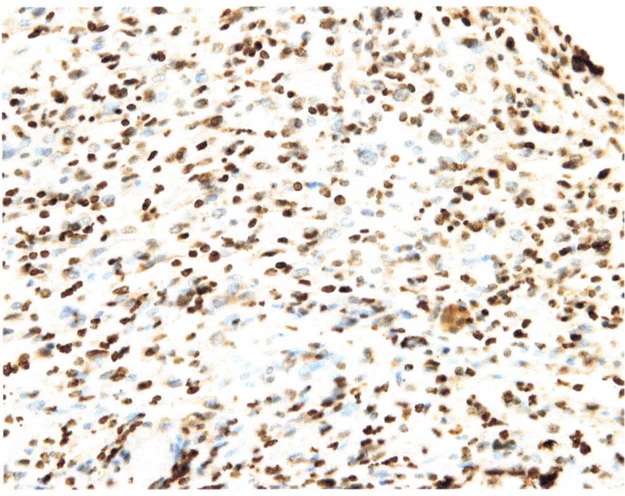

Fig. 15.9. Mosaic INI1 immunostaining (INI1 immunostain): partial loss (mosaic staining) of INI1 expression is common in NF-associated schwannomas

Neurofibromatosis Type 2 (NF2)

NF2 is an autosomal dominant disorder characterized by neoplastic and dysplastic lesions of Schwann cells, meningothelial cells, and glial cells. Patients are predisposed to develop multiple schwannomas, and the hallmark of the disease is bilateral VS. In addition, NF2 patients are predisposed to develop other tumors; multiple meningiomas and spinal ependymomas. Non-neoplastic lesions associated with the syndrome include meningioangiomatosis, glial hamartomas, retinal hamartomas, posterior subcapsular cataracts, epiretinal membranes, and polyneuropathies [1, 38].

The disease is rare, with an estimated incidence of 1 per 40,000 newborns [35]–1:25,000 [39] and is caused by a germline mutation in the NF2 gene on chromosome 22q that encodes the protein Merlin. *De novo* mutations (patients without family history) occur in 30 % of the patients. Particularly difficult to diagnose are patients with mosaic NF2 in which clinical manifestations may overlap with other forms of neurofibromatosis (NF1 or schwannomatosis) or may not fulfill the clinical criteria for the diagnosis of NF [40]. In these scenarios, the pathological diagnosis of nerve sheath tumors may be particularly helpful in supporting a suspected clinical diagnosis. Schwannomas associated with NF2 often present at an earlier age than sporadic, non-syndromic schwannomas [41, 42].

NF2-associated schwannomas frequently have a multilobular appearance ("bunch of grapes") which may be apparent macroscopically and/or microscopically [36]. In some cases, meningioma and schwannoma form a collision tumor, in which the two components are seen on the same slide (Fig. 15.8). Schwannoma/meningioma collision tumors are pathognomonic for NF2. In contrast to sporadic solitary schwannomas, the pattern of INI1 immunostaining of schwannomas associated with NF2 or schwannomatosis is a mosaic pattern, in which there is partial loss, with mixed positive and negative cells (Fig. 15.9); [37]. Therefore, the pattern of growth (multinodular) and the mosaic INI1 expression pattern may support the diagnosis of an NF-associated schwannoma in some cases. Plexiform cutaneous schwannomas may be seen in childhood in NF2 patients and should not be confused with neurofibromas (which would lead to the clinical diagnosis of NF1).

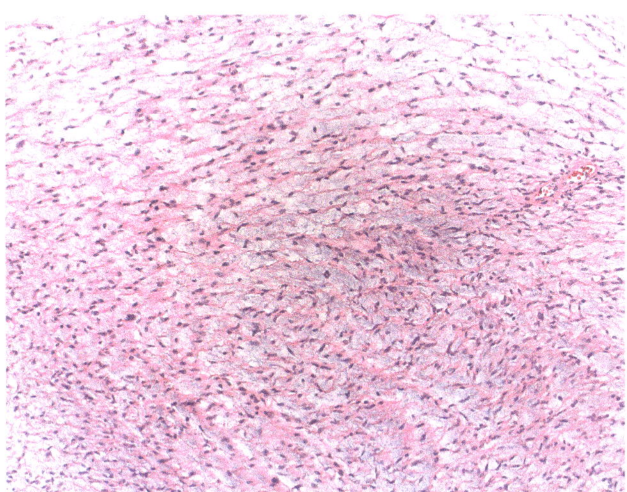

Fig. 15.10. Myxoid schwannoma (hybrid tumor): Schwannomas with abundant myxoid stroma may mimic neurofibroma (hybrid tumor) and are common in schwannomatosis

Schwannomatosis

Histologically, schwannomatosis-associated tumors often have prominent myxoid stroma, which may lead to a misdiagnosis of a neurofibroma [8, 11–13, 43–45]; (Fig. 15.10). Peripheral nerve sheath tumors with mixed features of schwannoma/neurofibroma are referred to as "hybrid tumors" [46] and may represent a myxoid schwannoma or a "Schwann cell rich" neurofibroma. Hybrid tumors are more common in the context of the neurofibromatoses [47] and misdiagnoses can be avoided by immunohistochemical stains that highlight the different components of the tumor (axons, Schwann cells, perineurial cells). Many of the schwannomatosis-associated tumors (especially familial schwannomatosis) have a mosaic (partial lack) pattern of expression of INI1 protein [37].

Carney's Complex

Schwannomas from patients with Carney's complex are pigmented and often calcified [18]. Histologically, they contain melanin and psammoma bodies and lack the classic features of conventional schwannomas. There is a risk of malignant transformation in 10 % of the cases. Although the histological criteria are not well defined, large nuclei with prominent nucleoli, brisk mitotic activity, and necrosis are worrisome signs of aggressive biological behavior.

Cytogenetics and Molecular Genetics

A number of studies to date have examined the cytogenetics and molecular genetics of schwannomas, including sporadic schwannomas and schwannomas associated with NF2 and schwannomatosis. A number of early studies demonstrated that loss of heterozygosity (LOH) is common in NF2-associated and sporadic schwannomas [48, 49], and subsequent work showed that both sporadic and NF2-related VS harbor mutational inactivation or loss of both alleles of the *NF2* gene [5, 50], consistent with Knudson's two hit model of tumorigenesis [51]. In the case of schwannomatosis, a four hit mechanism has been proposed, involving *NF2* and either *SMARCB1* [12] or *LZTR1* [15].

Studies in schwannomas using comparative genomic hybridization (CGH) [52–55] have identified loss on chromosome 22 (*NF2*) as the most common hit by far, detectable in up to 56 % of sporadic and 62 % of NF2-associated schwannomas, and LOH was caused by mitotic recombination in a subset [53]. Other genetic aberrations observed in subsets of tumors included gains involving 9q, 10q, 17q, 19p, and 19q, as well as losses involving 9p. Of note, and perhaps not surprising, some of the data indicate that genetic aberrations outside of chromosome 22 predominantly occur in tumors that were previously treated with radiotherapy [53]. Other investigators have looked at CpG island hypermethylation of the *NF2* gene as an alternate mechanism of gene silencing, but the results have been largely negative [56, 57].

Gene Expression Profiling

Several studies have been published on gene expression profiling in schwannomas, showing evidence of deregulation in the proto-oncogene *MET*, as well as *ITGA4*, *PLEXNB3/SEMA5, and CAV1* [58, 59]. In addition, upregulation of osteopontin (*SPP1*), a gene involved in the protein degradation of the NF2 gene product Merlin, was observed [58]. Gene regulation at the posttranscriptional level has been examined in a recent study, focusing on miRNA profiling of schwannomas [60]. In that study, 12 miRNAs were found to be significantly deregulated in tumors, including miR-7. Targets of miR-7 include several oncogenes relevant to schwannoma biology, including epidermal growth factor receptor (EGFR), p21-activated kinase (Pak1), and associated cdc42 kinase1 (Ack1).

Prognostic Stratification

Extent of resection is the strongest predictor of recurrence free survival. According to published data, recurrence risk for vestibular schwannomas ranges from 0 to 4 % after gross total resection, 9–29 % after near-total resection and 25–65 % after subtotal resection [61–63].

In NF2, a genotype-phenotype correlation exists and is of prognostic value. Compared to other hereditary disorders, NF2 has an unusually high rate of mosaicism of greater than 30 % amongst *de novo* patients [64], and clear associations between type of mutation and disease severity has been recognized. For example, while 5′ truncating mutations are associated with a high tumor burden, severe disease course and early mortality, missense mutations have been linked to a relatively mild phenotype [65, 66]. For individual tumors, it is presently not known whether the type of NF2 mutation present in the tumor, or any other genetic or molecular characteristics are prognostic or predictive of tumor aggressiveness or risk of recurrence after surgical resection.

Molecular Signaling Pathways

The molecular signaling pathways that drive tumor initiation and progression associated with loss of Merlin have been subject to intense research efforts over the past decades. It has become evident that rather than acting through a single pathway or at a single cellular compartment, Merlin regulates a wide variety of cellular processes, including contact inhibition, tumor suppression and growth through signaling at the cellular cortex and nucleus. Loss of Merlin has been linked to loss of contact inhibition and activation of a number of pro-growth signaling cascades, as recently reviewed by Li et al. [7]. These include the Rac-PAK

[67–70], mTORC [71–73], EGFR/PDGFR/c-kit RAS-RAF-ERK [74–82], PI3K-Akt [83], FAK-Src [84], and Hippo pathways [85–87]. In addition, Merlin has been shown to interact with α-catenin and Par3 at adherens junctions [88], and with the scaffold and signaling protein Angiomotin at tight junctions [89]. Recent studies showed that in addition to cortical functions, Merlin also translocates to the nucleus to alter gene expression through inhibition of the E3 ubiquitin ligase $CRL4^{DCAF1}$ [90, 91]. Several of these pathways have been validated in preclinical studies involving in vivo and/or in vitro schwannoma models.

The tumor microenvironment, including angiogenesis, has been recognized as an important aspect of schwannoma biology. VEGF and its receptors are expressed in schwannomas, and expression levels are associated with increased rates of tumor growth [92, 93]. Anti-VEGF(R)-directed therapy with bevacizumab and vandetanib normalized the vasculature of $NF2^{-/-}$ schwannoma xenografts in nude mice and decreased tumor growth [94]. Recent data suggest that Merlin regulates angiogenesis in schwannomas through Rac1-dependent semaphorin 3F expression [95].

Molecular Targeted Therapies

VEGF

The first "molecular targeted" therapy to show clinical success in treating VS in NF2 patients has been bevacizumab, a monoclonal anti-VEGF antibody. Based on retrospective data, bevacizumab may result in radiologic responses and/or hearing improvement in approximately 50 % of patients, although treatment effect is only maintained with continuous administration [96–99]. Recently completed and ongoing prospective clinical trials with bevacizumab (ClinicalTrials.gov identifiers NCT01207687 and NCT01767792) will provide additional data on the efficacy and safety of this therapy, including in children.

ErbB Receptor Family

Preclinical data implying overexpression and activation of ErbB family receptors in promoting schwannoma growth led to a clinical trial using lapatinib, a small-molecule inhibitor targeting EGFR and ErbB2. In this phase 2 study, 24 % of evaluable patients experienced a radiologic response. Median time to overall progression (i.e., volumetric progression or hearing loss) was 14 months, but only one transient hearing response was observed [100].

mTOR

Based on the observation that loss of Merlin leads to activation of mTORC1 signaling [71, 72], several phase 2 clinical trials with everolimus (RAD001) have been conducted. Results of one of these trials have been published recently, suggesting that everolimus is not clinically effective in treating NF2-related VS [101].

PDGFR and c-kit

Schwann cells express PDGFRα and PDGFRβ [76]. Signaling through these receptors activates the RAS-RAF-MEK-ERK and PI3K-AKT signaling pathways, and is important for Schwann cell proliferation in vivo and in vitro [77–79]. Overexpression of PDGFRβ has been observed in VS [74, 80, 81], and PDGFR inhibitors including AG1296, imatinib, and nilotinib are effective in preventing PDGFR-driven proliferation when tested in VS in vitro models [74, 82]. VS cells express activated c-KIT and are growth-inhibited by imatinib [81] and nilotinib [82]. Based on this preclinical data, a phase 2 clinical trial with nilotinib is ongoing (ClinicalTrials.gov identifier NCT01201538).

Other Targets and Future Outlook

Some of the key tumorigenic signaling pathways associated with loss of Merlin, such as the Hippo signaling pathway and activation of the E3 ubiquitin ligase $CRL4^{DCAF1}$, are not directly targetable with currently approved drugs, but of interest for future therapeutic development. Although it appears that loss of NF2 may be sufficient for tumor formation and progression, it is conceivable that other oncogenic drivers may cooperate with loss of Merlin. To identify such molecular genetic drivers in schwannomas, future studies using next-generation sequencing approaches, such as whole-exome/whole-genome sequencing and RNA-seq, could provide valuable information.

References

1. Stemmer-Rachamimov A, Wiestler OD, Louis DN. Neurofibromatosis type 2. In: Cavenee WK, editor. WHO classification of tumours of the central nervous system. Lyon, France: IARC Press; 2007. p. 210–4.
2. Bhatoe HS, Srinivasan K, Dubey AK. Intracerebral schwannoma. Neurol India. 2003;51:125–7.
3. Kimaya M, Hashizume Y. Pathological studies of aberrant peripheral nerve bundles of spinal cords. Acta Neuropathol (Berl). 1989;79:18–22.
4. Demyer W. Aberrant peripheral nerve fibers in the medulla oblongata of man. J Neurol Neurosurg Psychiatry. 1965;28: 121–3.
5. Rouleau GA, Merel P, Lutchman M, Sanson M, Zucman J, Marineau C, et al. Alteration in a new gene encoding a putative membrane-organizing protein causes neuro-fibromatosis type 2. Nature. 1993;363(6429):515–21.
6. Trofatter JA, MacCollin MM, Rutter JL, Murrell JR, Duyao MP, Parry DM, et al. A novel moesin-, ezrin-, radixin-like gene is a candidate for the neurofibromatosis 2 tumor suppressor. Cell. 1993;75(4):826.

7. Li W, Cooper J, Karajannis MA, Giancotti FG. Merlin: a tumour suppressor with functions at the cell cortex and in the nucleus. EMBO Rep. 2012;13(3):204–15.
8. MacCollin M, Chiocca EA, Evans DG, et al. Diagnostic criteria for schwannomatosis. Neurology. 2005;64(11):1838–45. Epub 2005/06/16.
9. Smith MJ, Kulkarni A, Rustad C, Bowers NL, Wallace AJ, Holder SE, et al. Vestibular schwannomas occur in schwannomatosis and should not be considered an exclusion criterion for clinical diagnosis. Am J Med Genet A. 2012;158A(1): 215–9. Epub 2011/11/23.
10. Bacci C, Sestini R, Provenzano A, Paganini I, Mancini I, Porfirio B, et al. Schwannomatosis associated with multiple meningiomas due to a familial SMARCB1 mutation. Neurogenetics. 2010;11(1):73–80. Epub 2009/07/08.
11. Hulsebos TJ, Plomp AS, Wolterman RA, Robanus-Maandag EC, Baas F, Wesseling P. Germline mutation of INI1/SMARCB1 in familial schwannomatosis. Am J Hum Genet. 2007;80(4):805–10. Epub 2007/03/16.
12. Sestini R, Bacci C, Provenzano A, Genuardi M, Papi L. Evidence of a four-hit mechanism involving SMARCB1 and NF2 in schwannomatosis-associated schwannomas. Hum Mutat. 2008;29(2):227–31. Epub 2007/12/12.
13. Hadfield KD, Newman WG, Bowers NL, et al. Molecular characterisation of SMARCB1 and NF2 in familial and sporadic schwannomatosis. J Med Genet. 2008;45:332–9. Epub 2008/02/21.
14. Smith MJ, Wallace AJ, Bowers NL, Rustad CF, Woods CG, Leschziner GD, et al. Frequency of SMARCB1 mutations in familial and sporadic schwannomatosis. Neurogenetics. 2012;13(2):141–5. Epub 2012/03/22.
15. Piotrowski A, Xie J, Liu YF, Poplawski AB, Gomes AR, Madanecki P, et al. Germline loss-of-function mutations in LZTR1 predispose to an inherited disorder of multiple schwannomas. Nat Genet. 2014;46(2):182–7. Epub 2013/12/24.
16. Carney JA. Psammomatous melanotic schwannoma. A distinctive heritable tumor with special associations including cardiac myxoma and the Cushing syndrome. Am J Surg Pathol. 1990;14(3):206–22.
17. Martin-Reay DG, Shauck MC, Guthrie Jr FW. Psammomatous melanotic schwannoma: an additional component of Carney's complex. Report of a case. Am J Clin Pathol. 1991;95(4):484–9. Epub 1991/04/01.
18. Handley J, Carson D, Sloan J, et al. Multiple lentigines, myxoid tumours and endocrine overactivity; four cases of Carney's complex. Br J Dermatol. 1992;126:367–71. Epub 1992/04/01.
19. Kirschner LS, Carney JA, Pack SD, Taymans SE, Giatzakis C, Cho YS, et al. Mutations of the gene encoding the protein kinase A type I-alpha regulatory subunit in patients with the Carney complex. Nat Genet. 2000;26(1):89–92. Epub 2000/09/06.
20. Vezzosi D, Vignaux O, Dupin N, Bertherat J. Carney complex: clinical and genetic 2010 update. Ann Endocrinol. 2010;71(6):486–93. Epub 2010/09/21.
21. Rowe JG, Radatz MW, Walton L, Soanes T, Rodgers J, Kemeny AA. Clinical experience with gamma knife stereotactic radiosurgery in the management of vestibular schwannomas secondary to type 2 neurofibromatosis. J Neurol Neurosurg Psychiatry. 2003;74(9):1288–93.
22. Mathieu D, Kondziolka D, Flickinger JC, Niranjan A, Williamson R, Martin JJ, et al. Stereotactic radiosurgery for vestibular schwannomas in patients with neurofibromatosis type 2: an analysis of tumor control, complications, and hearing preservation rates. Neurosurgery. 2007;60(3):460–8; discussion 468–70.
23. Evans DG, Birch JM, Ramsden RT, Sharif S, Baser ME. Malignant transformation and new primary tumours after therapeutic radiation for benign disease: substantial risks in certain tumour prone syndromes. J Med Genet. 2006;43(4): 289–94. Epub 2005/09/13.
24. Rowe J, Grainger A, Walton L, Radatz M, Kemeny A. Safety of radiosurgery applied to conditions with abnormal tumor suppressor genes. Neurosurgery. 2007;60(5):860–4; discussion 860–4.
25. Casadei GP, Scheithauer BW, Hirose T, Manfrini M, Van Houton C, Wood MB. Cellular schwannoma. A clinicopathologic, DNA flow cytometric and proliferation marker study of 70 patients. Cancer. 1995;75:1109–19.
26. Woodruff JM, Godwin TA, Erlandson RA, Susin M, Martini N. Cellular schwannoma: a variety of schwannoma sometimes mistaken for a malignant tumor. Am J Surg Pathol. 1981;5:733–44.
27. White W, Shiu MGH, Rosenblum MK, Erlandson RA, Woodruff JM. Cellular scwhannoma. A clinicaopathologic study of 57 patients and 58 tumors. Cancer. 1990;66:1266–75.
28. Woodruff JM, Marshall ML, Godwin TA, Funkhouser JW, Thompson NJ, Erlandson RA. Plexiform (multinodular) schwannoma. A tumor simulating the plexiform neurofibroma. Am J Surg Pathol. 1983;7:691–7.
29. Hebert-Blouin MN, Amrami KK, Scheithauer BW, Spinner RJ. Multinodular/plexiform (multifascicular) schwannomas of major peripheral nerves: an underrecognized part of the spectrum of schwannomas. J Neurosurg. 2010;112:372–82.
30. Megahed M. Plexiform schwannoma. Am J Dermatopathol. 1994;16(3):288–93.
31. Wechsler J, Lantieri L, Zeller J, et al. Aberrant axon neurofilaments in schwannomas associated with phacomatoses. Virchows Arch. 2003;443:768–73.
32. Val Bernal JF, Figols J, Vazquez-Barguero A. Cutaneous plexiform schwannoma associated with neurofibromatosis type 2. Cancer. 1995;76(7):1181–6.
33. Reith JD, Goldblum JR. Multiple cutaneous plexiform schwannomas. Report of a case and review of the literature with particular reference to the association with types 1 and 2 neurofibromatosis and schwannomatosis. Arch Pathol Lab Med. 1996;120(4):399–401.
34. Myers JL, Bernreuter W, Dunham W. Melanotic schwannoma. Clinicopathologic, immunohistochemical, and ultrastructural features of a rare primary bone tumor. Am J Clin Pathol. 1990;93(3):424–9.
35. Antiheimo J, Sankila R, Carpen O, et al. Population based analysis of sporadic and type 2 neurofibromatosis associated meningiomas and schwannomas. Neurology. 2000;54:71.
36. Sobel RA. Vestibular (acoustic) schwannomas: histological features in neurofibromatosis 2 and in unilateral cases. J Neuropathol Exp Neurol. 1993;52:106–13.
37. Patil S, Perry A, Maccollin M, et al. Immunohistochemical analysis supports a role for INI1/SMARCB1 in hereditary forms of schwannomas, but not in solitary, sporadic schwannomas. Brain Pathol. 2008;18:517–9.
38. Parry DM, Eldridge R, Kaiser-Kupfer MI, Bouzas EA, Pikus A, Patronas N. Neurofibromatosis 2 (NF2): clinical

characteristics of 63 affected individuals and clinical evidence for heterogeneity. Am J Med Genet. 1994;52:450–61.

39. Evans DG, Moran A, King A, Saeed S, Gurusinghe N, Ramsden R. Incidence of vestibular schwannoma and neurofibromatosis 2 in the North West of England over a 10-year period: higher incidence than previously thought. Otol Neurotol. 2005;26(1):93–7.
40. Evans DG. Neurofibromatosis type 2 (NF2): A clinical and molecular review. Orphanet J Rare Dis. 2009;4:16.
41. Martuza RL, Eldridge R. Neurofibromatosis 2 (bilateral acoustic neurofibromatosis). N Engl J Med. 1988;318:684–8.
42. Baser ME, Evans DGR, Gutmann DH. Neurofibromatosis 2. Curr Opin Neurol. 2003;16:27–33.
43. Smith MJ, Kulkarni A, Rustad C, Bowers NL, Wallace AJ, Holder SE, Heiberg A, Ramsden RT, Evans DG. Vestibular schwannomas occur in schwannomatosis and should not be considered an exclusion criterion for clinical diagnosis. Am J Med Genet. 2012;58A(1):215–9.
44. Wolkenstein P, Benchikhi H, Zeller J, Wechsler J, Revuz J. Schwannomatosis: a clinical entity distinct from neurofibromatosis type 2. Dermatology. 1997;195:228–31.
45. Merker VL, Esparza S, Smith MJ, Stemmer-Rachamimov A, Plotkin SR. Clinical features of schwannomatosis: a retrospective analysis of 87 patients. Oncologist. 2012;17(10):1317–22.
46. Feany MB, Anthony DC, Fletcher CD. Nerve sheath tumours with hybrid features of neurofi broma and schwannoma: a conceptual challenge. Histopathology. 1998;32:405–10.
47. Harder A, Wesemann M, Hagel C, Schittenhelm J, Fischer S, Tatagiba M, Nagel C, Jeibmann A, Bohring A, Mautner VF, Paulus W. Hybrid neurofibroma/schwannoma is overrepresented among schwannomatosis and neurofibromatosis patients. Am J Surg Pathol. 2012;36(5):702–9.
48. Seizinger BR, Martuza RL, Gusella JF. Loss of genes on chromosome 22 in tumorigenesis of human acoustic neuroma. Nature. 1986;322(6080):644–7. Epub 1986/08/14.
49. Bijlsma EK, Brouwer-Mladin R, Bosch DA, Westerveld A, Hulsebos TJ. Molecular characterization of chromosome 22 deletions in schwannomas. Genes Chromosomes Cancer. 1992;5(3):201–5. Epub 1992/10/01.
50. Irving RM, Moffat DA, Hardy DG, Barton DE, Xuereb JH, Maher ER. Somatic NF2 gene mutations in familial and nonfamilial vestibular schwannoma. Hum Mol Genet. 1994;3(2): 347–50. Epub 1994/02/01.
51. Knudson Jr AG, Hethcote HW, Brown BW. Mutation and childhood cancer: a probabilistic model for the incidence of retinoblastoma. Proc Natl Acad Sci U S A. 1975;72(12):5116–20. Epub 1975/12/11.
52. Antinheimo J, Sallinen SL, Sallinen P, Haapasalo H, Helin H, Horelli-Kuitunen N, et al. Genetic aberrations in sporadic and neurofibromatosis 2 (NF2)-associated schwannomas studied by comparative genomic hybridization (CGH). Acta Neurochir (Wien). 2000;142(10):1099–104; discussion 104–5. Epub 2000/12/29.
53. Warren C, James LA, Ramsden RT, Wallace A, Baser ME, Varley JM, et al. Identification of recurrent regions of chromosome loss and gain in vestibular schwannomas using comparative genomic hybridisation. J Med Genet. 2003;40(11):802–6. Epub 2003/11/25.
54. Ikeda T, Hashimoto S, Fukushige S, Ohmori H, Horii A. Comparative genomic hybridization and mutation analyses of sporadic schwannomas. J Neurooncol. 2005;72(3):225–30. Epub 2005/06/07.
55. DiazdeStahl T, Hansson CM, Debustos C, Mantripragada KK, Piotrowski A, Benetkiewicz M, et al. High-resolution array-CGH profiling of germline and tumor-specific copy number alterations on chromosome 22 in patients affected with schwannomas. Hum Genet. 2005;118(1):35–44. Epub 2005/08/04.
56. Kullar PJ, Pearson DM, Malley DS, Collins VP, Ichimura K. CpG island hypermethylation of the neurofibromatosis type 2 (NF2) gene is rare in sporadic vestibular schwannomas. Neuropathol Appl Neurobiol. 2010;36(6):505–14. Epub 2010/09/14.
57. Lee JD, Kwon TJ, Kim UK, Lee WS. Genetic and epigenetic alterations of the NF2 gene in sporadic vestibular schwannomas. PLoS One. 2012;7(1):e30418. Epub 2012/02/02.
58. Torres-Martin M, Lassaletta L, San-Roman-Montero J, De Campos JM, Isla A, Gavilan J, et al. Microarray analysis of gene expression in vestibular schwannomas reveals SPP1/MET signaling pathway and androgen receptor deregulation. Int J Oncol. 2013;42(3):848–62. Epub 2013/01/29.
59. Aarhus M, Bruland O, Saetran HA, Mork SJ, Lund-Johansen M, Knappskog PM. Global gene expression profiling and tissue microarray reveal novel candidate genes and down-regulation of the tumor suppressor gene CAV1 in sporadic vestibular schwannomas. Neurosurgery. 2010;67(4):998–1019; discussion 1019. Epub 2010/10/01.
60. Saydam O, Senol O, Wurdinger T, Mizrak A, Ozdener GB, Stemmer-Rachamimov AO, et al. miRNA-7 attenuation in schwannoma tumors stimulates growth by upregulating three oncogenic signaling pathways. Cancer Res. 2011;71(3):852–61. Epub 2010/12/16.
61. El-Kashlan HK, Zeitoun H, Arts HA, Hoff JT, Telian SA. Recurrence of acoustic neuroma after incomplete resection. Am J Otol. 2000;21(3):389–92. Epub 2000/05/23.
62. Sakaki S, Nakagawa K, Hatakeyama T, Murakami Y, Ohue S, Matsuoka K. Recurrence after incompletely resected acousticus neurinomas. Med J Osaka Univ. 1991;40(1–4):59–66. Epub 1991/03/01.
63. Seol HJ, Kim CH, Park CK, Kim DG, Chung YS, Jung HW. Optimal extent of resection in vestibular schwannoma surgery: relationship to recurrence and facial nerve preservation. Neurol Med Chir (Tokyo). 2006;46(4):176–80; discussion 80–1. Epub 2006/04/26.
64. Evans DG, Ramsden RT, Shenton A, Gokhale C, Bowers NL, Huson SM, et al. Mosaicism in neurofibromatosis type 2: an update of risk based on uni/bilaterality of vestibular schwannoma at presentation and sensitive mutation analysis including multiple ligation-dependent probe amplification. J Med Genet. 2007;44(7):424–8. Epub 2007/02/20.
65. Baser ME, Friedman JM, Aeschliman D, Joe H, Wallace AJ, Ramsden RT, et al. Predictors of the risk of mortality in neurofibromatosis 2. Am J Hum Genet. 2002;71(4):715–23. Epub 2002/09/18.
66. Selvanathan SK, Shenton A, Ferner R, Wallace AJ, Huson SM, Ramsden RT, et al. Further genotype–phenotype correlations in neurofibromatosis 2. Clin Genet. 2010;77(2):163–70. Epub 2009/12/09.
67. Okada T, Lopez-Lago M, Giancotti FG. Merlin/NF-2 mediates contact inhibition of growth by suppressing recruitment of Rac to the plasma membrane. J Cell Biol. 2005;171(2):361–71.

68. Kaempchen K, Mielke K, Utermark T, Langmesser S, Hanemann CO. Upregulation of the Rac1/JNK signaling pathway in primary human schwannoma cells. Hum Mol Genet. 2003;12(11):1211–21.
69. Kissil JL, Wilker EW, Johnson KC, Eckman MS, Yaffe MB, Jacks T. Merlin, the product of the Nf2 tumor suppressor gene, is an inhibitor of the p21-activated kinase, Pak1. Mol Cell. 2003;12(4):841–9. Epub 2003/10/29.
70. Shaw RJ, Paez JG, Curto M, Yaktine A, Pruitt WM, Saotome I, et al. The Nf2 tumor suppressor, merlin, functions in Rac-dependent signaling. Dev Cell. 2001;1(1):63–72. Epub 2001/11/13.
71. James MF, Han S, Polizzano C, Plotkin SR, Manning BD, Stemmer-Rachamimov AO, et al. NF2/merlin is a novel negative regulator of mTOR complex 1, and activation of mTORC1 is associated with meningioma and schwannoma growth. Mol Cell Biol. 2009;29(15):4250–61. Epub 2009/05/20.
72. Lopez-Lago MA, Okada T, Murillo MM, Socci N, Giancotti FG. Loss of the tumor suppressor gene NF2, encoding merlin, constitutively activates integrin-dependent mTORC1 signaling. Mol Cell Biol. 2009;29(15):4235–49. Epub 2009/05/20.
73. James MF, Stivison E, Beauchamp R, Han S, Li H, Wallace MR, et al. Regulation of mTOR complex 2 signaling in neurofibromatosis 2-deficient target cell types. Mol Cancer Res. 2012;10(5):649–59.
74. Ammoun S, Flaiz C, Ristic N, Schuldt J, Hanemann CO. Dissecting and targeting the growth factor-dependent and growth factor-independent extracellular signal-regulated kinase pathway in human schwannoma. Cancer Res. 2008; 68(13):5236–45.
75. Curto M, Cole BK, Lallemand D, Liu CH, McClatchey AI. Contact-dependent inhibition of EGFR signaling by Nf2/Merlin. J Cell Biol. 2007;177(5):893–903.
76. Eccleston PA, Funa K, Heldin CH. Expression of platelet-derived growth factor (PDGF) and PDGF alpha- and beta-receptors in the peripheral nervous system: an analysis of sciatic nerve and dorsal root ganglia. Dev Biol. 1993;155(2):459–70. Epub 1993/02/01.
77. Meier C, Parmantier E, Brennan A, Mirsky R, Jessen KR. Developing Schwann cells acquire the ability to survive without axons by establishing an autocrine circuit involving insulin-like growth factor, neurotrophin-3, and platelet-derived growth factor-BB. J Neurosci. 1999;19(10):3847–59. Epub 1999/05/11.
78. Peulve P, Laquerriere A, Paresy M, Hemet J, Tadie M. Establishment of adult rat Schwann cell cultures: effect of b-FGF, alpha-MSH, NGF, PDGF, and TGF-beta on cell cycle. Exp Cell Res. 1994;214(2):543–50. Epub 1994/10/01.
79. Monje PV, Rendon S, Athauda G, Bates M, Wood PM, Bunge MB. Non-antagonistic relationship between mitogenic factors and cAMP in adult Schwann cell re-differentiation. Glia. 2009;57(9):947–61. Epub 2008/12/05.
80. Fraenzer JT, Pan H, Minimo Jr L, Smith GM, Knauer D, Hung G. Overexpression of the NF2 gene inhibits schwannoma cell proliferation through promoting PDGFR degradation. Int J Oncol. 2003;23(6):1493–500.
81. Mukherjee J, Kamnasaran D, Balasubramaniam A, Radovanovic I, Zadeh G, Kiehl TR, et al. Human schwannomas express activated platelet-derived growth factor receptors and c-kit and are growth inhibited by Gleevec (Imatinib Mesylate). Cancer Res. 2009;69(12):5099–107. Epub 2009/06/11.
82. Ammoun S, Schmid MC, Triner J, Manley P, Hanemann CO. Nilotinib alone or in combination with selumetinib is a drug candidate for neurofibromatosis type 2. Neuro Oncol. 2011;13(7):759–66. Epub 2011/07/06.
83. Rong R, Tang X, Gutmann DH, Ye K. Neurofibromatosis 2 (NF2) tumor suppressor merlin inhibits phosphatidylinositol 3-kinase through binding to PIKE-L. Proc Natl Acad Sci U S A. 2004;101(52):18200–5. Epub 2004/12/16.
84. Poulikakos PI, Xiao GH, Gallagher R, Jablonski S, Jhanwar SC, Testa JR. Re-expression of the tumor suppressor NF2/merlin inhibits invasiveness in mesothelioma cells and negatively regulates FAK. Oncogene. 2006;25(44):5960–8. Epub 2006/05/03.
85. Hamaratoglu F, Willecke M, Kango-Singh M, Nolo R, Hyun E, Tao C, et al. The tumour-suppressor genes NF2/Merlin and Expanded act through Hippo signalling to regulate cell proliferation and apoptosis. Nat Cell Biol. 2006;8(1):27–36.
86. Zhao B, Wei X, Li W, Udan RS, Yang Q, Kim J, et al. Inactivation of YAP oncoprotein by the Hippo pathway is involved in cell contact inhibition and tissue growth control. Genes Dev. 2007;21(21):2747–61. Epub 2007/11/03.
87. Yin F, Yu J, Zheng Y, Chen Q, Zhang N, Pan D. Spatial organization of Hippo signaling at the plasma membrane mediated by the tumor suppressor Merlin/NF2. Cell. 2013;154(6):1342–55. Epub 2013/09/10.
88. Gladden AB, Hebert AM, Schneeberger EE, McClatchey AI. The NF2 tumor suppressor, Merlin, regulates epidermal development through the establishment of a junctional polarity complex. Dev Cell. 2010;19(5):727–39. Epub 2010/11/16.
89. Yi C, Troutman S, Fera D, Stemmer-Rachamimov A, Avila JL, Christian N, et al. A tight junction-associated Merlin-angiomotin complex mediates Merlin's regulation of mitogenic signaling and tumor suppressive functions. Cancer Cell. 2011;19(4):527–40. Epub 2011/04/13.
90. Li W, You L, Cooper J, Schiavon G, Pepe-Caprio A, Zhou L, et al. Merlin/NF2 suppresses tumorigenesis by inhibiting the E3 ubiquitin ligase CRL4(DCAF1) in the nucleus. Cell. 2010;140(4):477–90. Epub 2010/02/25.
91. Cooper J, Li W, You L, Schiavon G, Pepe-Caprio A, Zhou L, et al. Merlin/NF2 functions upstream of the nuclear E3 ubiquitin ligase CRL4DCAF1 to suppress oncogenic gene expression. Sci Signal. 2011;4(188):t6. Epub 2011/09/01.
92. Caye-Thomasen P, Baandrup L, Jacobsen GK, Thomsen J, Stangerup SE. Immunohistochemical demonstration of vascular endothelial growth factor in vestibular schwannomas correlates to tumor growth rate. Laryngoscope. 2003;113(12): 2129–34. Epub 2003/12/09.
93. Caye-Thomasen P, Werther K, Nalla A, Bog-Hansen TC, Nielsen HJ, Stangerup SE, et al. VEGF and VEGF receptor-1 concentration in vestibular schwannoma homogenates correlates to tumor growth rate. Otol Neurotol. 2005;26(1):98–101. Epub 2005/02/09.
94. Wong HK, Lahdenranta J, Kamoun WS, Chan AW, McClatchey AI, Plotkin SR, et al. Anti-vascular endothelial growth factor therapies as a novel therapeutic approach to treating neurofibromatosis-related tumors. Cancer Res. 2010;70(9): 3483–93. Epub 2010/04/22.

95. Wong HK, Shimizu A, Kirkpatrick ND, Garkavtsev I, Chan AW, di Tomaso E, et al. Merlin/NF2 regulates angiogenesis in schwannomas through a Rac1/semaphorin 3F-dependent mechanism. Neoplasia. 2012;14(2):84–94. Epub 2012/03/21.
96. Plotkin SR, Stemmer-Rachamimov AO, Barker 2nd FG, Halpin C, Padera TP, Tyrrell A, et al. Hearing improvement after bevacizumab in patients with neurofibromatosis type 2. N Engl J Med. 2009;361(4):358–67. Epub 2009/07/10.
97. Mautner VF, Nguyen R, Knecht R, Bokemeyer C. Radiographic regression of vestibular schwannomas induced by bevacizumab treatment: sustain under continuous drug application and rebound after drug discontinuation. Ann Oncol. 2010;21(11):2294–5. Epub 2010/09/24.
98. Mautner VF, Nguyen R, Kutta H, Fuensterer C, Bokemeyer C, Hagel C, et al. Bevacizumab induces regression of vestibular schwannomas in patients with neurofibromatosis type 2. Neuro Oncol. 2010;12(1):14–8. Epub 2010/02/13.
99. Plotkin SR, Merker VL, Halpin C, Jennings D, McKenna MJ, Harris GJ, et al. Bevacizumab for progressive vestibular schwannoma in neurofibromatosis type 2: a retrospective review of 31 patients. Otol Neurotol. 2012;33(6):1046–52.
100. Karajannis MA, Legault G, Hagiwara M, Ballas MS, Brown K, Nusbaum AO, et al. Phase II trial of lapatinib in adult and pediatric patients with neurofibromatosis type 2 and progressive vestibular schwannomas. Neuro Oncol. 2012;14(9):1163–70.
101. Karajannis MA, Legault G, Hagiwara M, Giancotti FG, Filatov A, Derman A, et al. Phase II study of everolimus in children and adults with neurofibromatosis type 2 and progressive vestibular schwannomas. Neuro Oncol. 2014;16(2):292–7. Epub 2013/12/07.

16 Malignant Peripheral Nerve Sheath Tumors

Brian Weiss, Amy Sheil, and Nancy Ratner

Malignant peripheral nerve sheath tumors (MPNSTs) (previously called neurogenic sarcomas, malignant schwannomas, or neurofibrosarcomas) are soft tissue sarcomas, which arise from a peripheral nerve or show nerve sheath differentiation. MPNSTs are associated with a high risk of local recurrence and predominantly hematogenous metastasis [1, 2]. They account for 10 % of all soft tissue sarcomas, and approximately half of these malignancies arise in patients with neurofibromatosis type 1 (NF1) [3]. MPNSTs occur in about 2–5 % of patients with NF1 compared with an incidence of 0.001 % in the general population [1]. In contrast, in a large population-based longitudinal study the lifetime risk of developing an MPNST in NF1 was 8–13 % [4]. In patients with NF1, the majority of MPNSTs arise in a previously clinically detectable plexiform neurofibroma, but MPNST may also develop as a primary tumor [5, 6].

The most frequent sites of metastasis of MPNSTs are lung, liver, brain, soft tissue, bone, regional lymph nodes, and retroperitoneum [1]. Early diagnosis of MPNSTs is crucial, as only complete surgical resection has been shown to be curative. However, the clinical diagnosis of MPNST in patients with NF1 can be difficult to establish, because clinical indicators of malignancy (mass and pain) may also be features of benign plexiform neurofibromas commonly seen in this patient population. For unresectable or metastatic disease, adjuvant or neoadjuvant radiation therapy and/or chemotherapy have been used, but are generally not curative. Therefore, novel molecular targeted agents are being evaluated in this difficulty to treat patient population.

Histopathology

MPNST are malignant tumors of neuroectodermal origin arising from a peripheral nerve with or without a preexisting benign nerve sheath tumor [7]. The diagnosis of MPNST is often challenging, due to a lack of standardized morphological criteria, specific immunohistochemical marker expression, or characteristic karyotypic aberrations. Sarcomas with involvement of a nerve and lacking features indicating an alternative line of differentiation (such as synovial sarcoma or angiosarcoma), or those sarcomas definitively arising from a preexisting benign nerve sheath tumor, are designated MPNST [8]. Malignant spindled tumors in patients with neurofibromatosis (NF1) are also considered to be MPNST unless proven otherwise. Spindled tumors that are unrelated to a major nerve are more difficult to classify. In order to establish a diagnosis, a combined analysis of histological features, immunohistochemical phenotype, and/or ultrastructural features of Schwann cell (basal lamina) or differentiation (such as intracytoplasmic vesicles) in perineurial-like cells is necessary [7, 8].

As noted above, the main recognizable benign precursor to MPNST is the plexiform neurofibroma common in the setting of NF1 (Figs. 16.1 and 16.2). Figures 16.1 and 16.2 are photomicrographs representative of plexiform neurofibroma [9]. Prior irradiation is also a risk factor for NF1 patients to develop MPNST [9]. Figures 16.3 and 16.4 represent the gross pathology of an MPNST arising from a plexiform neurofibroma of the vagus nerve [10].

Notable histological variation may be observed in MPNSTs. Common histological findings include fascicles of alternating cellularity (Fig. 16.5), whorls, palisading or rosette-like patterns, subendothelial condensation of tumor cells, and geographic necrosis [8, 11]. Occasionally, the tumors resemble primitive or undifferentiated sarcoma (Fig. 16.6). Less commonly, rhabdomyosarcomatous elements (malignant Triton tumor), angiosarcoma, melanin, neuroendocrine, or glandular structures are observed. The cell(s) of origin of these divergent features remain uncertain [7, 11].

MPNST grading is separated pathologically into low and high grade categories; the majority of MPNSTs are high grade [8]. Morphological criteria for a low grade MPNST include hypercellularity and nuclear enlargement (approximately 3× the size of a neurofibroma nucleus) and

M.A. Karajannis and D. Zagzag (eds.), *Molecular Pathology of Nervous System Tumors: Biological Stratification and Targeted Therapies*, Molecular Pathology Library 8,
DOI 10.1007/978-1-4939-1830-0_16,

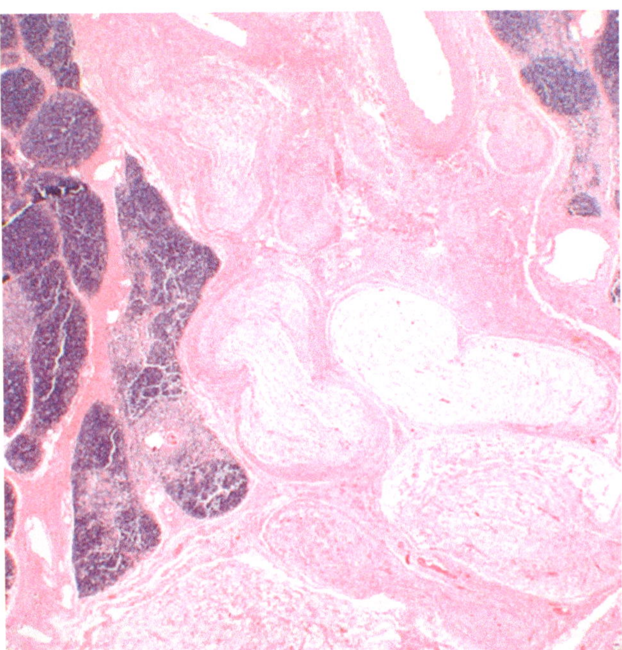

Fig. 16.1 Plexiform neurofibroma arising from the vagus nerve, involving the thymus gland

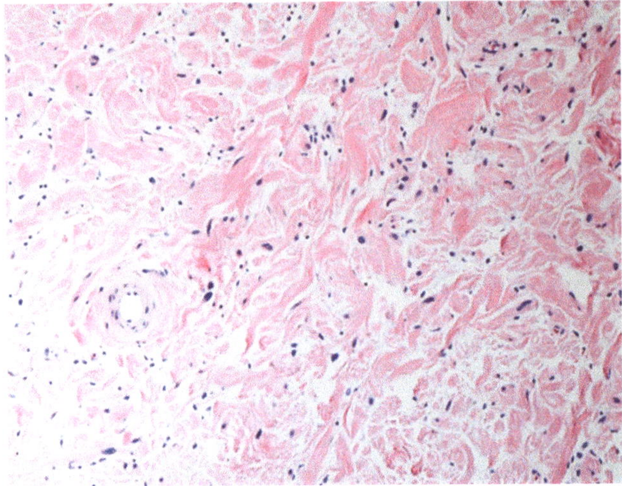

Fig. 16.2 Plexiform neurofibroma with low cellularity and "shredded carrot" collagen

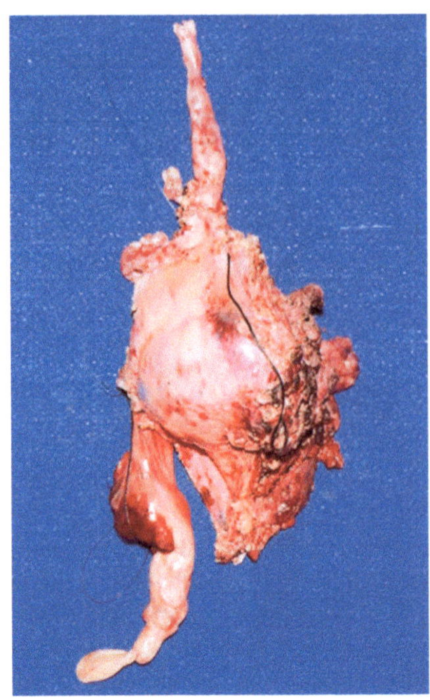

Fig. 16.3 Large mediastinal soft tissue mass (high grade MPNST) arising from vagus nerve (*top*) and encasing and eroding into the superior vena cava, with intravascular thrombosis (*bottom*) (Courtesy of Children's Hospital of Wisconsin, Milwaukee, WI)

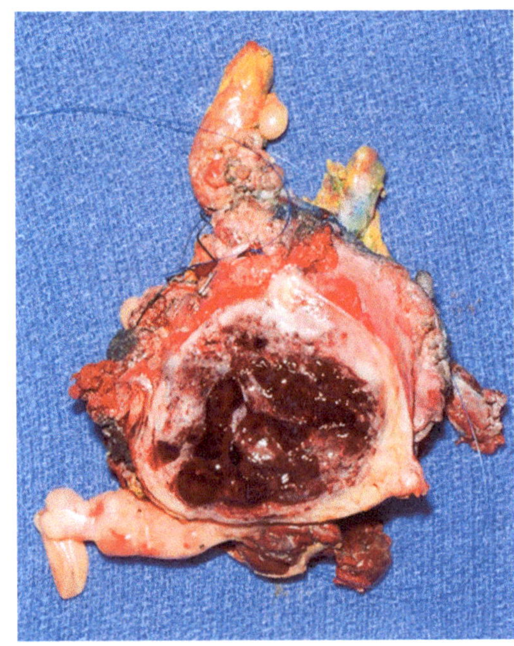

Fig. 16.4 Cut surface of MPNST depicted in Fig. 16.3 with peripheral rim of white-gray tumor and central hemorrhage and necrosis

hyperchromasia, features also seen in high grade MPNST; however, low grade MPNSTs exhibit little necrosis and show fewer than five mitoses per 10 high power fields [18, 12]. The isolated presence of one of these features in a neurofibroma is not adequate for a malignant diagnosis. Diagnostic difficulties arise due to the lack of objective criteria for hypercellularity, hyperchromasia, and the extent of changes required for a malignant diagnosis. Features concerning for malignant transformation include increased cellularity and a fascicular pattern of growth not usually seen in conventional neurofibromas (Fig. 16.7). Histological grading systems include the US National Cancer Institute (NCI) system [13], based on the tumor histological type, location, and degree of necrosis, as well as pleomorphism, cellularity, and mitotic activity. The Federation National des Centres de Lutte Contre

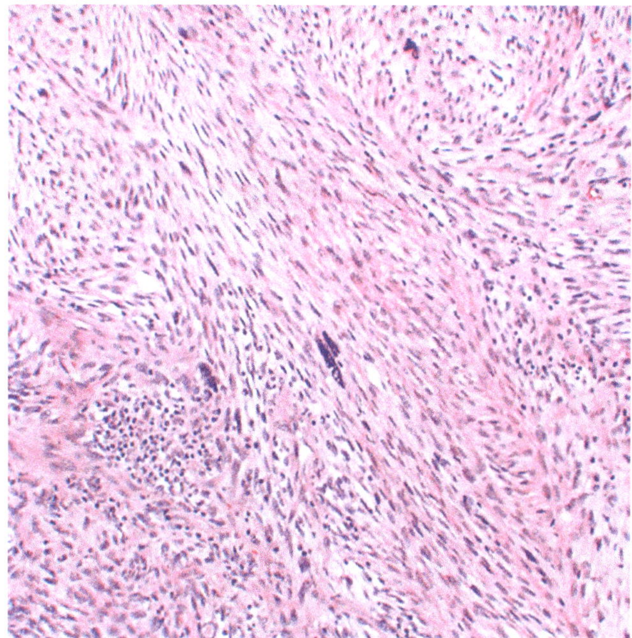

FIG. 16.5 High grade MPNST with spindled cells, fascicular pattern, and focal cytological atypia with nuclear enlargement and hyperchromasia

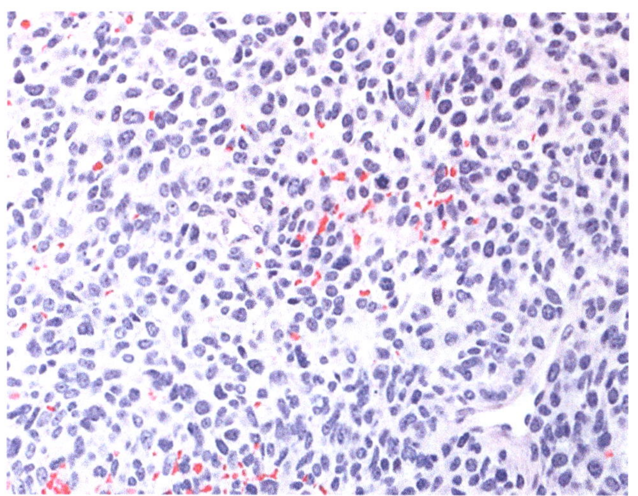

FIG. 16.6 High grade MPNST with appearance of undifferentiated, primitive sarcoma

le Cancer (FNCLCC) is a French grading system which uses a score generated by degree of tumor differentiation, mitotic activity, and extent of necrosis [14]. Neither of these grading systems has proven entirely useful in distinguishing low versus high grade MPNST and predicting clinical behavior. Information regarding the molecular biology of MPNST is anticipated to prove important for not only diagnosis but possible targeted therapy options.

Even more challenging is the separation of atypical neurofibroma (considered benign) from low grade MPNST (malignant), particularly in the setting of NF1. The term "atypical neurofibroma" has been applied to neurofibromas with degenerative nuclear changes [8]. This term, or alternatively, cellular neurofibroma, has also been used for nerve sheath tumors showing worrisome histological features, including high cellularity, few mitotic figures, monotonous cytomorphology, or fascicular growth, which do not fully meet criteria for malignancy. Atypical changes often develop in large, slowly growing neurofibromas [15]. Atypical neurofibromas have generally been regarded as benign. However, a study of NF1 patients suggests that atypical neurofibromas, defined as neurofibromas with increased cellularity and nuclear hyperchromasia and enlargement lacking mitotic figures (Figs. 16.8, 16.9, and 16.10), represent early malignant change in neurofibroma, with *CDKN2A* (p16) deletions (seen in MPNST) in the majority of studied cases [16, 17].

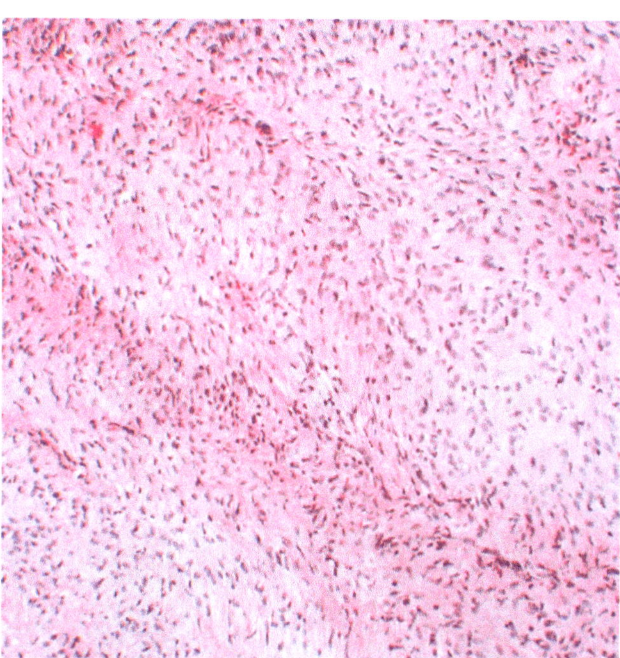

FIG. 16.7 Low grade MPNST with high cellularity and monotonous spindled cells arranged in long fascicles

Histological examination of a soft tissue lesion in which the differential comprises MPNST should include routine-stained H&E sections and possibly reticulin, to clearly outline nerve fibers. In addition, immunohistochemical stains for S100β protein, the skeletal muscle markers desmin and myogenin, and a proliferation marker (MIB-1 or KI-67) may be useful [1]. Increased MIB-1 (Ki-67) and p53 nuclear labeling by immunohistochemistry are seen in high grade MPNST [6, 18]. Genetic loss of the *CDKN2A* locus, and therefore loss of p16 immunoreactivity, are not found in neurofibroma, but are common in MPNST [16, 17]. Both p16 and p27 expression are typically present in neurofibromas and low grade MPNSTs but absent in high grade MPNSTs [6]; loss of expression may highlight foci of malignant

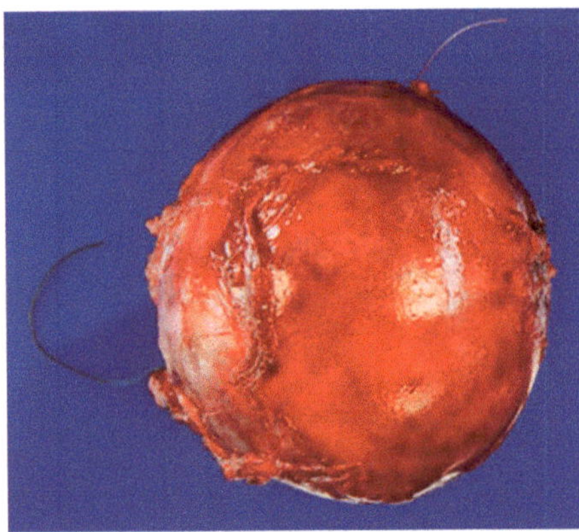

Fig. 16.8 Well-circumscribed, apparently encapsulated atypical neurofibroma

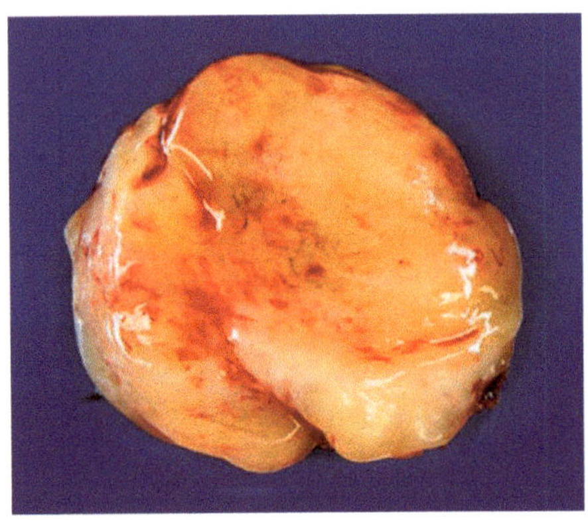

Fig. 16.9 Atypical neurofibroma shown in Fig. 16.8 with slightly gelatinous, yellow to white cut surfaces

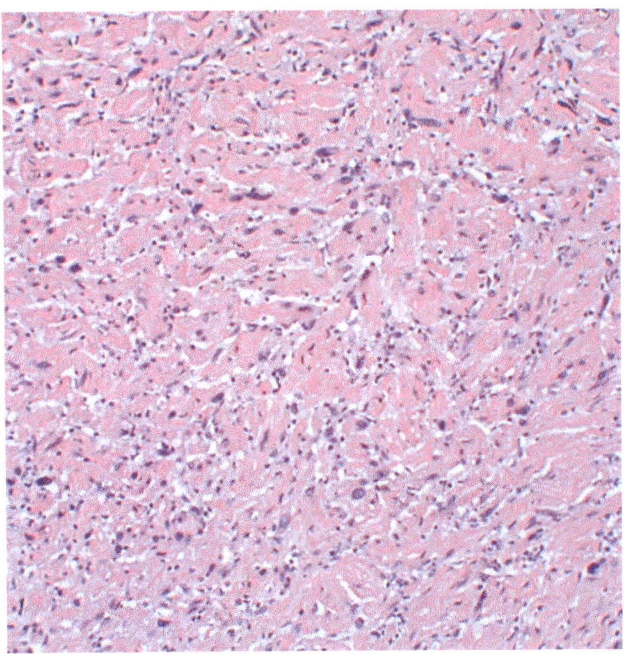

Fig. 16.10 Atypical neurofibroma with wavy collagenous stroma with increased cellularity, nuclear enlargement, and hyperchromasia; no mitotic activity was appreciated

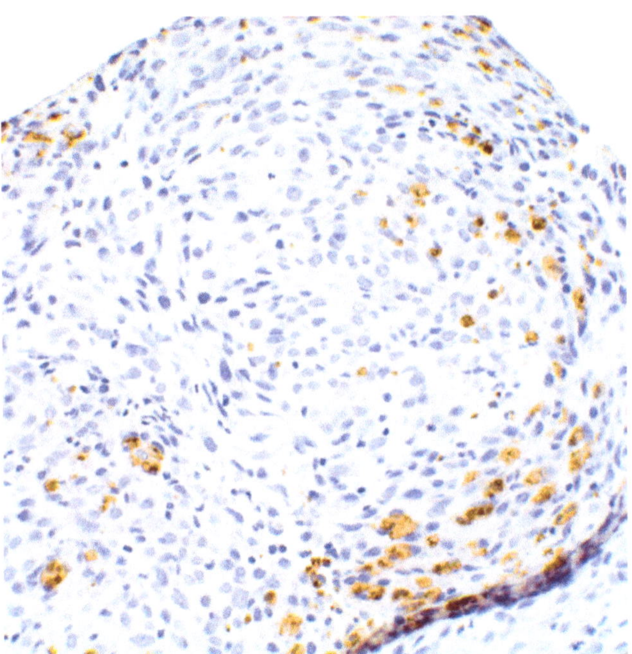

Fig. 16.11 Focal retention of S100β expression in high grade MPNST

transformation in neurofibromas, as may molecular alterations, including *EGFR* amplification [19].

The differential diagnosis of MPNST includes sarcomas, including adult-type fibrosarcoma, synovial sarcoma, rhabdomyosarcoma, leiomyosarcoma, dedifferentiated liposarcoma, and clear cell sarcoma. One useful distinction from benign Schwann cell tumors is the partial or complete loss of S100β expression in MPNST (Fig. 16.11). Conversely, isolated expression of S100β should not necessarily be diagnostic of MPNST, as S100β expression has been reported in leiomyosarcomas, rhabdomyosarcomas, and synovial sarcomas [6, 8, 18].

Synovial sarcoma, a high grade sarcoma of undetermined cell lineage, may occur in soft tissues in either biphasic (which includes a spindle cell component with interspersed glandular structures) or monophasic (spindle cell component only) forms. The monophasic variant may closely resemble MPNST, and may involve nerves or exhibit a plexiform growth pattern. Both synovial sarcoma and MPNST may show glandular differentiation. The only definitive histological feature used in the distinction of MPNST from synovial sarcoma is the presence of pleomorphic cells, not seen in synovial sarcoma (Fig. 16.12). Demonstration of *SS18-SSX1* or *SS18-SSX2* gene fusions, usually resulting from a characteristic X;18 translocation, may be required for definitive diagnosis of intraneural synovial sarcoma, as these gene fusions are limited to synovial sarcoma [8]. No specific chromosomal rearrangements in MPNST have been revealed by conventional cytogenetics, although a complex karyotype is characteristic (see below for details) [20].

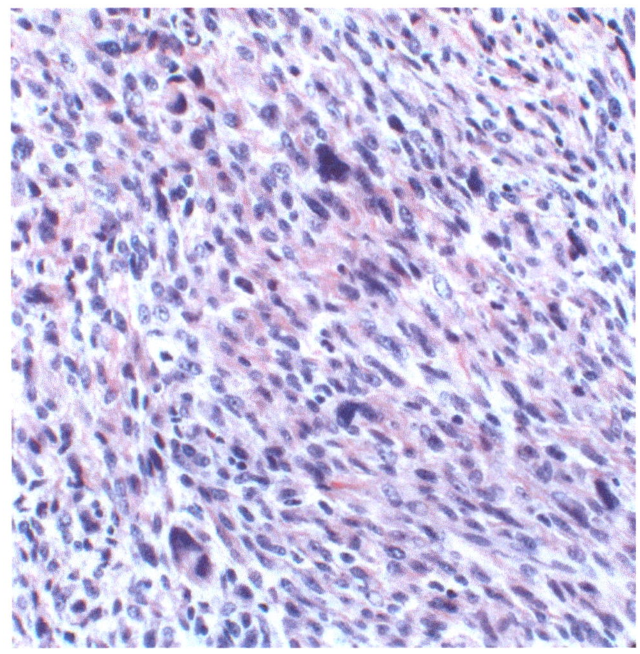

Fig. 16.12 High grade MPNST with eosinophilic stroma, elongated cells with vesicular nuclei, and cytological atypia

Epithelioid MPNST, a rare subtype of MPNST, is characterized by a predominance of large epithelioid cells. Epithelioid MPNSTs are more frequent in superficial sites and exhibit strong and usually diffuse expression of S100β protein [8]. The majority of MPNSTs arising within preexisting schwannomas, which occurs very rarely, are of epithelioid type [10]. The differential diagnosis of epithelioid MPNST includes epithelioid sarcoma, clear cell sarcoma, melanoma, and carcinoma. The absence of expression of melanocytic markers (MelanA, HMB45, MART-1) is useful in the differentiation of epithelioid MPNST from melanoma and clear cell sarcoma [8]. Absent cytokeratin expression distinguishes epithelioid MPNST from epithelioid sarcoma and carcinoma. Both epithelioid MPNST and epithelioid sarcoma may show loss of SMARCB1/INI1/BAF47 protein expression [21], a potential diagnostic pitfall in the consideration of rhabdoid tumor [6, 8, 13–15, 17, 18, 22].

Most MPNST are frankly high grade, aggressive tumors by histology and clinical behavior, and carry a dismal prognosis. Adverse prognosticators include truncal location, size >5 cm, incomplete resection, local recurrence, young age [7, 9], and high grade. According to some authors, histological grade is the most important prognostic factor for soft tissue sarcomas [13, 23] including MPNSTs. Past literature portended a worse prognosis for NF1-associated tumors as compared to sporadic MPNSTs [7, 24]. However, a large recent study indicates that while NF1 patients with MPNSTs demonstrate overall increased mortality compared to those patients with non-NF1-associated MPNSTs, decreased survival did not appear to be related to inherent tumor behavior [24].

Cytogenetics and Molecular Genetics

Primary among MPNST initiating mutations are mutations in the *NF1* gene. NF1 patients carry a constitutional mutation of the *NF1* tumor suppressor gene located on the long arm of chromosome 17 (17q11.2) [25], and mutation, or loss of the second allele, was found in 40 % of NF1 MPNST [26]. MPNST are particularly prevalent in NF1 patients whose constitutional mutations involve whole gene deletion, which can include contiguous genes that may contribute to tumor formation [27]. *NF1* mutations are also present in 41 % of sporadic MPNST [26], explaining why expression signatures and genomic changes overlap in NF1 and sporadic tumors [28–30]. Mutations in *RAS* or RAS pathway genes may also cause MPSNT tumor initiation in MPNST lacking *NF1* mutations; activating mutations in *N-RAS*(1/11), K-*RAS* (1/11) [31], and B-*RAF* (1/13 MPNST) [26] were identified in sporadic MPNST.

As discussed above, atypical neurofibromas represent an early stage in MPNST transformation from neurofibroma. Atypical neurofibromas (15/16) showed homozygous loss of the *CDKN2A* locus on chromosome 9p21.3 [17], and deletions of the *CDKN2A* locus are present in about 50 % of MPNSTs [16, 32]. The *CDKN2A* locus encodes two proteins: p16INK4A, which inhibits the cyclin-dependent kinases 4 (CDK4) and 6 (CDK6), and p14ARF, which inhibits the MDM2 ubiquitin ligase resulting in stabilization of tp53 [16, 32]. Mouse models support the importance of this locus in MPNST, as *Nf1+/−*; *Ink4a/Arf−/−* mice develop GEM-PNSTs resembling human MPNST [33].

Another tumor suppressor commonly inactivated in MPNST is TP53. An "inactivated p53-associated proliferation" gene expression signature was identified in 18/20 MPNST, and p53 inactivation caused downregulation of miR-34a, preventing MPNST cell apoptosis in tissue culture [34]. Estimates of MPNST with TP53 alterations (mutations or stabilized TP53) vary between 24 and 75 % [35–37], which is likely due to the variable sensitivity and specificity of different assays for assessing p53 expression and mutations, as well as intra-tumor heterogeneity [38–41]. TP53 stability can also be regulated through $p14^{ARF}$ so that if $p14^{ARF}$ is retained, TP53 is stabilized without TP53 mutation. While biallelic inactivation of the *TP53* locus is rare in MPNSTs [42] in mouse models, only complete loss of *tp53* and *Nf1* correlates with Genetically engineered mouse-Malignant Peripheral Nerve Sheath Tumor (GEM-MPNST) formation [43, 44].

The *PTEN* gene is an "off signal" for phosphoinositide 3-kinase (PI3K) signaling, and PTEN inactivation generally leads to activation of PI3K. Frequent monosomy of the *PTEN* locus was identified in MPNST without *PI3KCA* or *PTEN* mutations [31, 45]; *PTEN* methylation is detected in 45 % of MPNSTs, though not neurofibromas, and associated with early metastasis [46]. Co-deletion of *Nf1* and *Pte*n or expression of *RasG12D* or *EGFR* in combination with *Pten* deletion also resulted in GEM-PNST [47, 48]. In addition, expression of the retinoblastoma (*RB*) tumor suppressor, a molecule that impedes cell cycle progression, is lost in 25 % of MPNSTs [49, 50].

As in most sarcomas, chromosomal gains, losses, and rearrangements in MPNSTs are numerous and variable [51], and MPNSTs commonly have hypodiploid or near-triploid karyotypes. Combined genomic somatic copy number alteration (CNA) and loss of heterozygosity (LOH) analysis on sets of neurofibromas and MPNSTs verified that recurrent or overlapping copy number variations (CNVs) or CNAs are absent from neurofibromas, while MPNSTs showed 232 CNAs (encompassing >2,900 genes) and more than 500 genes showed consistent LOH [52]. The microRNA miR-10b can target *NF1* messenger RNA [53]; in principal miRs that target NF1 might also contribute to NF1 tumorigenesis.

Amplification of the epidermal growth factor receptor gene *EGFR* is frequent in MPNST [45, 54]. Perrone et al. found that *EGFR* was amplified in all sporadic MPNST and half of NF1 MPNST [31]. EGFR overexpression was correlated with a worse prognosis in one study [55], but not in another [56]. No activating mutations in *EGFR* have been detected in MPNST. Ligands that activate the EGFR including transforming growth factor (TGF)α and heparin binding epidermal growth factor (HBEGF) are expressed in 90 % of MPNST, suggesting the presence of an autocrine loop in MPNST cells [45, 57]. In 15 % of a small series of MPNST, the amplicon including *PDGFRA*, *KIT*, and *VEGFR-2/KDR* was present. Among the three genes, *PDGFRA* is most frequently amplified [49, 58, 59] and rarely mutant [59]. Hepatocyte growth factor is expressed and its c-Met receptor is expressed in 82 % of MPNST, and the *MET* gene is amplified in MPSNT [49, 60]. Short hairpin RNAs targeting *MET* and XL184, a multi-kinase inhibitor targeting MET and VEGFR2, decreased MPNST tumor growth and metastasis in tumor xenografts [61]. While in vitro studies in cell lines support roles for these receptors in MPNST, several histology-specific clinical trials with agents targeting PDGFR, C-KIT, and EGFR were completed, all without achieving responses or meaningful disease stabilization as single agents [62–65]. Possibly blocking one or more of these receptors will be useful in combination with other therapeutic agents.

Gene Expression Profiling

Sporadic and NF1 MPNST are indistinguishable by transcriptome analysis [30]. Transcriptome analysis comparing Schwann cells to MPNST found that expression of markers of neural crest cells is a prominent theme in human MPNST cell lines and tumors [29, 66]. Neural crest markers include *SOX9* and *TWIST1*, which are dramatically upregulated in MPNST [29, 66–68]. MPNST cells are dependent on expression of these genes, as downregulation of *SOX9* caused cell death and downregulation of *TWIST1* decreased cell migration [29, 66]. Increased expression of the neural crest markers FOXD3, PAX7, SOX5, and AP-2α in MPNST compared to neurofibroma was described in a series of 34 MPNSTs [68]. The placodal markers *EYA/SIX* are also upregulated in MPNST cells and tumors [69], and shRNA to diminish *EYA4* expression prevented tumor formation and caused necrosis. EYAs are phophatases that could in principle be targeted therapeutically.

Whole genome microRNA analysis of MPNST tumors identified downregulation of 14 miRs, and upregulation of two (miR-210 and miR-339-5p) [70]. There was no overlap with serum microRNAs in MPNST patients [71]. Serum miR expression distinguished patients with MPNST from those without MPNST. The authors identified miR-24 as upregulated in NF1 and MPNST, and MiR-214 and miR-801 as upregulated in serum of individuals with sporadic or NF1-related MPNST. The sensitivity (0.820) and specificity (0.844) of a three miR panel to identify NF1 MPNST supports a potential role in helping to diagnose MPNST and/or as a possible indicator of response to therapy [71].

On two-dimensional gel analysis of proteins, MPNST most closely resembled synovial sarcoma and clear cell carcinoma [72]. For this reason, a goal remains to identify the markers that distinguish MPNST from these tumors, and from surrounding neurofibroma. Several markers, each analyzed in relatively few tumors, may distinguish neurofibromas from MPNST. These include Tenascin-C and NNAT [73]; Cathepsin K [74]; and markers of an angiogenic switch: SMA, vWF, VEGF, and VEGF receptors Flt1 and Flk1 [75]. Many growing or atypical neurofibromas and MPNST stained positive for CD10 [76]. Some neurofibromas and MPNST express hTERT [77].

Prognostic Stratification

Complete surgical resection is the only known curative MPNST therapy, and predicts favorable prognosis in all MPNST patients [23, 78, 79]. In addition, survival is significantly better in female versus male MPNST patients [80, 81]. Gain/amplification of the CDK4 gene on chromosome 12q14.1 and upregulation of the FOXM1 gene on chromosome 12p13.3 were significant independent predictors of poor survival in 87 MPNST patients [82]. Chromosomal losses of 10q and Xq and gain of 16p were also associated with reduced MPNST patient survival [28]. In a large series, 93 % of MPNST showed positive staining for phospho-MEK, while about half expressed phospho-S6K, phospho-mTOR and/or phospho-AKT, and immunoreactivity toward all three mTOR pathway markers predicted significantly worse outcomes than in patients with tumors negative for the three markers [83]. Intriguingly, a single nucleotide polymorphisms in the microRNA biogenesis pathway gene *DROSHA* (rs1991401) significantly increased MPNST risk in NF1 patients, while SNPs in *AGO2* and

GEMIN4 in this pathway decreased risk [71]. To date, none of these indicators have been used to stratify patients for clinical trials.

Treatment of MPNSTS

Only complete MPNST surgical resection has been shown to be curative, and remains the cornerstone of therapy, but is rarely feasible due to tumor location or nerve association [23, 78, 79, 84, 85]. Radiotherapy is commonly used for local control in inoperable or incompletely resected MPNSTs, but when used as primary treatment, high doses of radiation are needed (median 50 Gy) [3]. The role of chemotherapy for adult and pediatric soft tissue sarcomas, including MPNSTs, is controversial. Only doxorubicin, dacarbazine, and ifosfamide are agents consistently associated with response rates of 20 % or more in patients with soft tissue sarcomas [23, 86, 87], and the combination of ifosfamide and doxorubicin has produced response rates as high as 46 % in these tumors [87, 88]. The response rate of MPNSTs to chemotherapy is unknown. Some investigators have suggested that they have intermediate chemosensitivity, less responsive than synovial sarcoma, but more responsive than refractory diseases such as alveolar soft part sarcoma [86]. However, recently others have questioned whether MPNSTs are at all chemosensitive [84]. Carli et al. summarized the 25-year experience of pediatric MPNSTs in German and Italian Groups [3]. The patients described encompass a span of three decades and were treated on standard sarcoma protocols. First, response to ifosfamide was significantly better than to cyclophosphamide (65 % vs. 17 %). Second, while chemotherapy increased overall and event-free survival over no chemotherapy, the 5-year overall survival for patients with unresectable and metastatic MPNST remained approximately 30 %. It may be that the addition of targeted agents to chemotherapy will improve response rate, and potentially improve outcome without undue morbidity.

Molecular Signaling Pathways

NF1 is an off signal for Ras GTPases [89]. Therefore, *NF1* loss activates signaling pathways downstream of Ras-GTP, and the Raf-MEK-ERK and mTOR-S6K-Akt pathways have been explored as potential therapeutic targets (Fig. 16.13). Targeting MEK with PD0325901 in a xenograft and in a genetically engineered mouse model transiently delayed MPNST growth, correlating with suppression of tumor vasculature and tumor cell proliferation [90, 91]. Using rapamycin or its analog RAD001 to target the mTOR/S6K pathway also transiently blocked MPNST growth in xenografts and a mouse model [92–94]. This effect of rapamycin was converted to cytotoxicity in combination with agents that promote proteotoxic/endoplasmic reticulum (ER) stress in a genetically engineered mouse model [95]. Based on these data, combinatorial clinical trials are being considered.

We have chosen to omit discussion of a host of studies focusing on effects in MPNST cell lines, pending confirmation of significant effects in in vivo model systems. In xenografts, hyaluronan oligomers suppressed drug transporter activity and inhibited growth of MPNST tumor growth, with synergy between oligomers and doxorubicin [96]. The effect of 4-hydroxytamoxifen on K-Ras degradation and MPNST cell autophagy correlated with decreased MPNST growth [57, 97]. Inhibition of Aurora kinases using MLN2036 caused prolonged MPNST growth arrest in the G2/M phase of the cell cycle [98]. The combination of histone deacetylase inhibitor PC-24791 (which promotes autophagy) and autophagy blockade with chloroquine abrogated MPNST xenograft growth and promoted cell apoptosis, although the durability of the response is not known [99]. Blocking STAT3 with FLLL32 or shSTAT3 prevented growth of MPNST xenografts but did not arrest growth of established tumors [100]. Whether these xenograft studies will translate to effects in immune-competent models or clinical trials remains to be tested.

An exciting recent development is a new link between MPNST and β-catenin signaling. Transposon-based

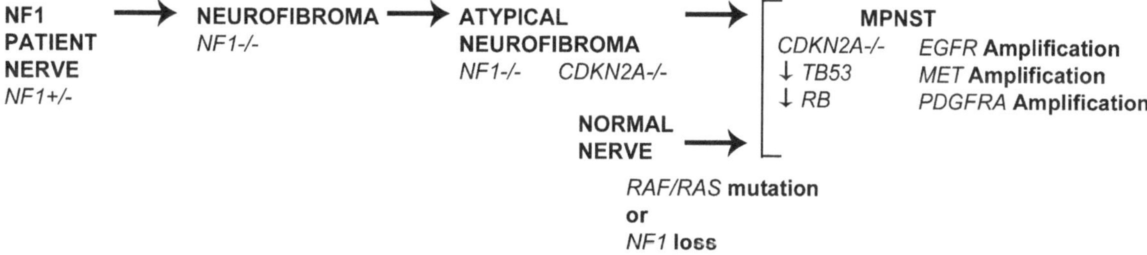

Fig. 16.13 Schematic illustration of some of the multiple genetic changes believed to contribute to NF1-related and sporadic MPNST. In NF1 patients, benign neurofibromas form when *NF1* haploinsufficient cells in the Schwann cell lineage lose remaining functional *NF1*. Subsequent progression toward MPNST is via an atypical neurofibroma intermediate, and is associated with loss of the tumor suppressor gene CDKN2A. MPNST also show mutation of additional tumor suppressor genes and amplification of several growth factor receptors. The bottom row shows that mutations in RAS genes, RAF genes, and *NF1* were recently identified in sporadic MPNST

mutagenesis screens identified many components of the β-catenin signaling pathway as potential driver mutations in MPNST [101, 102]. Strong evidence also supports the role for autocrine CXCL12 and CXCR4 signaling upstream of β-catenin [103]. Both blockade of CXCR4 with AMD3100 (which is already in clinical trials in other cancers) and treatment of MPNST cells with shβ-catenin decreased cell proliferation and MPNST tumor growth [102, 103].

Molecular Targeted Therapies

The outcome for patients with relapsed unresectable MPNST remains poor. Therapy options remain particularly limited in patients with NF-1 in the face of the increased risk of therapy-related monosomy 7 myelodysplastic syndrome and leukemia in NF-1 patients who had previously received alkylator-based chemotherapy or radiotherapy for solid tumors [104]. As elucidated above, several effector pathways have been interrogated in order to find a cure for resistant MPNST. Ohishi et al. analyzed the cytotoxic effects of imatinib mesylate blockade of PDGFRβ using six human MPNST cell lines [105]. They found that imatinib mesylate effectively suppressed cell growth in vitro at concentrations within the therapeutic range in three of the six human MPNST cell lines. In two of these three, imatinib mesylate-sensitive cell lines, imatinib mesylate also significantly suppressed tumor growth in a xenograft model. Others have seen similar results with the second-generation tyrosine kinase inhibitor nilotinib [106].

Another group identified bone morphogenetic protein 2 (BMP2) expression as neurofibromin regulated but independent of NRAS and MEK1/2. BMP2 belongs to the TGF-β superfamily and functions as a morphogen required for the development of lung, heart, and central nervous system. Overexpression of BMP2 promotes malignancy-related attributes such as migration and invasion and is found in NF1-related malignant tumors [107]. Inhibition of BMP2 signaling by the small molecule LDN-193189 or by BMP2 short hairpin RNA (shRNA) decreased the motility and invasion of Nf1-deficient MPNST cells in vitro.

Pigment epithelium-derived factor (PEDF) can induce differentiation and inhibit angiogenesis in several tumors, including MPNST. Demestre et al. determined that PEDF inhibited proliferation and augmented apoptosis in S462 MPNST cells in vitro, and suppressed MPNST tumor burden in a nude mouse model, mainly due to inhibition of angiogenesis [108]. These results demonstrate the inhibitory effects of PEDF on the growth of human MPNST via induction of anti-angiogenesis and apoptosis, and suggest a potential novel approach for future therapy against MPNST.

Chau et al. recently described a novel small chemical compound, Compound 21 (Cpd21) that inhibits tumor cell growth [109]. Cpd21 inhibits growth of all available in vitro models of MPNST and human MPNST cell lines, while remaining nontoxic to normally dividing Schwann cells or mouse embryonic fibroblasts by delaying the cell cycle, thereby leading to cellular apoptosis. While too early to determine if these findings will be replicable and transferable to treating human patients, Cpd21 certainly has potential as a novel chemotherapeutic agent.

Perhaps the most promising is the work done on the Ras/Raf/MEK/ERK signaling pathway in MPNST. Jessen et al. showed that the MEK inhibitor, PD0325901, had a robust, yet transient, in vivo effect on survival in MPNST xenografts, possibly due to effects on tumor vasculature [91]. Others have reported dramatic response in a patient with resistant *BRAF* V600E mutated MPNST to the second-generation B-Raf enzyme inhibitor, Vemurafenib [110]. There are many new BRAF and MEK inhibitors still to be investigated in this tumor type. In addition, due to the multiplicity of Ras effectors and complexity of negative feedback regulation, therapeutic strategies against more aggressive Ras-related tumors are likely to include combinations of compounds that target multiple points in the Ras signaling network [91].

References

1. Ferner RE, Gutmann DH. International consensus statement on malignant peripheral nerve sheath tumors in neurofibromatosis. Cancer Res. 2002;62(5):1573–7.
2. Woodruff JM. Pathology of tumors of the peripheral nerve sheath in type 1 neurofibromatosis. Am J Med Genet. 1999;89(1):23–30.
3. Carli M, Ferrari A, Mattke A, et al. Pediatric malignant peripheral nerve sheath tumor: the Italian and German soft tissue sarcoma cooperative group. J Clin Oncol. 2005;23(33):8422–30.
4. Evans DG, Baser ME, McGaughran J, Sharif S, Howard E, Moran A. Malignant peripheral nerve sheath tumours in neurofibromatosis 1. J Med Genet. 2002;39(5):311–4.
5. King AA, Debaun MR, Riccardi VM, Gutmann DH. Malignant peripheral nerve sheath tumors in neurofibromatosis 1. Am J Med Genet. 2000;93(5):388–92.
6. Zhou H, Coffin CM, Perkins SL, Tripp SR, Liew M, Viskochil DH. Malignant peripheral nerve sheath tumor: a comparison of grade, immunophenotype, and cell cycle/growth activation marker expression in sporadic and neurofibromatosis 1-related lesions. Am J Surg Pathol. 2003;27(10):1337–45.
7. Fletcher CDM, Bridge JA, Hogendoorn PCW, editors. WHO classification of tumours of soft tissue and bone. Lyon: International Agency for Research on Cancer; 2013.
8. Rodriguez FJ, Folpe AL, Giannini C, Perry A. Pathology of peripheral nerve sheath tumors: diagnostic overview and update on selected diagnostic problems. Acta Neuropathol. 2012;123(3): 295–319.
9. Stein-Wexler R. Pediatric soft tissue sarcomas. Semin Ultrasound CT MR. 2011;32(5):470–88.
10. Evans DG, Birch JM, Ramsden RT, Sharif S, Baser ME. Malignant transformation and new primary tumours after therapeutic radiation for benign disease: substantial risks in certain tumour prone syndromes. J Med Genet. 2006;43(4):289–94.
11. Guo A, Liu A, Wei L, Song X. Malignant peripheral nerve sheath tumors: differentiation patterns and immunohistochemical features—a mini-review and our new findings. J Cancer. 2012;3: 303–9.

12. Bernthal NM, Jones KB, Monument MJ, Liu T, Viskochil D, Randall RL. Lost in translation: ambiguity in nerve sheath tumor nomenclature and its resultant treatment effect. Cancer. 2013;5(2): 519–28.
13. Costa J, Wesley RA, Glatstein E, Rosenberg SA. The grading of soft tissue sarcomas. Results of a clinicohistopathologic correlation in a series of 163 cases. Cancer. 1984;53(3):530–41.
14. Trojani M, Contesso G, Coindre JM, et al. Soft-tissue sarcomas of adults; study of pathological prognostic variables and definition of a histopathological grading system. Int J Cancer. 1984;33(1): 37–42.
15. Ferner RE, Golding JF, Smith M, et al. [18F]2-fluoro-2-deoxy-D-glucose positron emission tomography (FDG PET) as a diagnostic tool for neurofibromatosis 1 (NF1) associated malignant peripheral nerve sheath tumours (MPNSTs): a long-term clinical study. Ann Oncol. 2008;19(2):390–4.
16. Nielsen GP, Stemmer-Rachamimov AO, Ino Y, Moller MB, Rosenberg AE, Louis DN. Malignant transformation of neurofibromas in neurofibromatosis 1 is associated with CDKN2A/p16 inactivation. Am J Pathol. 1999;155(6):1879–84.
17. Beert E, Brems H, Daniels B, et al. Atypical neurofibromas in neurofibromatosis type 1 are premalignant tumors. Genes Chromosomes Cancer. 2011;50(12):1021–32.
18. Brekke HR, Kolberg M, Skotheim RI, et al. Identification of p53 as a strong predictor of survival for patients with malignant peripheral nerve sheath tumors. Neuro Oncol. 2009;11(5): 514–28.
19. Li H, Velasco-Miguel S, Vass WC, Parada LF, DeClue JE. Epidermal growth factor receptor signaling pathways are associated with tumorigenesis in the Nf1:p53 mouse tumor model. Cancer Res. 2002;62(15):4507–13.
20. Mertens F, Dal Cin P, De Wever I, et al. Cytogenetic characterization of peripheral nerve sheath tumours: a report of the CHAMP study group. J Pathol. 2000;190(1):31–8.
21. Hollmann TJ, Hornick JL. INI1-deficient tumors: diagnostic features and molecular genetics. Am J Surg Pathol. 2011;35(10): e47–63.
22. Rodriguez FJ, Stratakis CA, Evans DG. Genetic predisposition to peripheral nerve neoplasia: diagnostic criteria and pathogenesis of neurofibromatoses, Carney complex, and related syndromes. Acta Neuropathol. 2012;123(3):349–67.
23. Cormier JN, Pollock RE. Soft tissue sarcomas. CA Cancer J Clin. 2004;54(2):94–109.
24. Kolberg M, Holand M, Agesen TH, et al. Survival meta-analyses for >1800 malignant peripheral nerve sheath tumor patients with and without neurofibromatosis type 1. Neuro Oncol. 2013;15(2):135–47.
25. Messiaen LM, Callens T, Mortier G, et al. Exhaustive mutation analysis of the NF1 gene allows identification of 95% of mutations and reveals a high frequency of unusual splicing defects. Hum Mutat. 2000;15(6):541–55.
26. Bottillo I, Ahlquist T, Brekke H, et al. Germline and somatic NF1 mutations in sporadic and NF1-associated malignant peripheral nerve sheath tumours. J Pathol. 2009;217(5):693–701.
27. Wimmer K, Yao S, Claes K, et al. Spectrum of single- and multiexon NF1 copy number changes in a cohort of 1,100 unselected NF1 patients. Genes Chromosomes Cancer. 2006;45(3):265–76.
28. Brekke HR, Ribeiro FR, Kolberg M, et al. Genomic changes in chromosomes 10, 16, and X in malignant peripheral nerve sheath tumors identify a high-risk patient group. J Clin Oncol. 2010; 28(9):1573–82.
29. Miller SJ, Rangwala F, Williams J, et al. Large-scale molecular comparison of human schwann cells to malignant peripheral nerve sheath tumor cell lines and tissues. Cancer Res. 2006;66(5): 2584–91.
30. Watson MA, Perry A, Tihan T, et al. Gene expression profiling reveals unique molecular subtypes of Neurofibromatosis Type I-associated and sporadic malignant peripheral nerve sheath tumors. Brain Pathol. 2004;14(3):297–303.
31. Perrone F, Da Riva L, Orsenigo M, et al. PDGFRA, PDGFRB, EGFR, and downstream signaling activation in malignant peripheral nerve sheath tumor. Neuro Oncol. 2009;11(6):725–36.
32. Kourea HP, Orlow I, Scheithauer BW, Cordon-Cardo C, Woodruff JM. Deletions of the INK4A gene occur in malignant peripheral nerve sheath tumors but not in neurofibromas. Am J Pathol. 1999;155(6):1855–60.
33. Joseph NM, Mosher JT, Buchstaller J, et al. The loss of Nf1 transiently promotes self-renewal but not tumorigenesis by neural crest stem cells. Cancer Cell. 2008;13(2):129–40.
34. Subramanian S, Thayanithy V, West RB, et al. Genome-wide transcriptome analyses reveal p53 inactivation mediated loss of miR-34a expression in malignant peripheral nerve sheath tumours. J Pathol. 2010;220(1):58–70.
35. Holtkamp N, Atallah I, Okuducu AF, et al. MMP-13 and p53 in the progression of malignant peripheral nerve sheath tumors. Neoplasia. 2007;9(8):671–7.
36. Upadhyaya M, Kluwe L, Spurlock G, et al. Germline and somatic NF1 gene mutation spectrum in NF1-associated malignant peripheral nerve sheath tumors (MPNSTs). Hum Mutat. 2008;29(1):74–82.
37. Verdijk RM, den Bakker MA, Dubbink HJ, Hop WC, Dinjens WN, Kros JM. TP53 mutation analysis of malignant peripheral nerve sheath tumors. J Neuropathol Exp Neurol. 2010;69(1): 16–26.
38. Thomas L, Mautner VF, Cooper DN, Upadhyaya M. Molecular heterogeneity in malignant peripheral nerve sheath tumors associated with neurofibromatosis type 1. Hum Genomics. 2012;6:18.
39. Birindelli S, Perrone F, Oggionni M, et al. Rb and TP53 pathway alterations in sporadic and NF1-related malignant peripheral nerve sheath tumors. Lab Invest. 2001;81(6):833–44.
40. Legius E, Dierick H, Wu R, et al. TP53 mutations are frequent in malignant NF1 tumors. Genes Chromosomes Cancer. 1994; 10(4):250–5.
41. Menon AG, Anderson KM, Riccardi VM, et al. Chromosome 17p deletions and p53 gene mutations associated with the formation of malignant neurofibrosarcomas in von Recklinghausen neurofibromatosis. Proc Natl Acad Sci U S A. 1990;87(14):5435–9.
42. Lothe RA, Smith-Sorensen B, Hektoen M, et al. Biallelic inactivation of TP53 rarely contributes to the development of malignant peripheral nerve sheath tumors. Genes Chromosomes Cancer. 2001;30(2):202–6.
43. Cichowski K, Shih TS, Schmitt E, et al. Mouse models of tumor development in neurofibromatosis type 1. Science. 1999; 286(5447):2172–6.
44. Vogel KS, Klesse LJ, Velasco-Miguel S, Meyers K, Rushing EJ, Parada LF. Mouse tumor model for neurofibromatosis type 1. Science. 1999;286(5447):2176–9.
45. Holtkamp N, Malzer E, Zietsch J, et al. EGFR and erbB2 in malignant peripheral nerve sheath tumors and implications for targeted therapy. Neuro Oncol. 2008;10(6):946–57.
46. Bradtmoller M, Hartmann C, Zietsch J, et al. Impaired Pten expression in human malignant peripheral nerve sheath tumours. PLoS One. 2012;7(11):e47595.
47. Gregorian C, Nakashima J, Dry SM, et al. PTEN dosage is essential for neurofibroma development and malignant transformation. Proc Natl Acad Sci U S A. 2009;106(46):19479–84.
48. Keng VW, Watson AL, Rahrmann EP, et al. Conditional inactivation of Pten with EGFR overexpression in Schwann cells models sporadic MPNST. Sarcoma. 2012;2012:620834.

49. Mantripragada KK, Spurlock G, Kluwe L, et al. High-resolution DNA copy number profiling of malignant peripheral nerve sheath tumors using targeted microarray-based comparative genomic hybridization. Clin Cancer Res. 2008;14(4):1015–24.
50. Mawrin C, Kirches E, Boltze C, Dietzmann K, Roessner A, Schneider-Stock R. Immunohistochemical and molecular analysis of p53, RB, and PTEN in malignant peripheral nerve sheath tumors. Virchows Arch. 2002;440(6):610–5.
51. Wallace MR, Rasmussen SA, Lim IT, Gray BA, Zori RT, Muir D. Culture of cytogenetically abnormal schwann cells from benign and malignant NF1 tumors. Genes Chromosomes Cancer. 2000; 27(2):117–23.
52. Upadhyaya M, Spurlock G, Thomas L, et al. Microarray-based copy number analysis of neurofibromatosis type-1 (NF1)-associated malignant peripheral nerve sheath tumors reveals a role for Rho-GTPase pathway genes in NF1 tumorigenesis. Hum Mutat. 2012;33(4):763–76.
53. Chai G, Liu N, Ma J, et al. MicroRNA-10b regulates tumorigenesis in neurofibromatosis type 1. Cancer Sci. 2010;101(9): 1997–2004.
54. Perry A, Kunz SN, Fuller CE, et al. Differential NF1, p16, and EGFR patterns by interphase cytogenetics (FISH) in malignant peripheral nerve sheath tumor (MPNST) and morphologically similar spindle cell neoplasms. J Neuropathol Exp Neurol. 2002;61(8):702–9.
55. Keizman D, Issakov J, Meller I, et al. Expression and significance of EGFR in malignant peripheral nerve sheath tumor. J Neurooncol. 2009;94(3):383–8.
56. Tabone-Eglinger S, Bahleda R, Cote JF, et al. Frequent EGFR positivity and overexpression in high-grade areas of human MPNSTs. Sarcoma. 2008;2008:849156.
57. Byer SJ, Brossier NM, Peavler LT, et al. Malignant peripheral nerve sheath tumor invasion requires aberrantly expressed EGF receptors and is variably enhanced by multiple EGF family ligands. J Neuropathol Exp Neurol. 2013;72(3):219–33.
58. Badache A, De Vries GH. Neurofibrosarcoma-derived Schwann cells overexpress platelet-derived growth factor (PDGF) receptors and are induced to proliferate by PDGF BB. J Cell Physiol. 1998;177(2):334–42.
59. Holtkamp N, Okuducu AF, Mucha J, et al. Mutation and expression of PDGFRA and KIT in malignant peripheral nerve sheath tumors, and its implications for imatinib sensitivity. Carcinogenesis. 2006;27(3):664–71.
60. Fan Q, Yang J, Wang G. Clinical and molecular prognostic predictors of malignant peripheral nerve sheath tumor. Clin Transl Oncol. 2013;16:191–9.
61. Torres KE, Zhu QS, Bill K, et al. Activated MET is a molecular prognosticator and potential therapeutic target for malignant peripheral nerve sheath tumors. Clin Cancer Res. 2011;17(12):3943–55.
62. Albritton K, Rankin C, Coffin C, et al. Phase II trial of erlotinib in metastatic or unresectable malignant peripheral nerve sheath tumor (MPNST). Journal of Clinical Oncology, 2006 ASCO Annual Meeting Proceedings (Post-Meeting Edition). Vol 24, No 18S (June 20 Supplement), 2006: 9518.
63. Chugh R, Wathen JK, Maki RG, et al. Phase II multicenter trial of imatinib in 10 histologic subtypes of sarcoma using a bayesian hierarchical statistical model. J Clin Oncol. 2009;27(19):3148–53.
64. Maki RG, D'Adamo DR, Keohan ML, et al. Phase II study of sorafenib in patients with metastatic or recurrent sarcomas. J Clin Oncol. 2009;27(19):3133–40.
65. Schuetze S, Wathen S, Choy E, et al. Results of a Sarcoma Alliance for Research through Collaboration (SARC) phase II trial of dasatinib in previously treated, high-grade, advanced sarcoma. ASCO. 2010. J Clin Oncol. 2010;28:15s (suppl; abstr 10009).
66. Miller SJ, Jessen WJ, Mehta T, et al. Integrative genomic analyses of neurofibromatosis tumours identify SOX9 as a biomarker and survival gene. EMBO Mol Med. 2009;1(4):236–48.
67. Carbonnelle-Puscian A, Vidal V, Laurendeau I, et al. SOX9 expression increases with malignant potential in tumors from patients with neurofibromatosis 1 and is not correlated to desert hedgehog. Hum Pathol. 2011;42(3):434–43.
68. Pytel P, Karrison T, Can G, Tonsgard JH, Krausz T, Montag AG. Neoplasms with schwannian differentiation express transcription factors known to regulate normal schwann cell development. Int J Surg Pathol. 2010;18(6):449–57.
69. Miller SJ, Lan ZD, Hardiman A, et al. Inhibition of Eyes Absent Homolog 4 expression induces malignant peripheral nerve sheath tumor necrosis. Oncogene. 2010;29(3):368–79.
70. Presneau N, Eskandarpour M, Shemais T, et al. MicroRNA profiling of peripheral nerve sheath tumours identifies miR-29c as a tumour suppressor gene involved in tumour progression. Br J Cancer. 2013;108(4):964–72.
71. Weng Y, Chen Y, Chen J, Liu Y, Bao T. Identification of serum microRNAs in genome-wide serum microRNA expression profiles as novel noninvasive biomarkers for malignant peripheral nerve sheath tumor diagnosis. Med Oncol. 2013;30(2):531.
72. Kawai A, Kondo T, Suehara Y, Kikuta K, Hirohashi S. Global protein-expression analysis of bone and soft tissue sarcomas. Clin Orthop Relat Res. 2008;466(9):2099–106.
73. Dugu L, Hayashida S, Nakahara T, et al. Aberrant expression of tenascin-c and neuronatin in malignant peripheral nerve sheath tumors. Eur J Dermatol. 2010;20(5):580–4.
74. Yan X, Takahara M, Dugu L, et al. Expression of cathepsin K in neurofibromatosis 1-associated cutaneous malignant peripheral nerve sheath tumors and neurofibromas. J Dermatol Sci. 2010;58(3):227–9.
75. Gesundheit B, Parkin P, Greenberg M, et al. The role of angiogenesis in the transformation of plexiform neurofibroma into malignant peripheral nerve sheath tumors in children with neurofibromatosis type 1. J Pediatr Hematol Oncol. 2010;32(7):548–53.
76. Cabibi D, Zerilli M, Caradonna G, Schillaci L, Belmonte B, Rodolico V. Diagnostic and prognostic value of CD10 in peripheral nerve sheath tumors. Anticancer Res. 2009;29(8):3149–55.
77. Patel RM, Folpe AL. Immunohistochemistry for human telomerase reverse transcriptase catalytic subunit (hTERT): a study of 143 benign and malignant soft tissue and bone tumours. Pathology. 2009;41(6):527–32.
78. Scaife CL, Pisters PW. Combined-modality treatment of localized soft tissue sarcomas of the extremities. Surg Oncol Clin N Am. 2003;12(2):355–68.
79. Abbas JS, Holyoke ED, Moore R, Karakousis CP. The surgical treatment and outcome of soft-tissue sarcoma. Arch Surg. 1981;116(6):765–9.
80. Ingham S, Huson SM, Moran A, Wylie J, Leahy M, Evans DG. Malignant peripheral nerve sheath tumours in NF1: improved survival in women and in recent years. Eur J Cancer. 2011;47(18): 2723–8.
81. Ren X, Wang J, Hu M, Jiang H, Yang J, Jiang Z. Clinical, radiological, and pathological features of 26 intracranial and intraspinal malignant peripheral nerve sheath tumors. J Neurosurg. 2013; 119(3):695–708.
82. Yu J, Deshmukh H, Payton JE, et al. Array-based comparative genomic hybridization identifies CDK4 and FOXM1 alterations as independent predictors of survival in malignant peripheral nerve sheath tumor. Clin Cancer Res. 2011;17(7):1924–34.
83. Endo M, Yamamoto H, Setsu N, et al. Prognostic significance of AKT/mTOR and MAPK pathways and antitumor effect of mTOR inhibitor in NF1-related and sporadic malignant peripheral nerve sheath tumors. Clin Cancer Res. 2013;19(2):450–61.

84. Zehou O, Fabre E, Zelek L, et al. Chemotherapy for the treatment of malignant peripheral nerve sheath tumors in neurofibromatosis 1: a 10-year institutional review. Orphanet J Rare Dis. 2013;8:127.
85. Amirian ES, Goodman JC, New P, Scheurer ME. Pediatric and adult malignant peripheral nerve sheath tumors: an analysis of data from the surveillance, epidemiology, and end results program. J Neurooncol. 2014;116(3):609–16.
86. Santoro A, Tursz T, Mouridsen H, et al. Doxorubicin versus CYVADIC versus doxorubicin plus ifosfamide in first-line treatment of advanced soft tissue sarcomas: a randomized study of the European Organization for Research and Treatment of Cancer Soft Tissue and Bone Sarcoma Group. J Clin Oncol. 1995; 13(7):1537–45.
87. Verma S, Bramwell V. Dose-intensive chemotherapy in advanced adult soft tissue sarcoma. Expert Rev Anticancer Ther. 2002; 2(2):201–15.
88. Fernberg JO, Wiklund T, Monge O, et al. Chemotherapy in soft tissue sarcoma. The Scandinavian Sarcoma Group experience. Acta Orthop Scand Suppl. 1999;285:62–8.
89. Donovan S, Shannon KM, Bollag G. GTPase activating proteins: critical regulators of intracellular signaling. Biochim Biophys Acta. 2002;1602(1):23–45.
90. Dodd RD, Mito JK, Eward WC, et al. NF1 deletion generates multiple subtypes of soft-tissue sarcoma that respond to MEK inhibition. Mol Cancer Ther. 2013;12:1906–17.
91. Jessen WJ, Miller SJ, Jousma E, et al. MEK inhibition exhibits efficacy in human and mouse neurofibromatosis tumors. J Clin Invest. 2013;123(1):340–7.
92. Bhola P, Banerjee S, Mukherjee J, et al. Preclinical in vivo evaluation of rapamycin in human malignant peripheral nerve sheath explant xenograft. Int J Cancer. 2010;126(2):563–71.
93. Johannessen CM, Johnson BW, Williams SMG, et al. TORC1 is essential for NF1-associated malignancies. Curr Biol. 2008; 18(1):56–62.
94. Johannessen CM, Reczek EE, James MF, Brems H, Legius E, Cichowski K. The NF1 tumor suppressor critically regulates TSC2 and mTOR. Proc Natl Acad Sci U S A. 2005;102(24):8573–8.
95. De Raedt T, Walton Z, Yecies JL, et al. Exploiting cancer cell vulnerabilities to develop a combination therapy for ras-driven tumors. Cancer Cell. 2011;20(3):400–13.
96. Slomiany MG, Dai L, Bomar PA, et al. Abrogating drug resistance in malignant peripheral nerve sheath tumors by disrupting hyaluronan-CD44 interactions with small hyaluronan oligosaccharides. Cancer Res. 2009;69(12):4992–8.
97. Kohli L, Kaza N, Coric T, et al. 4-Hydroxytamoxifen induces autophagic death through K-Ras degradation. Cancer Res. 2013; 73(14):4395–405.
98. Patel AV, Eaves D, Jessen WJ, et al. Ras-driven transcriptome analysis identifies aurora kinase A as a potential malignant peripheral nerve sheath tumor therapeutic target. Clin Cancer Res. 2012;18(18):5020–30.
99. Lopez G, Torres K, Liu J, et al. Autophagic survival in resistance to histone deacetylase inhibitors: novel strategies to treat malignant peripheral nerve sheath tumors. Cancer Res. 2011;71(1): 185–96.
100. Wu J, Patmore DM, Jousma E, et al. EGFR-STAT3 signaling promotes formation of malignant peripheral nerve sheath tumors. Oncogene. 2014;33(2):173–80.
101. Rahrmann EP, Watson AL, Keng VW, et al. Forward genetic screen for malignant peripheral nerve sheath tumor formation identifies new genes and pathways driving tumorigenesis. Nat Genet. 2013;45(7):756–66.
102. Watson AL, Rahrmann EP, Moriarity BS, et al. Canonical Wnt/beta-catenin signaling drives human schwann cell transformation, progression, and tumor maintenance. Cancer Discov. 2013; 3(6):674–89.
103. Mo W, Chen J, Patel A, et al. CXCR4/CXCL12 mediate autocrine cell-cycle progression in NF1-associated malignant peripheral nerve sheath tumors. Cell. 2013;152(5):1077–90.
104. Maris JM, Wiersma SR, Mahgoub N, et al. Monosomy 7 myelodysplastic syndrome and other second malignant neoplasms in children with neurofibromatosis type 1. Cancer. 1997;79: 1438–46.
105. Ohishi J, Aoki M, Nabeshima K, et al. Imatinib mesylate inhibits cell growth of malignant peripheral nerve sheath tumors in vitro and in vivo through suppression of PDGFR-beta. BMC Cancer. 2013;13:224.
106. Jiang W, Schnabel C, Spyra M, et al. Efficacy and selectivity of nilotinib on NF1-associated tumors in vitro. J Neurooncol. 2014; 116(2):231–6.
107. Sun D, Haddad R, Kraniak JM, Horne SD, Tainsky MA. RAS/MEK-independent gene expression reveals BMP2-related malignant phenotypes in the Nf1-deficient MPNST. Mol Cancer Res. 2013;11(6):616–27.
108. Demestre M, Terzi MY, Mautner V, Vajkoczy P, Kurtz A, Pina AL. Effects of pigment epithelium derived factor (PEDF) on malignant peripheral nerve sheath tumours (MPNSTs). J Neurooncol. 2013;115(3):391–9.
109. Chau V, Lim SK, Mo W, et al. Preclinical therapeutic efficacy of a novel pharmacologic inducer of apoptosis in malignant peripheral nerve sheath tumors. Cancer Res. 2014;74(2):586–97.
110. Kaplan HG. Vemurafenib treatment of BRAF V600E-mutated malignant peripheral nerve sheath tumor. J Natl Compr Cancer Netw. 2013;11(12):1466–70.

17 Meningiomas

Christian Mawrin and Michel Kalamarides

Meningiomas are brain tumors originating from meningeal coverings of the brain and spinal cord. Meningiomas are the most common intracranial tumors, with an incidence estimated at approximately 7.7/100,000 [1]. Meningiomas are predominantly tumors of the elderly, with a clear increase of incidence after the age of 65 years [1]. Among children, meningiomas are exceedingly rare (0.4–4.1 % of all pediatric tumors) [2]. However, pediatric meningiomas are an interesting subgroup because a high proportion is associated with germline alterations in the neurofibromatosis type 2 (*NF2*) gene and the diagnosis of a meningioma in a child therefore may represent the first clinical manifestation of NF2 [3]. Another hallmark of meningiomas is the preferential affection of women with a female:male ratio of 3.5:1 [4]. Other risk factors include ionizing radiation [5], presence of diabetes mellitus and arterial hypertension, and possibly smoking [6, 7]. In contrast, the use of mobile phones is not associated with increased meningioma development [8]. Radiation-induced meningiomas tend to present with aggressive histological features and are characterized by a more aggressive clinical course including frequent tumor recurrence [9]. Epidemiological data points to genetic susceptibilities to develop radiation-induced meningioma [10]. In children, radiation-induced meningiomas are often multiple on first presentation, and rare histological subtypes are encountered more frequently [11].

About 90 % of meningiomas can be found in the cranial meninges, while 10 % occur in the spinal meninges. Meningiomas may occur at multiple sites; in about 1 % multiple meningiomas are associated with NF2, while 4 % of cases are unrelated to NF2 [12]. Interestingly, individuals with a first-degree relative suffering from meningioma have a threefold higher risk of developing a tumor, suggesting underlying hereditary conditions [13]. Hereditary meningiomas in adults are again highly associated with *NF2* (see below), and at least 50–75 % of NF2 patients develop meningiomas during their lifetime [14]. Meningioma development in other familial tumor syndromes is uncommon. Few cases have been reported in the setting of Gorlin syndrome [15], Cowden syndrome [16], Li-Fraumeni syndrome [17], and multiple endocrine neoplasia type 1 (MEN1) [18].

Histopathology

Meningiomas are thought to originate from arachnoidal cap cells, which form the outer layer of the arachnoid mater and the arachnoid villi, the latter being responsible for cerebrospinal fluid (CSF) drainage into the dural sinuses and veins. Arachnoidal cap cells can appear normally as a single fibroblast-like cell layer, or as epithelioid nests consisting of several layers. With age, the arachnoidal cap cell clusters become increasingly prominent, forming whorls and psammoma bodies identical to those found in meningiomas. Based on cytological and functional similarities to meningioma cells, arachnoidal cap cells are favored as the most likely cell of origin [19]. Embryonically, the meninges at the skull base are derived from the mesoderm, while telencephalic meninges are neural crest derived [20].

As the neoplastic counterpart of cap cells, meningiomas display both mesenchymal and epithelial-like features. This is reflected by the histopathological appearance of the most frequent meningioma subtypes. Among the group of WHO (*World Health Organization*) grade I meningiomas which comprises about 80 %, meningothelial, fibrous, or mixed (transitional) tumors displaying both epithelial and mesenchymal characteristics are the dominating subtypes (Fig. 17.1a, b; Table 17.1). Interestingly, there is a preponderance of specific intracranial sites affected by meningiomas in association with certain histopathological subtypes. Meningothelial (epithelial) meningiomas are prone to develop at the skull base, while fibroblastic meningiomas are more likely to occur at the convexity of the brain [21, 22]. If the location is related to the grade of malignancy, the proportion of grade II/grade III meningiomas at the convexity or with parasagittal location is much higher than at the skull base, where grade I meningiomas

M.A. Karajannis and D. Zagzag (eds.), *Molecular Pathology of Nervous System Tumors: Biological Stratification and Targeted Therapies*, Molecular Pathology Library 8,
DOI 10.1007/978-1-4939-1830-0_17,

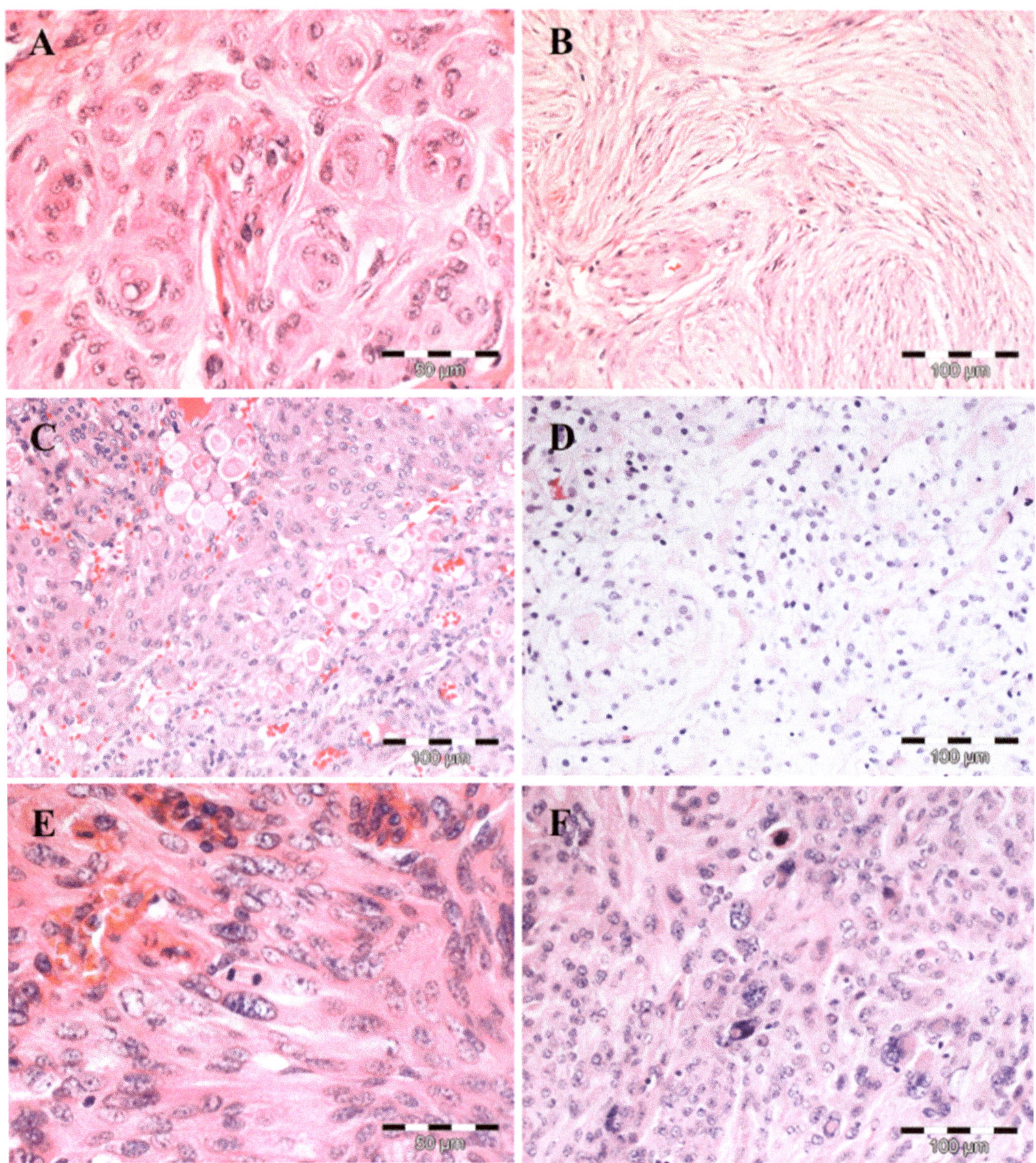

Fig. 17.1 Histopathological features of meningiomas. (**a**) Typical meningothelial meningioma WHO grade I with whorl formation. (**b**) Fibroblastic meningioma WHO grade I with spindle-shaped nuclei and fascicular growth. (**c**) Secretory meningioma WHO grade I with numerous inclusions. (**d**) Clear cell meningioma WHO grade II. (**e**) Atypical meningioma WHO grade II with increased nuclear polymorphisms and marked mitotic activity. (**f**) Anaplastic meningioma WHO grade III characterized by highly pleomorphic tumor cells and lack of typical meningioma features

dominate [23]. Rare meningioma variants designated as WHO grade I comprise psammomatous (calcified), angiomatous, secretory, microcystic, lymphoplasmacyte-rich, and metaplastic forms. Some variants, such as the secretory meningioma (Fig. 17.1c), have been recently related to characteristic molecular alterations (see below).

About 20 % of meningiomas belong to the group of atypical WHO grade II tumors. Atypical meningiomas have been

Table 17.1. Histopathological subtypes and grading of meningiomas in relation to genetic alterations and preferred sites affected by the tumor.

Histological subtype	WHO Grade	Molecular characteristics	Preferred site#	References
Meningothelial meningioma	I	(*NF2*), *TRAF7*, *AKT1*^{E17K}	Skull base	[43, 59, 60]
Fibroblastic meningioma	I	*NF2*	Convexity	[21]
Transitional (mixed) meningioma	I	*NF2*, *AKT1*^{E17K}	Convexity	[60]
Psammomatous meningioma	I	*NF2*	Spinal	[46, 59]
Angiomatous meningioma	I	?	–	
Microcystic meningioma	I	?	–	
Secretory meningioma	I	*KLF4/TRAF7*	–	[44, 59, 63]
Lymphoplasmacyte-rich meningioma	I	?	–	
Metaplastic meningioma	I	?	–	
Chordoid meningioma	II	?	–	
Clear cell meningioma	II	*SMARCE1*	Spinal	[74]
Atypical meningioma	II	*NF2*, *TRAF7*, *AKT1*^{E17K}	–	[59, 60]
Brain-invasive meningioma	II	?	–	
Papillary meningioma	III	?	–	
Rhabdoid meningioma	III	?	–	
Anaplastic meningioma	III	*NF2*	–	[43]

increasingly recognized in the last few years, mainly due to a shift in histopathological diagnosis from grade I to grade II meningiomas [24]. Atypical meningiomas are characterized by histopathological features indicating aggressiveness, including increased mitotic activity, nuclear atypia, and overall malignant biology (Fig. 17.1e, Table 17.1). Indeed, patients suffering from grade II meningiomas have a roughly eightfold increased risk of recurrence compared to benign WHO grade I tumors, and a slightly, but statistically significantly increased risk of mortality compared with age- and sex-matched controls. Within the group of atypical meningiomas, special attention is necessary for meningiomas characterized by brain invasion. It is now widely accepted that these patients are prone to increased risk of tumor recurrence, but the molecular mechanisms driving brain invasion are not well understood so far. Malignant meningiomas WHO grade III are rare, accounting for only 1–2 % of all meningiomas, but are associated with considerable risk of death from disease, with the average survival being less than 2 years [25–27]. While in atypical meningiomas the characteristic histopathological features of meningiomas (i.e., whorls, psammoma bodies) are at least focally present, malignant WHO grade III meningiomas sometimes completely lack any morphological hint of a meningeal origin and do require extensive immunohistochemical investigations to confirm the origin (Fig. 17.1f).

Cytogenetics and Molecular Genetics

Grade I Meningiomas

In 1967, Zang and Singer described loss of chromosome 22 in meningiomas [28]. This was the first report of genetic alterations in meningiomas, and chromosome 22 alterations are still by far among the most frequent findings in these tumors. Subsequently, a gene on chromosome 22 responsible for the hereditary tumor syndrome neurofibromatosis type 2 (NF2) was identified [29, 30]. Although bilateral vestibular schwannomas are the hallmark of the disorder, the majority of NF2 patients develop multiple meningiomas, implying a role for the *NF2* gene in meningioma development [31]. Indeed, several groups reported allelic losses of chromosome 22 including the *NF2* region in more than 50 % of sporadic meningiomas [32–35]. In meningiomas with allelic losses (LOH, *loss of heterozygosity*) at the *NF2* locus, point mutations in the remaining allele were found in a significant fraction of sporadic meningiomas, suggesting a complete inactivation of the gene [36, 37]. *NF2* mutations commonly result in a truncated, nonfunctional protein product. Aberrant promoter methylation in a fraction of tumors may represent an alternative mode of *NF2* inactivation in meningiomas [38, 39], or increased calpain-mediated proteolysis of merlin (also named schwannomin), the protein product of the *NF2* gene [40]. If the *NF2* gene is intact, promoter methylation is absent [41]. Merlin has significant sequence homology to members of the Ezrin/Radixin/Moesin (ERM) family of proteins, which link various cell adhesion receptors to the cortical actin cytoskeleton [42]. In keeping with *NF2* inactivation, protein expression of merlin is commonly reduced in meningiomas [37]. The frequency of *NF2* inactivation is roughly equal among different WHO grades, suggesting that it represents an important initiation rather than progression-associated alteration [26, 43–45]. Interestingly, differences in the frequency of *NF2* alterations have been noted based on variant histology, with higher rates in fibroblastic, transitional, and psammomatous than in meningothelial or secretory grade I meningiomas [39, 43, 46, 47]. Thus, *NF2* alterations appear to play a preferential role in the mesenchymal-like pathology. Accordingly, patients with non-NF2 familial multiple meningiomas are more likely to develop meningothelial tumors [48]. An association between the *NF2* gene and location has also been reported such that tumors of the convexity are more likely to harbor *NF2* alterations than anterior cranial-based tumors [21]. Excluding NF2 patients, about 4–10 % of meningioma patients experience multiple tumors [49]. Recurrent meningiomas often appear to have spread discontinuously along the dura. This has raised the question about the clonal origin of multiple meningiomas. Using clonality markers, it was demonstrated that *NF2*-mutated tumors within a patient are of clonal origin [48, 50, 51]. Somatic mosaicism is another issue in NF2 patients presenting with multiple meningiomas. Somatic mosaicism is caused by postzygotic mutations in the early stage of embryo development and results in only a subpopulation of normal cells carrying the constitutional mutation [52]. About a third of NF2 patients is affected by somatic mosaicism, which is associated with a milder phenotype [53]. Approximately 8 % of multiple meningiomas may be caused by mosaic *NF2* [54]. In contrast, patients with neurofibromatosis type 1 (NF1) only rarely present with meningiomas [55], and *NF1* gene mutations are absent in anaplastic meningiomas, suggesting that *NF1* alterations are not involved in meningioma development and/or progression [45].

Based on the clearly established role of *NF2* in meningiomas, it could be demonstrated that *Nf2* inactivation in leptomeningeal cells of conditional *Nf2* knockout mice (*Nf2*$^{flox/flox}$) by Cre-recombinase injection is sufficient to induce meningiomas [56]. Transorbital Cre-recombinase injection led to meningioma development in 29 % of mice, while subdural injection was efficient in 19 % of the animals. More interestingly, most of these tumors recapitulated the meningothelial, fibroblastic, or transitional subtype of human meningiomas, and tumors were characterized by reduced merlin expression. The knowledge concerning the mechanisms driving the development of the main histopathological subtypes among grade I meningiomas could be recently expanded by generating a mouse model with inactivation of meningeal *NF2* by using the prostaglandin D2 synthase (*PGDS*) gene promoter. PGDS is a specific marker of arachnoidal cells [57]. It was demonstrated that *Nf2* inactivation in PDGS-positive meningeal progenitor cells was capable to give rise to both meningothelial and fibroblastic meningiomas in 38 % of mice [58]. Moreover, it could be demonstrated that only during a critical pre- and perinatal time frame, *NF2* inactivation in mice led to the development of meningiomas. Surprisingly, additional knockout of *p16Ink4A* or *Tp53* did not result in an increase of meningioma frequency or aggressiveness in mice, but predisposed for the development of osteosarcomas and malignant peripheral nerve sheath tumors in these animals.

Besides the inactivation of *NF2*, few other recurrent genetic alterations have been identified in benign meningiomas, and these findings are largely based on recent whole genome-sequencing approaches. Three papers published in 2013 reported that four genes are affected in a small fraction of meningiomas: *TRAF7*, *KLF4*, *AKT1*, and *SMO* [44, 59, 60]. Interestingly, all reports emphasized the relation of these alterations to both tumor localization and *NF2* status. Moreover, the high frequency of *NF2* alterations was confirmed with inactivation in 43 % of tumors [44]. Probably the most important new mutation identified is related to the *AKT1* (*v-akt murine thymoma viral oncogene homolog 1*) gene. All three reports described a hotspot mutation (p.Glu17Lsy), also named *AKT1*^{E17K} mutation. This somatic mutation occurs in breast, ovarian, and colorectal cancers [61, 62]. The mutation activates *AKT1* due to pathological location to the plasma membrane, with subsequent growth factor-independent activation of the PI3K/Akt signaling pathway [61]. In meningioma, this mutation was found nearly exclusively in 7–12 % of WHO grade I meningiomas but was (exceptionally) rare in grade II meningiomas and absent in grade III meningiomas, respectively [59, 60]. Moreover, the *AKT1*^{E17K} mutation was predominantly found in the meningothelial or transitional subtype of grade I tumors, and meningiomas harboring the *AKT1*^{E17K} mutation were of *NF2* wildtype. The exact biological role, however, of the *AKT1*^{E17K} mutation for both tumor initiation and potential target for treatment using Akt inhibitors, remain to be determined.

The *AKT1*^{E17K} mutation was also found in about 65 % of meningiomas that harbor a mutation in the *TRAF7* (*TNF receptor-associated factor 7*) gene [59]. The *TRAF7* gene is located on chromosome 16p13. It encodes a proapoptotic protein which interacts with multiple signaling pathways. *TRAF7* mutations are mutually exclusive of *NF2* mutations and occur in about 24 % of meningiomas [59]. *TRAF7* mutations are present in 93–100 % of secretory meningiomas but also in meningothelial and atypical meningiomas [63]. In addition, meningiomas with *TRAF7* mutations are almost always characterized by the mutation K409Q in the gene for the transcription factor *KLF4* (*Kruppel-like factor 4*). *KLF4* gene, located on chromosome 9q, is involved in both transcriptional activation and repression, and both oncogenic activation and tumor suppression have been reported [64]. The combined *TRAF7*/*KLF4* mutation is highly characteristic for secretory meningiomas (Fig. 17.1c) [59, 63], providing a molecular marker for this grade I subtype that is characterized clinically by extensive peritumoral edema formation [65]. In contrast to *TRAF7*, *KLF4* mutations are absent in other meningioma subtypes [63]. KLF4 is known to co-regulate the bradykinin B2 receptor. Activation of bradykinin B2 mediates the formation of brain edema and may be targeted by specific antagonists [66]. Meningiomas with *TRAF7*/*KLF4* mutations are predominantly located at the medial/lateral skull base. Interestingly, based on retained merlin staining, an *NF2*-independent molecular background of secretory meningiomas was already suggested earlier [67].

Another non-*NF2*-associated mutation of meningiomas located at the skull base affects the *SMO* (Smoothened) gene

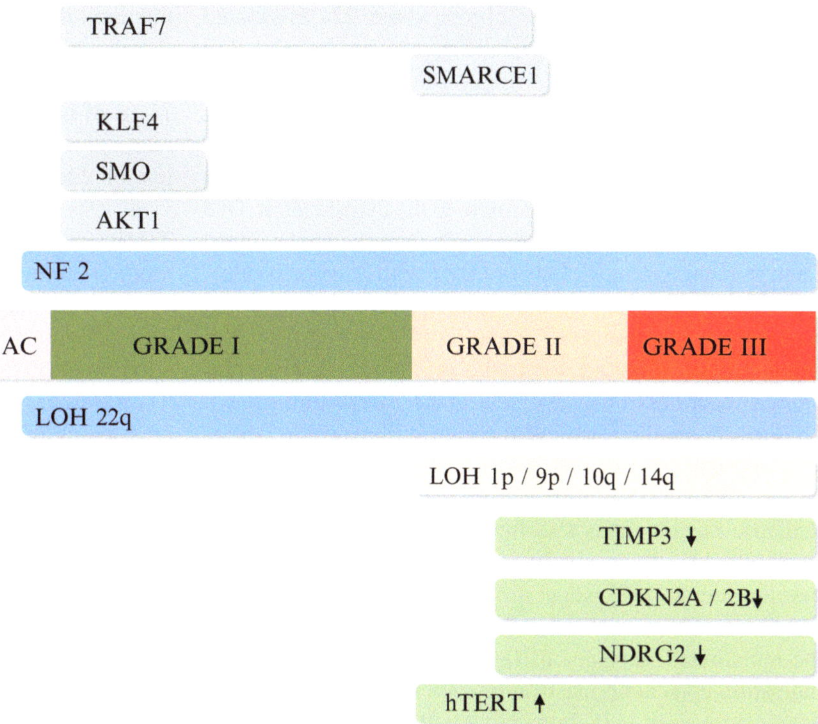

Fig. 17.2 Genetic alterations associated with meningioma development and progression. Bar lengths represent relative frequency of alterations in the given WHO group. See text for abbreviations. *AC* arachnoidal cap cell

which is a member of the hedgehog signaling pathway. *SMO* mutations occur in 4–5 % of grade I meningiomas and are restricted to the medial anterior skull base near the midline. Interestingly, *SMO* mutations are not only exclusive of *NF2* but also of *AKT1* and *TRAF7*/*KLF4* mutations, respectively [44, 59]. Although *SMO* affects only a minority of tumors, alterations of the hedgehog signaling pathway had been already reported in meningiomas. A family characterized by increased risk for meningiomas including multiple meningiomas with absent *NF2* mutations was described, in which meningiomas at different sites were associated with a mutation in the *SUFU* (*suppressor of fused homolog* [*Drosophila*]) tumor suppressor gene with dysregulated hedgehog signaling [68]. *SUFU* mutations have been found in meningiomas from patients with Gorlin syndrome [69].

While all of these mutations are mutually exclusive of *NF2* alterations, other relevant genetic alterations have been found in association with chromosome 22 in meningiomas. One interesting gene is *SMARCB1* (also named *INI1*/*hSNF5*/*BAF47*). *SMARCB1* is located on chromosome 22, and alterations are frequently found in pediatric malignant rhabdoid tumors. Screening a large group of sporadic meningiomas, including a fraction with LOH at chromosome 22, revealed that *SMARCB1* mutations occur with low frequency and might be cooperating with *NF2* mutations, because tumors harboring both *SMACRB1* and *NF2* mutations were identified [70, 71]. Meningiomas with SMARCB1 mutation are preferentially localized to the falx cerebri [72]. However, familial multiple meningiomas in non-NF2 patients are not associated with germline *SMARCB1* mutations [73].

In families with multiple spinal meningiomas and without *NF2* mutations, a loss-of-function mutation in the *SMARCE1* gene was recently identified [74]. *SMARCE1* is located on chromosome 17q21 and encodes for a 57-kDa subunit if the SWI/SNF complex which is involved in the regulation of chromatin structure by nucleosome remodeling. Loss of SMARCE1 expression was evident in immunohistochemical staining, suggesting a tumor suppressor mode of action similar to *SMARCB1*. Interestingly, the mutation only affected spinal meningiomas with histological features of clear-cell meningioma (Fig. 17.1d). This genetic alteration may be a hallmark of non-NF2 familial spinal meningiomas.

High-Grade (Malignant) Meningiomas

Meningiomas are generally thought to progress from low-grade to high-grade tumors, although this is not always easy to demonstrate clinically [75]. Histologically, progression from grade I to grade II can be confirmed in 17–38 % and from grade I/II to grade III in 54–70 %, respectively [76, 77]. At the cytogenetic level, a stepwise acquisition of chromosomal gains and losses during meningioma progression has been proposed (Fig. 17.2). As mentioned before, allelic losses at 22q12.2 (*NF2*) are regarded as an early event, and mouse models suggest that a restricted time window exists for loss of *NF2* to have tumorigenic potential [56, 58]. Comparing *NF2*-mutated and *NF2*-wildtype human meningiomas, overall chromosomal alterations are less frequent in *NF2*-wildtype compared to *NF2*-mutated tumors regardless of the histological grading, respectively [45]. This clearly indicates a greater chromosomal instability in meningiomas with *NF2* inactivation. This chromosome 22q-associated chromosomal instability has been suggested to be related to the tumor suppressor gene CHEK2, which is located near the *NF2* gene, but additional evidence will be needed to support this hypothesis [78].

The merlin protein belongs to the protein 4.1 family, with members linking membrane protein to the cytoskeleton. One gene of the protein 4.1 family has been suspected to be implicated in meningioma biology is *DAL1* with its gene product protein 4.1B. Allelic losses at 18p11.3 have been reported with frequencies between 20 and 70 % [79, 80]. Reduced protein 4.1B expression was found in about 60 % of meningiomas regardless of histological grade, suggesting protein 4.1B loss as another early event in meningioma pathogenesis [79, 81]. This is supported by the observation that nearly all tumors with *DAL-1* LOH have simultaneous *NF2* LOH [80]. Pediatric meningiomas also frequently show genetic losses of *DAL1* [3]. Interestingly, mice lacking *DAL1* do not develop tumors [82], suggesting *DAL1* alterations as early progression-associated rather than initiation steps. However, the mutational frequency of *DAL1* is low in meningiomas, indicating epigenetic inactivation as a more likely mode of gene inactivation [83]. In patients with multiple meningiomas, *DAL1* gene mutations were found in both tumor and paired blood samples, suggesting substantial differences between sporadic single and multiple meningioma patients with respect to *DAL1* [48].

Losses of 1p, 6q, 10q, 14q, 18q, as well as gains of 1q, 9q, 12q, 15q, 17q, and 20q have been proposed as important events in meningioma progression and recurrence [44, 84–88], and especially 1p and 14q loss are associated with meningioma progression [89–91]. The number of aberrations in 1p, 14q, and 22q correlates with meningioma cell proliferation index as determined by MIB1 immunohistochemical labeling, and also correlates with tumor growth and recurrence [92]. In grade I meningiomas, recurrent losses of 1p, 7p, 14p, and 19, as well as gains of chromosome 5 and 20 can be found [44]. Reduced expression of genes located on chromosome 1p, 6q, and 14q is a feature of recurrent meningiomas [93]. Of note, 1p loss is commonly found in tumors located at the convexity, but is rare in skull base or spinal meningiomas [23]. Moreover, 1p loss is associated with meningioma recurrence shorter overall survival [94]. Losses of 6q, 9p, 13 and 14 are exclusively found in highly proliferating meningiomas [95]. Loss of 18q is preferentially detected in women [91]. Comparing de novo atypical meningiomas and transformed atypical or anaplastic meningiomas, both groups share chromosome 14 and 22 alterations, while losses at chromosome 1, 10, and 18 are restricted to the progressive tumors [76]. Radiation-induced aggressive meningiomas show cytogenetic aberrations on chromosome 1p, 6q, and 22 [9].

Some of these chromosomal alterations have been associated with specific genes. Besides the *NF2* gene on chromosome 22, another tumor suppressor important for meningioma progression is the *TIMP3* (tissue inhibitor of metalloproteinase 3) gene located on 22q12. Hypermethylation of the *TIMP3* promoter was found in 17 % of benign, 22 % of atypical, and 67 % of anaplastic meningiomas and was exclusively associated with allelic loss on 22q12 [96] but seems to be not related to overall survival [94]. Comprehensive genomic studies also identified TIMP3 as a gene with significantly reduced expression in grade III compared to grade I meningiomas [97, 98]. TIMP3 protein inhibits matrix metalloproteinases, suggesting that epigenetic inactivation of TIMP3 by promoter hypermethylation might favor aggressive invasive tumor growth. TIPM3 has additional tumor suppressor activity, and in vitro overexpression of TIMP3 reduces tumor growth and induces apoptosis [99]. However, recently *TIMP3* hypermethylation was reported as not associated with tumor recurrence with no significant effect on overall survival [94].

Among other relevant candidate genes, alterations on 9p21 have been found to represent losses of the tumor suppressor genes *CDKN2A* (*p16*$^{\mathrm{INK4a}}$), *p14*^{ARF}, and *CDKN2B* (*p15*$^{\mathrm{INK4b}}$) in meningiomas [45, 100]. In anaplastic grade III meningiomas, deletions of *CDKN2A*/*CDKN2B* are associated with poorer survival [101]. However, the frequency of *CDKN2A*/*2B* promoter methylation appears to be low [100, 102, 103] and unrelated to the histological grade or risk of tumor recurrence [94].

In mouse models, deletion of *Cdkn2a*, together with *Nf2* inactivation, results in increased meningioma frequency, as well as development of grade II or grade III meningiomas, proving that loss of *CDKN2A* and *CDKN2B* is essential to generate aggressive meningiomas [104]. Interestingly, in this study the rate of pure meningothelial proliferation induced by inactivation of *Nf2* (50 %) dropped to 9 % in mice with combined *NF2*/*Cdkn2ab*, suggesting an accelerated tumorigenesis. Analysis of the *PATCH* (*Patched*) gene on chromosome 9q22 as an alternative candidate gene revealed only one mutation among nine meningiomas [105].

Amplification of the *S6 kinase* gene region on chromosome 17q23 is present in malignant meningiomas [106, 107], making the mTOR signaling pathway attractive for meningioma therapy [108]. The 14q32 region has been implicated in meningioma progression due to the maternally expressed gene 3 (*MEG3*) which has antiproliferative activity in meningiomas. *MEG3* encodes a noncoding RNA, and aggressive meningiomas show allelic losses, promoter hypermethylation, and reduced expression of MEG3 compared to normal arachnoidal cells [109, 110]. The important role of chromosome 14q loss was underlined by a study which identified *NDRG2* as a gene commonly inactivated in meningioma progression. *NDRG2* was found to be downregulated in anaplastic meningiomas, as well as in a small subset of lower-grade meningiomas and atypical meningiomas with aggressive clinical behavior. Recurrent meningiomas have also reduced NDRG2 expression levels. The reduced expression of NDRG2 is associated with promoter hypermethylation [111, 112].

LOH at chromosome 1p has been linked to few genes in meningioma. The *CDKN2C* gene was found to be deleted or mutated [100, 113]. Another candidate gene inactivated on 1p is the *TP73* gene, which was found to be aberrantly methylated in meningiomas [38]. However, these alterations are present in only a small fraction of tumors, leaving the relevant genes on chromosome 1p involved in progressive meningioma to be determined.

Hormone receptors, i.e., progesterone receptor (PR) and estrogen receptor (ER) are expressed in about 90 % and 40 % of meningiomas, respectively. Atypical and anaplastic meningiomas are characterized by a reduced incidence of ER or PR positivity, suggesting a progression-associated mechanism of hormone receptor loss [114]. Reduced expression of PR has been demonstrated in associated with increased recurrence rates and unfavorable prognosis [115]. ER-negative but PR-positive meningiomas have increased cytogenetic abnormalities on chromosome 14 and 22 [116], and meningiomas lacking PR have a higher rate of chromosome 22q loss than tumors with retained PR expression [117].

In normal cells, ends of chromosomal DNA strands are equipped with specialized DNA strands called telomeres. Telomeres are shortened during mitosis, thus limiting the life cycle of a cell. Telomerase is a reverse transcriptase using an RNA template encoded by the *hTR* gene to generate telomeric DNA. Therefore, maintenance of telomere length by telomerase activity is a prerequisite for continuous growth of tumor cells. The catalytic subunit of human telomerase is called hTERT. Telomerase activity has been reported to be another important mechanism of relevant for meningioma progression. Telomerase activity is rare in benign meningiomas, but is frequently detected in atypical and anaplastic meningiomas [118, 119]. Moreover, telomerase activity correlates with hTERT expression in meningiomas [120, 121]. Papillary meningiomas (WHO grade III) have higher hTR expression levels than atypical (grade II) or benign grade I meningiomas [122]. Clinically, telomerase activity is associated with shorter progression-free survival time [119]. Recurrent meningiomas have higher immunohistochemical hTERT expression levels compared to nonrecurrent tumors [123].

Recently, *hTERT* promoter mutations was found at high incidence exclusively in patients with meningiomas undergoing malignant histological progression (28 %), associated with a marked increase in TERT expression. *TERT* promoter mutations were found in both the lowest and the highest grade tumors [124].

DNA methylation and inactivation of gene promoters, resulting in reduced gene expression and function, represent additional mechanisms relevant to tumor growth, including meningiomas. The *O*^{6}*-methylguanine-DNA methyltransferase* (*MGMT*) promoter, which is frequently hypermethylated in malignant gliomas and associated with sensitivity to alkylating agents such as temozolomide [125], is rarely hypermethylated in meningiomas [126, 127]. In line with this observation, temozolomide has not shown any clinical activity in patients with meningiomas [128].

Recently, microRNAs (miRNAs) have been intensively studied in various tumor entities including meningiomas. Downregulation of miRNA-29c-3p, miRNA-219-5p, and miRNA-145 were found to be downregulated in aggressive meningiomas [129, 130]. Moreover, miRNA-145 expression could be clearly associated with meningioma cell invasion [130]. The miRNA-335 was attributed to meningioma cell proliferation targeting the Rb1 signaling pathway [131]. The miRNA-200a, which is downregulated in meningiomas, directly interacts with E-cadherin and the beta-catenin signaling pathway [132]. Regarding prognosis, high expression of miR-190a and low expression of miR-29c-3p and miR-219-5p was shown to be associated with increased recurrence rates in meningioma patients [129].

Gene Expression Profiling

The study of gene expression in tumors in general, and meningiomas in particular can be driven by various questions. Besides the detection of genes under- or overexpressed in meningiomas compared to non-tumoral meningeal tissue, unraveling of gene expression changes with increasing grade of malignancy is a key question to be addressed. Additional questions relate to differences between primary and recurrent meningiomas, including progressive meningiomas, or to differences between meningioma locations (spinal versus intracranial tumors). Finally, differences in gene expression depending on the primary genetic driver, predominantly *NF2*, are of high interest in meningiomas.

Starting from the earliest studies in 2002, a number of genes have been described to be associated with higher grades of malignancy in meningioma. In general, genes related to the insulin signaling pathway (IGF2, IGFBP-3, IGFBP-7, AKT3), the MAPK pathway, cell adhesion pathways, extracellular matrix remodeling-associated genes, Notch signaling, and the wingless (wnt) pathway were identified as overexpressed in high-grade meningiomas [98, 133–138]. In contrast, malignant meningiomas have been shown to have reduced expression of TGF-beta signaling components, TIMP3 and KCNMA1 [95, 97]. Moreover, the loss of NDRG2 as a feature of anaplastic meningiomas was identified by an Affymetrix U133A/B GenChip microarray [111]. Regardless of WHO grading, meningiomas can be separated into a "low-proliferative" and "high-proliferative" group based on the combination of gene expression profiling and array comparative genomic hybridization (aCGH). This is especially interesting because atypical meningiomas WHO grade II can fall in one or another of these group, while all grade I meningiomas are low proliferative and all grade III meningiomas are high proliferative [95]. Gene expression profile also differs between infiltrative and non-infiltrative meningiomas [139]. Combining data from gene expression profiling, copy number alterations, and clinicopathological information, five meningioma subgroups can be defined: while group 1 is characterized by benign histology and the absence of chromosomal losses, group 5 contains mainly grade II and grade III meningiomas and displays a high number of chromosomal losses. Interestingly, the designated group 3 contained meningiomas with all grades of malignancy but clustered especially with recurrent meningiomas. Group 2 and 4 consisted mainly of grade I or grade II/III meningiomas with variable degree of chromosomal losses, respectively. This study also showed for the first time that gene expression between meningiomas is highly variable in general [91].

One initial study reported different gene expression profiles between histological subtypes among grade I meningiomas. Additionally, an increased prevalence of *NF2* alterations in transitional/fibroblastic meningiomas was confirmed [47]. Compared to meningothelial meningiomas, fibroblastic meningiomas have a unique gene expression signature with differences in the genes BMPR1B, RAMP1, DMD, as well as genes involved in extracellular matrix remodeling like MMP-2 and Tenascin-C [98, 140]. Moreover, the expression profiles from infiltrative and non-infiltrative meningiomas appear to be different [139]. Moreover, there is an upregulation of genes related to the PI3K/AKT and TGF-beta signaling pathways in fibroblastic meningioma [138]. Different expression profiles between spinal and intracranial meningiomas have been reported, showing overexpression of transcription factors involved in cell proliferation and differentiation in spinal meningiomas [141].

Interestingly, the cytogenetically well-characterized prognostic groups, i.e., loss of chromosome 22 or deletion of 1p and 14q, can be matched with specific tumor-related gene expression profiles, and the expression profiles are more closely related to patient outcome than purely histology [142, 143]. In recurrent meningiomas, loss of chromosome 1p, 6q, and 14q is related to downregulation of genes involved in several pathways such as Notch, TGF-beta, WNT, PDGF, and PPAR signaling, as well as in cell cycle control and oxidative phosphorylation [93, 144]. Increased expression of Topoisomerase-2alpha in grade II meningiomas identified by gene expression analyses was found to be associated with reduced overall survival compared to patients with low Topoisomerase-2alpha expression levels [97]. Relapsing grade I meningiomas have reduced leptin receptor (LEPR) and cyclin-dependent kinases regulatory subunit 2 gene (CKS2) expression, and the C/L-index was proposed to define meningioma patients at risk for tumor relapse [145]. Altered expression of genes regulating tumor metabolism was identified as another risk factor influencing recurrence of histologically benign meningiomas [146]. Radiation-induced meningiomas, in contrast, do not appear to have a gene expression profile that can be distinguished from spontaneous meningiomas [147].

Prognostic Stratification

One of the strongest factors influencing tumor recurrence and overall prognosis is the histological tumor grading according to the WHO criteria [27]. High MIB-1 labeling index is another marker of poor prognosis [148]. Losses of 1p and 14q represent important steps for meningioma progression and, therefore, have poor prognostic implication [89–91, 94, 149–151]. Patients with tumor size over 50 mm and combined loss of 1p and 14q have been shown to represent a subgroup at high risk for early relapse [152]. Furthermore, relapse-free survival is negatively associated with male gender, presence of brain edema, intraventricular and anterior cranial base tumor location, age below 55 years, and tumor size larger than 50 mm [153]. Loss of progesterone receptor expression also indicates an unfavorable prognosis [115].

Molecular Signaling Pathways

Molecular signaling pathways, including those involved in mitogenic signal transduction, have been studied intensively in meningiomas. Nearly all of the growth factor receptors/kinases known to be involved in tumor growth have been described to be expressed in meningiomas, including epidermal growth factor receptor (EGFR), platelet-derived growth factor beta receptor (PDGFR), vascular endothelial growth factor receptor (VEGFR), and insulin-like growth factor receptor (IGFR) [154–157]. Activation of these receptors by their cognate ligands drives intracellular signaling cascades involved in a plethora of cellular functions. Mitogenic signals of EGFR and PDGFR are usually transduced by activation of the Ras-Raf-Mek-MAPK pathway. It was demonstrated that this signaling pathway is indeed activated in meningiomas [158, 159]. The PI3K-AKT/protein kinase B—p70 signaling pathway is another important mediator of growth-favoring signals in meningiomas [108, 159, 160]. The mTOR signaling pathway is of relevance for *NF2* mutant meningiomas, as well as meningiomas with other mechanisms of mTOR pathway activation, such as *S6K* gene amplification [106, 107]. Merlin (*NF2*) is a negative regulator of the mTORC1 kinase complex, and constitutive activation of mTORC1 signaling is present in meningioma cells from NF2 patients [161, 162]. Other signaling pathways shown to be activated in meningiomas include the phospholipase A2-arachidonic acid-cyclooxygenase pathway [163, 164] and the PLC-gamma1-PKC pathway [159, 165]. The TGF-beta–SMAD signaling pathway represents an inhibitory mechanism, and TGF-beta, as well as the TGF-beta receptor, are expressed in meningiomas [166–168].

Molecular Targeted Therapies

Due to the lack of efficacy of conventional chemotherapy in meningiomas, targeting signaling pathways by novel inhibitors offers therapeutic opportunities. These approaches are based on the characterization of signaling pathways and their growth factor receptors in meningiomas and meningioma cells. Indeed, some clinical trials have been performed already, however, with limited success thus far. The PDGF alpha/beta inhibitor imatinib mesylate was tested in a phase II study and was well tolerated, but had no significant activity [169]. Combining imatinib with hydroxyurea, a substance with a long history in meningioma chemotherapy, in recurrent or progressive meningiomas showed only very modest activity [170]. Gefitinib and erlotinib, both inhibitors of EGFR, were evaluated in recurrent meningiomas but failed to have significant anti-meningioma activity [171]. Inhibition of angiogenesis by targeting VEGF has been studied in a few retrospective series with encouraging results, but phase II trials have not been performed [172]. The tyrosine kinase inhibitor sunitinib, targeting both the VEGF and PDGF system, was studied in recurrent meningiomas, achieving disease stabilization. The same holds true for the combined VEGF/PDGF inhibitor vatalanib (summarized in [173]). No therapeutic clinical studies have been performed to test mTOR-inhibitors such as temsirolimus or everolimus, although preclinical data supports this approach [108]. A pharmacokinetic/pharmacodynamics "phase 0" study to explore the activity of everolimus in human meningiomas in vivo is ongoing (ClinicalTrials.gov identifier NCT01880749), and may provide valuable insights into mTOR inhibition as a potential clinical strategy. As of today, however, no chemotherapy or molecular targeted therapies have proven to be clinically active in meningiomas, leaving surgery and radiation therapy as the only standard treatment options [174].

The recently identified, novel mutations and activated signaling pathways in subsets of meningiomas provide opportunities for future development of targeted therapies, but the appropriate selection of target populations will require access to routine molecular genetic testing. It is also hoped that the ongoing efforts of developing therapies inhibiting oncogenic signaling pathways that are activated by the loss of Merlin (*NF2*) will be of benefit not only to NF2 patients, but also to the large subset of patients with sporadic meningiomas driven by *NF2* loss [175, 176].

References

1. Ostrom QT, Gittleman H, Farah P, Ondracek A, Chen Y, Wolinsky Y, et al. CBTRUS statistical report: primary brain and central nervous system tumors diagnosed in the United States in 2006–2010. Neuro Oncol. 2013;15 Suppl 2:ii1–56.
2. Tufan K, Dogulu F, Kurt G, Emmez H, Ceviker N, Baykaner MK. Intracranial meningiomas of childhood and adolescence. Pediatr Neurosurg. 2005;41(1):1–7.
3. Perry A, Giannini C, Raghavan R, Scheithauer BW, Banerjee R, Margraf L, et al. Aggressive phenotypic and genotypic features in pediatric and NF2-associated meningiomas: a clinicopathologic study of 53 cases. J Neuropathol Exp Neurol. 2001;60(10): 994–1003.
4. Klaeboe L, Lonn S, Scheie D, Auvinen A, Christensen HC, Feychting M, et al. Incidence of intracranial meningiomas in Denmark, Finland, Norway and Sweden, 1968–1997. Int J Cancer. 2005;117(6):996–1001.
5. Sadetzki S, Flint-Richter P, Ben-Tal T. Radiation induced meningioma: a descriptive study of 253 cases. J Neurosurg. 2002; 97:1078–82.
6. Schneider B, Pulhorn H, Rohrig B, Rainov NG. Predisposing conditions and risk factors for development of symptomatic meningioma in adults. Cancer Detect Prev. 2005;29(5):440–7.
7. Flint-Richter P, Mandelzweig L, Oberman B, Sadetzki S. Possible interaction between ionizing radiation, smoking, and gender in the causation of meningioma. Neuro Oncol. 2011;13(3):345–52.
8. Benson VS, Pirie K, Schuz J, Reeves GK, Beral V, Green J. Mobile phone use and risk of brain neoplasms and other cancers: prospective study. Int J Epidemiol. 2013;42(3):792–802.
9. Al-Mefty O, Topsakal C, Pravdenkova S, Sawyer JR, Harrison MJ. Radiation-induced meningiomas: clinical, pathological, cytokinetic, and cytogenetic characteristics. J Neurosurg. 2004;100(6): 1002–13.
10. Flint-Richter P, Sadetzki S. Genetic predisposition for the development of radiation-associated meningioma: an epidemiological study. Lancet Oncol. 2007;8(5):403–10.
11. Elbabaa SK, Gokden M, Crawford JR, Kesari S, Saad AG. Radiation-associated meningiomas in children: clinical, pathological, and cytogenetic characteristics with a critical review of the literature. J Neurosurg Pediatr. 2012;10(4):281–90.
12. Antinheimo J, Sankila R, Carpen O, Pukkala E, Sainio M, Jaaskelainen J. Population-based analysis of sporadic and type 2 neurofibromatosis-associated meningiomas and schwannomas. Neurology. 2000;54(1):71–6.
13. Hemminki K, Li X. Familial risks in nervous system tumors. Cancer Epidemiol Biomarkers Prev. 2003;12(11 Pt 1):1137–42.
14. Smith MJ, Higgs JE, Bowers NL, Halliday D, Paterson J, Gillespie J, et al. Cranial meningiomas in 411 neurofibromatosis type 2 (NF2) patients with proven gene mutations: clear positional effect of mutations, but absence of female severity effect on age at onset. J Med Genet. 2011;48(4):261–5.
15. Albrecht S, Goodman JC, Rajagopolan S, Levy M, Cech DA, Cooley LD. Malignant meningioma in Gorlin's syndrome: cytogenetic and p53 gene analysis. Case report. J Neurosurg. 1994; 81(3):466–71.
16. Lindboe CF, Helseth E, Myhr G. Lhermitte-Duclos disease and giant meningioma as manifestations of Cowden's disease. Clin Neuropathol. 1995;14(6):327–30.
17. De Moura J, Kavalec FL, Doghman M, Rosati R, Custodio G, Lalli E, et al. Heterozygous TP53stop146/R72P fibroblasts from a Li-Fraumeni syndrome patient with impaired response to DNA damage. Int J Oncol. 2010;36(4):983–90.
18. Marini F, Falchetti A, Del Monte F, Carbonell Sala S, Gozzini A, Luzi E, et al. Multiple endocrine neoplasia type 1. Orphanet J Rare Dis. 2006;1:38.
19. Mawrin C, Perry A. Pathological classification and molecular genetics of meningiomas. J Neurooncol. 2010;99(3):379–91.
20. Catala M. Embryonic and fetal development of structures associated with the cerebro-spinal fluid in man and other species. Part I: the ventricular system, meninges and choroid plexuses. Arch Anat Cytol Pathol. 1998;46(3):153–69.
21. Kros J, de Greve K, van Tilborg A, Hop W, Pieterman H, Avezaat C, et al. NF2 status of meningiomas is associated with tumour localization and histology. J Pathol. 2001;194(3):367–72.

22. Lee JH, Sade B, Choi E, Golubic M, Prayson R. Meningothelioma as the predominant histological subtype of midline skull base and spinal meningioma. J Neurosurg. 2006;105(1):60–4.
23. Ketter R, Rahnenfuhrer J, Henn W, Kim Y, Feiden W, Steudel W, et al. Correspondence of tumor localization with tumor recurrence and cytogenetic progression in meningiomas. Neurosurgery. 2008;62(1):61–9.
24. Pearson BE, Markert JM, Fisher WS, Guthrie BL, Fiveash JB, Palmer CA, et al. Hitting a moving target: evolution of a treatment paradigm for atypical meningiomas amid changing diagnostic criteria. Neurosurg Focus. 2008;24(5):E3.
25. Durand A, Labrousse F, Jouvet A, Bauchet L, Kalamarides M, Menei P, et al. WHO grade II and III meningiomas: a study of prognostic factors. J Neurooncol. 2009;95(3):367–75.
26. Perry A, Scheithauer BW, Stafford SL, Lohse CM, Wollan PC. "Malignancy" in meningiomas: a clinicopathologic study of 116 patients, with grading implications. Cancer. 1999;85(9):2046–56.
27. Perry A, Stafford S, Scheithauer B. Meningioma grading: an analysis of histologic parameters. Am J Surg Pathol. 1997;22:1482–90.
28. Zang KD, Singer H. Chromosomal constitution of meningiomas. Nature. 1967;216(5110):84–5.
29. Rouleau GA, Merel P, Lutchman M, Sanson M, Zucman J, Marineau C, et al. Alteration in a new gene encoding a putative membrane-organizing protein causes neuro-fibromatosis type 2. Nature. 1993;363(6429):515–21.
30. Trofatter JA, MacCollin MM, Rutter JL, Murrell JR, Duyao MP, Parry DM, et al. A novel moesin-, ezrin-, radixin-like gene is a candidate for the neurofibromatosis 2 tumor suppressor. Cell. 1993;72(5):791–800.
31. Evans DG, Huson SM, Donnai D, Neary W, Blair V, Teare D, et al. A genetic study of type 2 neurofibromatosis in the United Kingdom. I. Prevalence, mutation rate, fitness, and confirmation of maternal transmission effect on severity. J Med Genet. 1992; 29(12):841–6.
32. Seizinger BR, de la Monte S, Atkins L, Gusella JF, Martuza RL. Molecular genetic approach to human meningioma: loss of genes on chromosome 22. Proc Natl Acad Sci U S A. 1987;84(15): 5419–23.
33. Dumanski JP, Carlbom E, Collins VP, Nordenskjold M. Deletion mapping of a locus on human chromosome 22 involved in the oncogenesis of meningioma. Proc Natl Acad Sci U S A. 1987; 84(24):9275–9.
34. Ruttledge MH, Xie YG, Han FY, Peyrard M, Collins VP, Nordenskjold M, et al. Deletions on chromosome 22 in sporadic meningioma. Genes Chromosomes Cancer. 1994;10(2):122–30.
35. Dumanski JP, Rouleau GA, Nordenskjold M, Collins VP. Molecular genetic analysis of chromosome 22 in 81 cases of meningioma. Cancer Res. 1990;50(18):5863–7.
36. Ruttledge MH, Sarrazin J, Rangaratnam S, Phelan CM, Twist E, Merel P, et al. Evidence for the complete inactivation of the NF2 gene in the majority of sporadic meningiomas. Nat Genet. 1994;6(2):180–4.
37. Gutmann DH, Giordano MJ, Fishback AS, Guha A. Loss of merlin expression in sporadic meningiomas, ependymomas and schwannomas. Neurology. 1997;49(1):267–70.
38. Lomas J, Bello MJ, Arjona D, Alonso ME, Martinez-Glez V, Lopez-Marin I, et al. Genetic and epigenetic alteration of the NF2 gene in sporadic meningiomas. Genes Chromosomes Cancer. 2005;42(3):314–9.
39. Hansson CM, Buckley PG, Grigelioniene G, Piotrowski A, Hellstrom AR, Mantripragada K, et al. Comprehensive genetic and epigenetic analysis of sporadic meningioma for macro-mutations on 22q and micro-mutations within the NF2 locus. BMC Genomics. 2007;8:16.
40. Kimura Y, Koga H, Araki N, Mugita N, Fujita N, Takeshima H, et al. The involvement of calpain-dependent proteolysis of the tumor suppressor NF2 (merlin) in schwannomas and meningiomas. Nat Med. 1998;4(8):915–22.
41. van Tilborg AA, Morolli B, Giphart-Gassler M, de Vries A, van Geenen DA, Lurkin I, et al. Lack of genetic and epigenetic changes in meningiomas without NF2 loss. J Pathol. 2006;208(4): 564–73.
42. Curto M, McClatchey AI. Nf2/Merlin: a coordinator of receptor signalling and intercellular contact. Br J Cancer. 2008;98(2): 256–62.
43. Wellenreuther R, Kraus JA, Lenartz D, Menon AG, Schramm J, Louis DN, et al. Analysis of the neurofibromatosis 2 gene reveals molecular variants of meningioma. Am J Pathol. 1995;146(4): 827–32.
44. Brastianos PK, Horowitz PM, Santagata S, Jones RT, McKenna A, Getz G, et al. Genomic sequencing of meningiomas identifies oncogenic SMO and AKT1 mutations. Nat Genet. 2013;45(3): 285–9.
45. Goutagny S, Yang HW, Zucman-Rossi J, Chan J, Dreyfuss JM, Park PJ, et al. Genomic profiling reveals alternative genetic pathways of meningioma malignant progression dependent on the underlying NF2 status. Clin Cancer Res. 2010;16(16):4155–64.
46. Hartmann C, Sieberns J, Gehlhaar C, Simon M, Paulus W, von Deimling A. NF2 mutations in secretory and other rare variants of meningiomas. Brain Pathol. 2006;16(1):15–9.
47. Wada K, Maruno M, Suzuki T, Kagawa N, Hashiba T, Fujimoto Y, et al. Chromosomal and genetic aberrations differ with meningioma subtype. Brain Tumor Pathol. 2004;21(3):127–33.
48. Heinrich B, Hartmann C, Stemmer-Rachamimov AO, Louis DN, MacCollin M. Multiple meningiomas: investigating the molecular basis of sporadic and familial forms. Int J Cancer. 2003; 103(4):483–8.
49. Nahser HC, Grote W, Lohr E, Gerhard L. Multiple meningiomas. Clinical and computer tomographic observations. Neuroradiology. 1981;21(5):259–63.
50. Larson JJ, Tew Jr JM, Simon M, Menon AG. Evidence for clonal spread in the development of multiple meningiomas. J Neurosurg. 1995;83(4):705–9.
51. Stangl AP, Wellenreuther R, Lenartz D, Kraus JA, Menon AG, Schramm J, et al. Clonality of multiple meningiomas. J Neurosurg. 1997;86(5):853–8.
52. Goutagny S, Kalamarides M. Meningiomas and neurofibromatosis. J Neurooncol. 2010;99(3):341–7.
53. Kluwe L, Mautner V, Heinrich B, Dezube R, Jacoby LB, Friedrich RE, et al. Molecular study of frequency of mosaicism in neurofibromatosis 2 patients with bilateral vestibular schwannomas. J Med Genet. 2003;40(2):109–14.
54. Evans DG, Watson C, King A, Wallace AJ, Baser ME. Multiple meningiomas: differential involvement of the NF2 gene in children and adults. J Med Genet. 2005;42(1):45–8.
55. Hsieh HY, Wu T, Wang CJ, Chin SC, Chen YR. Neurological complications involving the central nervous system in neurofibromatosis type 1. Acta Neurol Taiwan. 2007;16(2):68–73.
56. Kalamarides M, Niwa-Kawakita M, Leblois H, Abramowski V, Perricaudet M, Janin A, et al. Nf2 gene inactivation in arachnoidal cells is rate-limiting for meningioma development in the mouse. Genes Dev. 2002;16(9):1060–5.
57. Kawashima M, Suzuki SO, Yamashima T, Fukui M, Iwaki T. Prostaglandin D synthase (beta-trace) in meningeal hemangiopericytoma. Mod Pathol. 2001;14(3):197–201.
58. Kalamarides M, Stemmer-Rachamimov AO, Niwa-Kawakita M, Chareyre F, Taranchon E, Han ZY, et al. Identification of a progenitor cell of origin capable of generating diverse meningioma histological subtypes. Oncogene. 2011;30(20):2333–44.

59. Clark VE, Erson-Omay EZ, Serin A, Yin J, Cotney J, Ozduman K, et al. Genomic analysis of non-NF2 meningiomas reveals mutations in TRAF7, KLF4, AKT1, and SMO. Science. 2013; 339(6123):1077–80.
60. Sahm F, Bissel J, Koelsche C, Schweizer L, Capper D, Reuss D, et al. AKT1E17K mutations cluster with meningothelial and transitional meningiomas and can be detected by SFRP1 immunohistochemistry. Acta Neuropathol. 2013;2013:6.
61. Carpten JD, Faber AL, Horn C, Donoho GP, Briggs SL, Robbins CM, et al. A transforming mutation in the pleckstrin homology domain of AKT1 in cancer. Nature. 2007;448(7152):439–44.
62. Bleeker FE, Felicioni L, Buttitta F, Lamba S, Cardone L, Rodolfo M, et al. AKT1(E17K) in human solid tumours. Oncogene. 2008;27(42):5648–50.
63. Reuss DE, Piro RM, Jones DT, Simon M, Ketter R, Kool M, et al. Secretory meningiomas are defined by combined KLF4 K409Q and TRAF7 mutations. Acta Neuropathol. 2013;125(3):351–8.
64. Rowland BD, Peeper DS. KLF4, p21 and context-dependent opposing forces in cancer. Nat Rev Cancer. 2006;6(1):11–23.
65. Kamp MA, Beseoglu K, Eicker S, Steiger HJ, Hanggi D. Secretory meningiomas: systematic analysis of epidemiological, clinical, and radiological features. Acta Neurochir (Wien). 2011; 153(3):457–65.
66. Stover JF, Dohse NK, Unterberg AW. Significant reduction in brain swelling by administration of nonpeptide kinin B2 receptor antagonist LF 16-0687Ms after controlled cortical impact injury in rats. J Neurosurg. 2000;92(5):853–9.
67. Buccoliero AM, Gheri CF, Castiglione F, Ammannati F, Gallina P, Taddei A, et al. Merlin expression in secretory meningiomas: evidence of an NF2-independent pathogenesis? Immunohistochemical study. Appl Immunohistochem Mol Morphol. 2007;15(3):353–7.
68. Aavikko M, Li SP, Saarinen S, Alhopuro P, Kaasinen E, Morgunova E, et al. Loss of SUFU function in familial multiple meningioma. Am J Hum Genet. 2012;91(3):520–6.
69. Kijima C, Miyashita T, Suzuki M, Oka H, Fujii K. Two cases of nevoid basal cell carcinoma syndrome associated with meningioma caused by a PTCH1 or SUFU germline mutation. Fam Cancer. 2012;11(4):565–70.
70. Schmitz U, Mueller W, Weber M, Sevenet N, Delattre O, von Deimling A. INI1 mutations in meningiomas at a potential hotspot in exon 9. Br J Cancer. 2001;84(2):199–201.
71. Rieske P, Zakrzewska M, Piaskowski S, Jaskolski D, Sikorska B, Papierz W, et al. Molecular heterogeneity of meningioma with INI1 mutation. Mol Pathol. 2003;56(5):299–301.
72. van den Munckhof P, Christiaans I, Kenter SB, Baas F, Hulsebos TJ. Germline SMARCB1 mutation predisposes to multiple meningiomas and schwannomas with preferential location of cranial meningiomas at the falx cerebri. Neurogenetics. 2012;13(1):1–7.
73. Hadfield KD, Smith MJ, Trump D, Newman WG, Evans DG. SMARCB1 mutations are not a common cause of multiple meningiomas. J Med Genet. 2010;47(8):567–8.
74. Smith MJ, O'Sullivan J, Bhaskar SS, Hadfield KD, Poke G, Caird J, et al. Loss-of-function mutations in SMARCE1 cause an inherited disorder of multiple spinal meningiomas. Nat Genet. 2013;45(3):295–8.
75. Al-Mefty O, Kadri PA, Pravdenkova S, Sawyer JR, Stangeby C, Husain M. Malignant progression in meningioma: documentation of a series and analysis of cytogenetic findings. J Neurosurg. 2004;101(2):210–8.
76. Krayenbuhl N, Pravdenkova S, Al-Mefty O. De novo versus transformed atypical and anaplastic meningiomas: comparisons of clinical course, cytogenetics, cytokinetics, and outcome. Neurosurgery. 2007;61(3):495–503; discussion 503–4.
77. Yang SY, Park CK, Park SH, Kim DG, Chung YS, Jung HW. Atypical and anaplastic meningiomas: prognostic implications of clinicopathological features. J Neurol Neurosurg Psychiatry. 2008;79(5):574–80.
78. Yang HW, Kim TM, Song SS, Shrinath N, Park R, Kalamarides M, et al. Alternative splicing of CHEK2 and codeletion with NF2 promote chromosomal instability in meningioma. Neoplasia. 2012;14(1):20–8.
79. Gutmann C, Donahoe J, Perry A. Loss of DAL-1, a second protein 4.1 tumor suppressor, is an important early event in the pathogenesis of meningioma. Hum Mol Genet. 2000;9:1495–500.
80. Nunes F, Shen Y, Niida Y, Beauchamp R, Stemmer-Rachamimov AO, Ramesh V, et al. Inactivation patterns of NF2 and DAL-1/4.1B (EPB41L3) in sporadic meningioma. Cancer Genet Cytogenet. 2005;162(2):135–9.
81. Perry A, Cai D, Scheithauer B, Swanson P, Lohse C, Newsham I, et al. Merlin, DAL-1, and progesterone receptor expression in clinicopathologic subsets of meningioma: a correlative immunohistochemical study of 175 cases. J Neuropathol Exp Neurol. 2000;59(10):872–9.
82. Yi C, McCarty JH, Troutman SA, Eckman MS, Bronson RT, Kissil JL. Loss of the putative tumor suppressor band 4.1B/Dal1 gene is dispensable for normal development and does not predispose to cancer. Mol Cell Biol. 2005;25(22):10052–9.
83. Martinez-Glez V, Bello MJ, Franco-Hernandez C, De Campos JM, Isla A, Vaquero J, et al. Mutational analysis of the DAL-1/4.1B tumour-suppressor gene locus in meningiomas. Int J Mol Med. 2005;16(4):771–4.
84. Simon M, von Deimling A, Larson JJ, Wellenreuther R, Kaskel P, Waha A, et al. Allelic losses on chromosomes 14, 10, and 1 in atypical and malignant meningiomas: a genetic model of meningioma progression. Cancer Res. 1995;55(20):4696–701.
85. Weber RG, Bostrom J, Wolter M, Baudis M, Collins VP, Reifenberger G, et al. Analysis of genomic alterations in benign, atypical, and anaplastic meningiomas: toward a genetic model of meningioma progression. Proc Natl Acad Sci U S A. 1997; 94(26):14719–24.
86. Gabeau-Lacet D, Engler D, Gupta S, Scangas GA, Betensky RA, Barker II FG, et al. Genomic profiling of atypical meningiomas associates gain of 1q with poor clinical outcome. J Neuropathol Exp Neurol. 2009;68(10):1155–65.
87. Krupp W, Holland H, Koschny R, Bauer M, Schober R, Kirsten H, et al. Genome-wide genetic characterization of an atypical meningioma by single-nucleotide polymorphism array-based mapping and classical cytogenetics. Cancer Genet Cytogenet. 2008; 184(2):87–93.
88. Lee JY, Finkelstein S, Hamilton RL, Rekha R, King Jr JT, Omalu B. Loss of heterozygosity analysis of benign, atypical, and anaplastic meningiomas. Neurosurgery. 2004;55(5):1163–73.
89. Ishino S, Hashimoto N, Fushiki S, Date K, Mori T, Fujimoto M, et al. Loss of material from chromosome arm 1p during malignant progression of meningioma revealed by fluorescent in situ hybridization. Cancer. 1998;83(2):360–6.
90. Sulman EP, White PS, Brodeur GM. Genomic annotation of the meningioma tumor suppressor locus on chromosome 1p34. Oncogene. 2004;23(4):1014–20.
91. Lee Y, Liu J, Patel S, Cloughesy T, Lai A, Farooqi H, et al. Genomic landscape of meningiomas. Brain Pathol. 2010;20(4): 751–62.
92. Pfisterer WK, Coons SW, Aboul-Enein F, Hendricks WP, Scheck AC, Preul MC. Implicating chromosomal aberrations with meningioma growth and recurrence: results from FISH and MIB-I analysis of grades I and II meningioma tissue. J Neurooncol. 2008; 87(1):43–50.
93. Perez-Magan E, Rodriguez de Lope A, Ribalta T, Ruano Y, Campos-Martin Y, Perez-Bautista G, et al. Differential expression profiling analyses identifies downregulation of 1p, 6q, and 14q

genes and overexpression of 6p histone cluster 1 genes as markers of recurrence in meningiomas. Neuro Oncol. 2010;12(12):1278–90.

94. Linsler S, Kraemer D, Driess C, Oertel J, Kammers K, Rahnenfuhrer J, et al. Molecular biological determinations of meningioma progression and recurrence. PLoS One. 2014;9(4):e94987.
95. Carvalho LH, Smirnov I, Baia GS, Modrusan Z, Smith JS, Jun P, et al. Molecular signatures define two main classes of meningiomas. Mol Cancer. 2007;6(64):64.
96. Barski D, Wolter M, Reifenberger G, Riemenschneider MJ. Hypermethylation and transcriptional downregulation of the TIMP3 gene is associated with allelic loss on 22q12.3 and malignancy in meningiomas. Brain Pathol. 2010;20(3):623–31.
97. Stuart JE, Lusis EA, Scheck AC, Coons SW, Lal A, Perry A, et al. Identification of gene markers associated with aggressive meningioma by filtering across multiple sets of gene expression arrays. J Neuropathol Exp Neurol. 2011;70(1):1–12.
98. Fevre-Montange M, Champier J, Durand A, Wierinckx A, Honnorat J, Guyotat J, et al. Microarray gene expression profiling in meningiomas: differential expression according to grade or histopathological subtype. Int J Oncol. 2009;35(6):1395–407.
99. Bian J, Wang Y, Smith MR, Kim H, Jacobs C, Jackman J, et al. Suppression of in vivo tumor growth and induction of suspension cell death by tissue inhibitor of metalloproteinases (TIMP)-3. Carcinogenesis. 1996;17(9):1805–11.
100. Bostrom J, Meyer-Puttlitz B, Wolter M, Blaschke B, Weber RG, Lichter P, et al. Alterations of the tumor suppressor genes CDKN2A (p16(INK4a)), p14(ARF), CDKN2B (p15(INK4b)), and CDKN2C (p18(INK4c)) in atypical and anaplastic meningiomas. Am J Pathol. 2001;159(2):661–9.
101. Perry A, Banerjee R, Lohse CM, Kleinschmidt-DeMasters BK, Scheithauer BW. A role for chromosome 9p21 deletions in the malignant progression of meningiomas and the prognosis of anaplastic meningiomas. Brain Pathol. 2002;12(2):183–90.
102. Tse JY, Ng HK, Lo KW, Chong EY, Lam PY, Ng EK, et al. Analysis of cell cycle regulators: p16INK4A, pRb, and CDK4 in low- and high-grade meningiomas. Hum Pathol. 1998;29(11):1200–7.
103. Liu Y, Pang JC, Dong S, Mao B, Poon WS, Ng HK. Aberrant CpG island hypermethylation profile is associated with atypical and anaplastic meningiomas. Hum Pathol. 2005;36(4):416–25.
104. Peyre M, Stemmer-Rachamimov A, Clermont-Taranchon E, Quentin S, El-Taraya N, Walczak C, et al. Meningioma progression in mice triggered by Nf2 and Cdkn2ab inactivation. Oncogene. 2013;32(36):4264–72.
105. Xie J, Johnson RL, Zhang X, Bare JW, Waldman FM, Cogen PH, et al. Mutations of the PATCHED gene in several types of sporadic extracutaneous tumors. Cancer Res. 1997;57(12):2369–72.
106. Cai DX, James CD, Scheithauer BW, Couch FJ, Perry A. PS6K amplification characterizes a small subset of anaplastic meningiomas. Am J Clin Pathol. 2001;115(2):213–8.
107. Surace EI, Lusis E, Haipek CA, Gutmann DH. Functional significance of S6K overexpression in meningioma progression. Ann Neurol. 2004;56(2):295–8.
108. Pachow D, Andrae N, Kliese N, Angenstein F, Stork O, Wilisch-Neumann A, et al. mTORC1 inhibitors suppress meningioma growth in mouse models. Clin Cancer Res. 2013;19(5):1180–9.
109. Zhang X, Gejman R, Mahta A, Zhong Y, Rice KA, Zhou Y, et al. Maternally expressed gene 3, an imprinted noncoding RNA gene, is associated with meningioma pathogenesis and progression. Cancer Res. 2010;70(6):2350–8.
110. Balik V, Srovnal J, Sulla I, Kalita O, Foltanova T, Vaverka M, et al. MEG3: a novel long noncoding potentially tumour-suppressing RNA in meningiomas. J Neurooncol. 2013;112(1):1–8.
111. Lusis EA, Watson MA, Chicoine MR, Lyman M, Roerig P, Reifenberger G, et al. Integrative genomic analysis identifies NDRG2 as a candidate tumor suppressor gene frequently inactivated in clinically aggressive meningioma. Cancer Res. 2005;65(16):7121–6.
112. Skiriute D, Tamasauskas S, Asmoniene V, Saferis V, Skauminas K, Deltuva V, et al. Tumor grade-related NDRG2 gene expression in primary and recurrent intracranial meningiomas. J Neurooncol. 2011;102(1):89–94.
113. Santarius T, Kirsch M, Nikas DC, Imitola J, Black PM. Molecular analysis of alterations of the p18INK4c gene in human meningiomas. Neuropathol Appl Neurobiol. 2000;26(1):67–75.
114. Korhonen K, Salminen T, Raitanen J, Auvinen A, Isola J, Haapasalo H. Female predominance in meningiomas can not be explained by differences in progesterone, estrogen, or androgen receptor expression. J Neurooncol. 2006;80(1):1–7.
115. Maiuri F, De Caro MB, Esposito F, Cappabianca P, Strazzullo V, Pettinato G, et al. Recurrences of meningiomas: predictive value of pathological features and hormonal and growth factors. J Neurooncol. 2007;82(1):63–8.
116. Pravdenkova S, Al-Mefty O, Sawyer J, Husain M. Progesterone and estrogen receptors: opposing prognostic indicators in meningiomas. J Neurosurg. 2006;105(2):163–73.
117. Claus EB, Park PJ, Carroll R, Chan J, Black PM. Specific genes expressed in association with progesterone receptors in meningioma. Cancer Res. 2008;68(1):314–22.
118. Langford LA, Piatyszek MA, Xu R, Schold Jr SC, Wright WE, Shay JW. Telomerase activity in ordinary meningiomas predicts poor outcome. Hum Pathol. 1997;28(4):416–20.
119. Leuraud P, Dezamis E, Aguirre-Cruz L, Taillibert S, Lejeune J, Robin E, et al. Prognostic value of allelic losses and telomerase activity in meningiomas. J Neurosurg. 2004;100(2):303–9.
120. Simon M, Park TW, Leuenroth S, Hans VH, Loning T, Schramm J. Telomerase activity and expression of the telomerase catalytic subunit, hTERT, in meningioma progression. J Neurosurg. 2000;92(5):832–40.
121. Simon M, Park TW, Koster G, Mahlberg R, Hackenbroch M, Bostrom J, et al. Alterations of INK4a(p16-p14ARF)/INK4b(p15) expression and telomerase activation in meningioma progression. J Neurooncol. 2001;55(3):149–58.
122. Rushing EJ, Colvin SM, Gazdar A, Miura N, White III CL, Coimbra C, et al. Prognostic value of proliferation index and expression of the RNA component of human telomerase (hTR) in papillary meningiomas. J Neurooncol. 1999;45(3):199–207.
123. Maes L, Lippens E, Kalala JP, de Ridder L. The hTERT-protein and Ki-67 labelling index in recurrent and non-recurrent meningiomas. Cell Prolif. 2005;38(1):3–12.
124. Goutagny S, Nault JC, Mallet M, Henin D, Rossi JZ, Kalamarides M. High incidence of activating TERT promoter mutations in meningiomas undergoing malignant progression. Brain Pathol. 2014;24:184–9.
125. Hegi ME, Diserens AC, Gorlia T, Hamou MF, de Tribolet N, Weller M, et al. MGMT gene silencing and benefit from temozolomide in glioblastoma. N Engl J Med. 2005;352(10):997–1003.
126. de Robles P, McIntyre J, Kalra S, Roldan G, Cairncross G, Forsyth P, et al. Methylation status of MGMT gene promoter in meningiomas. Cancer Genet Cytogenet. 2008;187(1):25–7.
127. Brokinkel B, Fischer BR, Peetz-Dienhart S, Ebel H, Sepehrnia A, Rama B, et al. MGMT promoter methylation status in anaplastic meningiomas. J Neurooncol. 2010;100(3):489–90.
128. Chamberlain MC, Tsao-Wei DD, Groshen S. Temozolomide for treatment-resistant recurrent meningioma. Neurology. 2004;62(7):1210–2.

129. Zhi F, Zhou G, Wang S, Shi Y, Peng Y, Shao N, et al. A microRNA expression signature predicts meningioma recurrence. Int J Cancer. 2013;132(1):128–36.
130. Kliese N, Gobrecht P, Pachow D, Andrae N, Wilisch-Neumann A, Kirches E, et al. miRNA-145 is downregulated in atypical and anaplastic meningiomas and negatively regulates motility and proliferation of meningioma cells. Oncogene. 2013;32(39):4712–20.
131. Shi L, Jiang D, Sun G, Wan Y, Zhang S, Zeng Y, et al. miR-335 promotes cell proliferation by directly targeting Rb1 in meningiomas. J Neurooncol. 2012;110(2):155–62.
132. Saydam O, Shen Y, Wurdinger T, Senol O, Boke E, James MF, et al. Downregulated microRNA-200a in meningiomas promotes tumor growth by reducing E-cadherin and activating the Wnt/beta-catenin signaling pathway. Mol Cell Biol. 2009;29(21):5923–40.
133. Watson MA, Gutmann DH, Peterson K, Chicoine MR, Kleinschmidt-DeMasters BK, Brown HG, et al. Molecular characterization of human meningiomas by gene expression profiling using high-density oligonucleotide microarrays. Am J Pathol. 2002;161(2):665–72.
134. Wrobel G, Roerig P, Kokocinski F, Neben K, Hahn M, Reifenberger G, et al. Microarray-based gene expression profiling of benign, atypical and anaplastic meningiomas identifies novel genes associated with meningioma progression. Int J Cancer. 2005; 114(2):249–56.
135. Fathallah-Shaykh HM, He B, Zhao LJ, Engelhard HH, Cerullo L, Lichtor T, et al. Genomic expression discovery predicts pathways and opposing functions behind phenotypes. J Biol Chem. 2003;278(26):23830–3.
136. Cuevas I, Slocum A, Jun P, Costello J, Bollen A, Riggins G, et al. Meningioma transcript profiles reveal deregulated Notch signaling pathway. Cancer Res. 2005;65(12):5070–5.
137. Keller A, Ludwig N, Backes C, Romeike BF, Comtesse N, Henn W, et al. Genome wide expression profiling identifies specific deregulated pathways in meningioma. Int J Cancer. 2008; 124:346–51.
138. Wang X, Gong Y, Wang D, Xie Q, Zheng M, Zhou Y, et al. Analysis of gene expression profiling in meningioma: deregulated signaling pathways associated with meningioma and EGFL6 overexpression in benign meningioma tissue and serum. PLoS One. 2012;7(12):e52707.
139. Gay E, Lages E, Ramus C, Guttin A, El Atifi M, Dupre I, et al. The heterogeneity of meningioma revealed by multiparameter analysis: infiltrative and non-infiltrative clinical phenotypes. Int J Oncol. 2011;38(5):1287–97.
140. Aarhus M, Bruland O, Bredholt G, Lybaek H, Husebye ES, Krossnes BK, et al. Microarray analysis reveals down-regulation of the tumour suppressor gene WWOX and up-regulation of the oncogene TYMS in intracranial sporadic meningiomas. J Neurooncol. 2008;88(3):251–9.
141. Sayagues JM, Tabernero MD, Maillo A, Trelles O, Espinosa AB, Sarasquete ME, et al. Microarray-based analysis of spinal versus intracranial meningiomas: different clinical, biological, and genetic characteristics associated with distinct patterns of gene expression. J Neuropathol Exp Neurol. 2006;65(5):445–54.
142. Tabernero MD, Maillo A, Gil-Bellosta CJ, Castrillo A, Sousa P, Merino M, et al. Gene expression profiles of meningiomas are associated with tumor cytogenetics and patient outcome. Brain Pathol. 2009;19(3):409–20.
143. Martinez-Glez V, Alvarez L, Franco-Hernandez C, Torres-Martin M, de Campos JM, Isla A, et al. Genomic deletions at 1p and 14q are associated with an abnormal cDNA microarray gene expression pattern in meningiomas but not in schwannomas. Cancer Genet Cytogenet. 2010;196(1):1–6.
144. Perez-Magan E, Campos-Martin Y, Mur P, Fiano C, Ribalta T, Garcia JF, et al. Genetic alterations associated with progression and recurrence in meningiomas. J Neuropathol Exp Neurol. 2012;71(10):882–93.
145. Menghi F, Orzan FN, Eoli M, Farinotti M, Maderna E, Pisati F, et al. DNA microarray analysis identifies CKS2 and LEPR as potential markers of meningioma recurrence. Oncologist. 2011;16(10):1440–50.
146. Serna E, Morales JM, Mata M, Gonzalez-Darder J, San Miguel T, Gil-Benso R, et al. Gene expression profiles of metabolic aggressiveness and tumor recurrence in benign meningioma. PLoS One. 2013;8(6):e67291.
147. Lillehei KO, Donson AM, Kleinschmidt-DeMasters BK. Radiation-induced meningiomas: clinical, cytogenetic, and microarray features. Acta Neuropathol. 2008;116(3):289–301.
148. Yamaguchi S, Terasaka S, Kobayashi H, Asaoka K, Motegi H, Nishihara H, et al. Prognostic factors for survival in patients with high-grade meningioma and recurrence-risk stratification for application of radiotherapy. PLoS One. 2014;9(5):e97108.
149. Ketter R, Henn W, Niedermayer I, Steilen-Gimbel H, Konig J, Zang KD, et al. Predictive value of progression-associated chromosomal aberrations for the prognosis of meningiomas: a retrospective study of 198 cases. J Neurosurg. 2001;95(4): 601–7.
150. Maillo A, Orfao A, Sayagues JM, Diaz P, Gomez-Moreta JA, Caballero M, et al. New classification scheme for the prognostic stratification of meningioma on the basis of chromosome 14 abnormalities, patient age, and tumor histopathology. J Clin Oncol. 2003;21(17):3285–95.
151. Kim YJ, Ketter R, Henn W, Zang KD, Steudel WI, Feiden W. Histopathologic indicators of recurrence in meningiomas: correlation with clinical and genetic parameters. Virchows Arch. 2006;449(5):529–38.
152. Maillo A, Orfao A, Espinosa AB, Sayagues JM, Merino M, Sousa P, et al. Early recurrences in histologically benign/grade I meningiomas are associated with large tumors and coexistence of monosomy 14 and del(1p36) in the ancestral tumor cell clone. Neuro Oncol. 2007;9(4):438–46.
153. Domingues PH, Sousa P, Otero A, Goncalves JM, Ruiz L, de Oliveira C, et al. Proposal for a new risk stratification classification for meningioma based on patient age, WHO tumor grade, size, localization, and karyotype. Neuro Oncol. 2014;16(5): 735–47.
154. Weisman AS, Raguet SS, Kelly PA. Characterization of the epidermal growth factor receptor in human meningioma. Cancer Res. 1987;47(8):2172–6.
155. Maxwell M, Galanopoulos T, Hedley-Whyte ET, Black PM, Antoniades HN. Human meningiomas co-express platelet-derived growth factor (PDGF) and PDGF-receptor genes and their protein products. Int J Cancer. 1990;46(1):16–21.
156. Baumgarten P, Brokinkel B, Zinke J, Zachskorn C, Ebel H, Albert FK, et al. Expression of vascular endothelial growth factor (VEGF) and its receptors VEGFR1 and VEGFR2 in primary and recurrent WHO grade III meningiomas. Histol Histopathol. 2013;28(9):1157–66.
157. Lichtor T, Kurpakus MA, Gurney ME. Expression of insulin-like growth factors and their receptors in human meningiomas. J Neurooncol. 1993;17(3):183–90.
158. Johnson MD, Woodard A, Kim P, Frexes-Steed M. Evidence for mitogen-associated protein kinase activation and transduction of mitogenic signals by platelet-derived growth factor in human meningioma cells. J Neurosurg. 2001;94(2):293–300.
159. Mawrin C, Sasse T, Kirches E, Kropf S, Schneider T, Grimm C, et al. Different activation of mitogen-activated protein kinase and Akt signaling is associated with aggressive phenotype of human meningiomas. Clin Cancer Res. 2005;11(11):4074–82.
160. Johnson MD, Okedli E, Woodard A, Toms SA, Allen GS. Evidence for phosphatidylinositol 3-kinase-Akt-p7S6K pathway activation and transduction of mitogenic signals by platelet-derived growth factor in meningioma cells. J Neurosurg. 2002; 97(3):668–75.

161. Lopez-Lago MA, Okada T, Murillo MM, Socci N, Giancotti FG. Loss of the tumor suppressor gene NF2, encoding merlin, constitutively activates integrin-dependent mTORC1 signaling. Mol Cell Biol. 2009;29(15):4235–49.
162. James MF, Han S, Polizzano C, Plotkin SR, Manning BD, Stemmer-Rachamimov AO, et al. NF2/merlin is a novel negative regulator of mTOR complex 1, and activation of mTORC1 is associated with meningioma and schwannoma growth. Mol Cell Biol. 2009;29(15):4250–61.
163. Castelli MG, Chiabrando C, Fanelli R, Martelli L, Butti G, Gaetani P, et al. Prostaglandin and thromboxane synthesis by human intracranial tumors. Cancer Res. 1989;49(6):1505–8.
164. Kang HC, Kim IH, Park CI, Park SH. Immunohistochemical analysis of cyclooxygenase-2 and brain fatty acid binding protein expression in grades I-II meningiomas: correlation with tumor grade and clinical outcome after radiotherapy. Neuropathology. 2014 Apr 30. doi: 10.1111/neup.12128. [Epub ahead of print].
165. Johnson MD, Horiba M, Winnier AR, Arteaga CL. The epidermal growth factor receptor is associated with phospholipase C-gamma 1 in meningiomas. Hum Pathol. 1994;25(2):146–53.
166. Johnson MD, Shaw AK, O'Connell MJ, Sim FJ, Moses HL. Analysis of transforming growth factor beta receptor expression and signaling in higher grade meningiomas. J Neurooncol. 2011;103(2):277–85.
167. Nagashima G, Asai J, Suzuki R, Fujimoto T. Different distribution of c-myc and MIB-1 positive cells in malignant meningiomas with reference to TGFs, PDGF, and PgR expression. Brain Tumor Pathol. 2001;18(1):1–5.
168. Johnson MD, O'Connell MJ, Vito F, Pilcher W. Bone morphogenetic protein 4 and its receptors are expressed in the leptomeninges and meningiomas and signal via the Smad pathway. J Neuropathol Exp Neurol. 2009;68(11):1177–83.
169. Wen PY, Yung WK, Lamborn KR, Norden AD, Cloughesy TF, Abrey LE, et al. Phase II study of imatinib mesylate for recurrent meningiomas (North American Brain Tumor Consortium study 01-08). Neuro Oncol. 2009;11(6):853–60.
170. Reardon DA, Norden AD, Desjardins A, Vredenburgh JJ, Herndon II JE, Coan A, et al. Phase II study of Gleevec((R)) plus hydroxyurea (HU) in adults with progressive or recurrent meningioma. J Neurooncol. 2012;106(2):409–15.
171. Norden AD, Raizer JJ, Abrey LE, Lamborn KR, Lassman AB, Chang SM, et al. Phase II trials of erlotinib or gefitinib in patients with recurrent meningioma. J Neurooncol. 2009; 27:15s.
172. Nayak L, Iwamoto FM, Rudnick JD, Norden AD, Lee EQ, Drappatz J, et al. Atypical and anaplastic meningiomas treated with bevacizumab. J Neurooncol. 2012;109(1):187–93.
173. Moazzam AA, Wagle N, Zada G. Recent developments in chemotherapy for meningiomas: a review. Neurosurg Focus. 2013; 35(6):E18.
174. Kaley T, Barani I, Chamberlain M, McDermott M, Panageas K, Raizer J, et al. Historical benchmarks for medical therapy trials in surgery- and radiation-refractory meningioma: a RANO review. Neuro Oncol. 2014;16:829–40.
175. Ammoun S, Hanemann CO. Emerging therapeutic targets in schwannomas and other merlin-deficient tumors. Nat Rev Neurol. 2011;7(7):392–9.
176. Li W, Cooper J, Karajannis MA, Giancotti FG. Merlin: a tumour suppressor with functions at the cell cortex and in the nucleus. EMBO Rep. 2012;13(3):204–15.

Index

M.A. Karajannis and D. Zagzag (eds.), *Molecular Pathology of Nervous System Tumors: Biological Stratification and Targeted Therapies*, Molecular Pathology Library 8,
DOI 10.1007/978-1-4939-1830-0, © Springer Science+Business Media New York 2015

H

I

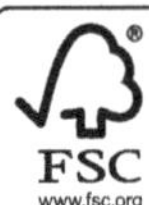

MIX
Papier aus verantwortungsvollen Quellen
Paper from responsible sources
FSC® C105338

If you have any concerns about our products,
you can contact us on
ProductSafety@springernature.com

In case Publisher is established outside the EU,
the EU authorized representative is:
Springer Nature Customer Service Center GmbH
Europaplatz 3, 69115 Heidelberg, Germany

Printed by Libri Plureos GmbH
in Hamburg, Germany